FEMALE REPRODUCTIVE SYSTEM: DYNAMICS OF SCAN AND TRANSMISSION ELECTRON MICROSCOPY

FEMALE REPRODUCTIVE SYSTEM: DYNAMICS OF SCAN AND TRANSMISSION ELECTRON MICROSCOPY

ALEX FERENCZY, M.D.

Instructor in Pathology, Columbia University, New York, New York

RALPH M. RICHART, M.D.

Professor of Pathology, College of Physicians and Surgeons, Columbia University; Director of Pathology and Cytology Laboratories of the Obstetrical and Gynecological Service (The Sloane Hospital for Women) of the Presbyterian Hospital, New York City; and the International Institute for the Study of Human Reproduction

A WILEY BIOMEDICAL-HEALTH PUBLICATION

JOHN WILEY & SONS, New York • London • Sydney • Toronto

Library of Congress Cataloging in Publication Data:

Ferenczy, Alex.
Female reproductive system.

(A Wiley biomedical health publication)
Includes bibliographies.
1. Generative organs, Female—Diseases—Diagnosis.
2. Radioisotope scanning. I. Richart, Ralph M., joint author. II. Title. [DNLM: 1. Genitalia, Female—Cytology—Atlases. 2. Microscopy, Electron, Scanning—Atlases. WP17 F349s 1974]

RG107.5.R3F47 618.1'07'575 73-17486
ISBN 0-471-25730-3

Printed in the United States of America

10 9 8 7 6 5 4 3 2 1

PREFACE

In the study of the structure and function of cells, tissues, and organs, few breakthroughs have proven as valuable as the development of transmission electron microscopy. Scanning electron microscopy may be equally valuable. Although industry has made extensive use of the scanning electron microscope, investigators have only recently applied this new tool to the study of biological systems and the many unresolved questions concerning the structure and function of cell surfaces.

Much remains to be done. As yet neither scanning nor transmission electron microscopy have been widely applied to the study of the female genital trade. More significantly, the work that has been done in this area is scattered among isolated publications and is largely inaccesible to the general scientific community. We felt that the compilation of various studies in a single volume would be a useful contribution to the field of human reproduction, and thus produced this atlas as an aid to those persons interested in this field or in diseases of the human female genital tract.

Our goal in preparing this book was to gather the best electron microphotographs available and to arrange them by organ system, with textual descriptions linking the subunits. Rather than using a textbook approach with prose predominating or a photojournalistic approach with minimal text, we have combined the two methods by putting emphasis on the photographs, but accompanying them with an abbreviated discussion and pertinent references. In most instances light microscope photographs are included in the plates for reference purposes.

ALEX FERENCZY
RALPH M. RICHART

New York, New York
January 15, 1974

ACKNOWLEDGMENTS

We are grateful to the investigators who kindly contributed their excellent photographs to sections of this book, all of whom are acknowledged individually in the legend credits. We are also indebted to the excellent technical assistance of Mrs. Arline Albala Cormons, Mr. Khalid Khan, and Mr. George A. Cottral; the collaboration of Dr. Hiroshi Nakazawa and Miss Judith Anderson; the assistance in manuscript preparation and bibliographic work of Mrs. Hartley Humphreys, Mrs. Karen Mishler, and Mrs. Awilda Pinero; the photographic skills of Mr. Dennis Chrisbaum; and the assistance in specimen procurement of Miss M. V. Peterson, R.N.

A. F.
R. M. R.

CONTENTS

FEMALE REPRODUCTIVE SYSTEM: DYNAMICS OF SCAN AND TRANSMISSION ELECTRON MICROSCOPY

MATERIALS AND METHODS

Although transmission electron microscopy is a widely used and accepted technique in a great variety of investigative fields, the scanning electron microscope (SEM) represents a relatively new tool in biological research. In contrast to the transmission electron microscope, the electrons emitted from the gun of the SEM are demagnified by a series of lenses, resulting in a fine electron probe, which is then deflected by a set of scanning coils in a square raster fashion over the surface of the specimen. To avoid electron, or heat, buildup a film of conductive metal of varying thickness is evaporated over the surface of the specimen. The image is formed by low-energy, secondary electrons emitted from the atoms of the target (upon excitation by the primary electrons) colliding with incident electrons to produce a signal that is transmitted as variations in brightness to the cathode ray tube. The image appears on a fluorescent screen by a process similar to that taking place in the human eye. The stereoscopic reproduction of the image is due primarily to the considerable depth of focus, which permits sharp delineation of "summits" and "valleys" on the surfaces with a resolving power of 100 to 150 Å. With scanning microscopy, specimens up to 2 in. in diameter can rapidly be prepared and the samples can be rotated and tilted in the specimen chamber in all four directions, providing considerable observational ease. The artifacts that occur in SEM consist principally of degeneration, compression, fracture, collapse, and surface coatings, all of which are most likely to occur before and during the preparative procedures.

The material presented in this atlas has been prepared principally from human tissue and has been collected over a period of 4 years from the operating rooms and clinics of the Sloane Hospital for Women. All specimens were thoroughly washed in physiological saline at room or body temperature to eliminate surface coatings from secretions or other materials. The samples were divided into three portions to be used for light, transmission, and scanning electron microscopy. They were fixed in 10% buffered formalin for light microscopy and 2.5% glutaraldehyde, in 0.1 *M* phosphate buffer, at pH 7.4 for both transmission and scanning microscopy. The use of a mucolytic agent in preference to isotonic saline offered no significant advantage in obtaining "clear" cell surfaces for scanning electron microscopy.

The following factors are critical in obtaining acceptable specimens: (1) wherever possible, they should be removed by biopsy, to avoid prolonged anoxia and degeneration, even if the biopsy is taken from what eventually becomes a "major" surgical specimen; and (2) they should be washed as soon as possible and fixed within a few minutes of their acquisition.

LIGHT MICROSCOPY

Specimens for light microscopy were processed in the usual manner, and various histochemical reactions were used when needed.

TRANSMISSION ELECTRON MICROSCOPY

Blocks of tissue, measuring 1 × 1 mm, were postfixed in 2% osmium tetroxide, dehydrated in an ethyl alcohol series of ascending concentrations from 30 to 100%, and embedded in Epon. Thin sections were stained with uranyl acetate and Reynold's lead citrate and examined in a Jeolco-7A transmission electron microscope at 80 kV.

SCANNING ELECTRON MICROSCOPY

Samples of various sizes, measuring up to 4 cm in greatest dimension, were washed for several hours with phosphate buffer at pH 7.4 and then dehydrated and dried by either freeze-drying or critical-point drying (CPD) techniques. When freeze-drying was used, the samples were frozen with liquid Freon, chilled with liquid nitrogen, and then dried while frozen at −50°C for 12 hours. When CPD was used, specimens were dehydrated in ethanol and amyl acetate of ascending concentrations from 50 to 100% and dried in a CPD apparatus. Dried specimens were examined with a dissecting microscope to ensure proper surface orientation and were cemented onto specimen holders with conductive silver paint. These mounted samples were then coated with an approximately 150-Å-thick layer of gold–palladium in a high vacuum evaporator and examined in a JEOL JSM-U3 scanning electron microscope at 25 kV.

Although both drying methods produce acceptable results, the CPD technique offers a better preserved surface architecture, relatively free of surface tension artifacts, than does the freeze-drying method.

REFERENCES

1. Ayres, A., J. M. Allen, and A. E. Williams. A method for obtaining conventional histological sections from specimens after examination by scanning electron microscopy. *J. Microsc.* **93**: 247 (1971).
2. Barber, V. C. and A. Boyde. Scanning electron microscopic studies of cilia. *Z. Zellforsch.* **84**: 269 (1968).
3. Boyde, A. Direct recording of stereoscopic images with the scanning electron microscope by the Anaglyph Colour Technique. *Med. Biol. III.* **21**: 130 (1971).
4. Boyde, A. and V. C. Barber. Freeze-drying methods for the scanning electron-microscopical study of the protozoon *Spirostomum ambiguum* and the statocyst of the cephalopod mollusc *Loligo vulgaris*. *J. Cell Sci.* **4**: 223 (1969).
5. Boyde, A. and C. Wood. Preparation of animal tissue for surface-scanning electron microscopy. *J. Microsc.* **90**: 221 (1969).
6. Carr, K. E. Applications of scanning electron microscopy in biology. In *International Review of Cytology*, G. H. Bourne and J. F. Danielli (Eds.). Academic Press, New York, 1971, pp. 183-255.
7. Clarke, J. A., A. J. Salsbury, and G. F. Rowland. The scanning electron microscope. *Science* **4**: 54 (1968).
8. Cosslett, V. E. Scanning microscopy with electrons and X-rays. *J. Electronmicrosc. (Tokyo)* **16**: 51 (1967).
9. Everhart, T. E. and T. L. Hayes. The scanning electron microscope. *Am. Sci.* **226**: 55 (1972).
10. Fujita, T., J. Tokunaga, and H. Inoue. *Atlas of Scanning Electron Microscopy in Medicine*, Igaku Shoin Ltd. (Ed.). Elseiver, New York, 1971.
11. Fujita, T., J. Tokunaga, and H. Inoue. Scanning electron microscopy of the skin using celluloid impressions. *Arch. Histol. Jap.* **30**: 321 (1969).
12. Fujita, T., M. Miyoshi, and J. Tokunaga. Scanning and transmission electron microscopy of human ejaculate spermatozoa with special reference to their abnormal forms. *Z. Zellforsch.* **105**: 483 (1970).
13. Hayes, T. L., R. F. W. Pease, and L. W. McDonald. Applications of the scanning electron microscope to biological investigations. *Lab Invest.* **15**: 1320 (1966).
14. Jaques, W. E., J. Coalson, and A. Zervins. Application of the scanning electron microscope to human tissues. A preliminary study. *Exp. Mol. Pathol.* **4**: 576 (1965).
15. Murakami, T., M. Miyoshi, and T. Fujita. Glomerular vessels of the rat kidney with special reference to double efferent arterioles. A scanning electron microscope study of corrosion casts. *Arch. Histol. Jap.* **33**: 179 (1971).
16. Pease, R. F. W. and T. L. Hayes. Scanning electron microscopy of biological material. *Nature* **5040**: 1049 (1966).
17. *Scanning Electron Microscopy/1972 Proceedings of the Fifth Annual Scanning Electron Microscope Symposium*, Ô. Johari (Symposium Director). IIT Research Institute, Chicago, 1972.
18. Watters, W. B. and R. C. Buck. An improved simple method of specimen preparation for replicas or scanning electron microscopy. *J. Microsc.* **94**: 185 (1971).
19. Kanagawa, H., E. S. E. Hafez, C. A. Baechler, W. C. Pitchford, and M. I. Barnhart. Improved methodology for scanning electron microscopy of the female reproductive tract. *Int. J. Fertil.* **17**: 75 (1972).

VULVA

1

Normal Vulvar Skin

The vulva is covered by a keratinizing, stratified, squamous epithelium of ectodermal origin.

Detailed observations dealing with the scanning electron microscopic appearance of human and animal skin and hair have been reported.[1-11]

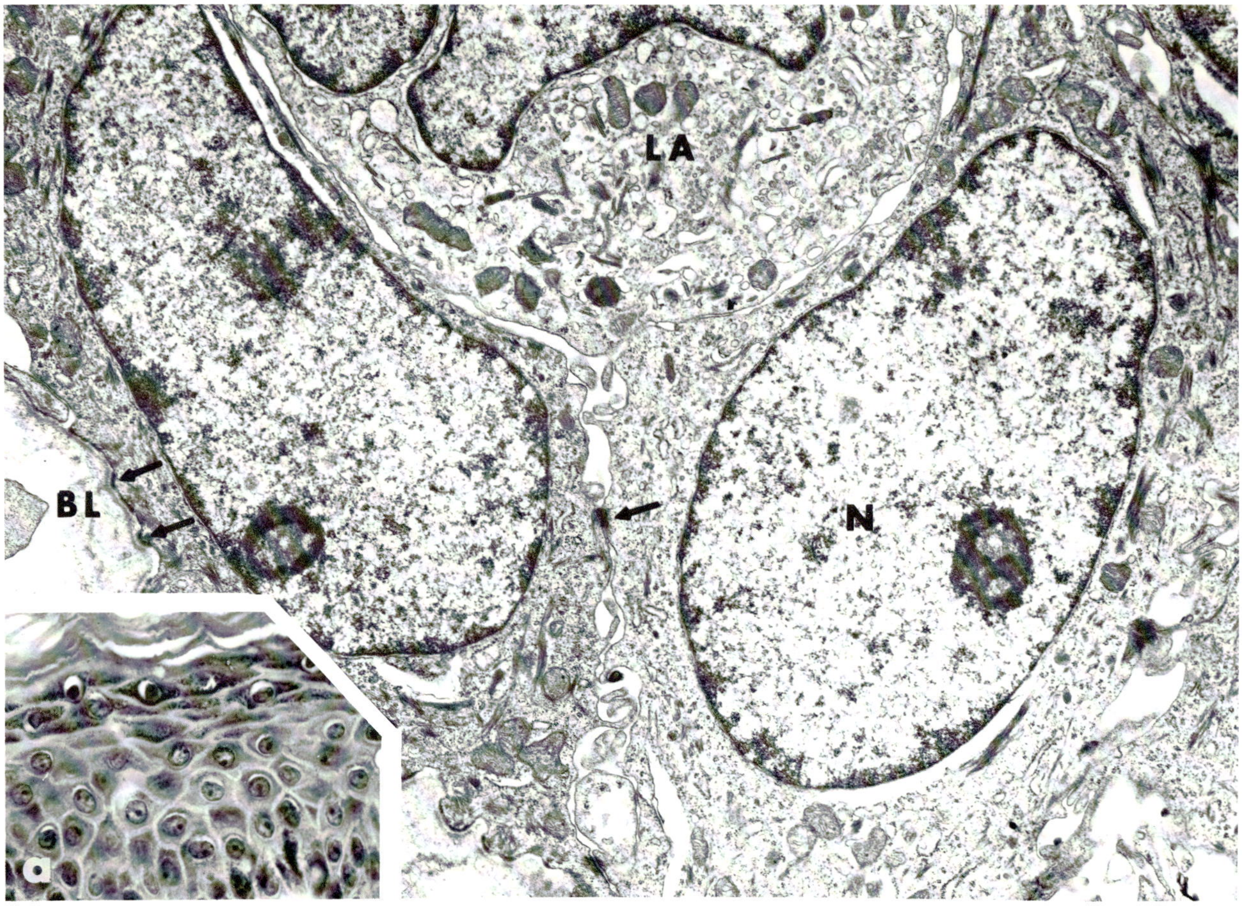

Figure 1a. *Histologically,* the deepest layer consists of a single row of elongated, mitotically active, basal cells that form the *stratum germinativum*. The overlying and predominant zone, called the *stratum spinosum,* contains several layers of polyhedral cells attached to one another by prominent intercellular bridges. These maturing cells produce tonofilaments, keratohyaline granules, and other precursor elements of keratin. The next layer, the *stratum granulosum,* is a narrow zone of one or two layers of large granular cells with conspicuous keratohyaline granules, and the most superficial layer, the *stratum corneum,* is composed of a lamellated layer of horny cells devoid of nuclei, representing the final stage of differentiation. (H & E stain, × 125.)

Figure 1. *Ultrastructurally, the basal cells* have large nuclei (N) and are attached by desmosomes (arrow) to the neighboring cells and by hemidesmosomes (arrows) to the limiting basal lamina (BL). The plasma membrane is highly convoluted, and the cytoplasm contains centrioles, dispersed tonofilaments, abundant free ribosomes, and mitochondria, a reflection of active protein synthesis. Langerhans cells (LA), with their characteristic cytoplasmic inclusions, are often[1] seen in this region or some distance above. They are regarded as thymus-dependent macrophages[2] and are presumably related to primary antigen phagocytosis.[3] × 9800.

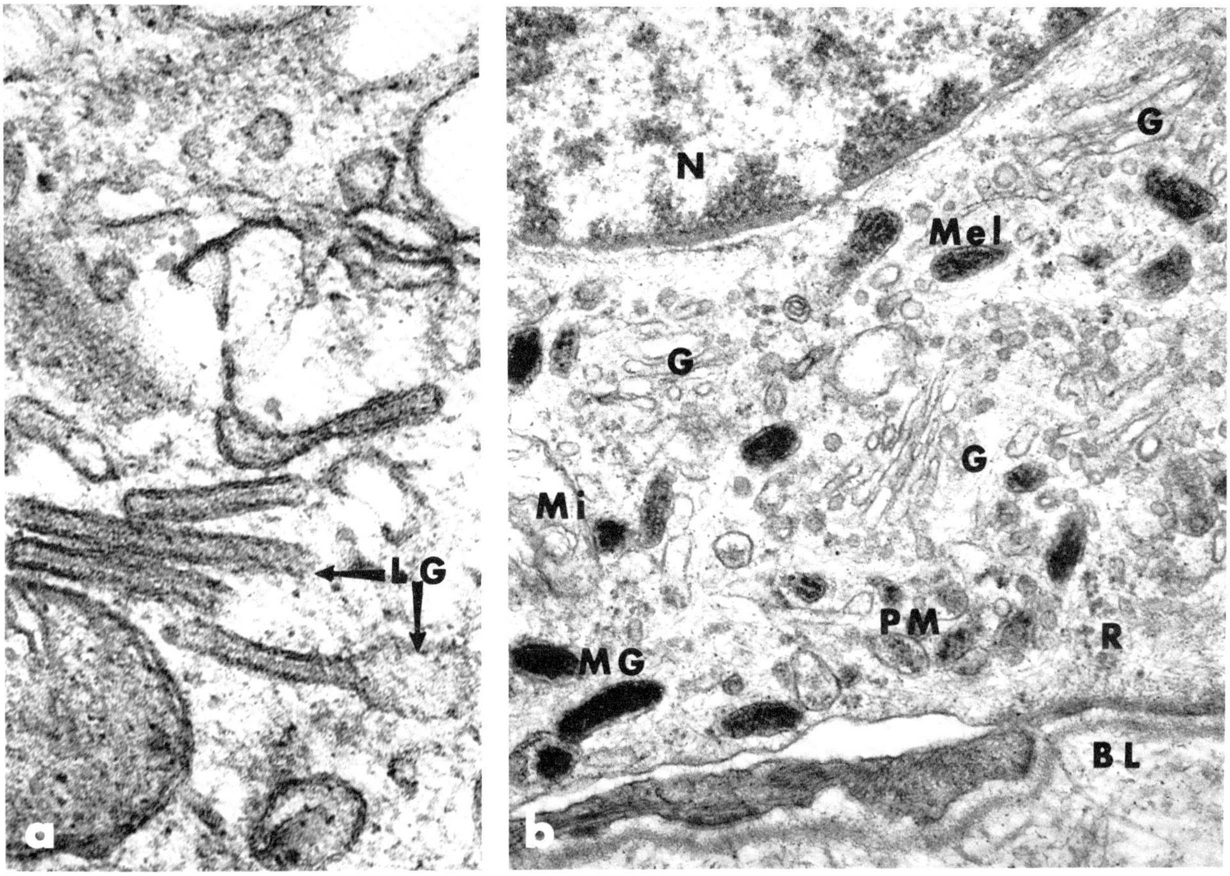

Figure 2a. *Higher magnification of Langerhans granules* (LG). They are thought to be derived either from the Golgi apparatus[1] or by endocytosis of closely apposed plasma membranes of Langerhans cells and are believed to participate in the intracellular transport system.[3] The latter suggestion seems to be supported by the transmission electron microscopic demonstration of exogenous peroxidase within the Langerhans cell granules.[3] × 135,000.

Figure 2b. *Vulvar melanocyte.*[1] Well-developed Golgi apparatuses (G) are associated with numerous premelanosomes (PM), melanosomes (Mel), and melanin granules (MG). Characteristically, neither the Langerhans cells nor the melanocytes have desmosomal attachments with the adjacent epidermal cells. × 41,000. Mi: mitochondrion; N: nucleus; BL: basal lamina, R: free ribosomes.

REFERENCES (Figures 1–2b)

1. Zelickson, A. S. Melanocyte, melanin granule, and Langerhans cells. In *Ultrastructure of Normal and Abnormal Skin,* A. S. Zelickson (Ed.). Lea & Febiger, Philadelphia, 1967, pp. 163-187.
2. Kuwahara, H.: Electron microscopic studies on dendritic cells of the epidermis, especially on the function of Langerhans cells and etiology of certain leucodermas. *Jap. J. Dermatol.* **80:** 69 (1970).
3. Hashimoto, K. Langerhans' cell granule. An endocytic organelle. *Arch. Dermatol.* **104:** 148 (1971).

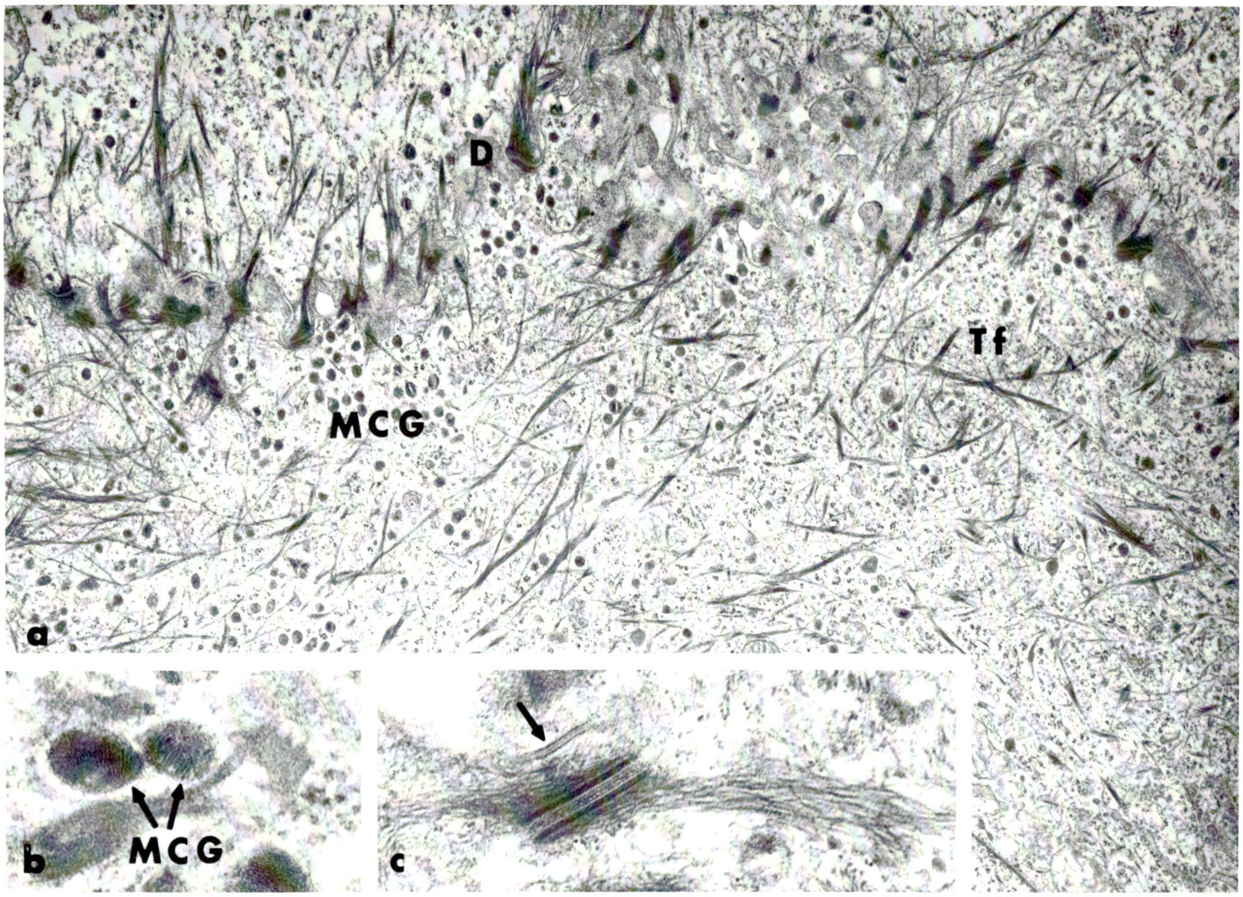

Figure 3a. *The cells from the stratum spinosum* are characterized by a gradually increasing cytoplasmic volume, accompanied by an increase in the Golgi, granular endoplasmic reticulum, and tonofilaments. As maturation advances, polysaccharides and lipid-containing, lamellated keratinosomes or membrane-bound granules (MCG) and keratohyaline granules appear,[1] and tonofilaments (Tf) become more numerous. The less convoluted plasma membranes are reinforced by numerous well-developed desmosomal plaques (D). × 9800.

Figure 3b. *High-power view* of the lamellated matrix of membrane-bound granules (MCG). × 60,750.

Figure 3c. *Detail* of a tonofilament–desmosome complex and of a pentalaminar nexus (arrow). × 46,125.

REFERENCE (Figures 3a–4a)

1. Matoltsy, A. G. and P. M. Parakkal. Keratinization. In *Ultrastructure of Normal and Abnormal Skin*, A. S. Zelickson (Ed.). Lea & Febiger, Philadelphia, 1967, pp. 76-104.

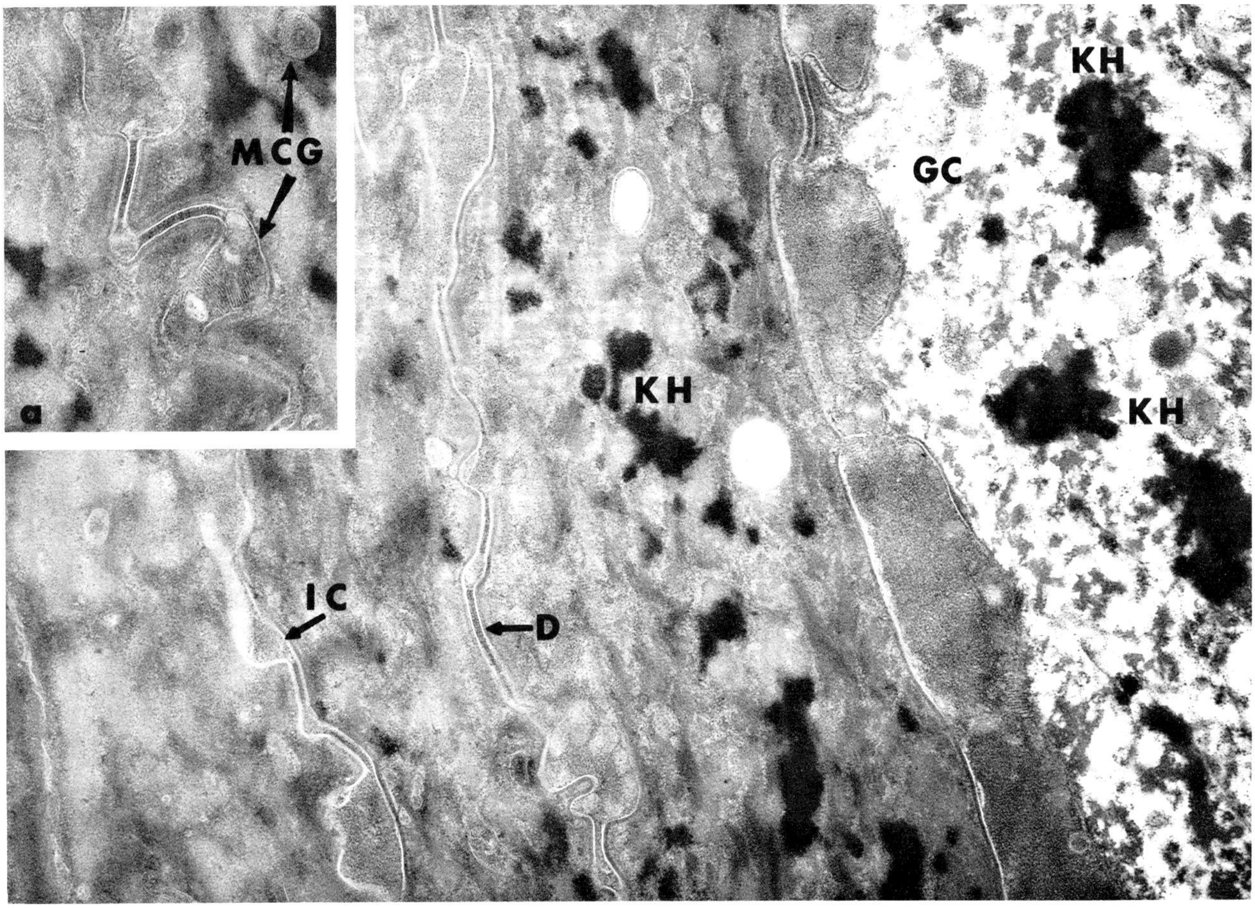

Figure 4. *The granular cells* (GC) contain large bundles of tonofilaments associated with coalescing masses of keratohyaline granules (KH). The latter represent condensed sulfur-negative filaments and ribosomes, presumably contributing sulfur-poor fibrous and amorphous proteins to the horny layer.[1] After the extracellular discharge of lamellar, membrane-bound granules (keratinosomes) (MCG, Figure 4*a*), the plasma membranes become coated with sulfur-rich, lipoproteinic, amorphous substances of an intracellular origin (IC). This newly acquired cellular envelope contributes to cell stability. At the same time, a progressive disintegration of the cytoplasmic organelles and nuclei takes place, and a marked condensation of low-density filaments, which is responsible for the fibrillar pattern of the keratin, occurs. The cohesiveness of the complexly convoluted and interdigitating horny cells is maintained by desmosomal belts (D). The final stage is characterized by loss of water and dissolution of desmosomal attachments, resulting in widening of the intercellular spaces and eventual desquamation. It has been suggested that the sulfur-poor, fibrofilamentous component of the horny layer assures flexibility, whereas the interfilamentous matrix, rich in disulfide bonds, provides stability.[1] × 35,000.

Figure 4a. *Horny layer* with intra- and intercellular membrane-bound granules (MGG). × 54,000.

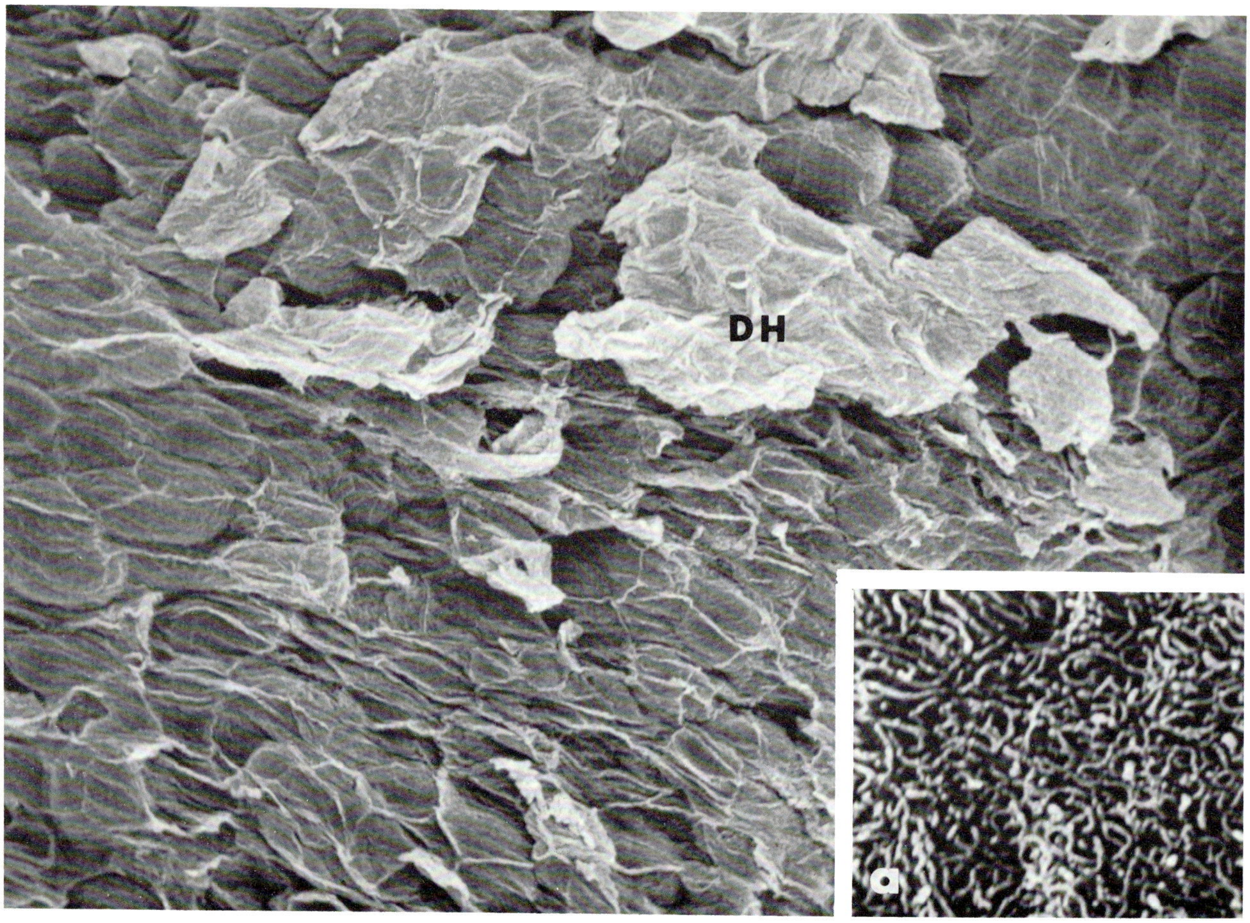

Figure 5. *Stratum corneum.* The convoluted surface pattern and the well-defined polygonal contour of horny cells can better be appreciated with the scanning electron microscope. The most superficial horny cells form large aggregates that appear partly detached from the surface, representing desquamating horny (DH) cells. × 480.

Figure 5a. *The surface of horny cells* contains a prominent, labyrinthine system of microridges, similar in structure to those found in the nonkeratinizing vaginal or cervical mucous membranes. × 3200.

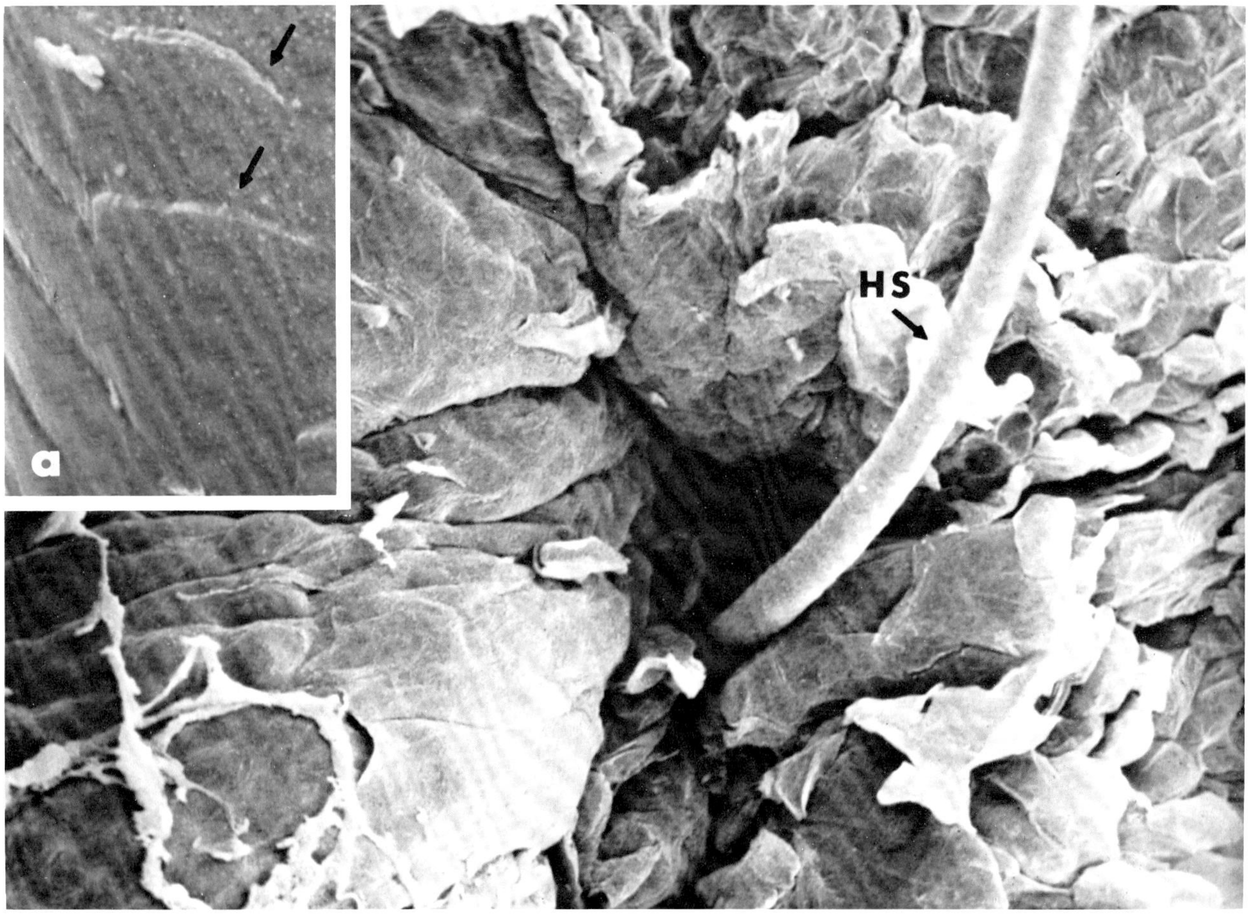

Figure 6. *Surface topographic appearance of vulvar skin and hair shaft (HS).* × 350.

Figure 6a. *The outer layer of the hair shaft* is composed of flat epicuticules (arrows). × 3680.

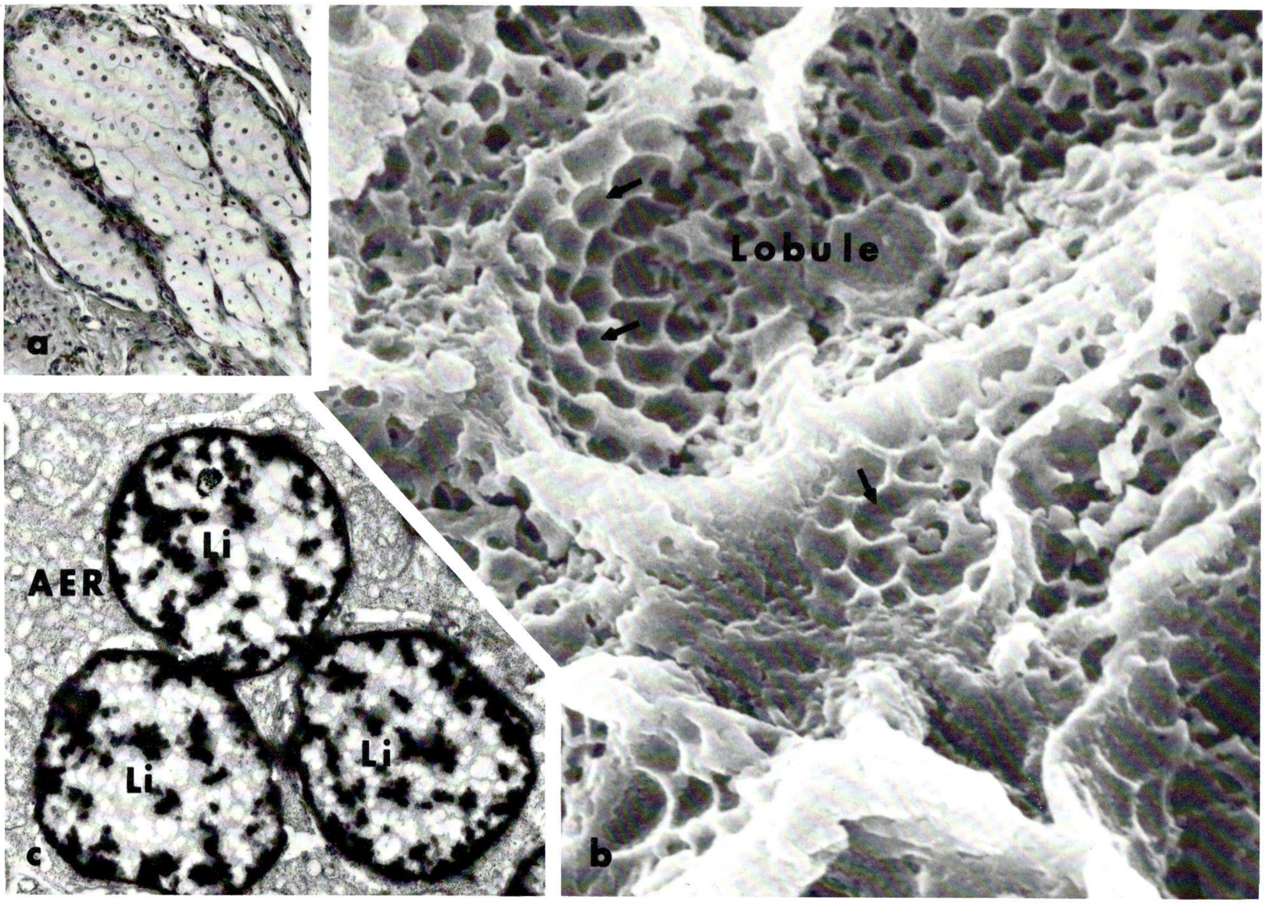

Figure 7a. *Histologic appearance of sebaceous glands* representing the secretory unit of the pilosebaceous system. The lobules are composed of large, polyhedral, clear cells with granular cytoplasm and centrally placed round nuclei. (H & E stain, × 30.)

Figure 7b. *Scanning electron microscopic view of sebaceous lobules* (lobule) in which the cells (arrows) have a honeycomb pattern, probably due to vacuum compression artifact (specimen prepared by freeze-drying technique). × 1600.

Figure 7c. *At the transmission electron microscopic level,* the mature sebaceous cells are packed with vesicular agranular endoplasmic reticulum (AER), associated with prominent Golgi and lipid droplets (Li).[1] × 12,000.

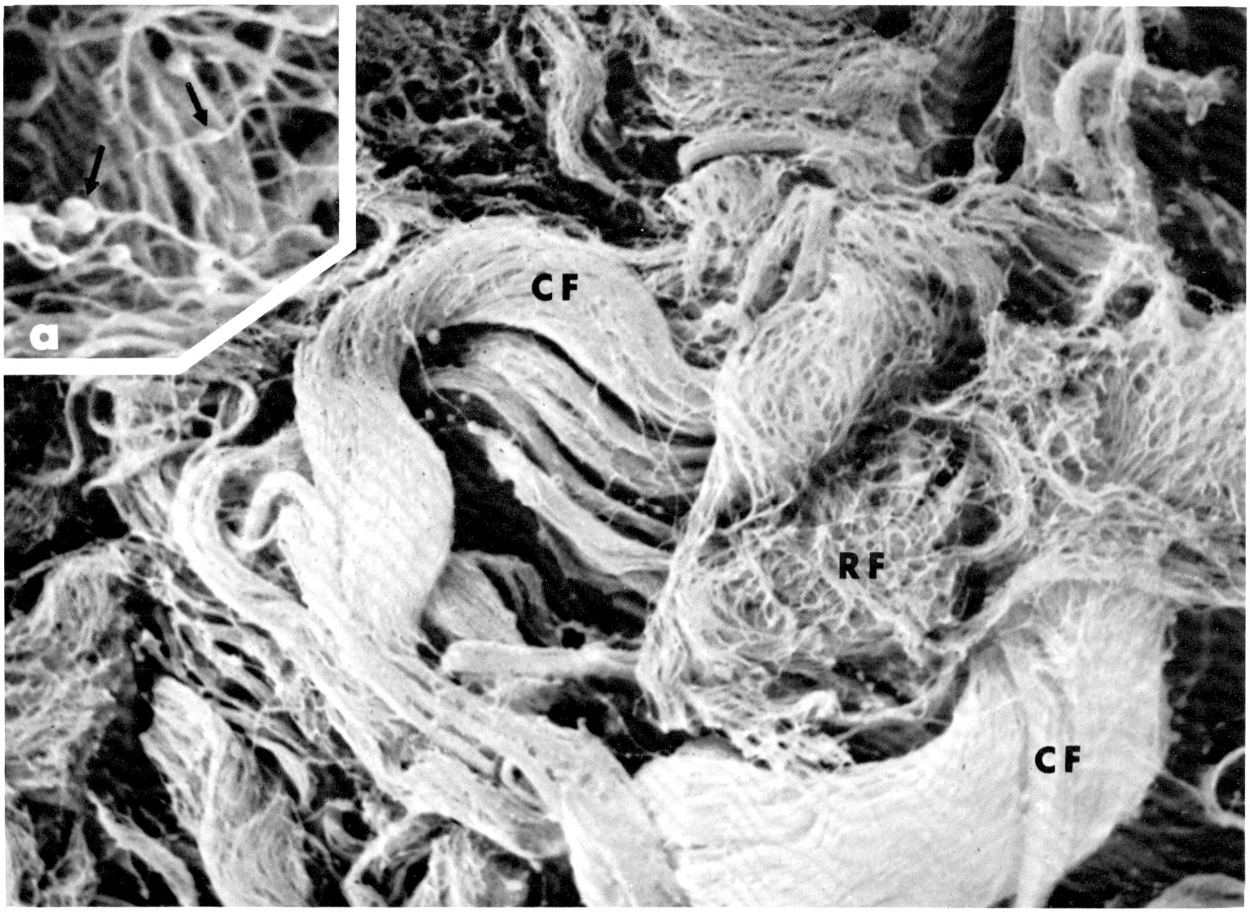

Figure 8. *Scanning electron microscopy of dermal collagen.* The collagen fibers are arranged either in voluminous and tortuous bundles (CF) or in an interlacing fibrous network (RF). × 3200.

Figure 8a. *Individual collagen fibers* often contain randomly distributed nodular thickenings (arrow) of various sizes. × 8000.

REFERENCE (Figures 7a–8a)

1. Ellis, R. A. Eccrine, sebaceous and apocrine glands. In *Ultrastructure of Normal and Abnormal Skin,* A. S. Zelickson (Ed.). Lea & Febiger, Philadelphia, 1967, pp. 132-162.

REFERENCES

1. Amelunxen, F. K., K. Morgenroth, and T. Picksak. Investigations on the epidermis with the stereoscan electron microscope. *Z. Pflanzenphysiol.* **57:** 79 (1967).
2. Bernstein, E. O. and C. B. Jones. Skin replication procedure for the scanning electron microscope. *Science* **166:** 252 (1969).
3. Caputo, R. and B. Ceccarelli. Study of normal hair and some malformations with a scanning electron microscope. *Arch. Klin. Exp. Dermatol.* **234:** 242 (1969).
4. Carteaud, A. J. P. Present status of scanning electron microscopy in dermatology. In *Proceedings of the Third Annual Scanning Electron Microscope Symposium,* Ô. Johari (Ed.) IIT Research Institute, Chicago, 1970, pp. 217-224.
5. Dawber, R., and S. Comaish. Scanning electron microscopy of normal and abnormal hair shafts. *Arch. Dermatol.* **101:** 316 (1970).
6. Finlay, J. B. and J. A. Hunter. Visualization of collagen cross-banding in the scanning electron microscope. *J. Microsc.* **93:** 241 (1971).
7. Finlay, J. B., J. A. Hunter and F. S. Steven. Preparation of human skin for high resolution scanning electron microscope using phosphate buffered crude bacterial c-amylase. *J. Microsc.* **93:** 73 (1971).
8. Fujita, T., J. Tokunaga and H. Inoue. Scanning electron microscopy of the skin using celluloid impressions. *Arch. Histol. Jap.* **30:** 321 (1969).
9. Goldman, L., J. Vahl, R. J. Rockwell, R. Meyer, M. Franzen, P. Owens, and S. Hyatt. Replica microscopy and scanning electron microscopy of laser impacts on the skin. *J. Invest. Dermatol.* **52:** 18 (1969).
10. Millington, P. F. and I. A. Brown. Scanning electron microscope studies of some internal surfaces in human skin. *Z. Zellforsch.* **106:** 209 (1970).
11. Papa, C. M. and B. Farber. Direct scanning electron microscopy of human skin. *Arch. Dermatol.* **104:** 262 (1971).

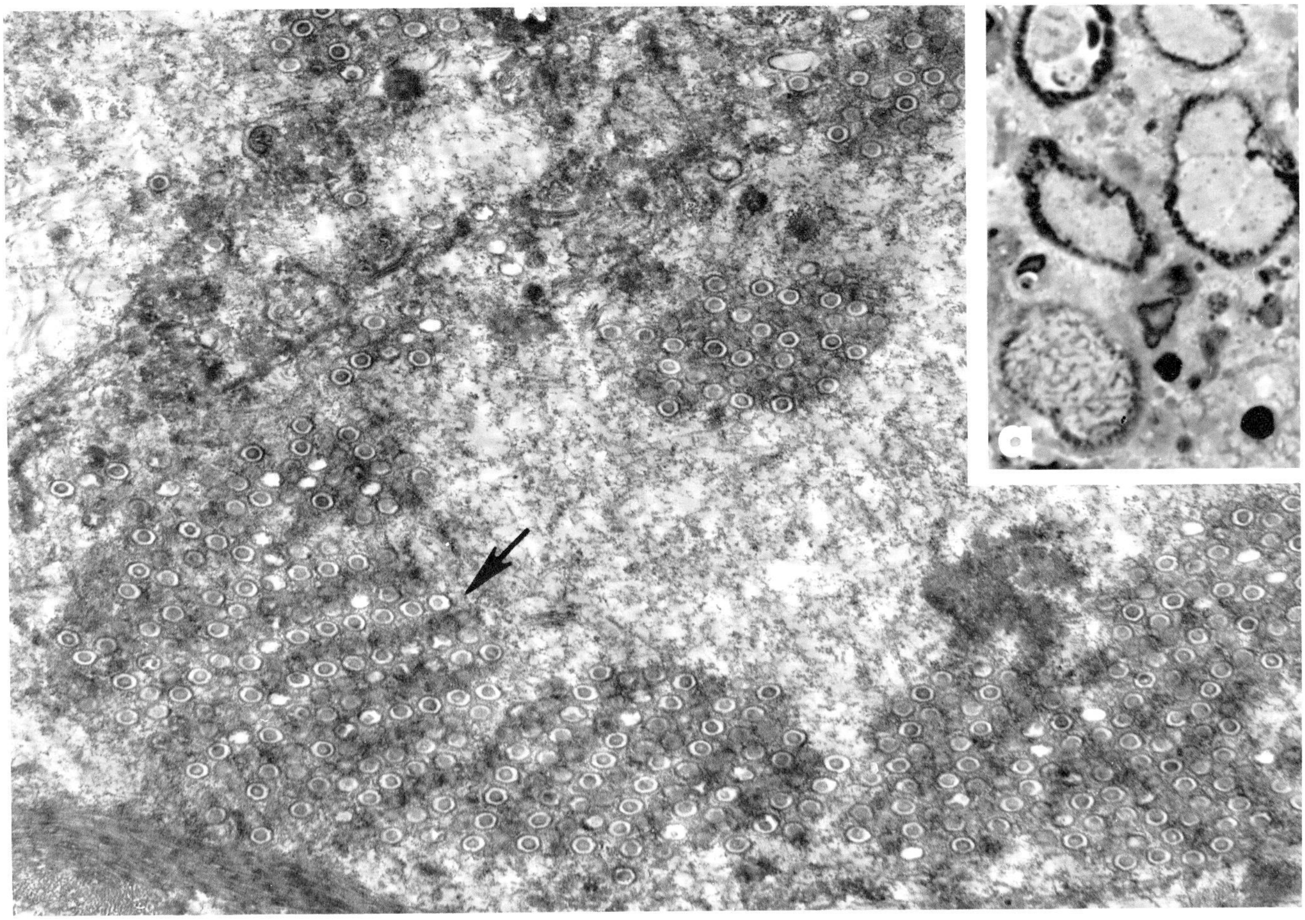

2

Herpetic Vulvitis

Herpes simplex genitalis occurs as painful vesicles or ulcers on the labia. The responsible pathogen is the herpes simplex virus (herpesvirus hominis) type II, a member of the poxvirus group. The virus can be demonstrated by neutralizing antibodies, serologic techniques, and by viral growth in monkey kidney and human amniotic cells. Corneal inoculation of the virus produces keratoconjunctivitis in rabbits, and it can be grown on the chorioallontoic membrane of chick embryos.

Figure 9a. *The characteristic histologic findings* consist of a suprabasal intraepidermal vesicle, filled with serum, degenerated epidermal cells, and multinucleated giant cells, some of them containing acidophilic, intranuclear inclusions surrounded by a clear halo. × 1200.[1]

Figure 9. *Ultrastructurally,*[1] the pattern of cellular degeneration includes dissolution of cytoplasmic organelles, clumping of tonofilaments, loss of desmosomal attachments, widening of the intercellular spaces, and increased lysosomal activity. The herpes simplex virions are incorporated into the cytoplasm through pinocytotic vesicles and transported to the nucleus, where they are uncoated.[2] Intranuclear viral particles are absent in the basal cells but are numerous in the superficial cells. The mature virions are often found in a crystal-like arrangement (arrow) and have a DNA core 400 to 500 Å in diameter, surrounded by an inner halo and an outer hexagonal-shaped capsid 500 to 950 Å thick. "Naked" viruses are occasionally found in the cytoplasm after their expulsion from the nucleus, or in phagocytotic vacuoles of intraepithelial leukocytes.[1] The presence of intranuclear fibrils, with or without associated viral particles, has been reported.[1] × 39,000. *From* E. R. Freidrich, W. Cole, and J. N. Middlekamp. Herpes simplex. Clinical aspects and electron microscopic findings. *J. Obstet. Gynecol.* **104:** 758-779 (1969).

3

Vulvar Warts

Vulvar warts are relatively common, rapidly growing, and highly contagious verruciform lesions. Genital warts, like the common skin warts (verruca vulgaris), are viral-induced lesions, and the two lesions probably have a common viral etiology.[3,4] The responsible agent has been identified as a DNA-containing, human, papilloma virus that is a member of the papovirus group. The spherical virions have a cubic capsid with either 42 or 72 subunits, and measure from 480 to 580 Å in diameter in the genital warts,[4] and from 450 to 550 Å in the skin warts,[2] depending on the preparative procedures employed: conventional thin sections or negative staining techniques. The virions are found in the nuclei and nuceoli of the upper stratum spinosum, granulosum, and corneum.[2,4] Viral particles are thought to replicate within the host cell nuclei but are not found in the deeper Malpighian layer or in basal cells. The typical histologic features are papillomatosis with marked acanthosis, hyperkeratosis, the presence of large vacuolated cells in the upper part of the epidermis, and intracytoplasmic, acidophilic inclusion bodies which, fine structurally, are composed of giant ketratohyaline granules.

REFERENCES (Figures 9–10)

1. Friedrich, E. R., W. Cole and J. N. Middlekamp. Herpes simplex. Clinical aspects and electron microscopic findings. *Am. J. Obstet. Gynecol.* **104:** 758(1969).
2. Lutzner, M. A. Virus diseases. In *Ultrastructure of Normal and Abnormal Skin,* A. C. Zelickson (Ed.). Lea & Febiger, Philadelphia, 1967, pp. 365–387.
3. Melczer, N. Uber die atiologische Identitat der gewohnlichen Warzen und spitzen Kondylome. *Hautarzt* **16:** 150 (1965).
4. Oriel, J. D. and J. D. Almeida. Demonstration of virus particles in human genital warts. *Brit. J. Vener. Dis.* **46:** 37 (1970).

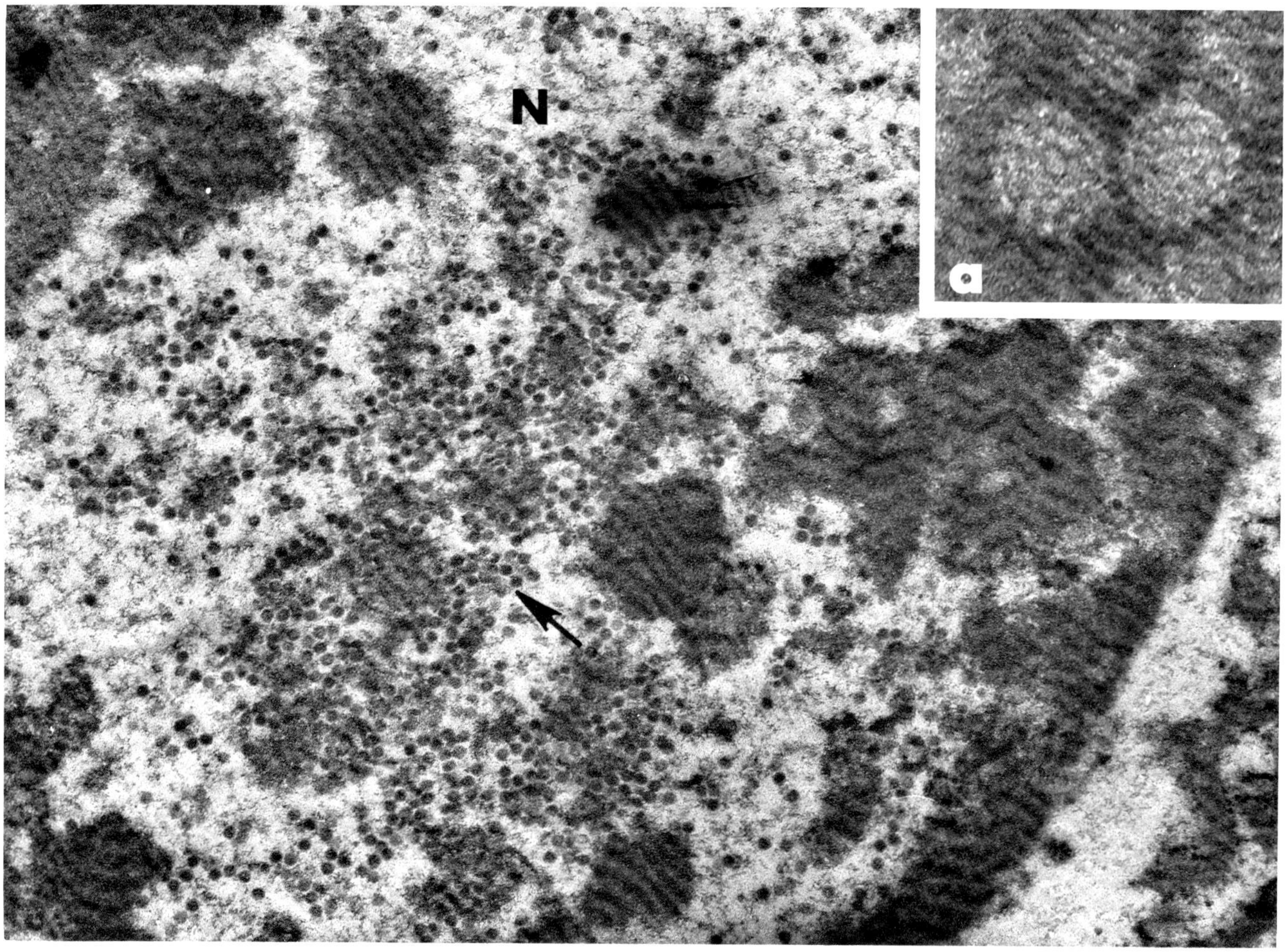

Figure 10. *Portion of nucleus (N) from the stratum granulosum of a vulvar wart,* containing a high concentration of virus particles (arrow). This type of virus distribution is frequently found in common skin warts. × 41,000.

Figure 10a. When *genital warts* were lightly disrupted, more numerous virus particles were present and could easily be identified against the rather greater amount of background material. × 300,000. *From* J. D. Oriel and J. D. Almeida. Demonstration of virus particles in human genital warts. *Brit. J. Venr. Dis.* **46:** 37-42 (1970).

4

Molluscum Contagiosum

Molluscum contagiosum is a viral-induced, often venereally transmitted, hyperkeratotic and acanthotic epidermal lesion. Characteristically, the epidermal cells of the middle and upper strata contain large intracytoplasmic inclusions (molluscum bodies), which are more prominent in the upper, horny layer. These inclusions are not released from the cells but are expelled within the desquamated epidermal cells. The latter, when viewed with the scanning electron microscope, appear as clusters of prominent, dome-shaped cells, distorted by viral inclusions.[1,2] This particular topographic configuration contrasts sharply with the large (300 × 300 × 100 mμ), rectangular molluscum contagiosum virions, which belong to the poxvirus group.[3] The DNA core of the mature virion has an hourglass appearance, is surrounded by a protein capsule, and has an outer tubular envelope.[4] The immature virions are membrane-bound, spherical structures with central, granular nucleoids. Viral replication occurs in the viroplasmic, cytoplasmic foci of the middle and upper spinous cells.[3] Immature viruses are numerous near these regions.

The morphobiochemical aspects of the cytoplasmic receptor sites, the intracytoplasmic phagocytosis, and the uncoating of the DNA core of the molluscum contagiosum virus are unknown, but are thought to be similar to those of the early phases of the host-cell vaccina virus (also a member of the pox group) relationship. In vaccina virus-infected cells, the host DNA is inhibited after the release of viral DNA, and new viral (messenger) RNA appears. Viral DNA synthesis is completed in about 7 hours.[3]

Figure 11. *Section through a lesion of molluscum contagiosum.* The epidermis is normal (Q) on either side of the lesion. Several acanthotic lobules of epidermis are seen (L). Cells at the basal cell level (Ba) appear normal. Abnormal cells are seen in the stratum spinosum (Sp) and throughout the granular layer (Gr). The dense material surrounding these cells is keratohyaline (K). Virus-containing cells are exfoliating at (Co). (H & E stain, approximately × 80.) *From* M. A. Lutzner. Virus diseases. In *Ultrastructure of Normal and Abnormal Skin,* A. C. Zelickson (Ed.). Lea & Febiger, Philadelphia, 1967, pp. 365–387.

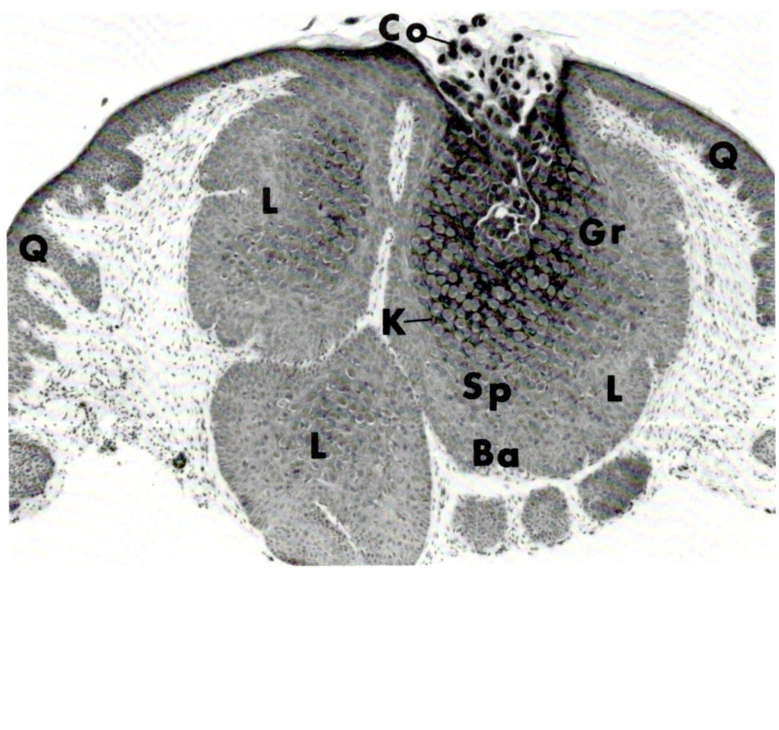

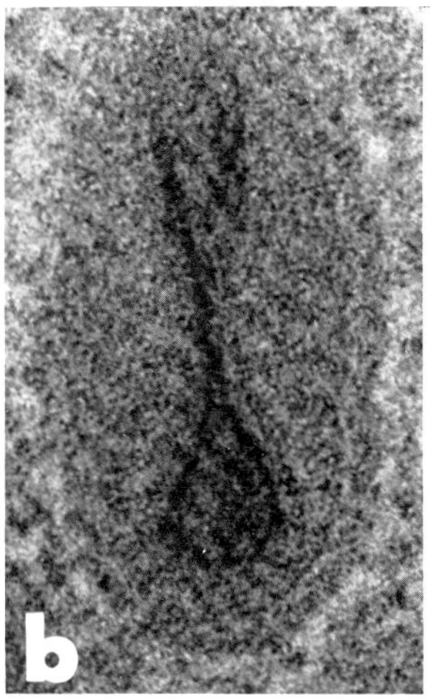

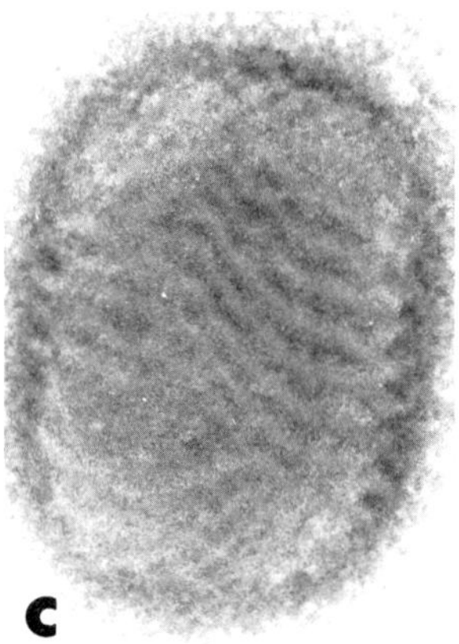

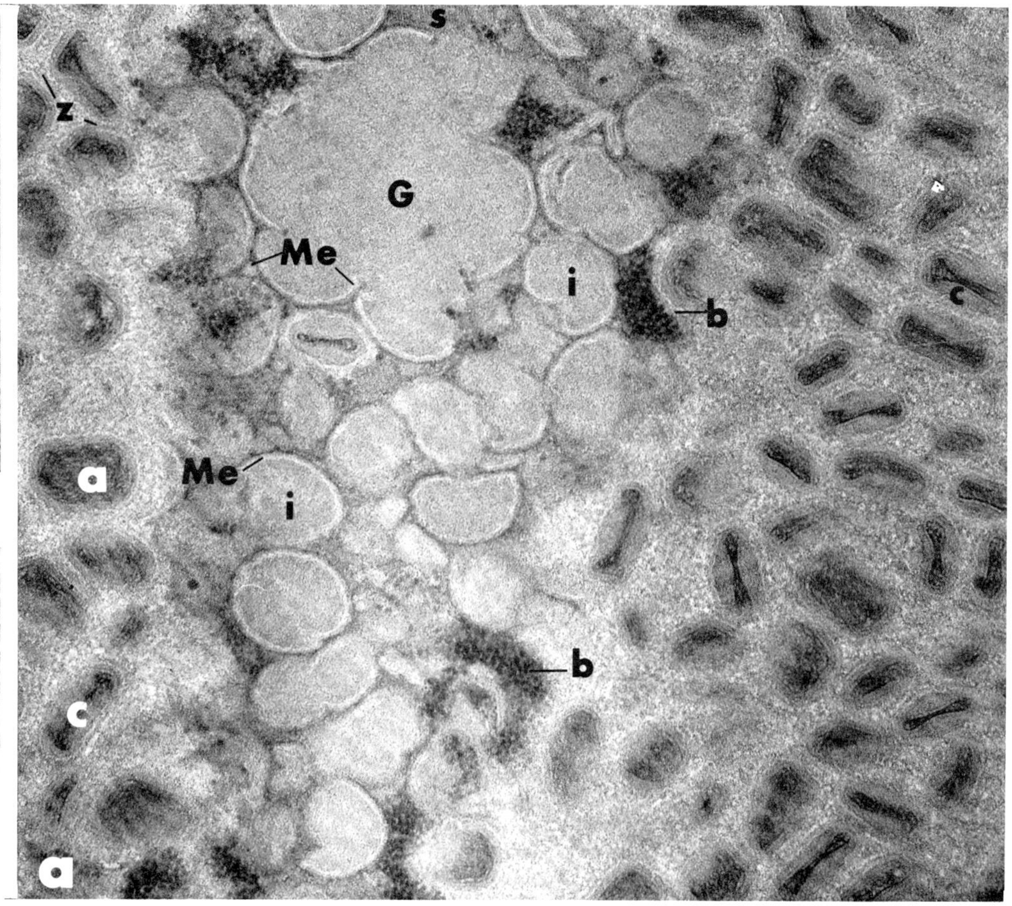

Figure 12a. *Portion of an epidermal cell of the upper stratum spinosum from a lesion of molluscum contagiosum.* An area of viroplasm (G), composed of finely granular material, is present in the cytoplasm. This viroplasmic area is delineated by viral membranes (Me) composed of electron-dense and electron-lucid layers. Immature, spherical virions (i), delineated by viral membranes (Me), lie near this viroplasmic area. Interspersed with these immature virions are clusters of electron-dense particles (b), which may be ribosomal in nature. Mature virions are seen, recognizable by their brick-shaped contours (a) or their dumbbell-shaped nucleoids (c). The material between mature virions is composed of granular densities that appear to run in linear arrays (z) and may follow the contour of virions. Striated patterns (s) are occasionally seen near sites of virus formation. Approximately × 57,200. *From* M. A. Lutzner. Virus diseases. In *Ultrastructure of Normal and Abnormal Skin,* A. C. Zelickson (Ed.). Lea & Febiger, Philadelphia, 1967, pp. 365–387.

Figure 12b. *Electron micrograph* of the molluscum contagiosum virion. Approximately × 175,000. *From* M. A. Lutzner. Virus diseases. In *Ultrastructure of Normal and Abnormal Skin,* A. C. Zelickson (Ed.). Lea & Febiger, Philadelphia, 1967, pp. 365–387.

Figure 12c. *Electron micrograph* illustrating negatively stained molluscum contagiosum virion. *From* M. A. Lutzner. Virus diseases. In *Ultrastructure of Normal and Abnormal Skin,* A. C. Zelickson (Ed.). Lea & Febiger, Philadelphia, 1967, pp. 365–387.

REFERENCES (Molluscum contagiosum–Figure 12c)

1. Carteaud, A. J. P. I. Possibilities of the scanning electron microscope in dermatology. II. Aspects of molluscum contagiosum under the scanning electron microscope. *Bull. Soc. Fr. Dermatol. Syphiligr.* **75:** 800 (1968).
2. Carteaud, A. J. P. Scanning electron microscopy in dermatology. *Brit. Med. J.* **3:** 239 (1969).
3. Lutzner, M. A. Virus diseases. In *Ultrastructure of Normal and Abnormal Skin,* A. C. Zelickson (Ed.). Lea & Febiger, Philadelphia, 1967, pp. 365–387.
4. Howatson, A. F. Viruses connected with tumours and warts. *Brit. Med. Bull.* **18:** 193 (1962).

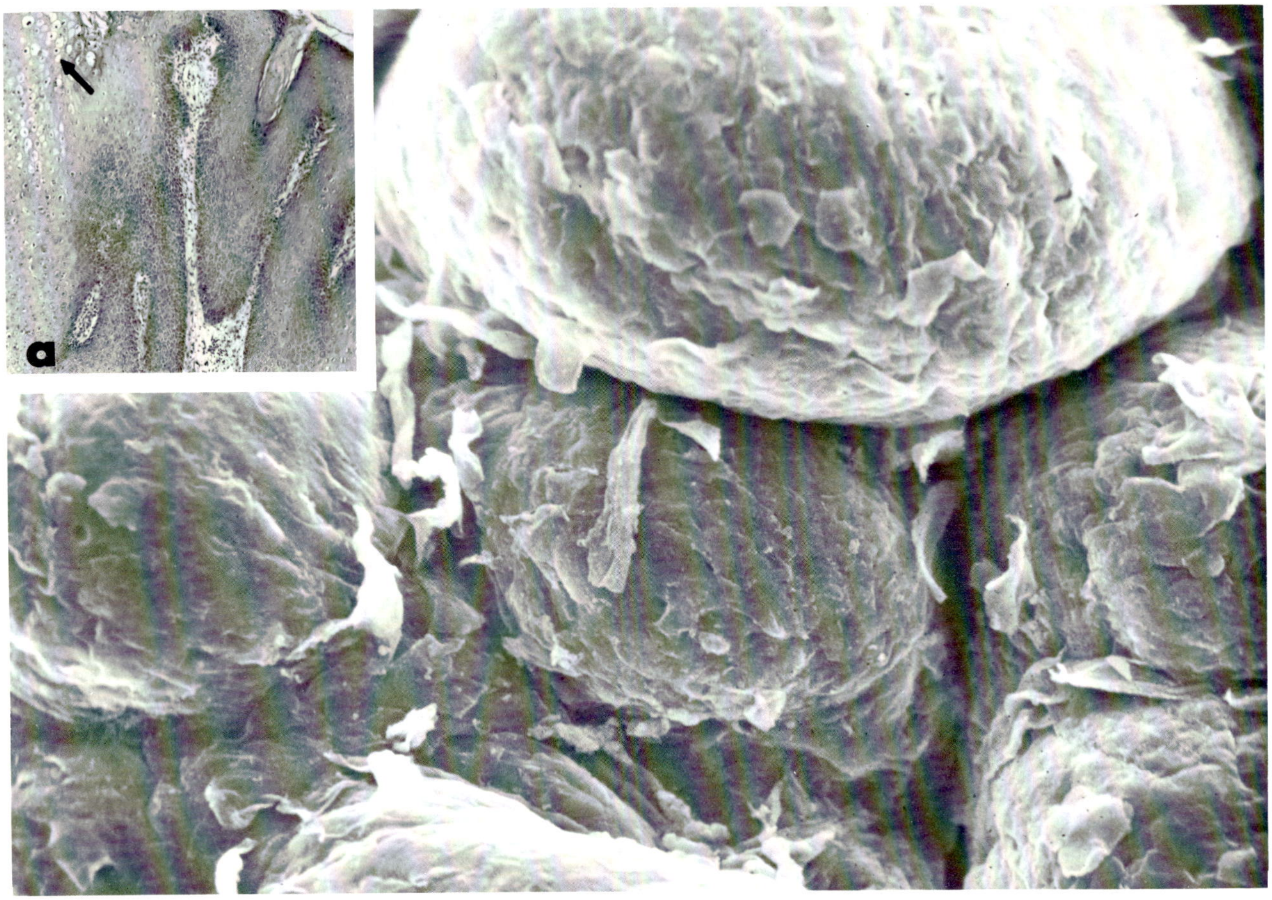

5

Condyloma Acuminatum

Condyloma acuminata are benign, cauliflowerlike, verruciform lesions usually found on the vulvar vestibule and labial folds. They occur primarily during the reproductive period and may enlarge rapidly during pregnancy. The lesions are generally considered to be viral-induced, and viral particles of the presumed human papilloma virus type have been found by electron microscopy.[1,2] Although the exact mode of transmission is unknown, the venereal route is the most likely possibility.

Figure 13a. *Microscopically,* there is prominent acanthosis, with elongation and clubbing of the rete ridges, accompanied by papillomatosis and parakeratosis. Characteristically, hyperkeratosis is minimal or lacking, and, in addition to cytoplasmic vacuolization of the upper cell layers (arrow), nuclear atypia and mitotic figures are prominent. A well-defined basal lamina separates the epithelial cells from the chronically inflammed upper dermis. (H & E stain, × 12.)

Figure 13. *The surface configuration of desquamated condylomatous lesions* contains prominent, club-shaped papillae with numerous desquamated cells. At a higher magnification the superficial cells are large, polygonal, and covered by well-developed microridges. × 160.

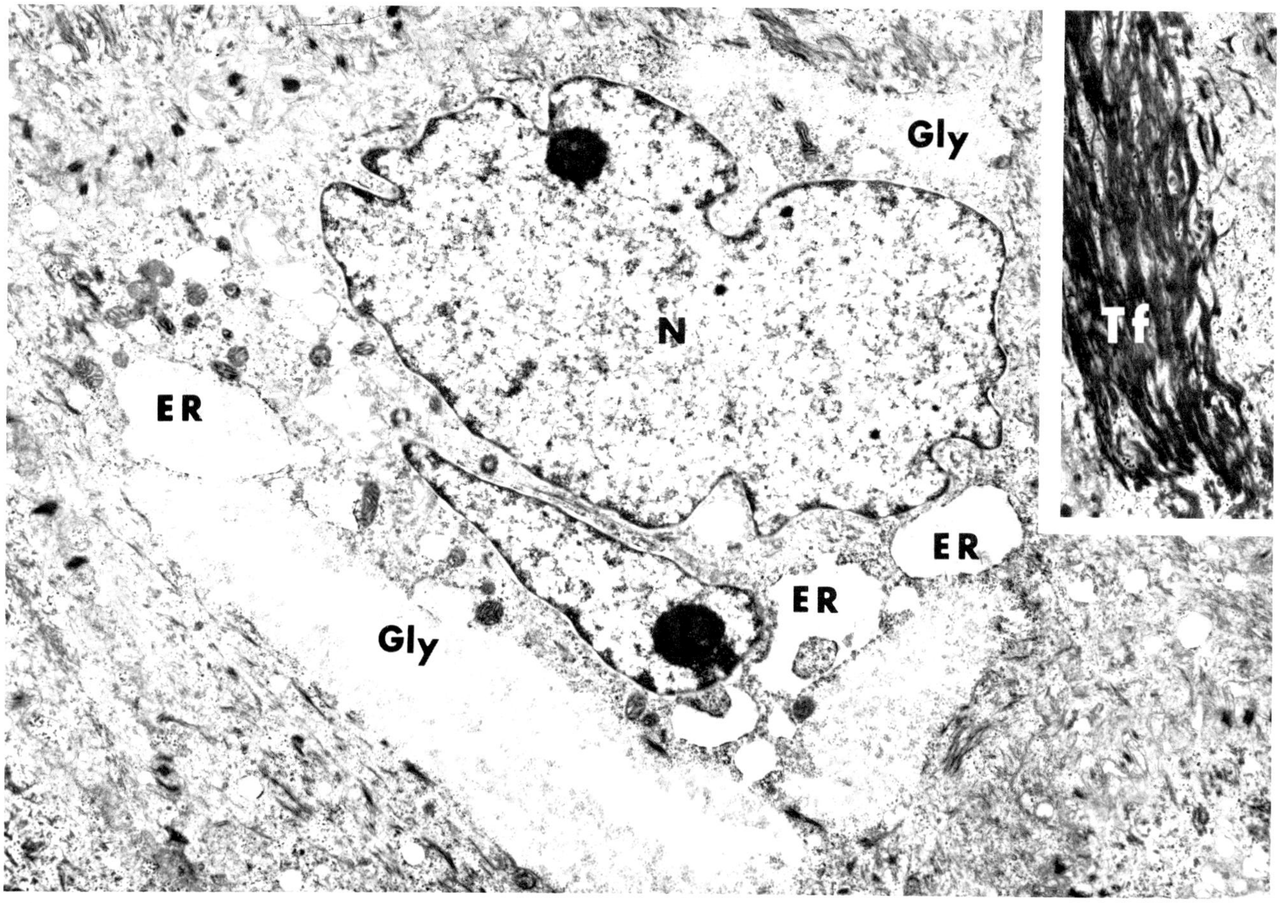

Figure 14. *Ultrastructurally,* keratinization is incomplete and the parakeratotic cells are dark and slender, with small, degenerating nuclei. The cells in the *upper strata* contain pools of glycogen particles (Gly) with central vacuolar degeneration. As a result, the Golgi, mitochondria, endoplasmic reticulum (ER), and tonofilaments are displaced to the periphery of the cytoplasm. The significance of the conspicuous accumulation of glycogen in condyloma accuminatum is not known, but it is thought to be responsible for the vacuolated appearance of the superficial epidermal keratinocytes by light microscopy. Binucleated (N) cells are frequently seen, and many nuclei contain two or more prominent nucleoli. × 5400.

Figure 14a. *In the deeper and mid-Malpighian layers,* aggregated bundles of tonofilaments (Tf), with an occasional whorl formation, are seen but the general architecture and number of desmosomal attachments are unaltered. Viral particles were not found in our material. × 6600.

REFERENCES (Condyloma acuminatum—Figure 14a)

1. Zimmer, S. Morphologic virus demonstration in condyloma, acuminatum. *Zentralbl. Gynaekol.* **86:** 1116 (1964).
2. Dunn, A. E. G. and M. M. Ogilvie. Intranuclear virus particles in human genital wart tissue: observations on the ultrastructure of the epidermal layer. *J. Ultrastruct. Res.* **22:** 282 (1968).

6 Lymphogranuloma Venerum

Lymphogranuloma venerum (lymphogranuloma inguinale) is a highly contagious, venereal disease which is prevalent largely in women living in tropical countries and in recent immigrants from such countries to more temperate climes. The disease involves primarily the regional lymphatic system and produces inguinal and perirectal, necrotizing lymphadenitis with characteristic stellate microabscesses. Pronounced scarring of the advanced lesions results in anorectal strictures and vulvar elephantiasis. Clinically, the intradermal Frei test and the complement fixation test, using lymphogranuloma venerum agent antigen recovered from inguinal buboes and infected chick yolk-sac membranes, respectively, are usually positive.

Contrary to the general belief, the lesion is caused not by a virus, but by a DNA–RNA-containing micro-organism of the Chlamydiaceae group. Characteristically, the Chlamydiaceae undergo three successive phases of development in phagocytic vacuoles of infected cells e.g., (HeLa).[1] The immature or "elementary" particles (0.3 μ) are composed of a DNA-containing nucleoid, surrounded by ribosomes and double limiting membranes. These are transformed into larger (1– 2 μ) "initial" bodies with central, fibrillar nucleoids that multiply by binary division and multiple cytoplasmic buddings within the phagocytic vacuoles, forming polymorphic, intracytoplasmic inclusions. The subsequent condensation of "initial" bodies results in "intermediary" corpuscles, which, in turn, are transformed into "elementary" bodies, and a new cycle is initiated. Since the presence of a glycogen matrix is inconsistent, the differentiation of the lymphogranuloma venerum agent, *Chlamydia trachomatis,* from organisms of the ornithosis-psittacosis species cannot be established at the ultrastructural level.

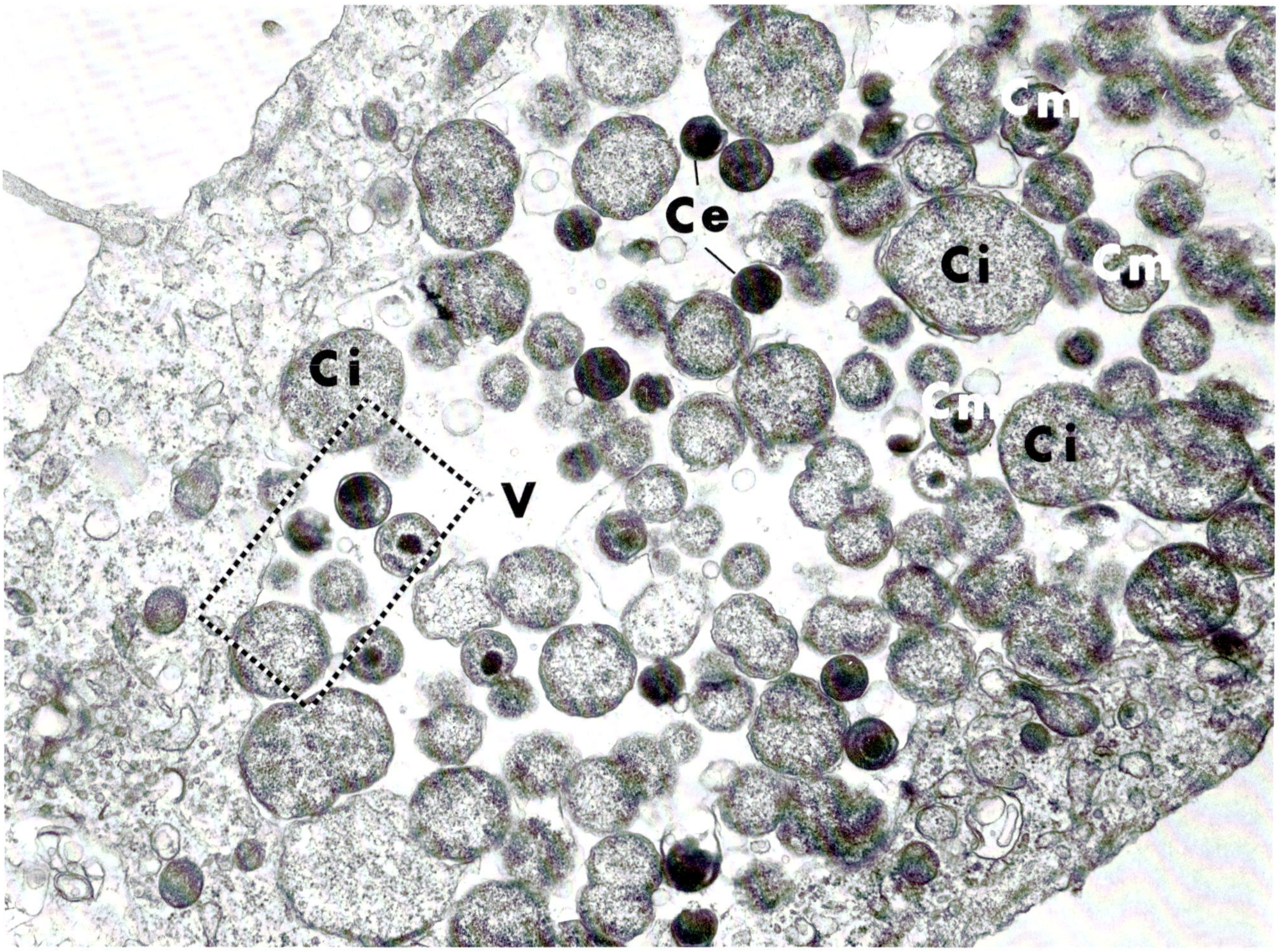

Figure 15. *HeLa cell infected by the agent of lymphogranuloma venerum.* Electron micrograph illustrating the development of chlamydiae 48 hours after penetration into the cell: several different bodies are present within the host's phagocytic vacuole (V). Reticulate bodies (Ci), elementary bodies (Ce), and intermediate forms (Cm) are seen. Some reticulate bodies are dividing by binary fission. × 23,400. *From* F. Eb, G. Devauchelle, and J. Orfila. Etude ultrastructurale de l'agent de la lymphogranulomatose vénérienne (Rickettsiales, Chlamydiaceae). *J. Microsc.* **13:** 47-56 (1972).

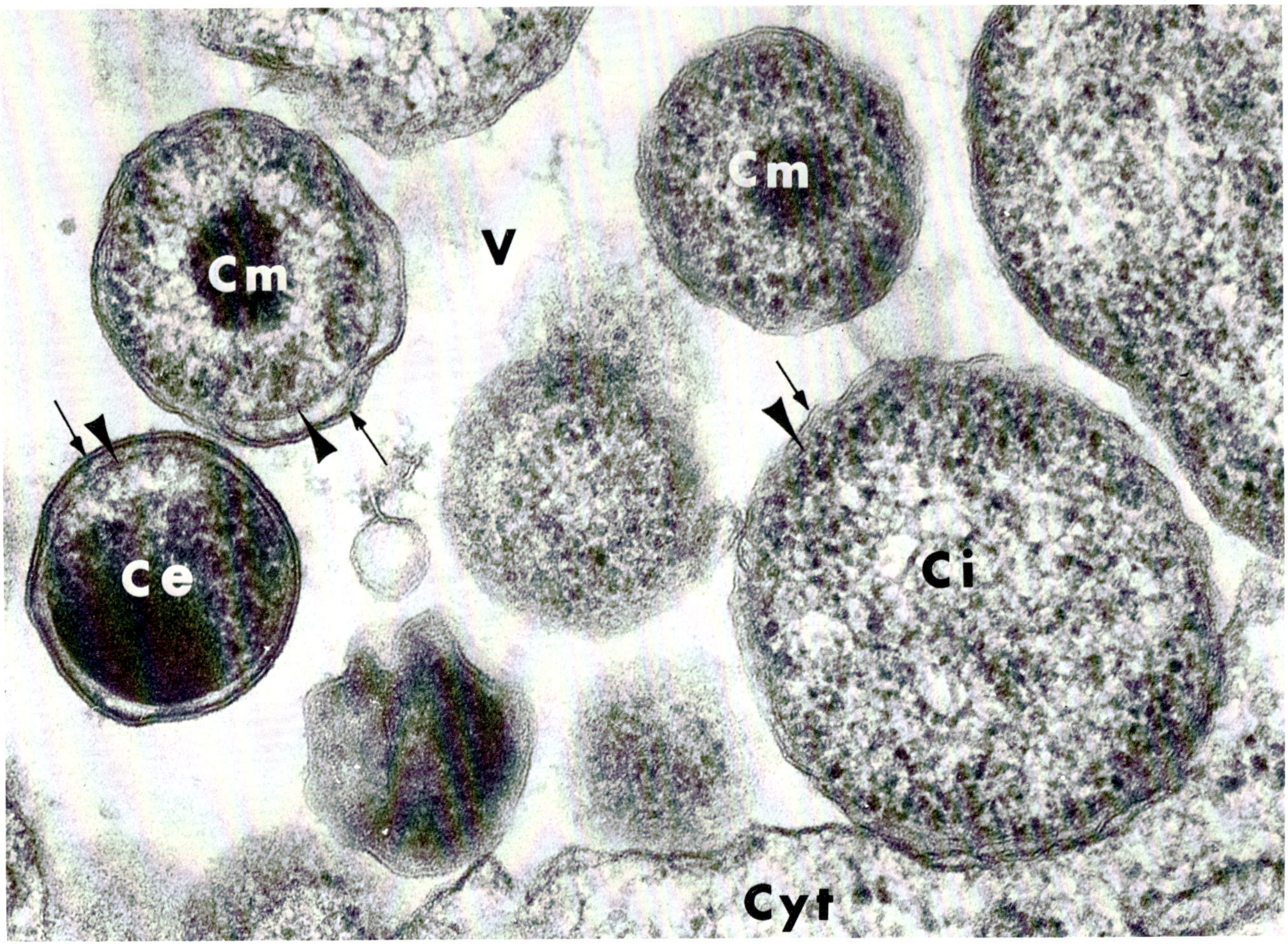

Figure 16. *Ce: elementary body of the lymphogranuloma venerum agent.* This is the smallest chlamydial cell (0.3 μ in diameter), limited by a cell wall (arrow head) and a plasma membrane (arrow). The nucleoid is eccentric. *Ci: initial body of the lymphogranuloma venerum agent.* Each reticulate body is surrounded by two trilaminar membranes separated by diffuse material. They contain granular components. *Cm: the Intermediate form of the lymphogranuloma venerum agent* has a dense, central nucleoid. × 112,000. V: vacuole; Cyt: cytoplasm. *From* F. Eb, G. Devauchelle, and J. Orfila. Etude ultrastructurale de l'agent de la lymphogranulomatose vénérienne (Rickettsiales, Chlamydiaceae). *J. Microsc.* **13:** 47-56 (1972).

REFERENCE (Lymphogranuloma venerum—Figure 16)

1. Eb, F., G. Devauchelle, and J. Orfila. Etude ultrastructurale de l'agent de la lymphogranulomatose vénérienne (Rickettsiales, Chlamydiaceae). *J. Microsc.* **13:** 47 (1972).

7

Bartholin's Duct, Glands, and Duct Cyst

Figure 17a. *Bartholin's duct.* The proximal two-thirds of the major excretory duct of Bartholin's gland is lined by a stratified transitional epithelium, which is gradually replaced by a stratified squamous epithelium as the duct approaches the vulvovestibular ostium. Similar transitional-type epithelium lines the secondary ducts and ductules. × 120.

Figure 17b. *The fine structure of the transitional ductal lining* is identical to the transitional epithelium of the urinary tract.[1] The cells near the basal lamina are low columnar and contain relatively few organelles. In the middle layer, the cells are enlarged and are rich in cytoplasmic free and bound ribosomes. Some cells contain numerous perinuclear bundles of tonofilaments (arrows), and the microvillous plasma membranes are interconnected by well-developed desmosomes, resembling the spinous cells of stratified squamous mucous membranes.[1] In general, the intercellular spaces (ICS) are dilated, and there are numerous microvillous projections. Desmosomes (D) between transitional cells are small and are randomly distributed. In the upper zone, the cells have abundant smooth, and rough, endoplasmic reticulum, Golgi (G), and prominent autophagic lysosomes (telolysosomes). The most superficial cells contain numerous lysosomes (long arrow) and covered by stubby, irregular microvilli; pinocytotic vesicles are numerous. These surface specializations, together with the abundant cytoplasmic organelles, are probably related to the transport of water, proteins, and electrolytes. × 7200. Lu: ductal lumen.

Figure 17c. *Detail of membrane-bound dense bodies,* which are concentrated beneath the luminal plasma membranes. × 22,000.

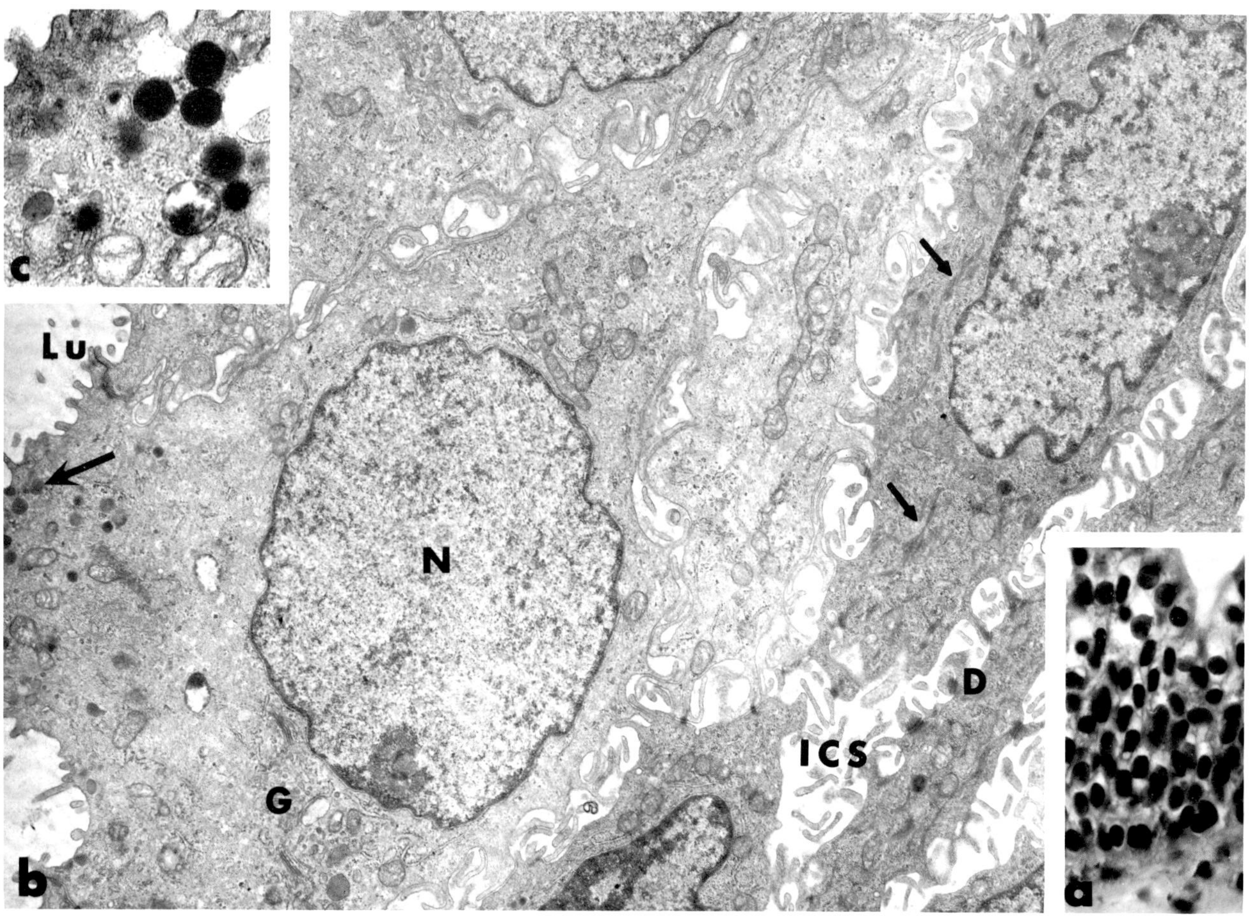

Occasionally, the transitional epithelium is covered by a single layer of secretory cells which are rich in secretory vacuoles and Golgi. These cells are attached by desmosomes to the underlying cells, which contain abundant Golgi and scattered supranuclear secretory vesicles, suggesting a cell type intermediate between the transitional and secretory cells.[1] These submicroscopic observations support the concept that the secretory cells in the Bartholin's duct transitional epithelium, like the urothelium of the Brenner tumor and Walthard's cell nest epithelia, are derived through a metaplastic process.[2] The presence of squamous spinous cells within the Bartholin's duct transitional lining is also a common finding in normal, and especially in neoplastic, urothelia. Their increasing number toward the distal third of the duct suggests a progressive metaplastic transformation from the transitional lining epithelium.

REFERENCES (Figures 17a–18d)

1. Ferenczy, A. and R. M. Richart. Unpublished data.
2. Bransilver, B., A. Ferenczy, and R. M. Richart. Brenner tumors and Walthard cell nests. A comparative study, in preparation.

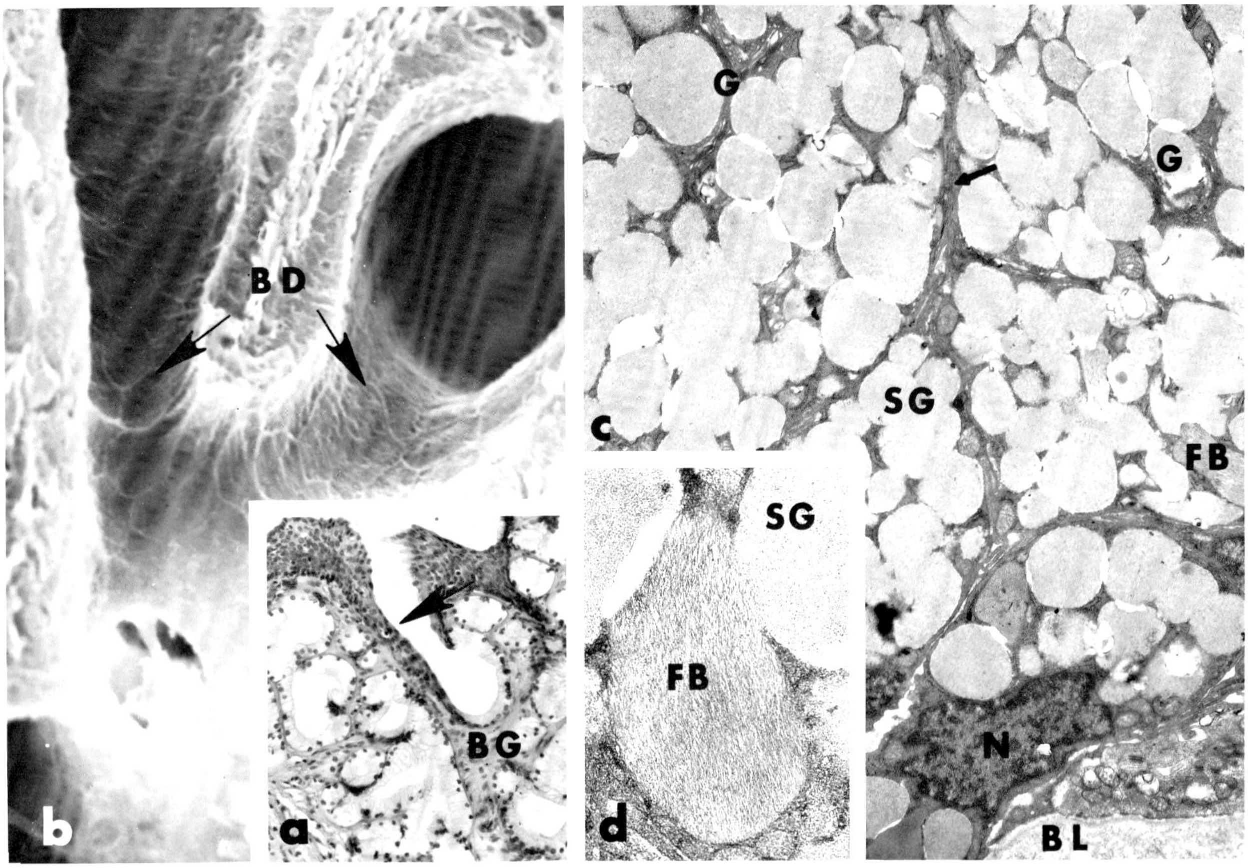

Figure 18a. *Light micrograph of a ductule* (arrow) in which the "low" transitional cell epithelium is in direct continuity with the underlying glandular epithelium. *Bartholin's glands* are arranged in lobules of mucus-secreting, columnar, acinar epithelium (BG). (H & E stain, × 30.)

Figure 18b. *Scanning electron micrograph* of two merging ductules (BD). The superficial cells of the transitional epithelium have a regular hexagonal outline. × 1160.

Figure 18c. *Ultrastructurally,* the nucleus (N) is relatively small, triangular, and basally located. The entire cytoplasmic substance is occupied by tightly packed secretory granules (SG), intermingled with clusters of fibrillar bodies (FB). The Golgi (G) are prominent with numerous peripheral vesicles. The formation of secretory products occurs, as in other secretory glandular epithelia, through the ribosome–endoplasmic reticulum–Golgi complex, and secretion is of the apocrine type.[1] The intercellular spaces are narrow, and small desmosomes are found along adjacent plasma membranes (arrow). The luminal portions, however, are closely maintained by tight junctional complexes. The surface boundary membrane contains microvilli of various sizes, and ciliated cells are not seen. Myoepithelial cells are not encountered in either acinar or ductular epithelium. × 5600 BL: Basal lamina.

Figure 18d. The frequent interrelationship between *fibrillar bodies* (FB) and secretory granules (SG) suggests that the former are derived from the latter and represent a fibrillar or proteinaceous storage form of mucopolysaccharides. × 34,200.

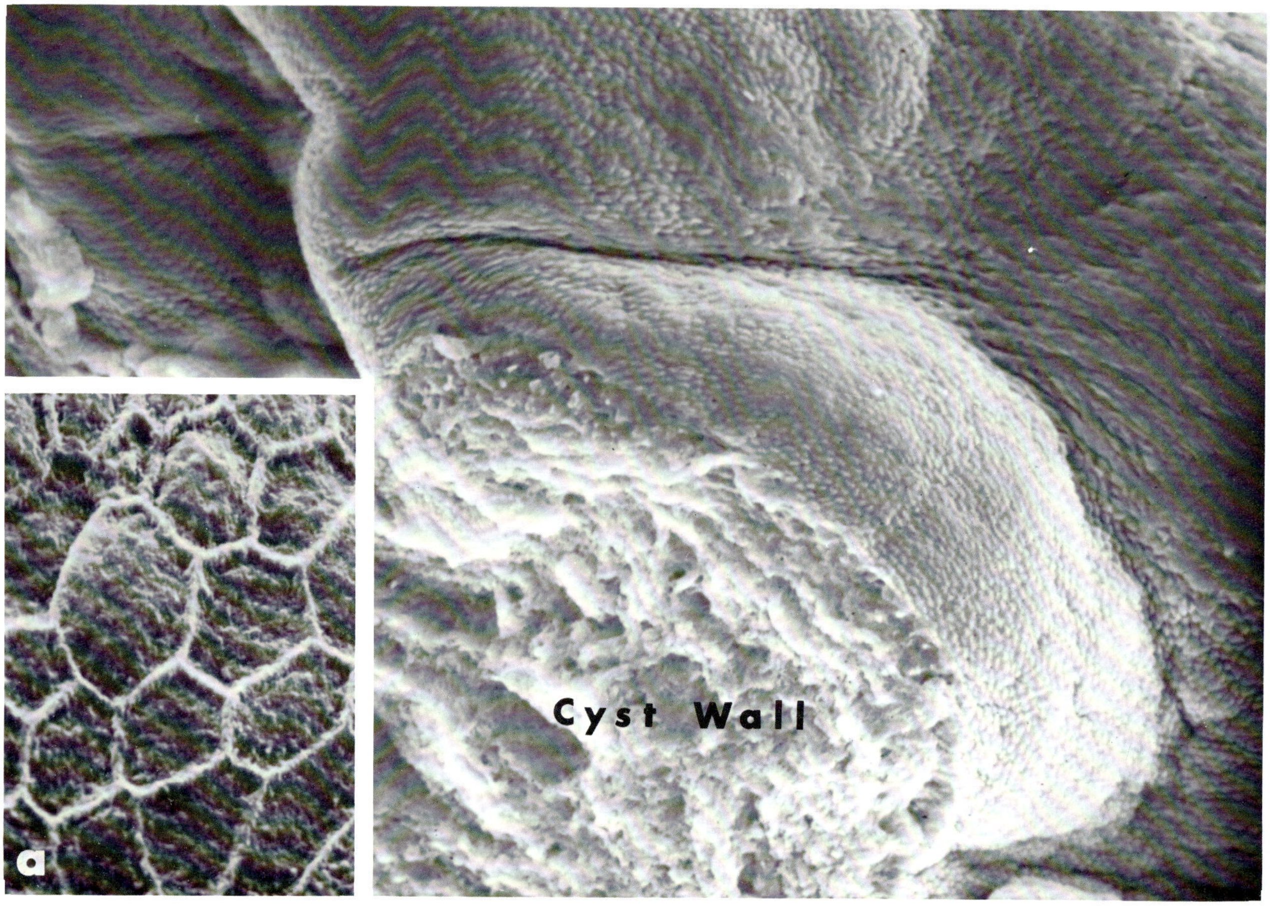

Bartholin's duct cyst is the most common clinically observed vulvar cystic lesion. These cysts are usually located in the labia majora and arise after obstruction of the duct due to gonorrheal infections, congenital stenosis, inspissated mucus, or squamous metaplasia. The cyst is lined by stratified transitional or squamous epithelium, according to the site of obstruction, and is distended by mucus, secreted by Bartholin's glands.

Certain foci contain an intermixture of large transitional cells and smaller dome-shaped, sponge-like, secretory cells,[1] and the submicroscopic characteristics of the cyst lining are identical to those of the transitional cell epithelium of the normal excretory duct, including the presence of squamous and mucinous metaplastic foci.

Figure 19. *Scanning electron microscopy* of the epithelial surface reveals a uniform cell population with a cobblestone pattern. Several ductular openings are seen.[1] × 160.

Figure 19a. *The cells have pentagonal or hexagonal outlines,* and the apical cytoplasmic membrane is slightly collapsed and covered by numerous short microvilli. × 3040.

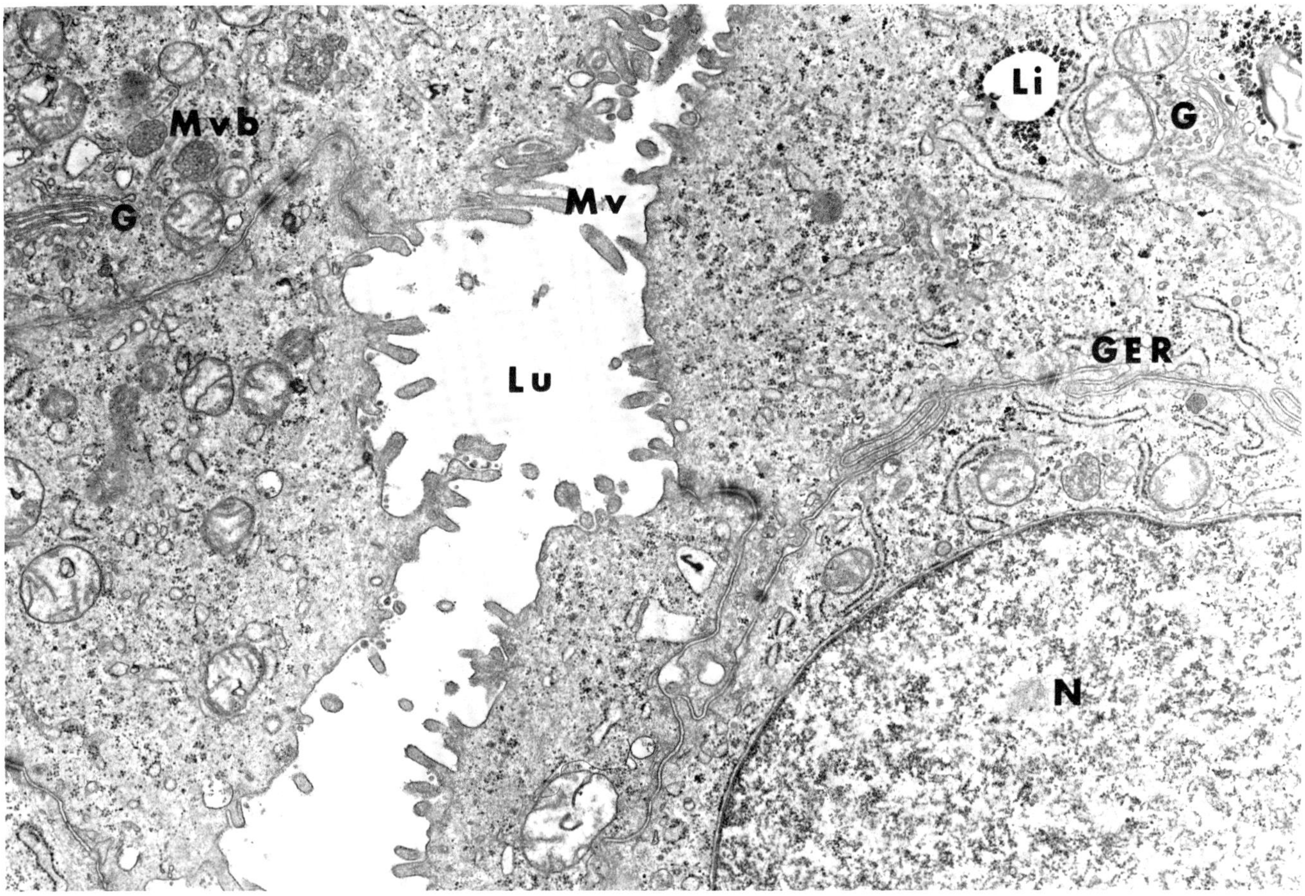

8

Adenocarcinoma of Bartholin's Gland

An uncommon neoplasm, *Bartholin's gland adenocarcinoma* has the histological appearance of an adenocarcinoma, usually with a cribriform pattern (adenoid cystic) and usually lacking evidence of mucus secretion.

REFERENCE (Figures 19–20)

1. Ferenczy, A. and R. M. Richart. Unpublished data.

Figure 20. *At the ultrastructural level,* the malignant glandular cells have the dedifferentiated features commonly found in malignant epithelial neoplasms, the most prominent of which are numerous luminal microvilli (Mv), abundant free and bound ribosomes (GER), Golgi (G), and an absence of specialized cell products, including mucus-containing secretory vacuoles. Accumulation of glycogen particles, especially around lipid droplets (Li), is seen. × 1500. Lu: neoplastic glandular lumen Mvb: multivesicular bodies; N: nucleus. *From* H. M. Shingleton, Associate Professor, Department of Obstetrics and Gynecology, University of Alabama, 1919 Seventh Avenue South, Birmingham, Ala. 35233.

9

Paget's Disease

Paget's disease is a rare vulvar disorder in which the epidermis is invaded by characteristic large, pale, often signet-ring-shaped cells referred to as Paget's cells.

Paget's cells, regardless of whether they are of mammary or extramammary origin, are essentially identical in their fine structure,[1] and the cytophotometric demonstration of an aneuploid nuclear DNA content[2] is consistent with the contention that they are malignant cells. Two distinct cell types can be identified: secretory and nonsecretory, according to the presence or absence of secretory vacuoles. The secretory products are associated with prominent Golgi and, histochemically, contain PAS- and alcian blue-positive, hyaluronidase-resistant, mucicarmine-positive material. The intraepidermal Paget cells are attached by small, irregularly distributed desmosomes to the adjacent normal squamous epidermal cells and by rare hemidesmosomes to the epidermal basal lamina.[1]

Despite numerous electron microscopic observations, opinion is still divided concerning the origin of extramammary Paget's cells. In approximately 50% of the cases of vulvar Paget's disease an underlying carcinoma of sweat gland or, occasionally, Bartholin's gland[3] origin is present. For such patients the prognosis is poor and is essentially that of the underlying carcinoma. When no underlying lesion is found, the prognosis is much better. In these cases, the disease is said to arise autochthonously and there is disagreement over the cell of origin. Although some investigators believe that the Paget cells in autochthonous disease are derived from in-situ malignant transformation of epidermal squamous cells [4-8] or from intraepidermal neoplastic transformation of the sweat gland apparatus,[7,9] others favor an extraepidermal glandular origin from either the apocrine[10-12] or eccrine[1,13,14] dermal sweat gland apparatus. An eccrine, rather than apocrine, derivation is supported by the histochemical demonstration of a similar pattern of amylophosphorylase, leucine aminopeptidase, and oxidative enzymes in Paget's cells and in the eccrine epithelium,[14] a distribution dissimilar to that found in the eccrine sweat gland cells.

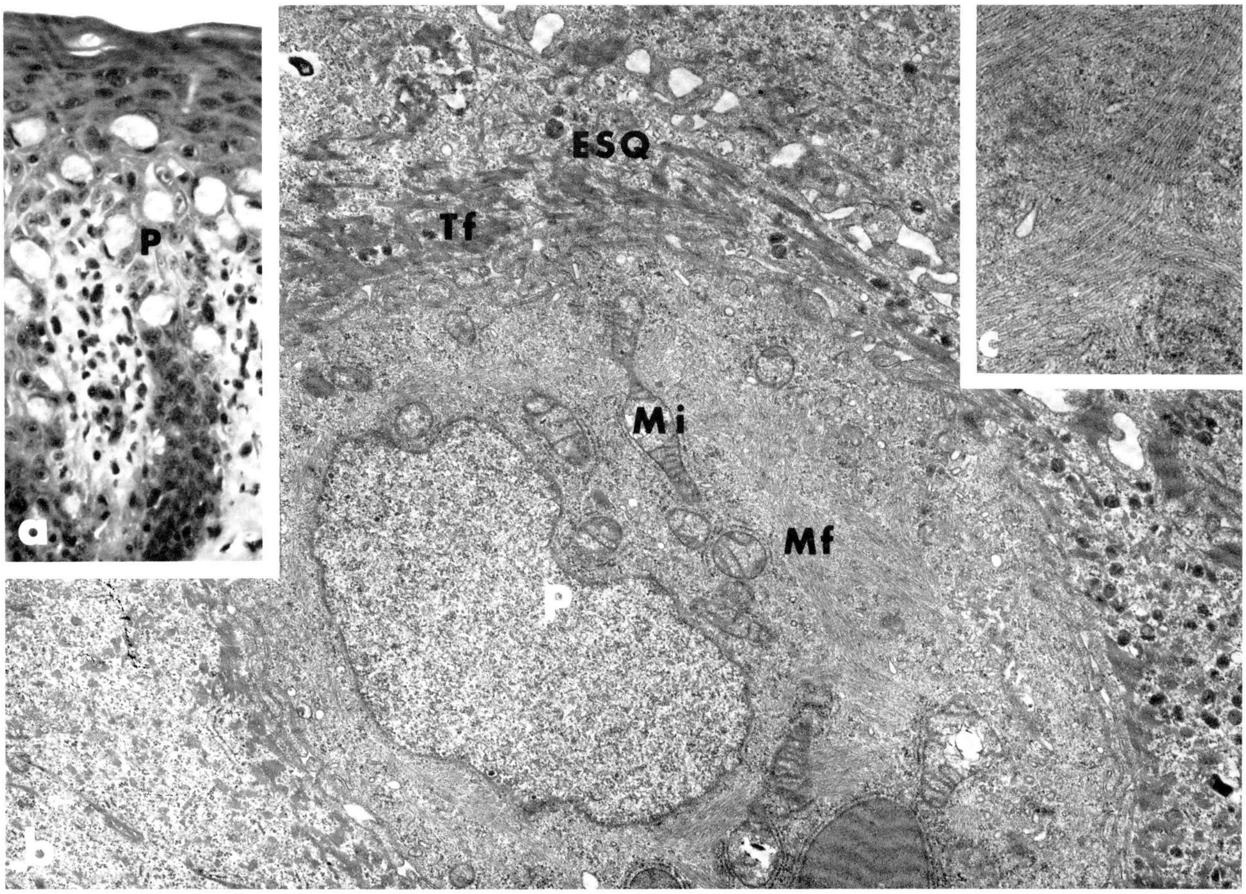

Figure 21a. *Histologic appearance of signet-ring-shaped Paget's cells* (P), which may occur singly or in clusters, may form acini, and may be present along the epithelial root sheath of hair follicles. (HPS × 160).

Figure 21b. *A nonsecretory Paget's cell* (P) in the upper Malpighian layer is completely surrounded by epidermal squamous cells (ESQ) in which tonofilaments (Tf) are aggregated. The peculiar concentration of tonofilaments in the neighboring keratinocytes is interpreted as a compression effect by Paget's cells upon the adjacent cells.[1] The cytoplasm of the Paget cell is packed with interlacing bundles of microfilaments (Mf), and the mitochondria (Mi) appear pleomorphic. The plasma membrane contains numerous interdigitating microvillous processes. × 4600.

Figure 21c. *Higher-power view* of microfilaments. × 22,000.

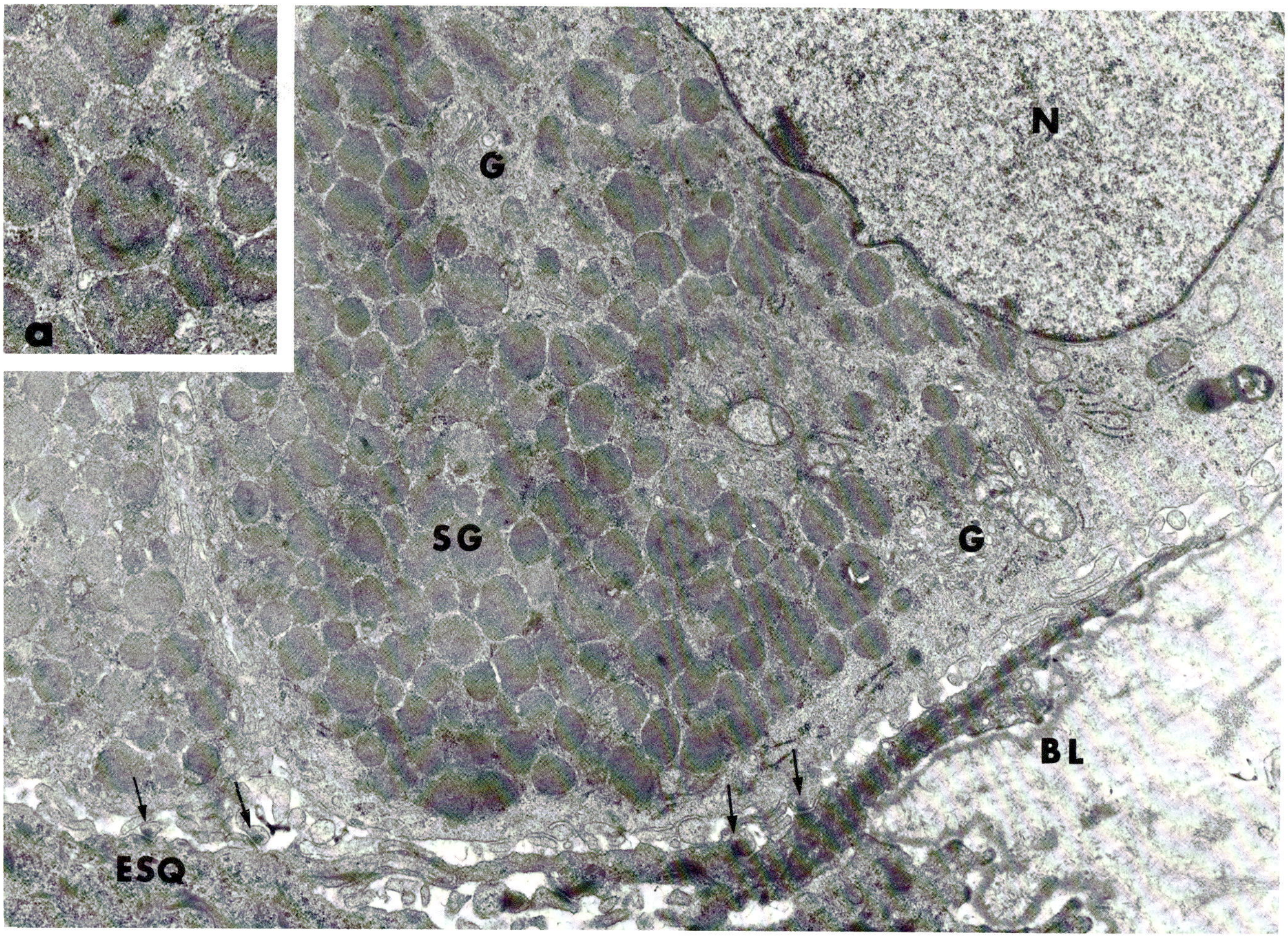

Figure 22. *The signet-ring-shaped secretory Paget cell* has an eccentrically placed nucleus (N), and most of the cytoplasmic substance is occupied by tightly packed secretory granules (SG), associated with rows of juxtanuclear Golgi (G). Contacts between Paget cells and keratinocytes (ESQ) are established by small desmosomes (arrows). Slender cytoplasmic extensions from the adjacent keratinocytes are often found between Paget cells and the epidermal basal lamina (BL). × 6200.

Figure 22a. *The content* of the secretory granules is filamentous. × 16,500.

REFERENCES (Paget's Disease–Figure 22)

1. Ferenczy, A. and R. M. Richart, Ultrastructure of perianal Paget's disease. *Cancer* **29:** 1141 (1972).
2. Sachs, H. Cytophotometric DNA determination of Paget's cells of the mamillary region and the vulva. *Arch. Gynakol.* **209:** 256 (1970).
3. Tchang, F., T. Okagaki, and R. M. Richart. Adenocarcinoma of Bartholin's gland associated with Paget's disease of vulvar area. *Cancer* **31:** 221 (1973).
4. Sagami, S. Electron microscopic studies in Paget's disease. *Med. J. Osaka Univ.* **14:** 173 (1963).
5. Pierard, J. and A. Kint. Maladie de Paget extrammaire. *Arch. Belges Dermatol. Syphil.* **24:** 335 (1968).
6. Yshibashi, Y. and G. Jager. Elektronenmickroskipische untersuchung eines extramammaren Morbus Paget. *Arch. Klin. Exp. Dermatol.* **234:** 293 (1969).
7. Fetherston, W. C. and E. G. Friedrich, Jr. The origin and significance of vulvar Paget's disease. *Obstet. Gynecol.* **39:** 735 (1972).
8. Medinica, M. and T. Sahihi. Ultrastructural study of a case of extrammary Paget's disease of the vulva. *Arch. Dermatol.* **105:** 236 (1972).
9. Helwig, E. B. and J. H. Graham. Anogenital (extramammary) Paget's disease. A clinicopathological study. *Cancer* **16:** 387 (1963).
10. Caputo, R. and A. Califano. Ultrastructural features of extramammary Paget's disease. *Arch. Klin. Exp. Dermatol.* **236:** 121 (1970).
11. Demopoulos, R. I. Fine structure of the extrammary Paget's cell. *Cancer* **27:** 1202 (1971).
12. Neilson, D. and J. D. Woodruff. Electron microscopy in in situ and invasive vulvar Paget's disease. *Am. J. Obstet. Gynecol.* **113:** 719 (1972).
13. Koss, L. G. and A. Brockunier, Jr. Ultrastructural aspects of Paget's disease of the vulva. *Arch. Pathol.* **87:** 592 (1969).
14. Belcher, R. W. Extramammary Paget's disease. Enzyme histochemical and electron microscopic study. *Arch. Pathol.* **94:** 59 (1972).

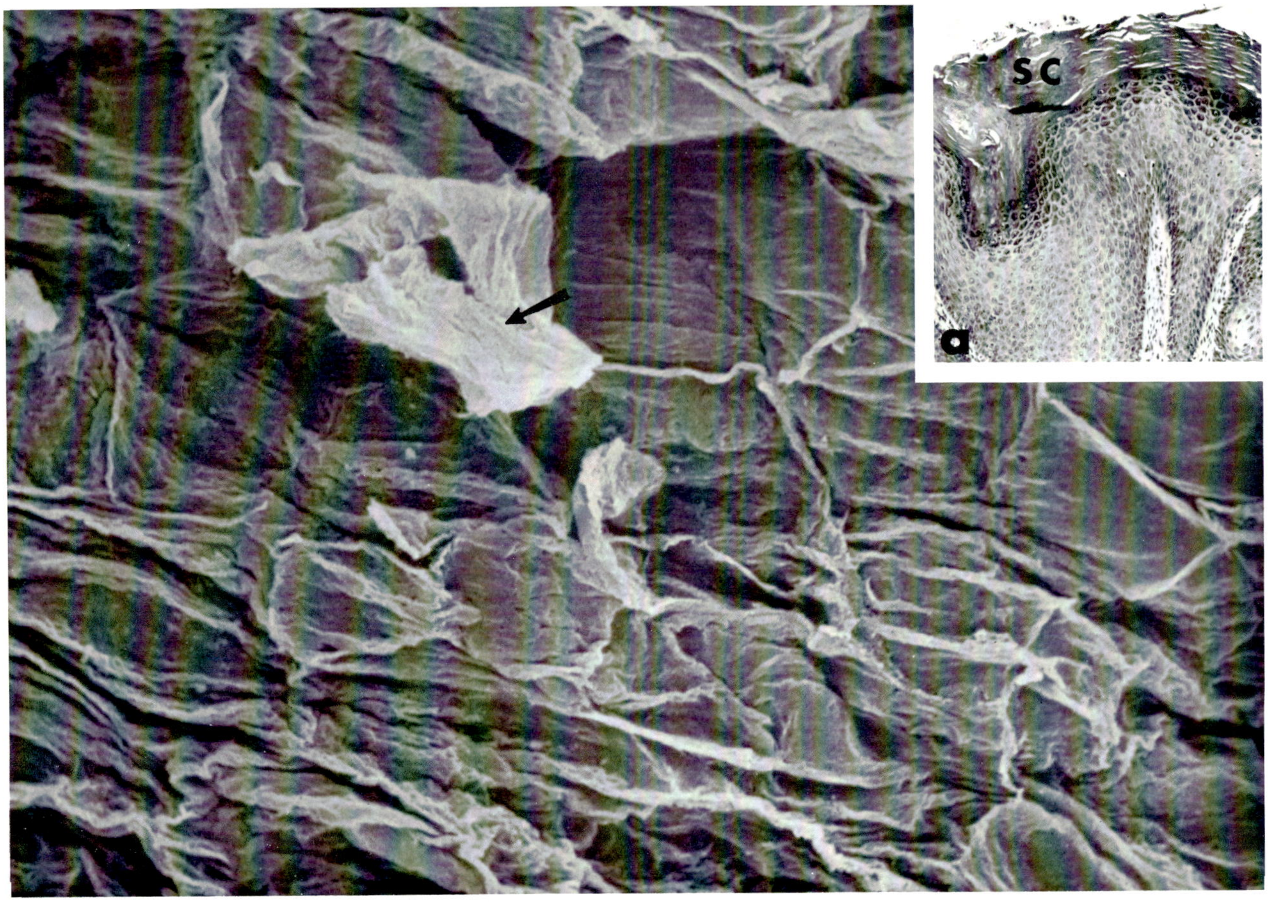

Figure 23a. *Histologically,* the whitish plaque corresponds to a pronounced thickening of the stratum corneum (SC). The epidermis is often acanthotic with a well-developed granular cell layer and elongated rete ridges. Cytological atypicality is generally absent in vulvar hyperkeratosis, whether associated with chronic vulvitis or not. Characteristically, the upper dermis contains dense fibrosis and exhibits a conspicuous chronic inflammatory reaction. (H & E stain, × 19.)

Figure 23. *The stereoscopic surface pattern of the horny cells* is similar to that of normal skin and includes the presence of interlacing microridges. Superficial cells are desquamating from the surface (arrow). × 1600.

10

Vulvar Hyperkeratosis

Vulvar hyperkeratosis has the clinical appearance of a whitish, indurated plaque (leukoplakia), which corresponds to a thickened horny layer. This layer, however, appears normal in its structural organization, and there is no evidence of defective formation of intercellular cement or desmosomal attachments, which would lead to precocious or exaggerated desquamation. Increased mitotic activity and binucleated epidermal cells are not observed, suggesting that hyperkeratosis occurs secondarily to accelerated keratin formation and that there is a relative decrease in the shedding of horny cells, rather than an increase in the turnover rate of epidermal cells, such as is seen in other hyperkeratotic conditions (e.g., psoriasis, Darier's disease, and epidermolytic hyperkeratosis).[1,2]

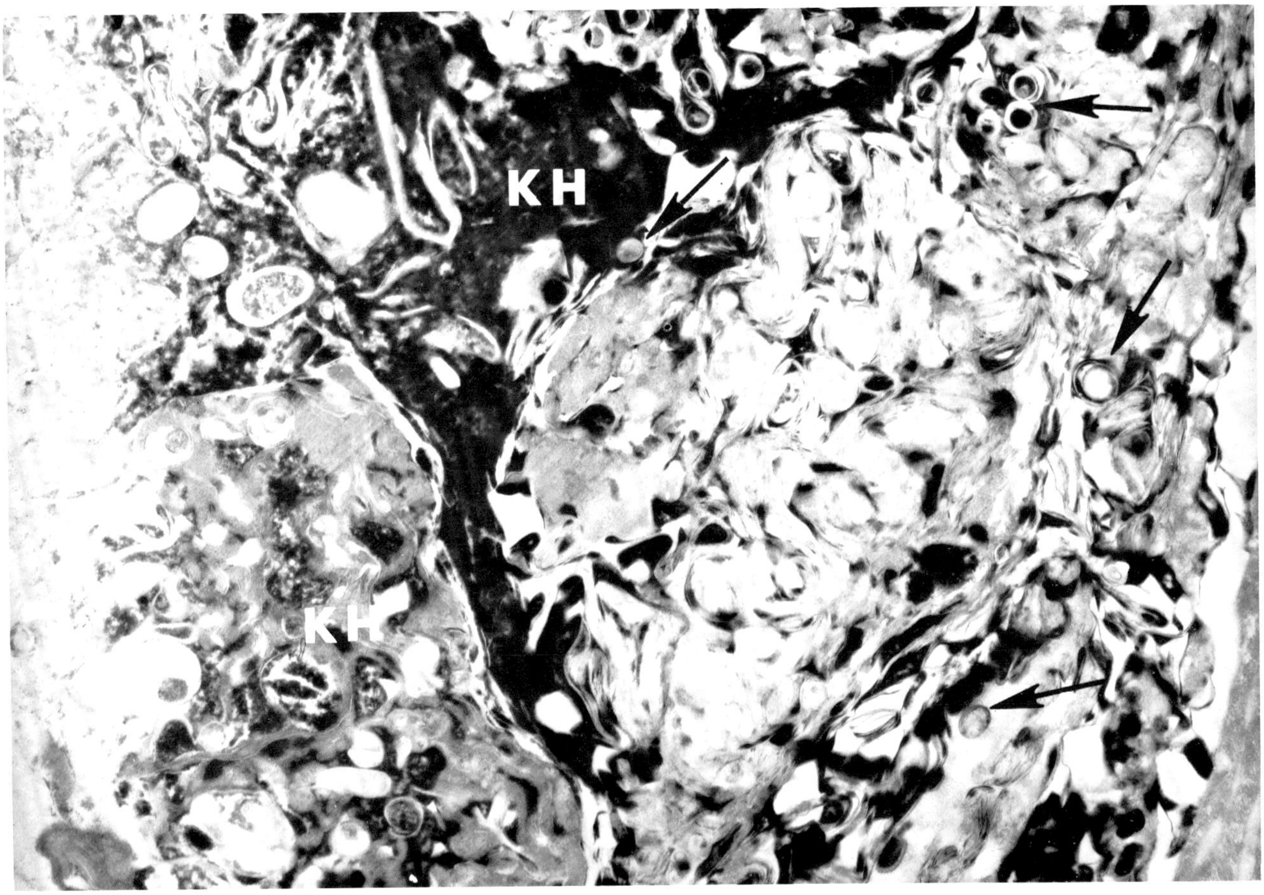

Figure 24. *Ultrastructurally, the epidermal cells of the upper strata* have an increased number of cytoplasmic organelles, membrane-coated granules (keratinosomes:arrows), keratohyaline granules (KH), and tonofilaments. × 8400

REFERENCES (Vulvar hyperkeratosis–Figure 24)

1. Wilgram, G. F, E. G. Madgic, and J. B. Caulfield. Electron microscopic studies of genetic errors in keratinization. In *The Biology of Skin and Hair Growth,* E. Lyne (Ed.). Oxford University Press, New York, 1965.
2. Wilgram, G. F. and J. B. Caulfield. An electron microscopic study of epidermolytic hyperkeratosis. *Arch. Dermatol.* **94:** 127 (1966).

11

Intraepithelial Carcinoma (Bowen's Disease)

Intraepithelial carcinoma (Bowen's disease) occurs in the vulvar skin as a slowly growing, pruritic, reddish, scaling plaque. The lesion may be multifocal and may be associated with vaginal, cervical, or systemic malignancy. Spherical, viruslike particles 800 to 1100 Å in diameter were demonstrated extruding from plasma membranes of altered keratinocytes by Nordquist et al.,[1] but their significance is unknown. Herpes simplex virus type II has been isolated from vulvar carcinoma in situ, and a positive type II antibody titer was found in a case of reversible Bowenoid vulvar atypia associated with pregnancy.[2]

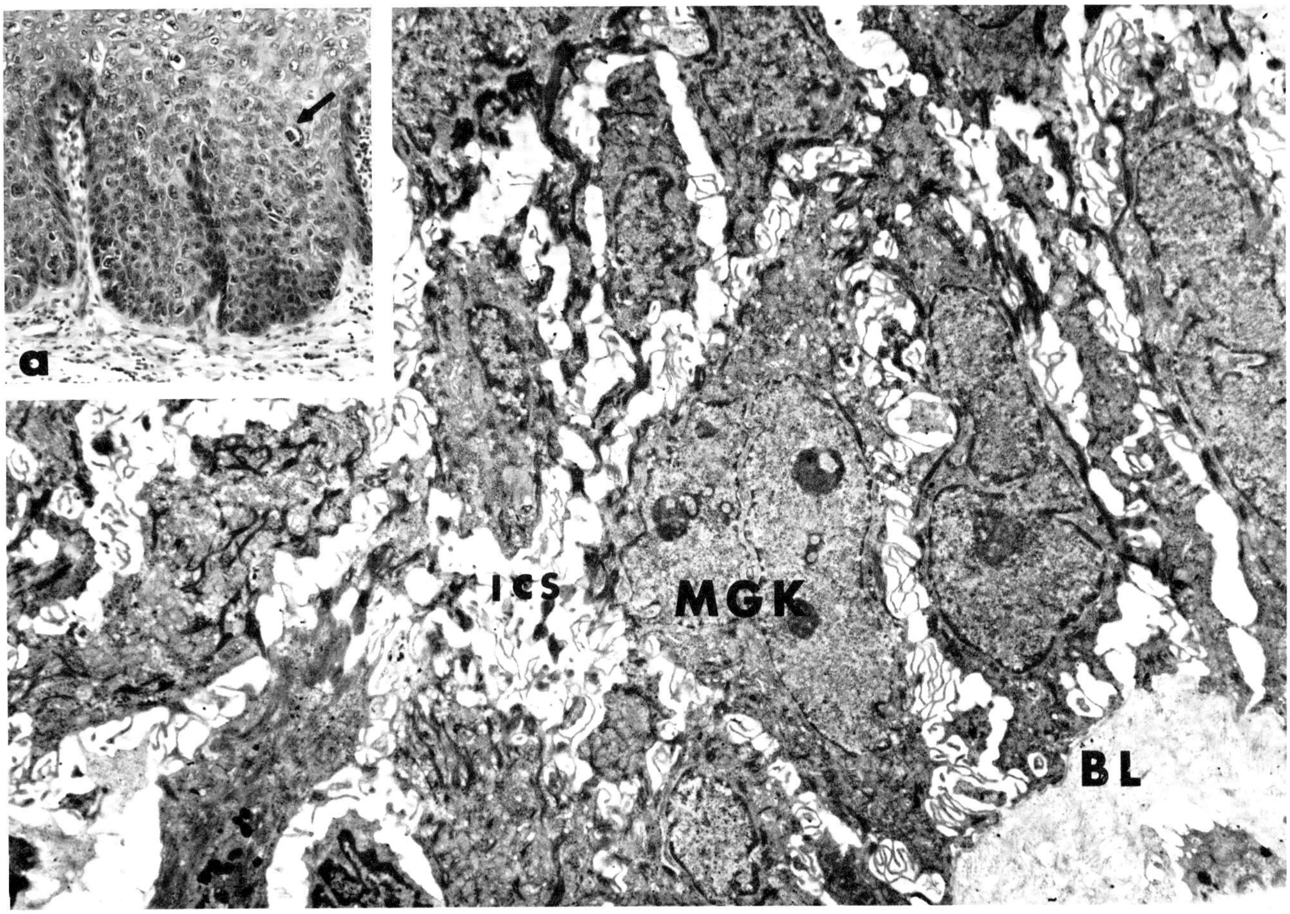

Figure 25a. *Histologically,* the acanthotic Malpighian layer contains a disorganized, pleomorphic cell population with prominent neoplastic, dyskeratotic (individual cell keratinization) (arrow), frequently multinucleated cells and a large number of mitotic figures. The upper dermis usually contains a lymphoplasmacytic infiltrate. (H & E stain, × 40.)

Figure 25. *The giant multinucleated epidermal cells (MGK)* have a condensed nuclear substance occasionally mixed with tonofilaments.[3] There is often abnormal segregation of nucleolar RNA, which is similar to the nucleolar changes produced by actinomycin-D and similar compounds, suggesting an impairment of RNA synthesis.[4] Other pertinent findings include widened intercellular spaces (ICS), pleomorphic mitochondria, decreased quantities of glycogen, and focal dissolution of the basal lamina (BL).[3,5,6] × 8320. *From* J. Karasek, J. Pitha, W. Oehlert, and B. Konrad. Dyskeratosis in Bowen's disease: the ultrastructure and fate of keratinocytes with altered tonofilament–desmosome complexes. *Brit. J. Dermatol.* **85:** 348-356 (1971).

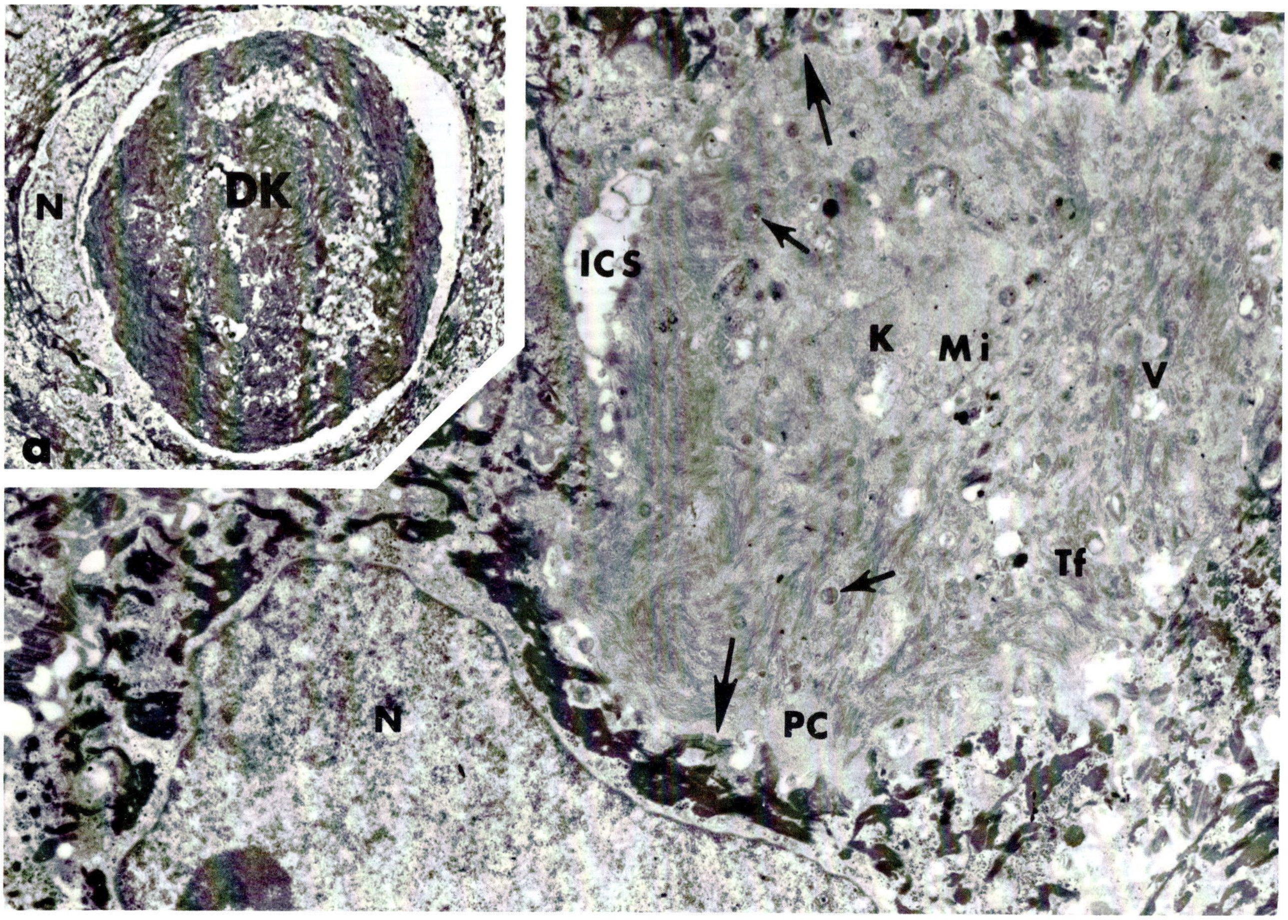

Figure 26. *Altered keratinocyte* (K), largely filled with bundles and clumps of loosely aggregated tonofilaments (TF), mostly separated and retracted from the desmosomes (arrows). Sparse, irregular, smooth vesicles (V), altered mitochondria (Mi), dense bodies (small arrows), and melanin granules are present within this keratinocyte. (× 13,000) PC: peripheral cytoplasm free of tonofilaments; ICS: widened intercellular space; N: nucleus. *From* J. Karasek, J. Pitha, W. Oehlert, and B. Konrad. Dyskeratosis in Bowen's disease: the ultrastructure and fate of keratinocytes with altered tonofilament-desmosome complexes. *Brit. J. Dermatol.* **85:** 348-356 (1971).

Figure 26a. *At the ultrastructural level, the dyskeratotic cells* (DK) or *corps ronds* are uniformly devoid of keratohyaline granules, contain prominent aggregates of tonofilaments, and have a decreased number of desmosomal-tonofilamentous attachments.[3,5,6] Separation and retraction of tonofilaments from altered desmosomal complexes result in tonofilamentous aggregation,[5] peripheral displacement of the nucleus (N), disappearance of desmosomes, and eventual acantholysis of the abnormal cells.[6] The presence of abundant acid phosphatase activity denotes the presence of the enzyme system necessary for individual cell keratinization.[5] × 8000. *From* J. Karasek and A. Hrdlicka. Dyskeratosis in Bowen's disease: the ultrastructure and origin of most frequent type of dyskeratotic cells. In preparation.

REFERENCES (Intraepithelial carcinoma–Figure 25–26a)

1. Nordquist, R. E., R. L. Olson, M. A. Everett, and P. T. Condit. Virus-like particles in Bowen's disease. *Cancer Res.* **30:** 288 (1970).
2. Friedrich, E. G. Jr. Reversible vulvar atypia. *Obstet. Gynecol.* **39:** 173 (1972).
3. Seiji, M. and F. Mizuno. Electron microscopic study of Bowen's disease. *Arch. Dermatol.* **99:** 3 (1969).
4. Karasek, J., K. Smetana, W. Oehlert, and B. Konrad. The ultrastructure of Bowen's disease: nuclear and nucleolar lesions. *Cancer Res.* **30:** 2791 (1970).
5. Olson, R. L., R. Nordquist, and M. A. Everett. An electron microscope study of Bowen's disease. *Cancer Res.* **28:** 2078 (1968).
6. Karasek, J., J. Pitha W. Oehlert, and B. Konrad. Dyskeratosis in Bowen's disease: the ultrastructure and fate of keratinocytes with altered tonofilament–desmosome complexes. *Brit. J. Dermatol.* **85:** 248 (1971).

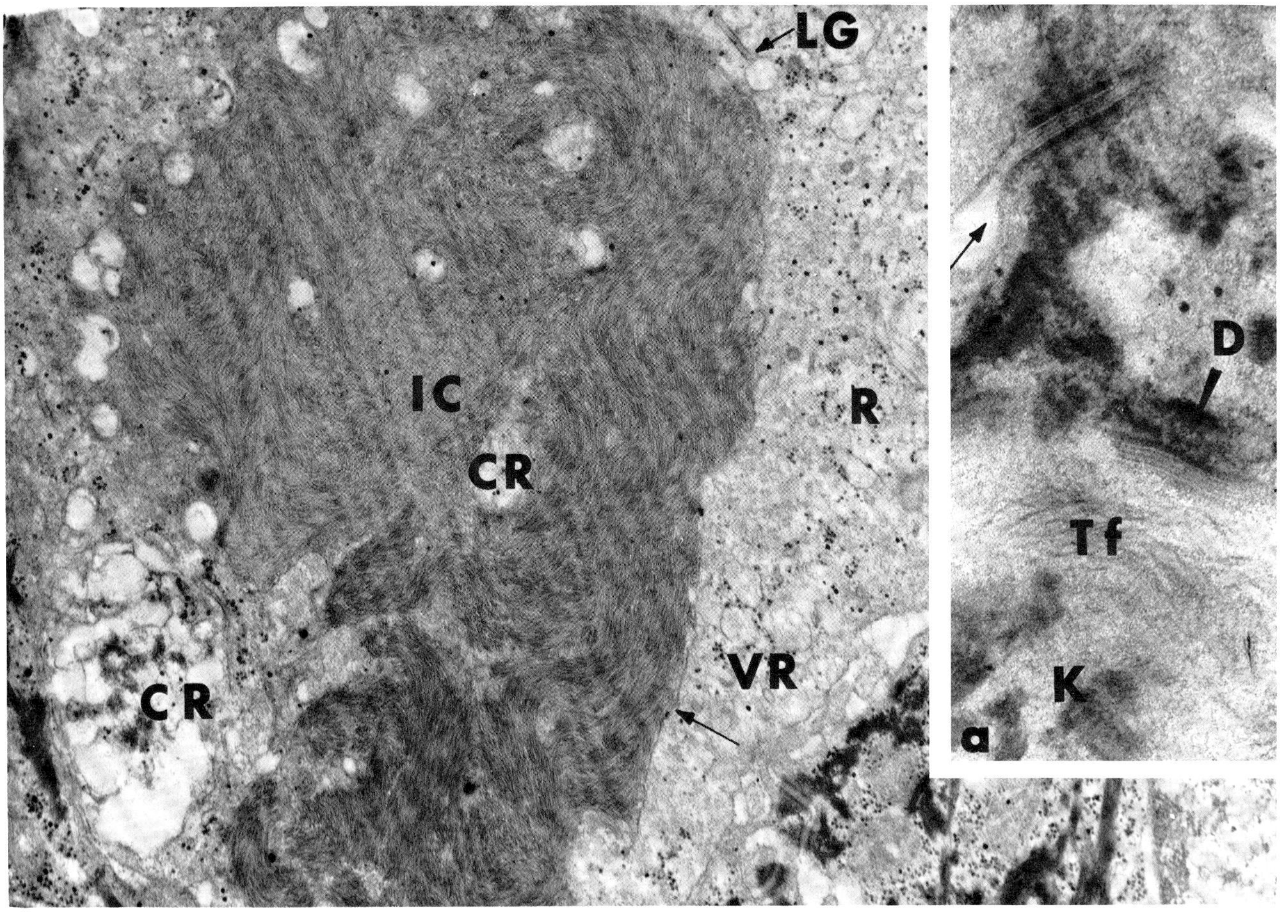

Figure 27. The *intracellulary-located convolute* of loosely aggregated tonofilaments (IC) seems to be partially delineated by a single membrane (arrow). Remnants of cytoplasmic organelles (CR) within and at the periphery of this convolute are evident. The cell containing this convolute has no desmosomes, and its cytoplasm contains ribosomes (R), smooth vesicles, vesicles partially covered with ribosomes (VR), and a structure resembling the Langerhans granule (LG). × 14,000. *From* J. Karasek, J. Pitha, W. Oehlert, and B. Konrad. Dyskeratosis in Bowen's disease the ultrastructure and fate of keratinocytes with altered tonofilament-desmosome complexes. *Brit. J. Dermatol.* **85:** 348-356 (1971).

Figure 27a. In *Bowen's disease* desmosomes are reduced in number and occasionally occur within the cytoplasmic matrix.[1] In an advanced stage of tonofilament–desmosome complex alteration, the tonofilaments (Tf) of the altered keratinocyte (K) are separated and retracted from the desmosomes (D). The attachment plaque as well as the intermediate dense and intercellular contact layers of the desmosome are indistinct. Arrow: plasma membrane. × 80,000. *From* J. Karasek, J. Pitha, W. Oehlert and B. Konrad. Dyskeratosis in Bowen's disease: the ultrastructure and fate of keratinocytes with altered tonofilament-desmosome complexes. *Brit. J. Dermatol.* **85:** 348-356 (1971).

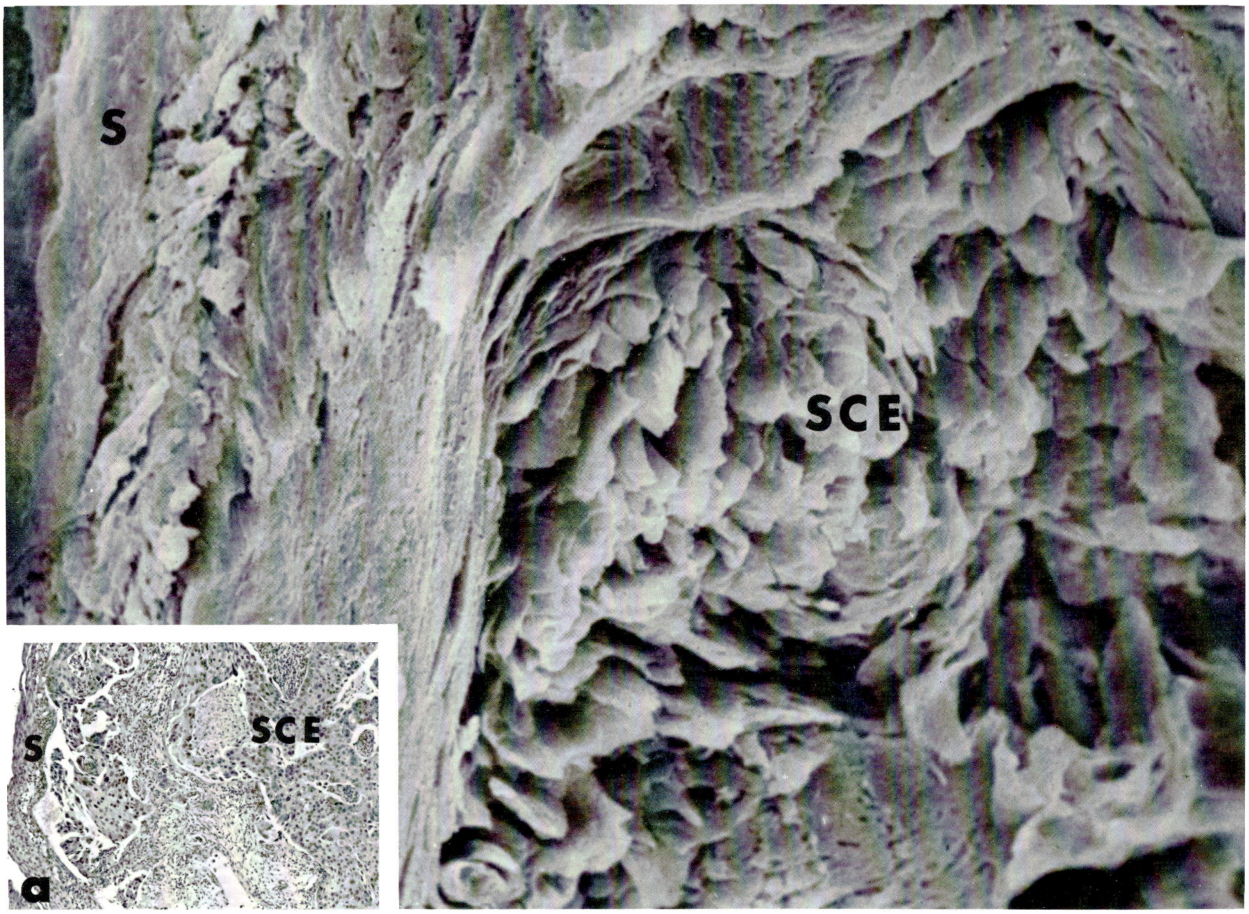

12

Invasive Epidermoid Carcinoma

Epidermoid carcinoma of the vulva accounts for about 3% of all genital cancers and is primarily a disease of postmenopausal women. The lesion is frequently fungating and ulcerated and most commonly occurs in the labia majora. Perineal extension and lymphatic metastases are common findings. To date, no etiologic agents have been identified, although the frequent association with cervical and vaginal neoplasia suggests a common carcinogen.

In experimental animals riboflavin deficiency leads to epidermal atrophy with decreased tritiated thymidine uptake,[2] followed by hyperkeratosis and hyperplasia.[3] Temporary riboflavin deficiency in young mice enhances chemically induced skin carcinogenesis.[2]

REFERENCES (Figures 27–28)

1. Seiji, M. and F. Mizuno. Electron microscopic study of Bowen's disease. *Arch. Dermatol.* **99:** 3 (1969).
2. Wynder, E. L. and P. C. Chan. The possible role of riboflavin deficiency in epithelial neoplasia. II. Effect of skin tumor development. *Cancer* **26:** 1221 (1970).
3. Wynder, E. L. and U. E. Klein. The possible role of riboflavin deficiency in epithelial neoplasia. I. Epithelial changes of mice in simple deficiency. *Cancer* **18:** 167 (1965).

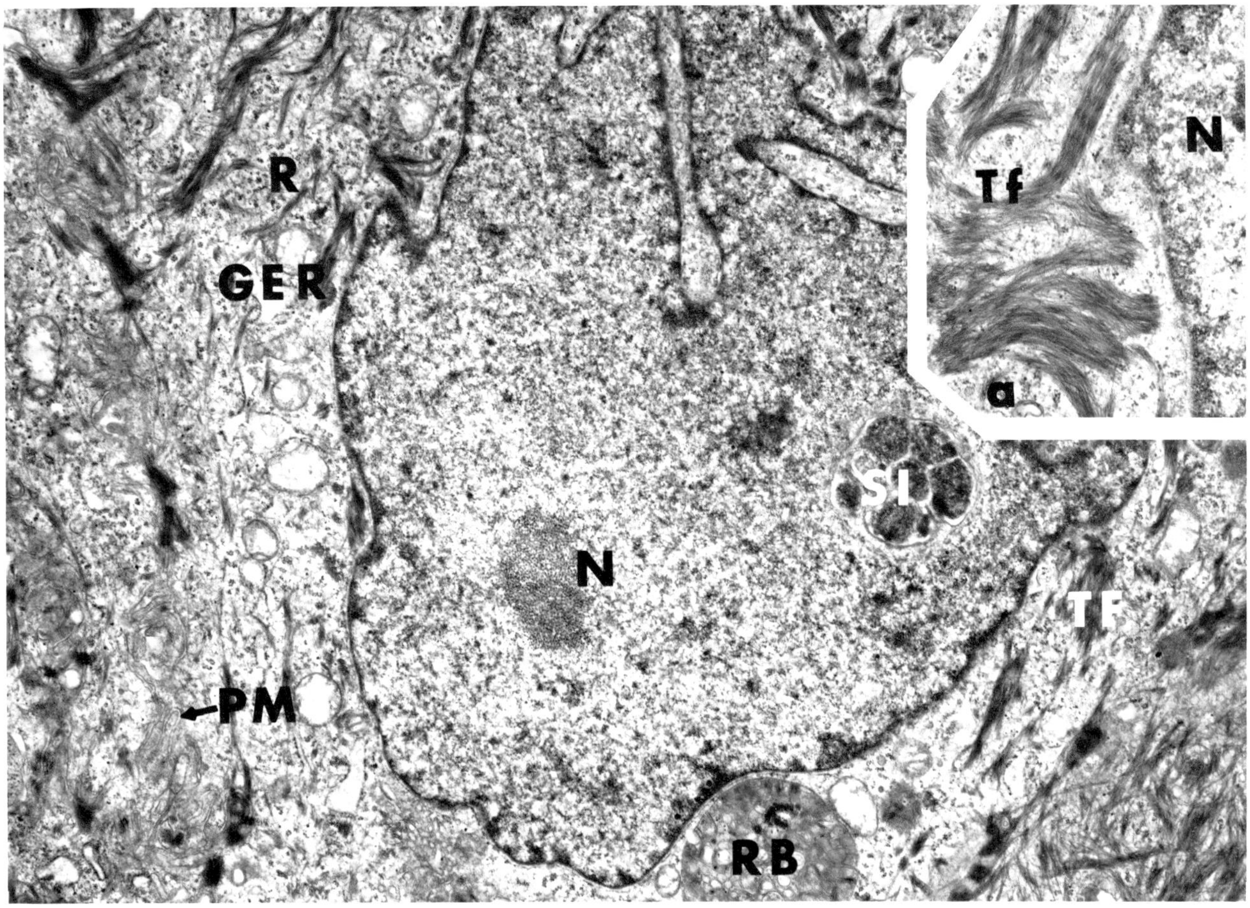

Figure 28a. *Microscopically,* the cancer is most commonly well differentiated and keratinizing, although more anaplastic lesions also occur. The photomicrograph illustrates a moderately well-differentiated epidermoid carcinoma (SCE) infiltrating the subepidermal dermis. (H & E stain, × 12.) S: epidermal surface.

Figure 28. *With the scanning electron microscope,* the invasive neoplastic squamous cells (SCE) are disposed in a disorganized fashion and overlap one another. Although the well-differentiated cancer cells contain cytoplasmic microridges, stubby microvilli cover the immature cells. Keratin pearls appear as concentric masses of multilamellated horny cells. × 288. S: epidermal surface.

Figure 29. *Ultrastructurally,* in addition to nuclear (N) and nucleolar enlargement, cytoplasmic and plasma membrane abnormalities are observed. As in intraepithelial carcinoma (Bowen's disease), the neoplastic keratinocytes in invasive vulvar cancer contain aggregates of tonofilaments (Tf), decreased tonofilament–desmosome complexes, numerous residual bodies (RB), free ribosomes (R), convoluted plasma membranes (PM), and incomplete formation of basal lamina.[1,2] The granular endoplasmic reticulum (GER) undergoes dilatation, fragmentation, and lamellar organization.[3] These morphological aberrations of the endoplasmic reticulum in neoplastic cells are thought to reflect impaired metabolic and enzymatic reactions.[4] In contrast to normal epidermal cells, neoplastic squamous cells have comparatively fewer desmosomes and gap junctions (nexuses) are generally absent.[5,6] These intercellular abnormalities may be responsible for the reduced cellular adhesiveness, cell contact inhibition,[7] and altered intercellular electrical coupling[8,9] that have been reported to occur between malignant neoplastic cells. × 9800. SI: intranuclear cytoplasmic inclusion.

Figure 29a. *Note the prominent perinuclear aggregation of* tonofilaments (Tf). × 9600. N: nucleus.

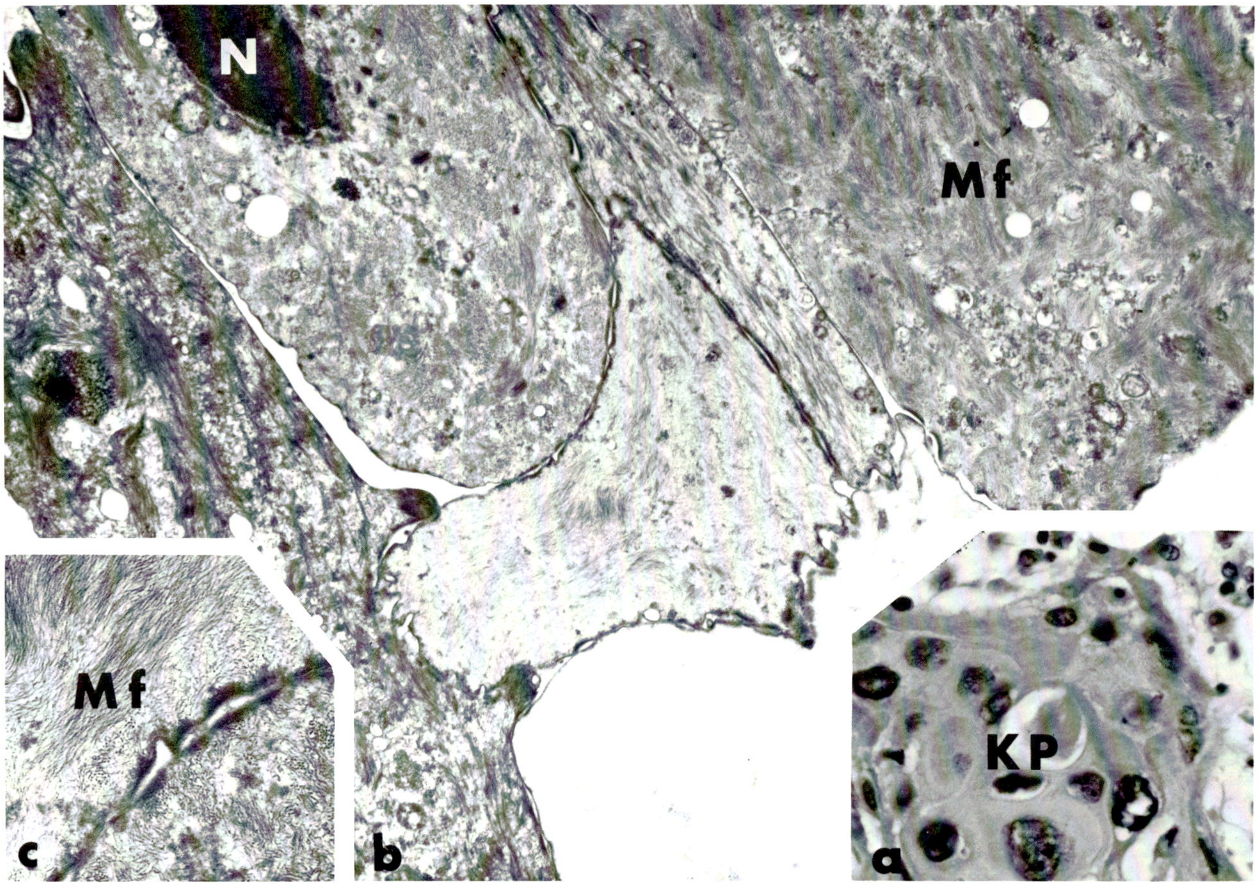

Figure 30a. *Histologic appearance* of well-differentiated invasive epidermoid carcinoma cells with early attempt at keratin pearl (KP) formation. (H & E stain, × 120.)

Figure 30b. *Transmission electron micrograph of tightly apposed, well-differentiated neoplastic cells* exhibiting keratinization, which corresponds to the classic keratin pearl formation seen at the light microscopic level. Like the horny cells of normal epidermis, keratin pearl-forming neoplastic cells are also packed with fine intracytoplasmic tonofibrils (Mf). × 7300. N: degenerated nucleus.

Figure 30c. *Detail of tonofibrils* (Mf) in keratinized neoplastic squamous cells. × 31,600.

REFERENCES (Figures 29–30c)

1. Hirone, T. and Y. Eryu. Fine structure of squamous cell carcinoma. *Skin Res. (Osaka)* **12:** 352 (1970).
2. Borland, R. and A. J. Webber. An electron microscope study of squamous cell carcinoma in Merino sheep associated with keratin-filled cells of the skin. *Cancer Res.* **26:** 172 (1966).
3. Klehr, H. U. and G. Klingmuller. Different forms of endoplasmic reticulum in neoplastic keratinocytes. Investigations on the squamous cell carcinoma. *Arch. Dermatol. Forsch.* **242:** 111 (1972).
4. Wallach, D. F. H. Generalized membrane defects in cancer. *New Engl. J. Med.* **280:** 761 (1969).
5. McNutt, N. S. and R. S. Weinstein. Carcinoma of the cervix: deficiency of nexus intercellular junctions. *Science* **165:** 597 (1969).
6. Martinez-Paloma, A. Ultrastructural modifications of intercellular junctions in some epithelial tumors. *Lab. Invest.* **22:** 605 (1970).
7. Abercrombie, M. and E. J. Ambrose. The surface properties of cancer cells. Review. *Cancer Res.* **22:** 525 (1962).
8. Lowenstein, W. R. Permeability of membrane junctions. *Ann. N. Y. Acad. Sci.* **137:** 441 (1966).
9. Jamakosmanovic, A. and W. R. Lowenstein. Intercellular communication and tissue growth. III. Thyroid cancer. *J. Cell Biol.* **38:** 556 (1968).

13

Granular Cell Tumor

The granular cell tumor is a rare, benign, subepithelial vulvar neoplasm, first described by Abrikosoff, who coined the term granular cell myoblastoma. Ultrastructurally,[1-5] the neoplastic cells contain numerous fibrillar bodies and lysosome- and cytosegrosomelike structures of varying sizes. These bodies are responsible for the AB–PAS-positive, diastase-resistant, granular appearance seen by light microscopy. Occasionally, unmyelinated axonal arrangements have been described.

The histogenetic origin of the granular cell lesion is the subject of considerable controversy, and various theories, including myogenous, histiocytic, and neurogenous derivations, have been proposed. Although most histochemical, biochemical, and fine structural studies have favored a neurogenic origin,[1-4] tissue cultures of granular cell tumors do not yield the typical Schwannian growth pattern, and recently myofilaments were demonstrated, suggesting a myogenous origin.[5] In the light of these observations it seems possible that this peculiar lesion may have several different cellular origins,[4,5] the common feature being intense autophagic activity, the significance of which remains obscure.

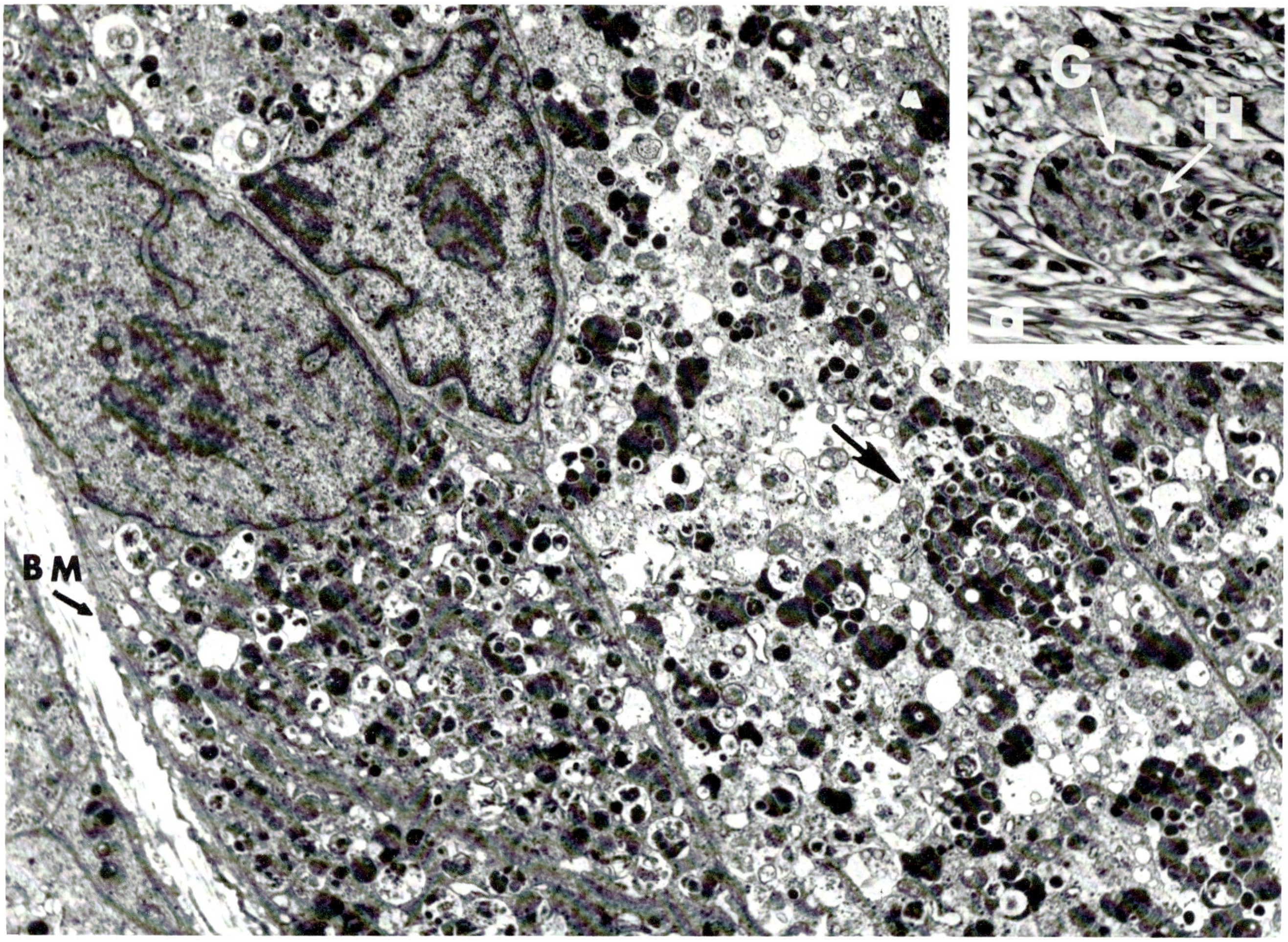

Figure 31a. *Histologic appearance of granular cell tumor cells.* Note the clusters of cells with finely granular, poorly defined cytoplasmic particles and occasional more sharply defined, coarse granules. Some of the coarse granules are homogeneous (H) and correspond to myelin figures. Others are composed of clumps of fine granules (G) and are autophagosomes. (H & S stain, × 350). From H. J. Sobel, E. Marquet, E. Avrin, and R. Schwartz. Granular cell myoblastoma. An electron microscopic and cytochemical study illustrating the genesis of granules and aging of myoblastoma. *Am. J. Pathol.* **65:** 59 (1971).

Figure 31. *Electron micrograph of a granular cell tumor of the vulva,* illustrating mature neoplastic cells with prominent basement membranes (BM) surrounding groups of cells. These cell nests are also bounded by collagen and fibroblasts that do not have basement membranes. The cells are packed with membrane-bound large and small granules (arrow). Endoplasmic reticulum, mitochondria, and other cell organelles are scanty. × 7000. *From* H. J. Sobel, E. Marquet, E. Avrin, and R. Schwarz. Granular cell myoblastoma. An electron microscopic and cytochemical study illustrating the genesis of granules and aging of myoblastoma. *Am. J. Pathol.* **65:** 59 (1971).

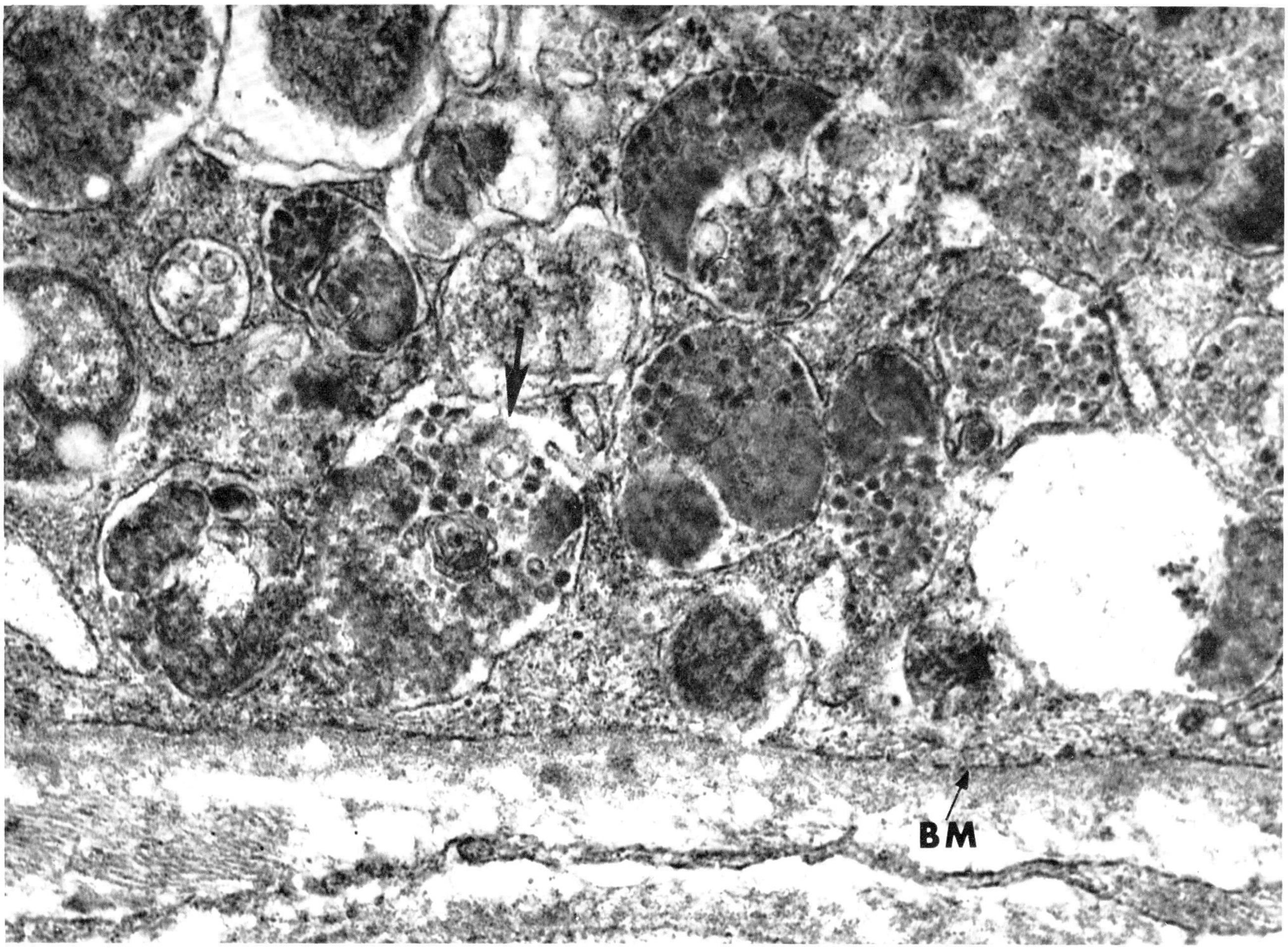

Figure 32. *Detailed view from Figure 31.* Note prominent basement membrane at surface (BM). Mitochondria are not seen. Profiles of endoplasmic reticulum are rare. Complex, poorly preserved, membrane-bound granules containing fine vesicles and particles with apparently solid core and unidentifiable dense material are noted (arrow). × 47,500. From H. J. Sobel, E. Marquet, E. Avrin, and R. Schwarz. Granular cell myoblastoma. An electron microscopic and cytochemical study illustrating the genesis of granules and aging of myoblastoma. *Am. J. Pathol.* **65:** 59 (1971).

REFERENCES (The granular cell tumor—Figure 32)

1. Fisher, E. R. and H. Wechsler. Granular cell myoblastoma—a misnomer. *Cancer* **15:** 936 (1962).
2. Carstens, H. B. Ultrastructure of granular cell myoblastoma. *Acta Pathol. Microbiol. Scand.* **78:** 685 (1970).
3. Garancis, J. C., R. A. Komorowski, and J. F. Kuzma. Granular cell myoblastoma. *Cancer* **25:** 242 (1970).
4. Sobel, H. J., E. Marquet, E. Avrin, and R. Schwarz. Granular cell myoblastoma. An electron microscopic and cytochemical study illustrating the genesis of granules and aging of myoblastoma cells. *Am. J. Pathol.* **65:** 59 (1971).
5. Christ, M. L. and L. Ozzello. Myogenous origin of a granular cell tumor of the urinary bladder. *Am. J. Clin. Pathol.* **56:** 736 (1971).

14

Malignant Melanoma

Malignant melanoma is a rare, highly malignant, invasive vulvar neoplasm, thought to arise from epidermal melanoblasts or, rarely, from junctional melanogenic nevoblasts.[1]

At the ultrastructural level, melanoma cells have a considerably increased number of Golgi and mitochondria and contain melanosomes that differ morphologically from those found in normal melanocytes.[2,3] Melanogenesis within vulvar melanoma cells was demonstrated to involve the Golgi–endoplasmic reticulum system.[4] A similar pathway for melanization has been described in extragenital[3,5] melanoma cells. Electron microscopic studies,[5-8] combined with histochemistry[9] and autoradiography,[10] have suggested that both the enzyme (tyrosinase) and the precursor protein fibrils are synthetized by ribosomes[11] and are transferred to dilated agranular endoplasmic reticulum (early premelanosomes) through the granular endoplasmic reticulum–Golgi–agranular endoplasmic reticulum complex. Melanin formation occurs in late premelanosomes only[7,12] when the intermembranous structure is established. The fully formed, stage IV melanosome consists of a uniformly dense structure devoid of internal membranes. Both the premelanosomes and the melanosomes in malignant melanomas contain acid phosphatase activity and are therefore considered to be lysosomes[3] or modified lysosomes.[10] In this regard, the neoplastic melanocytes differ from their normal counterparts in that the melanosomes in the latter are acid phosphatase negative. The significance of enzymatically active melanosomes in melanoma is not known.

REFERENCES (Malignant melanoma–Figure 33)

1. Mishima, Y., Melanotic tumors. In *Ultrastructure of Normal and Abnormal Skin,* A. S. Zelickson (Ed.). Lea & Febiger, Philadelphia, 1967, pp. 388–424.
2. Clark. W. H. and R. Bretton. Four kinds of melanocytes seen in electron micrographs of primary human malignant melanomas. *Fed. Proc.* **29:** 758 (1970).
3. Maul, G. G. and M. M. Romsdahl. Ultrastructural comparison of two human malignant melanoma cell lines. *Cancer Res.* **30:** 2782 (1970).
4. Overbeck, L. and E. Philipp. Elektronenmikroscopische Untersuchungen am Melanomalignom der Vulva. *Z. Geburtsh. Gynaekol.* **168:** 167 (1968).
5. Maul, G. G. Golgi-melanosome relationships in human melanomas in vitro. *J. Ultrastruct. Res.* **26:** 163 (1969).
6. Mishima, Y. Electron microscopy of melanin synthesis in intradermal nevus cells. *J. Invest. Dermatol.* **39:** 369 (1962).
7. Birbeck, M. S. C. Electron microscopy of melanocytes: the fine structure of hair bulb premelanosomes. *Ann. N. Y. Acad. Sci.* **100:** 540 (1963).
8. Seiji, M., T. B. Fitzpatrick, and M. S. C. Birbeck. The melanosome: a distinct subcellular particle of mammalian melanocytes and the site of melanogenesis. *J. Invest. Dermatol.* **36:** 243 (1961).
9. Hunter, J. A. A., J. H. Mottaz, and A. S. Zelickson. Melanogenesis: ultrastructural histochemical observations on ultraviolet irradiated human melanocytes. *J. Invest. Dermatol.* **54:** 213 (1970).
10. Novikoff, A., A. Albala, and L. Biempica. Ultrastructural and cytochemical observations on B-16 and Harding-Passey mouse melanomas: the origin of premelanosomes and compound melanosomes. *J. Histochem. Cytochem.* **16:** 299 (1968).
11. Duchon, J., T. B. Fitzpatrick, and M. Seiji. Melanin 1968: some definitions and problems. In *Yearbook of Dermatology, 1967–1968.* Yearbook Medical Publishers, Chicago.
12. Moyer, F. H. Melanosome fine structure and ontogeny. *Ann. N. Y. Acad. Sci.* **100:** 584 (1963).

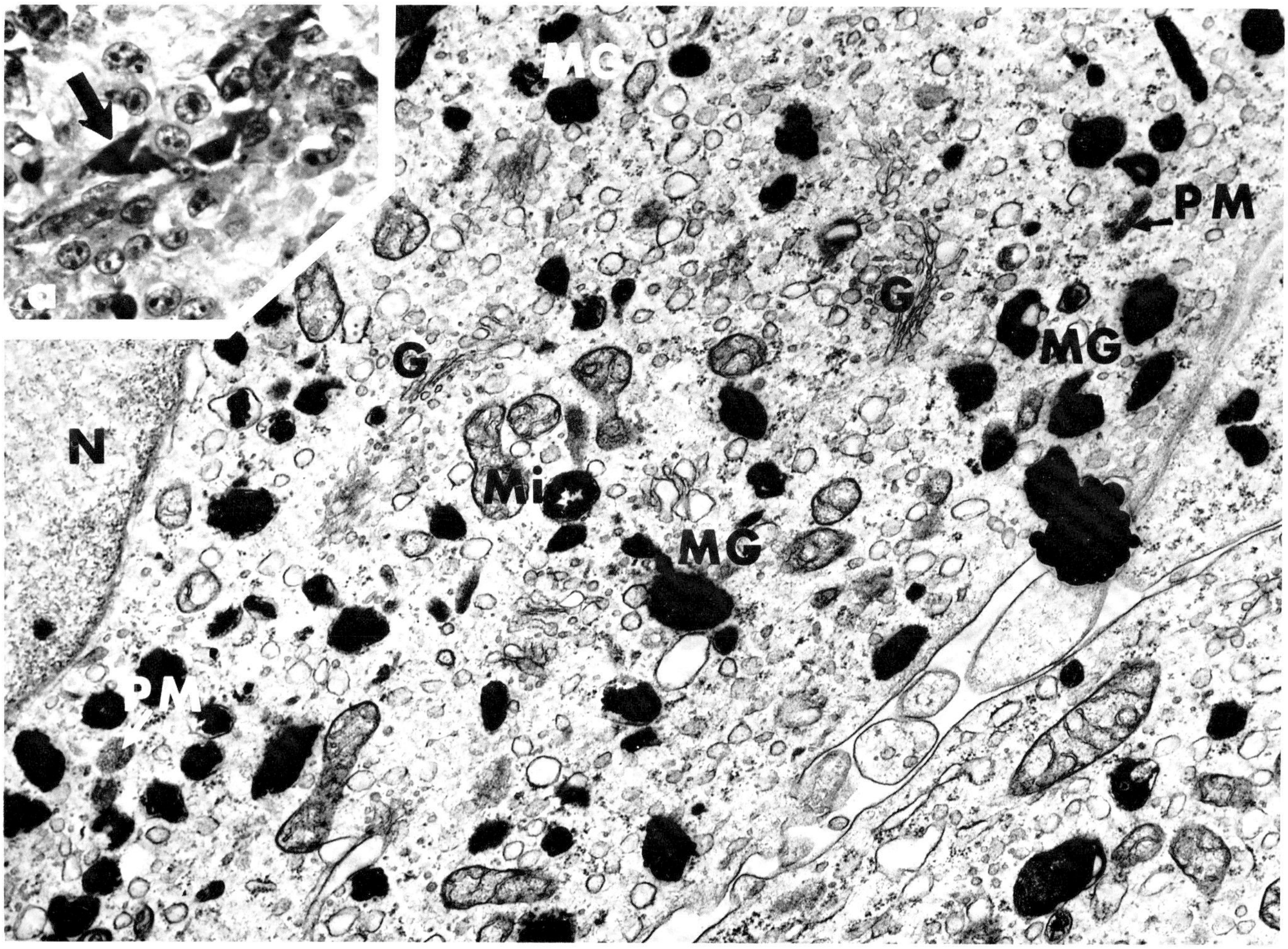

Figure 33a. The *typical lesion* consists of nests of large cuboidal cells with conspicuous nuclear and nucleolar pleomorphism, numerous mitotic figures, and a varying quantity of cytoplasmic melanin pigment granules (arrow). In addition to dermal invasion, the Malpighian layer is invaded by clusters of neoplastic cells or by individual neoplastic cells. In the latter instance, as in lentigo maligna melanoma, the melanoma cells may resemble Paget's cells, but a mucicarmine stain will usually lead to the correct diagnosis, as Paget's cells are mucicarminophilic whereas melanoma cells are not (see **Paget's Disease**). In addition, regardless of the histologic presence or absence of melanin pigment, the DOPA and tyrosinase reactions are strongly positive in melanomas. (H & E stain, × 120.)

Figure 33. *Malignant melanoma cell* with numerous melanin granules (MG) and occasional premelanosomes (PM). The Golgi (G), as well as the granular and agranular endoplasmic reticulum system, are prominent. × 26,000. M: mitochondria; N: nucleus. *From* L. Overbeck and E. Philipp. Elektronen mikroscopische Untersuchungen am Melanomalignom der Vulva. *Z. Geburtsh. Gynaekol.* **168:** 167 (1968).

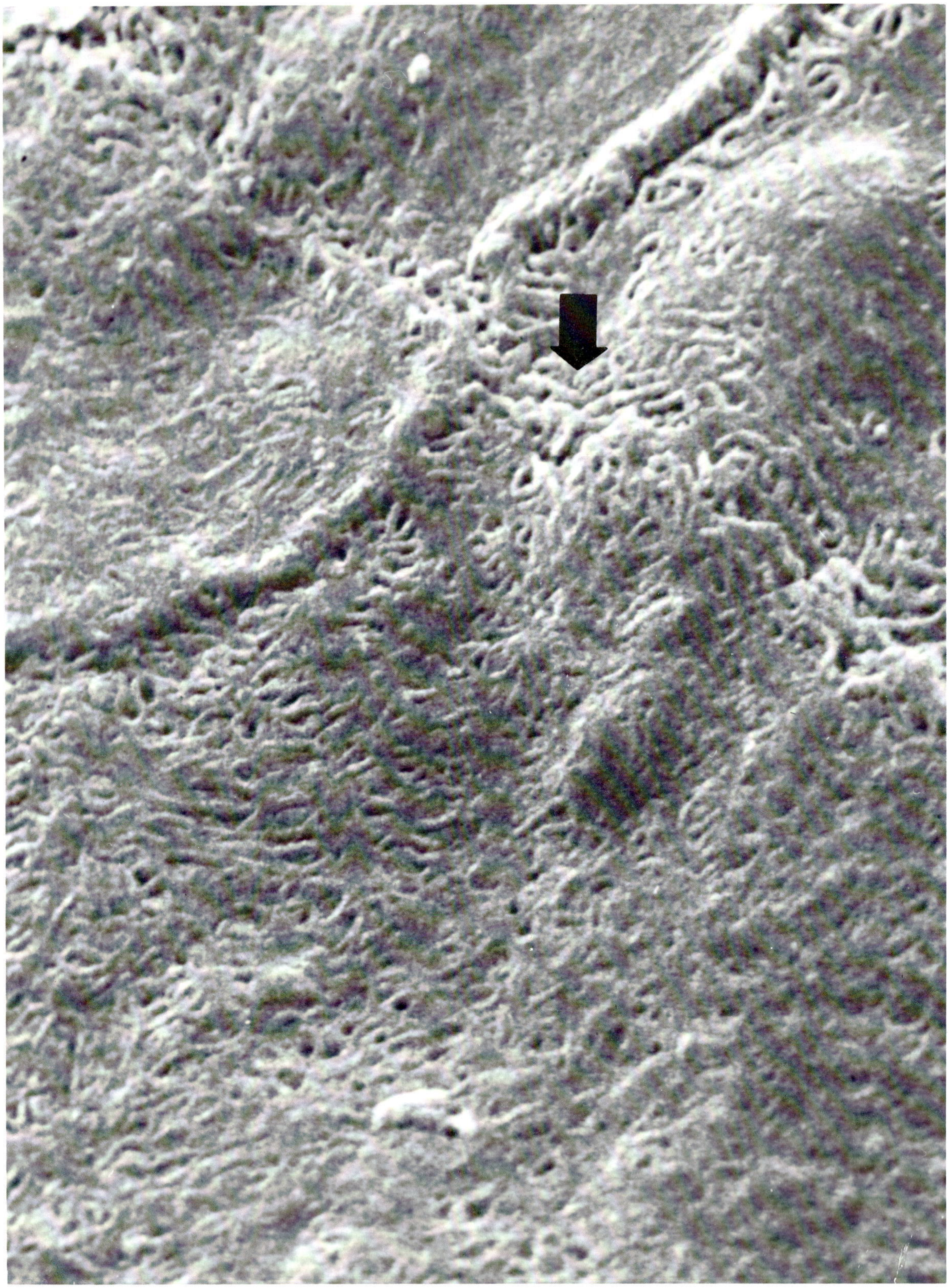

Mucous Membrane of Vagina. Scanning electron micrograph of the complex network of surface microridges (arrow) that characterizes the most superficial squamous cells of the vagina. × 9000.

VAGINA

15

Normal Vaginal Epithelium

The steroid sex hormones of ovarian origin produce a cyclic response in the vaginal epithelium. Estrogen initiates proliferation, maturation, and "cornification," and progesterone induces either a partial proliferation (up to the end of the intermediate cells) or epithelial regression. Conversely, a lack of estrogenic activity generally results in epithelial atrophy. During pregnancy, with high levels of progesterone, glycogen-rich intermediate cells predominate, producing the appearance of an "exaggerated" luteal phase. The mechanism of hormonal effect on the vaginal epithelium, although still uncertain, seems to be similar to that acting on the other target cells of the female genital tract and to take place through the stimulation of nucleolar RNA synthesis.

Cells other than squamous epithelium may be encountered in the vaginal mucosa, including intercellular, emperiopoietic lymphocytes, which are especially numerous during the mid-luteal phase of the menstrual cycle.[1] The significance of these intraepithelial, migrating, inflammatory cells remains obscure. Langerhans cells, similar in structure to those found in the epidermis, are also encountered.[2]

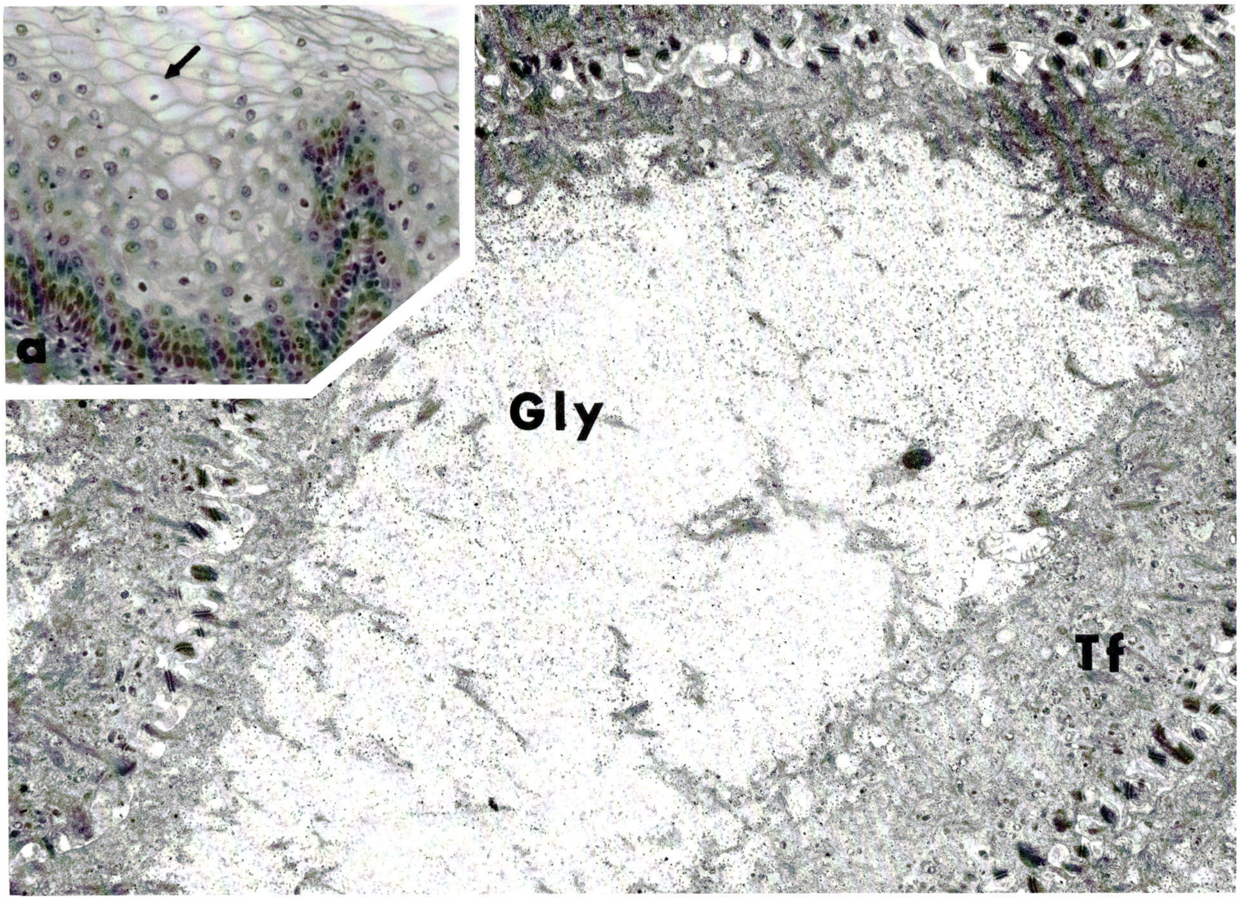

Figure 34a. *Histologically, the vaginal mucosa* is composed of a nonkeratinizing, squamous, stratified epithelium. *The stratum germinativum, or basal zone,* is composed of a single layer of elliptical cells with oval nuclei, characteristically oriented perpendicular to the underlying basal lamina. Epithelial renewal is the major function of the basal cells, and their general structural organization is that of a metabolically active cell population[1] with a high rate of replication.[1-4] The suprabasal layer, or *parabasal zone,* contains larger cells with a comparatively more abundant cytoplasm. With ascending epithelial maturation, the amount of cytoplasm progressively increases, whereas the absolute nuclear size decreases. These cells often have a glycogen-rich cytoplasmic matrix (arrow) and are equivalent to the *intermediate cells* of exfoliate cytology. The *superficial zone* is composed of several layers of large, flattened cells with small pyknotic nuclei. (H & E stain, × 48.)

Figure 34. *Ultrastructurally,* both the parabasal and the *intermediate cells* are bound by numerous well-developed desmosomes, tight and intermediate junctions.[2] Bundles of tonofilaments (Tf), as well as cytoplasmic organelles and massive aggregates of glycogen (Gly), are dispersed throughout the cytoplasm and are most prominent during the luteal phase of the menstrual cycle.[1] The nuclei become disposed parallel to the surface, and numerous stubby microvilli project into the intercellular space. In the superficial zone, desmosomal attachments become less numerous and the intercellular spaces are wider.[1] Large masses of glycogen and scattered keratohyaline granules are seen.[1,4] × 7200.

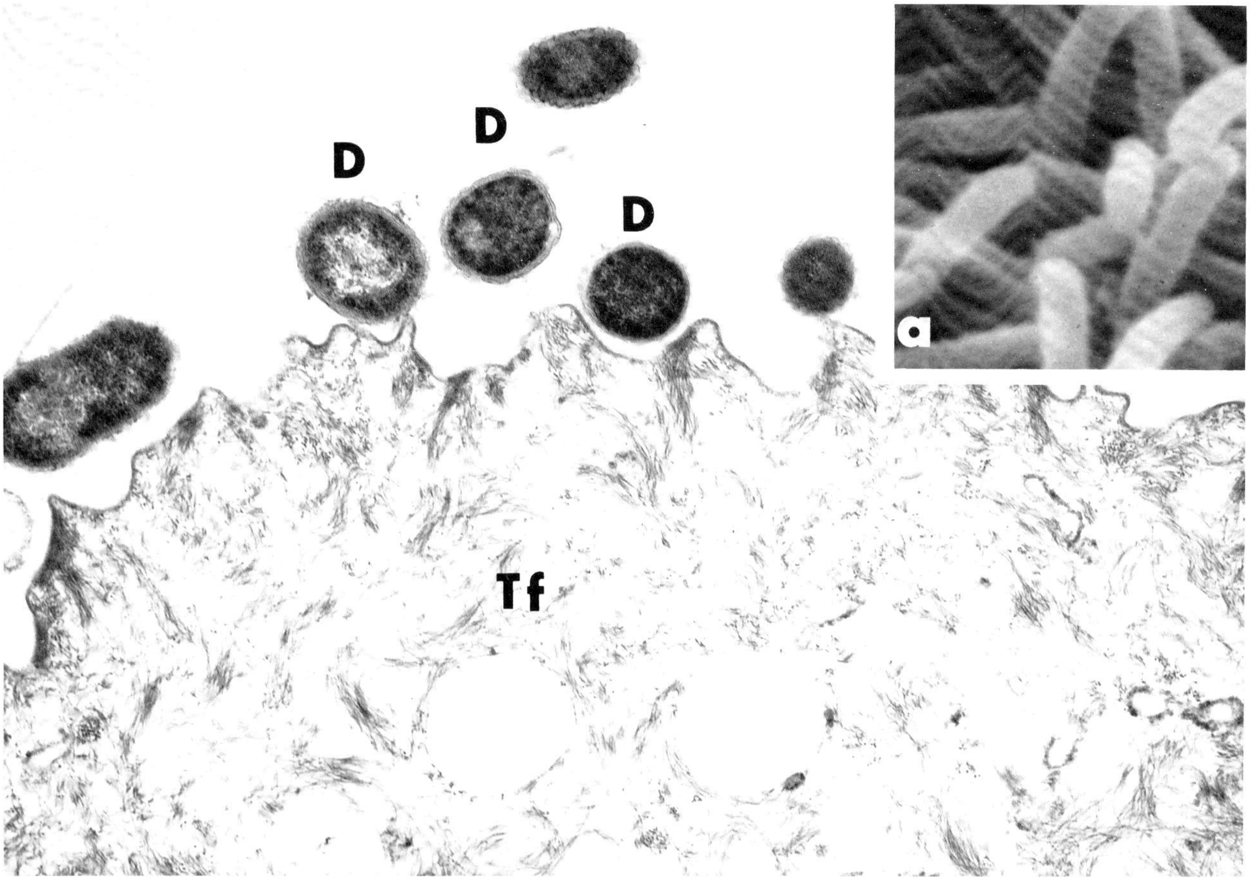

Figure 35. *The most superficial cells* of the vaginal mucosa have irregular and stubby surface plasma projections, and the cytoplasm contains scattered bundles of tonofilaments (Tf). Several gram-positive, membrane-coated Doderlein bacilli (D) are found near or on the superficial cells. × 30,400.

Figure 35a. *Scanning electron microscopic* appearance of Donderlein bacilli, which are found as short cylindrical rods, occurring singly or in chains, often over large areas of the cell surface. × 23,800.

REFERENCES (Figures 34–35a)

1. Leonardi, R. and A. Regano. Sull'ultrastruttura dell'epitelia vaginale umana. *Arch. Ostet. Ginecol.* **67:** 715 (1962).
2. Burgos, M. H. and C. E. Roig de Vargas-Linares. Cell junctions in the human vaginal epithelium. *Am. J. Obstet. Gynecol.* **108:** 565 (1970).
3. Capria, V. and R. Sermann. Ultrastruttura dell'epitelia della portio vaginalis umana. *Arch. Ostet. Ginecol.* **68:** 459 (1963).
4. Jaeger, J. New light and electron microscopic studies on cervical and vaginal epithelium. *Arch. Gynaekol.* **207:** 55 (1969).

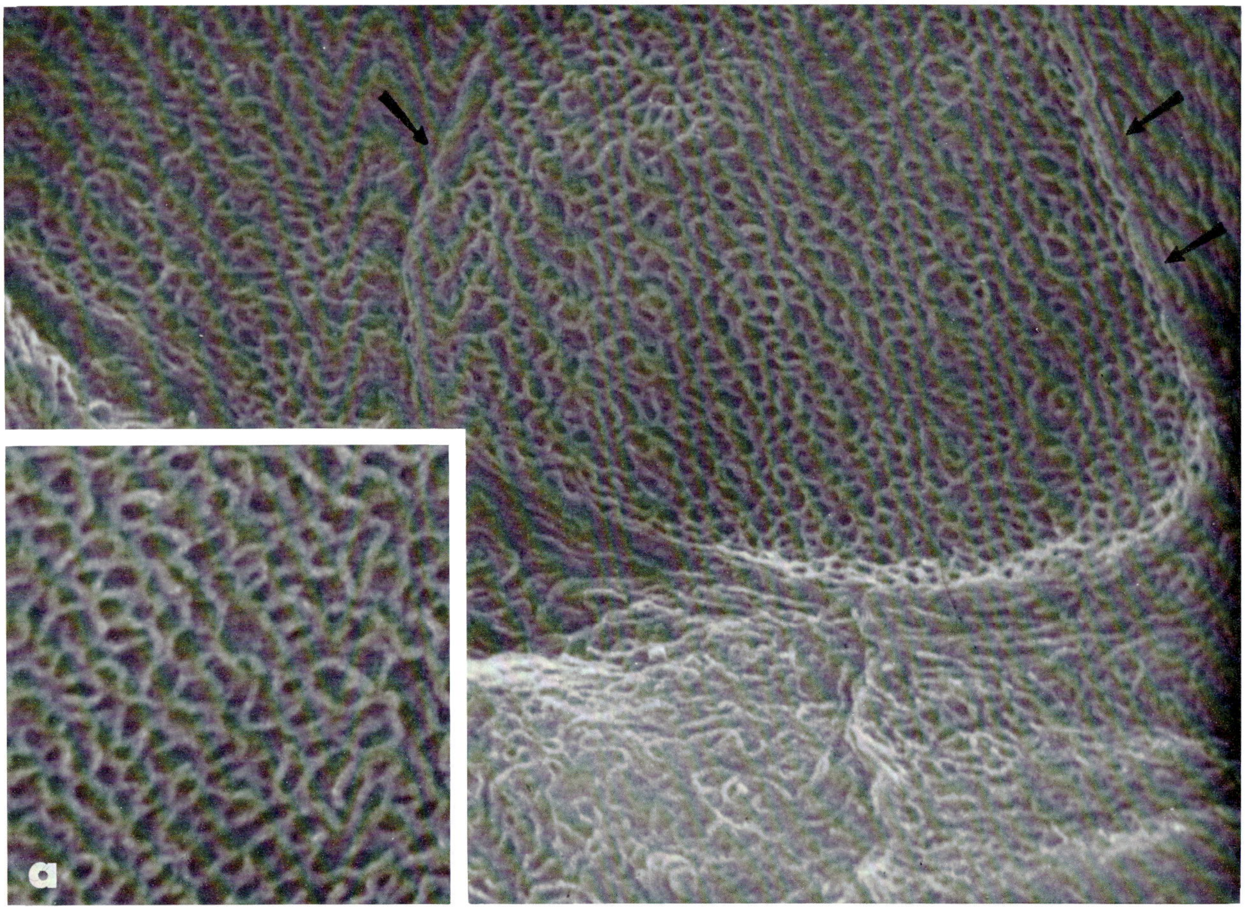

Figure 36. *Vaginal epithelium. By scanning electron microscopy,* the surface of the most superficial epithelium shows a complicated, interlacing system of cytoplasmic microridges, and the cells have prominent, nodular outlines (arrow). This peculiar surface configuration is probably due to the "cornified" nature of the superficial cells, which, histochemically, contain disulfide-rich, cytoplasmic proteins, probably representing keratin precursors. Keratinization, however, does not occur under normal conditions in the vaginal mucous membrane. × 4800.

Figure 36a. *Higher magnification of microridges,* which correspond to the evaginations of the surface plasma membrane, seen in Figure 35. × 7500.

16

Candidiasis (Moniliasis)

Genital candidiasis, the most common vulvovaginal fungal disease, is caused by the genus *Candida,* the most frequently occurring species being *albicans.* This mucocutaneous inflammatory condition is frequently found associated with pregnancy, diabetes, administration of oral contraceptives, corticosteroids, and antibiotics. In all these conditions, the vaginal secretions, intraepithelial glycogen, and nonpathogenic bacterial flora are thought to be altered. Histologically, the fungi remain on the epithelial surface, and the underlying, nonspecific, inflammatory exudate, if any, is due either to a secondary bacterial infection or to the fermentation or allergenic products produced by the fungal organisms.[3] The conidia (spores) and hyphea of the fungus are easily recognized in Papanicolaou smears or in gentian violet-or gram-stained smears.

Ultrastructurally, the blastospores are enveloped by a 1000- to 1300-Å-thick coat of glycoprotein.[4] Antibodies against mannon, a polysaccharide found in the blastospore wall, have been demonstrated in patients with localized, systemic, or subclinical candidiasis.[5] The cytoplasm is poor in organelles and contains several invaginations, presumably to increase the cytoplasmic surface and to facilitate cellular metabolic activity.

REFERENCES (Figures 36–37)

1. Roig de Vargas-Linares, C. E. and M. H. Burgos. Migration of lymphocytes in the normal human vagina. *Am. J. Obstet. Gynecol.* **102:** 1094 (1968).
2. Hoffmeister, H. and M. Rupec. Electron microscopic demonstration of Langerhans cells in the epithelium of the vagina. *Experientia* **24:** 168 (1968).
3. Montes, L. F. Fungi and fungal infections. In *Ultrastructure of Normal and Abnormal Skin,* A. S. Zelickson (Ed.). Lea & Febiger, Philadelphia, 1967, pp. 347–364.
4. Chew, W. and T. L. Theus. *Candida precipitins. Clin. Res.* **14:** 55 (1966).
5. Gardner, H. L. and R. H. Kaufman. *Benign Diseases of the Vulva and Vagina.* C. V. Mosby, St. Louis, 1969, pp. 149–163.

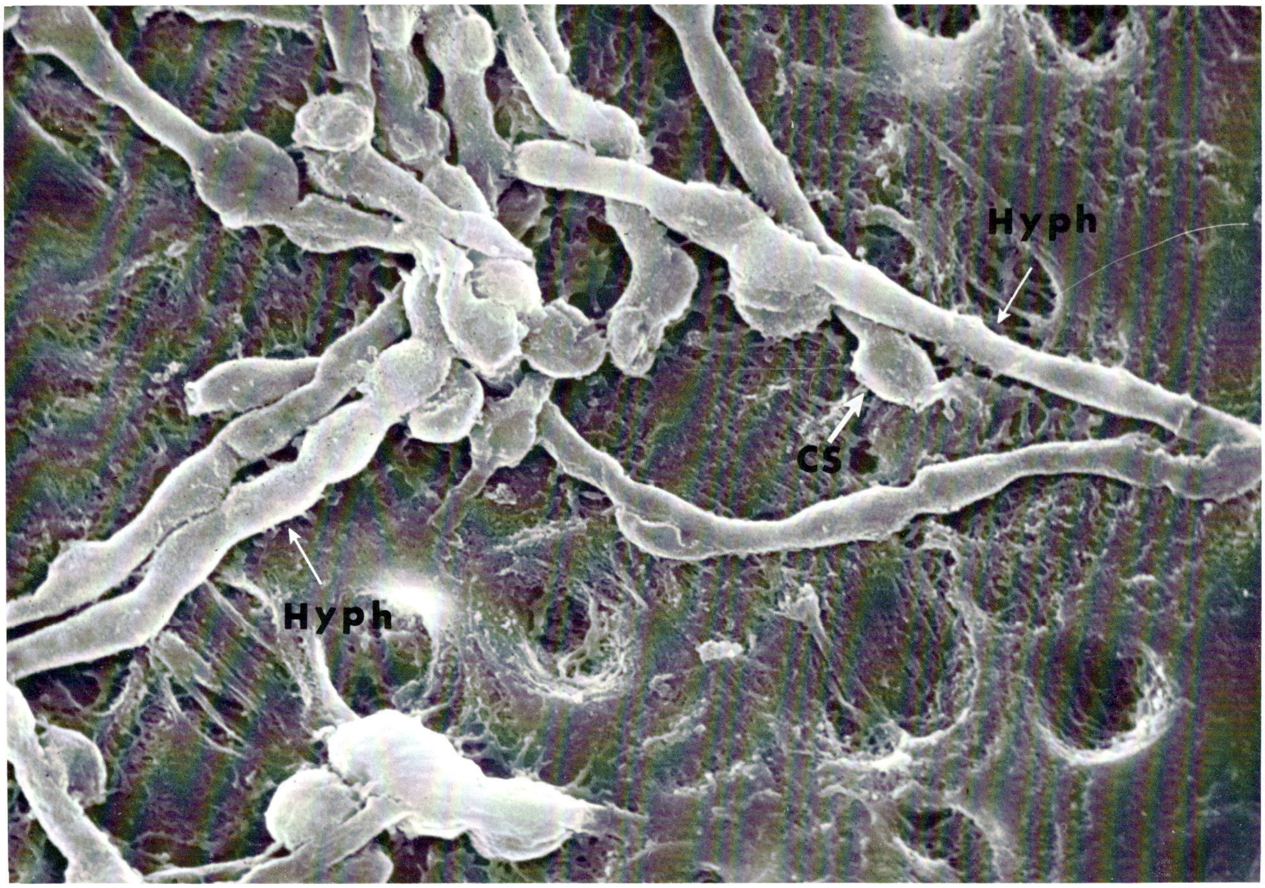

Figure 37. *The high-resolution stereoscopic characteristics* of the septate hyphae (Hyph) and chlamydospores (CS) are illustrated.

17

Invasive Epidermoid Carcinoma

Epidermoid carcinoma of the vagina is a rare neoplasm that has a close similarity, both histologically and ultrastructurally, to invasive epidermoid carcinoma arising in the vulvar skin or cervical mucous membranes.

Figure 38. *Scanning electron micrograph* of a circumscribed focus of tangentially sectioned invasive epidermoid carcinoma (SCE), penetrating deep into the subepithelial connective tissue stroma (D). The somewhat flat neoplastic cells are in tight apposition and lack organization and cellular cohesion. × 3200.

Figure 38a. *The surface* of the most superficial neoplastic cells contains numerous microvilli (Mv). × 9600.

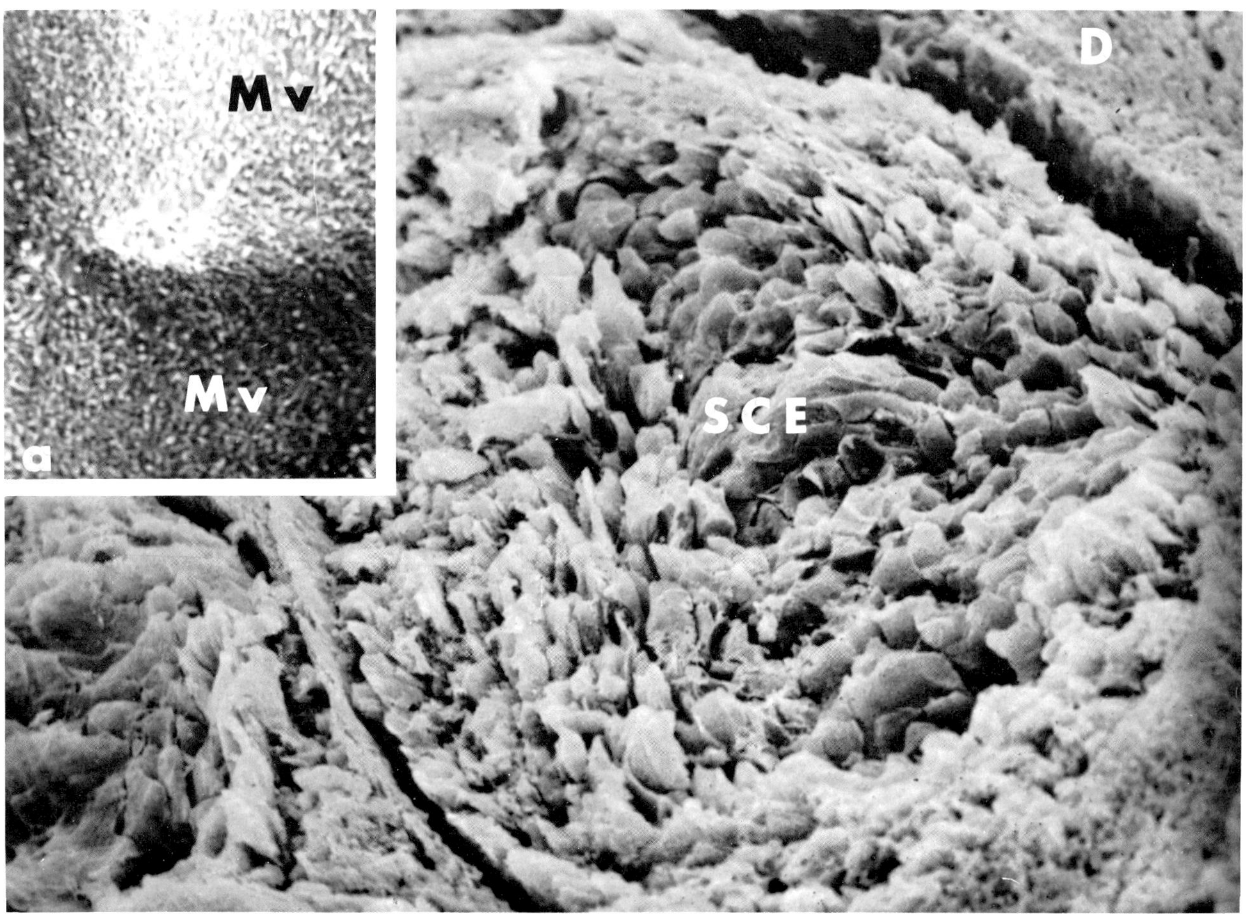

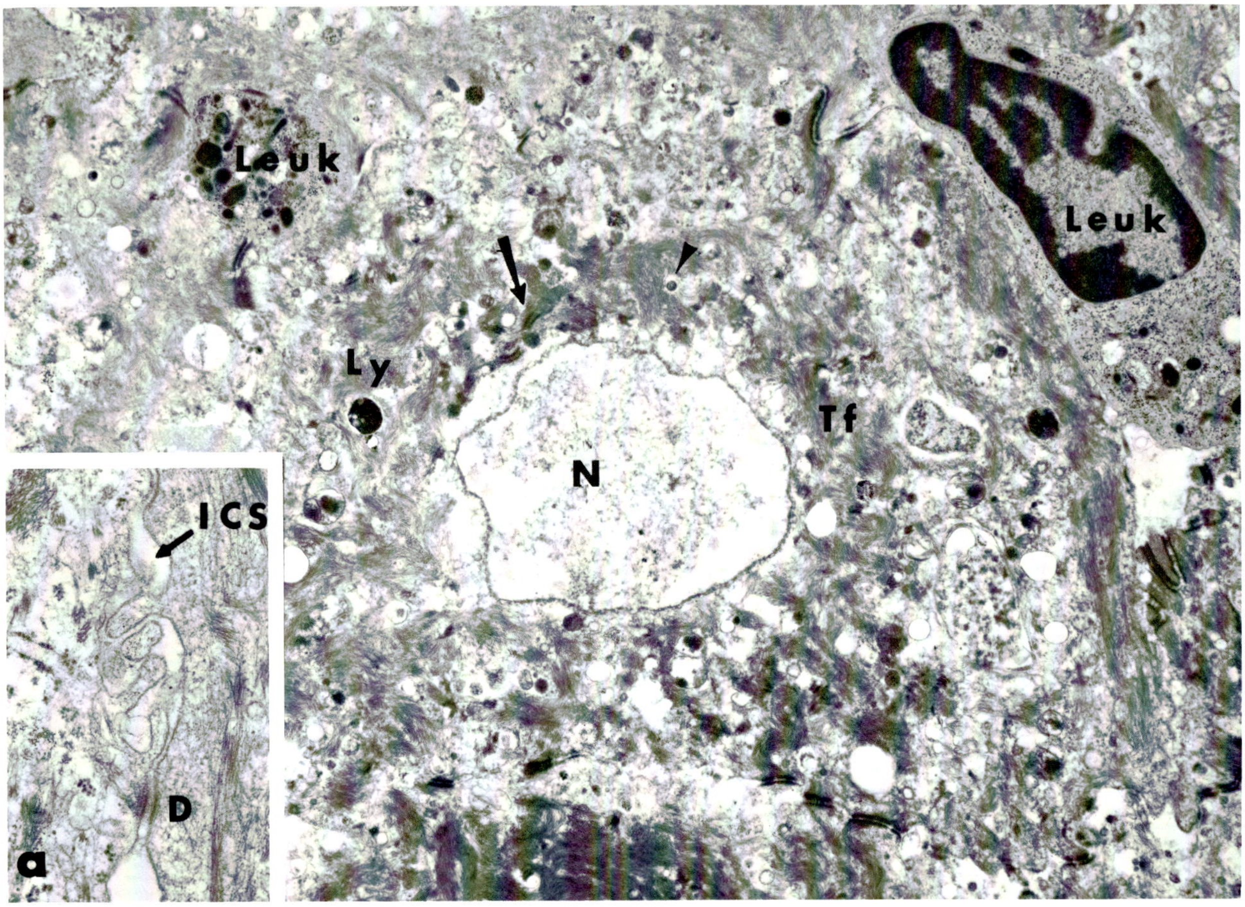

Figure 39. *Transmission electron micrograph* of a degenerating neoplastic squamous cell, in which the nuclear substance (N) underwent karyolysis but the nuclear membrane remains intact. There is marked retraction of desmosome–tonofilament complexes (arrow), resulting in the perinuclear aggregation of tonofilaments (Tf). Lysosomes (Ly), membrane-coated granules (arrow head), and organellar vacuolization are seen throughout. Several leukocytes (Leuk) are present in the intercellular spaces. × 6400.

Figure 39a. *The intercellular space* (ICS) contains stubby interdigitating microvilli, and the closely apposed plasma membranes are attached by poorly developed desmosomes (D) devoid of tonofilaments. × 9800.

18

Clear Cell Adenocarcinoma

Abundant evidence has recently been presented[1] to support a close association between the maternal ingestion of diethylstilbestrol (DES), a synthetic nonsteroid estrogen, during the early stages of pregnancy and the subsequent development of *clear cell adenocarcinoma* of the vagina and cervix in young (8–25 years) female offspring. In this population at risk, additional stilbestrol-related, nonneoplastic abnormalities include vaginal adenosis, cervical "erosion," and transverse vaginal and cervical ridges.[1] Histologically, most of the neoplasms are of the clear cell adenocarcinoma type, forming tubules, solid nests, papillae, or cysts which are lined by large, clear cells with occasional hobnail cytonuclear patterns.[1] Histochemically and ultrastructurally,[2] there is abundant intracytoplasmic glycogen, which is thought to be responsible for the clear cytoplasmic appearance of the neoplastic cells. The presently available morphologic and experimental[3] data favor a Müllerian, rather than a mesonephric, origin for these neoplasms.[1] This is supported by the frequent association of clear cell adenocarcinoma and Müllerian-derived[3] vaginal adenosis and cervical eversion, and the observation of histologically and electron microscopically similar neoplasms in the endometrium[4] and ovary.[5,6]

In contrast to the generally anterior location of DES-related clear cell adenocarcinoma, mesonephric carcinomas are usually found deep in the lateral wall of the vagina, in a site corresponding to the general location of mesonephric (Wolffian or Gartner's) duct remnants. In addition, the cells of mesonephric adenocarcinomas are not clear and contain little or no glycogen.[6]

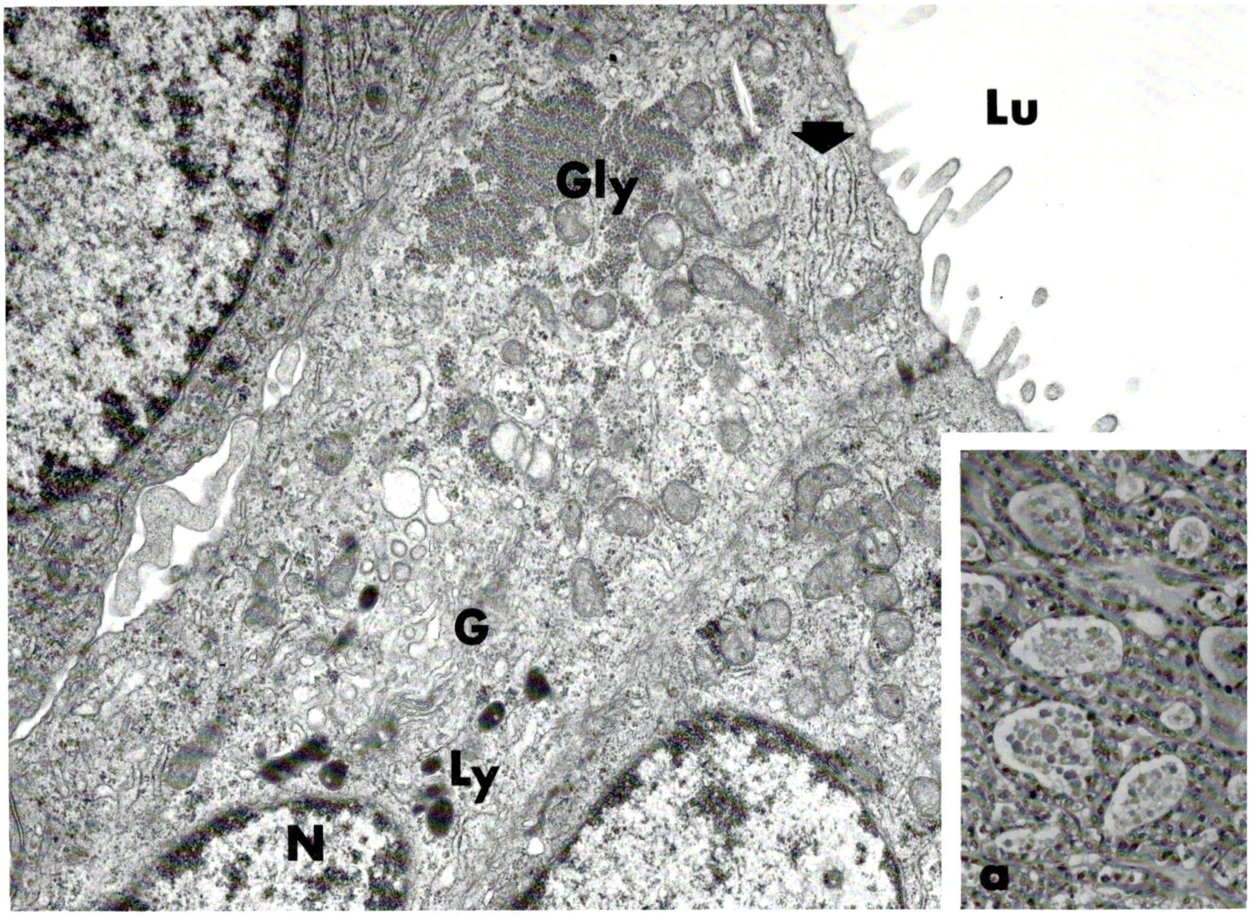

Figure 40a. *Clear cell adenocarcinoma of the vagina in a 21-year-old girl with a history of diethylstilbestrol exposure in utero.* The neoplasm is composed of tubules and nests of large, clear cells with prominent, irregular, and hyperchromatic nuclei and acidophilic nucleoli. Characteristically, mitoses are rare. The intraluminal secretions stain faintly with mucicarmine and may partly be digested with diastase. (H & E stain, × 12.)

Figure 40. *Ultrastructurally,* the neoplastic clear cells contain large collections of supranuclear (N) glycogen particles (Gly) in close association with parallel membranes of granular endoplasmic reticulum (arrow), free ribosomes, and mitochondria. The Golgi (G) are well developed with numerous peripheral vesicles and membrane-bound, electron-dense lysosomes (Ly). × 17,000. Lu: glandular lumen.

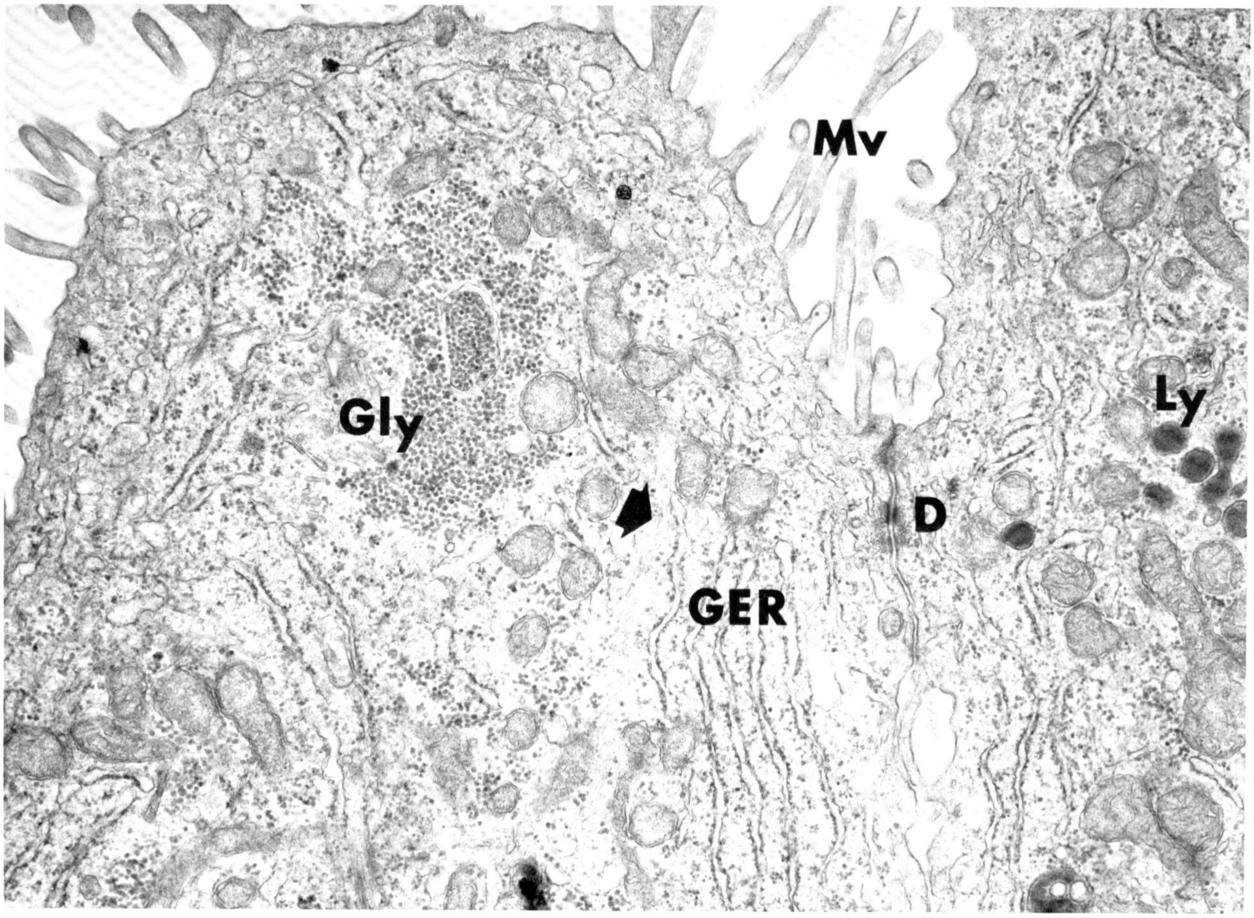

Figure 41. *Higher magnification of neoplastic clear cells,* illustrating their well-differentiated organellar content. Pools of supranuclear glycogen particles (Gly) are surrounded by mitochondria and cisternae of granular endoplasmic reticulum (GER). Agranular vesicles, microtubules (arrow), and microfilaments are also seen. The plasma membranes near the lumen are apposed by tight junctional complexes (D), and well-developed microvilli (Mv) project into the glandular lumen. The precise significance of this intense organellar development and glycogen accumulation in clear cell neoplasms of the vagina, as well as those arising in various other parts of the female genital tract, is presently unclear. × 21,000. Ly: lysosomes.

REFERENCES (Abundant evidence–Figure 41)

1. Herbst, A. L., R. J. Kurman, R. E. Scully, and D. C. Poskanzer. Clear-cell adenocarcinoma of the genital tract in young females. Registry report. *New Engl. J. Med.* **287:** 1259 (1972).
2. Silverberg, S. G. and L. S. DeGiorgi. Clear cell carcinoma of the vagina. A clinical, pathologic, and electron microscopic study. Cancer **29:** 1680 (1972).
3. Forsberg, J. G. Estrogen, vaginal cancer, and vaginal development. *Amer. J. Obstet. Gynecol.* **113:** 83 (1972).
4. Rorat, E., A. Ferenczy, and R. M. Richart. The ultrastructure of clear cell adenocarcinoma of endometrium. *Cancer* (in press).
5. Okagaki, T. and R. M. Richart. "Mesonephroma ovarii (hypernephroid carcinoma)": light microscopic and ultrastructural study of a case. *Cancer* **26:** 453 (1970).
6. Changus, G. W., J. E. Towne, C. J. Smith, and T. N. Yonan. Fine structure of the so-called mesonephric carcinoma (abstract). *Lab. Invest.* **20:** 579 (1969).

19

Juvenile Sarcoma Botryoides

Juvenile sarcoma botryoides is a highly malignant, soft, polyploid growth resembling a cluster of grapes. The tumor is most commonly seen in infancy or in early childhood. Ultrastructurally,[1,2] many of the immature or undifferentiated cells are recognized as rhabdomyoblasts by the identification of intracellular striated muscle fibrils, which are produced with varying degrees of success by many of the malignant cells. Although myogenic differentiation generally remains in an abortive state, occasionally a high degree of maturation may occur, resulting in the formation of scattered bundles of striated myofilaments closely resembling those seen in adult skeletal muscle. These cells are the ones that are recognized by light microscopy as embryonal rhabdomyoblasts.

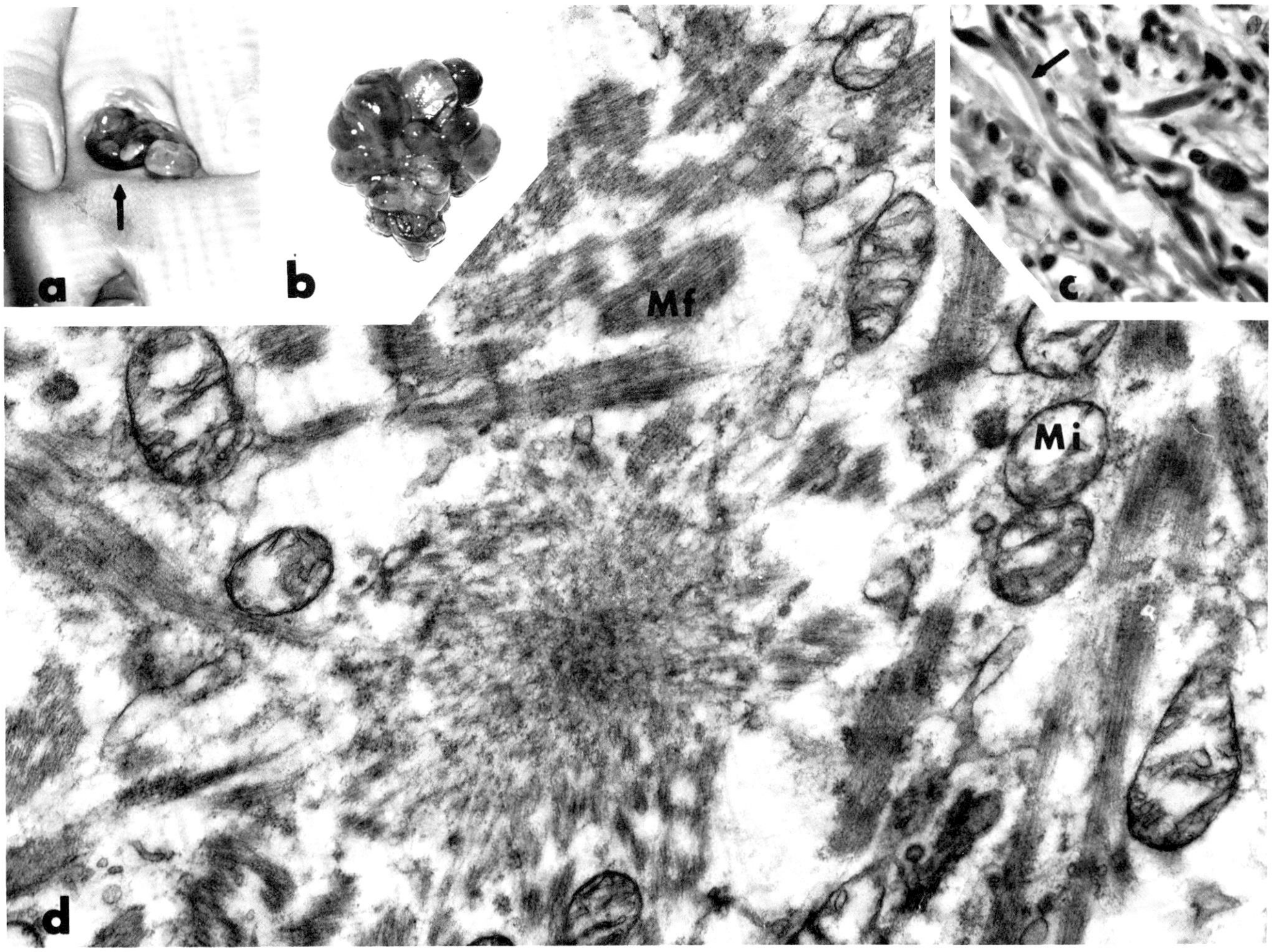

Figures 42a and b. *Sarcoma botryoides of the vagina in a 9-month-old infant.* The macroscopic grapelike appearance of sarcoma botryoides, attached to the base by a small pedicle (arrow), is obvious. *From* L. Overbeck. Das Sarcomas Botryoides oder Traubeusarkom der Vagina beim Kind. *Z. Geburtsh. Gynaekol.* **166:** 225–243 (1967).

Figure 42c. *Histologically,* the neoplasm has a fibromyxoid appearance and contains immature mesenchymal cells, some of which are recognizable as embryonal rhabdomyoblasts (arrow). Characteristically, the vaginal epithelium is invaded, and the submucosal region of the neoplasm contains a band of closely packed, primitive mesenchymal cells, referred to as the "cambium layer." (H & E stain, × 120.)

Figure 42d. *Primitive rhabdomyosarcoma cell* with disorganized rudimentary cross-striated myofibrils (Mf). Coinciding with the increase in myofibrils there is an increase in the mitochondria (Mi), providing the necessary energy for myofibrillogenesis. × 35,000. *From* L. Overbeck. Elektronenmikroskopische Untersuchungen des embryonalen Rhabdomyosarkoms. *Frankf. Z. Pathol.* **77:** 49-60 (1967).

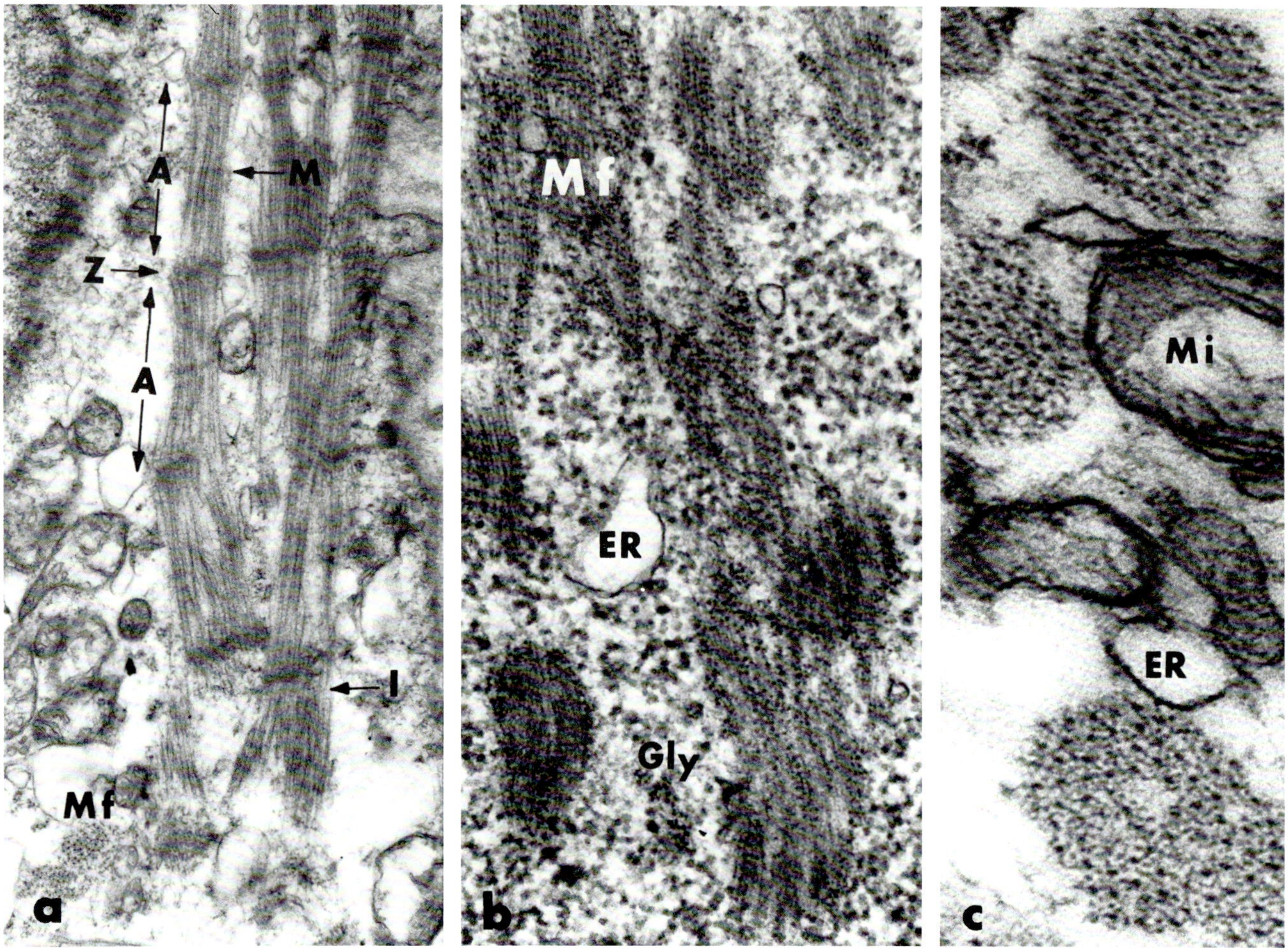

Figure 43a. *Sarcoma botryoides of vagina. Embryonal rhabdomyosarcoma cell* with well-differentiated myofibrils, containing regularly distributed sarcomeres delimited by *Z* lines. Whereas the *A* band with its central *M* band is easily recognized, the narrow isotropic *I* band is only occasionally visualized and the *H* band is not seen. × 27,000. Mf: transverse section of myofibrils. *From* L. Overbeck. Die Ultrastruktur des Sarcoma Botryoides oder Traubeusarkoms der Vagina beim Kind. *Z. Geburtsh. Gynaekol.* **167:** 13-28 (1967).

Figure 43b. *Sarcoma botryoides of vagina. Embryonal rhabdomyosarcoma cell* rich in sarcoplasmic glycogen (Gly). Free ribosomes are abundant between myofilaments (Mf). × 40,000. ER: endoplasmic reticulum. *From* L. Overbeck. Elektronenmikroskopische Untersuchungen des embryonalen Rhabdomyosarkoms. *Frankf. Z. Pathol.* **77:** 49-60 (1967).

Figure 43c. *Transverse section of the A band of three myofibrils of an embryonal rhabdomyosarcoma cell,* illustrating the regular hexagonal arrangement of thick (approx. 100 Å) and thin (approx. 50 Å) filaments. × 100,000. Mi: mitochondria; ER: endoplasmic reticulum. *From* L. Overbeck. Elektronenmikroskopische Untersuchungen des embryonalen Rhabdomyosarkoms. *Frankf. Z. Pathol.* **77:** 49-60 (1967).

REFERENCES (Juvenile sarcoma botryoides—Figure 43c)

1. Overbeck, L. Die Ultrastruktur des Sarcoma Botryoides oder Traubeusarkoms der Vagina beim Kind. *Z. Geburtsh. Gynaekol.* **167:** 13 (1967).
2. Overbeck, L. Elektronenmikroskopische Untersuchungen des embryonalen Rhabdomyosarkoms. *Franf. Z. Pathol.* **77:** 49 (1967).

CERVIX

20

Native Portio Epithelium (Ectocervix)

The cervix uteri has a complex epithelial covering that is highly responsive to ovarian hormones and is in a state of constant flux during the reproductive years. The exposed, or vaginal, portion of the cervix is generally covered by a nonkeratinizing, squamous epithelium continuous with the vaginal epithelium, which is referred to as the "native portio epithelium." At birth the portio epithelium is usually mature and glycogenated because of the influence of maternal estrogens, but it rapidly becomes atrophic as the hormones are cleared from the infant's circulation and does not begin maturation again until the time of menarche.

REFERENCES (Figures 44–45a)

1. Fluhman, C. F. *The Cervix Uteri and Its Diseases*. W. B. Saunders, Philadelphia, 1961.
2. Richart, R. M. A radioautographic analysis of cellular proliferation in dysplasia and carcinoma-in-situ of the uterine cervix. *Am. J. Obstet. Gynecol.* **86:** 925 (1963); *Fed. Proc.* **22** (Abstract) (1963).
3. Shingleton, H. M., R. M. Richart, J. Wiener, and D. Spiro. Human cervical intraepithelial neoplasia: fine structure of dysplasia and carcinoma in situ. *Cancer Res.* **28:** 695 (1968).
4. Ashworth, C. T., F. Luibel, and E. Sanders. Epithelium of normal cervix uteri studied with electron microscopy and histochemistry. *Am. J. Obstet. Gynecol.* **79:** 1149 (1960).
5. Davies, J. and R. B. Woolf. Histology and fine structure of the adult human cervix uteri. *Clin. Obstet Gynecol.* **6:** 265 (1963).
6. Younes, M. S. Electron microscope observations on carcinoma in situ of the cervix. *Obstet. Gynecol. Surv.* **24:** 768 (1969).
7. Hashimoto, K. Langerhans' cell granule. An endocytic organelle. *Arch. Dermatol.* **104:** 148 (1971).
8. Kuwahara, H. Electron microscopic studies on dendritic cells of the epidermis, especially on the function of Langerhans cells and etiology of certain leucodermas. *Jap. J. Dermatol.* **80:** 69 (1970).
9. McNutt, N. S. and R. S. Weinstein. Carcinoma of the cervix: deficiency of nexus intercellular junctions. *Science* **165:** 597 (1969).

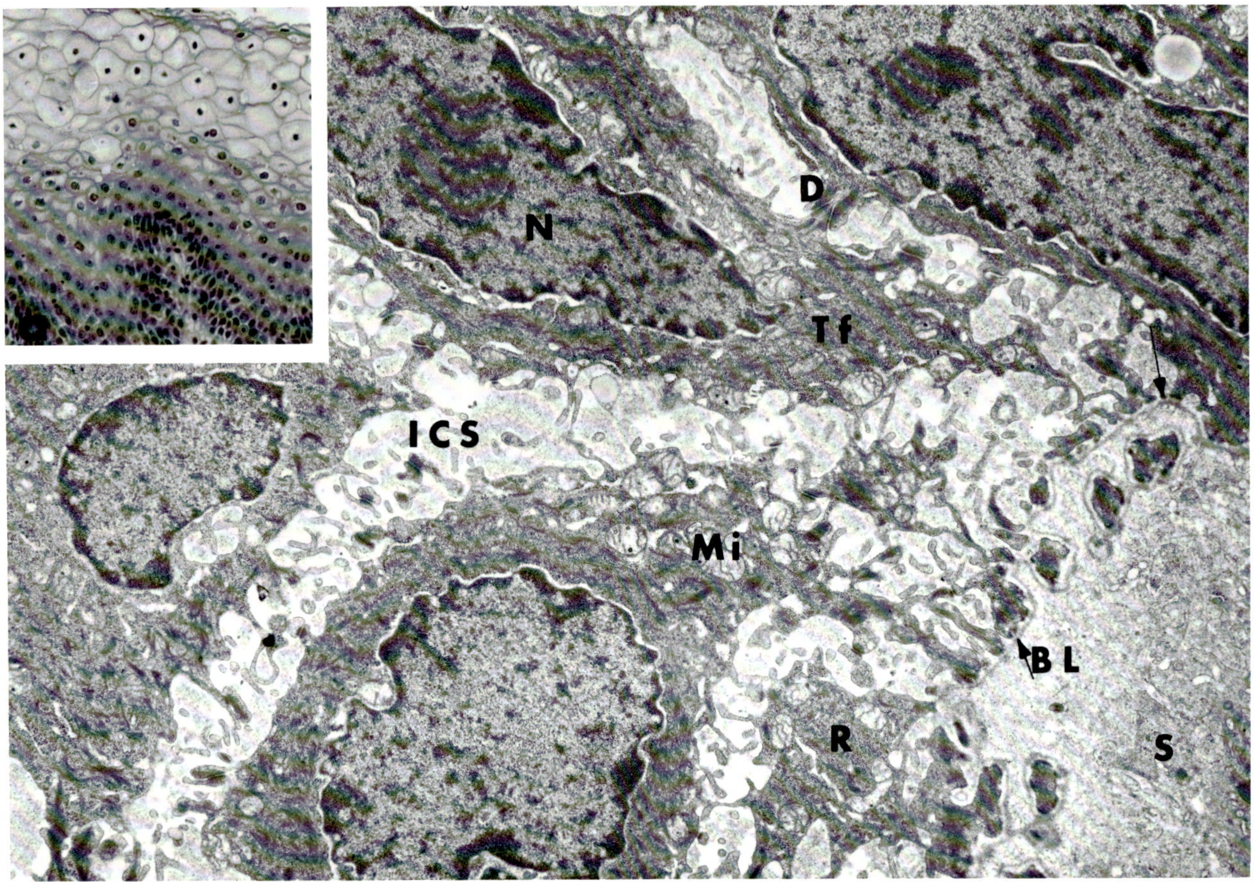

Figure 44a. *Histologically,*[1] the mature cervical squamous epithelium is similar to the vaginal epithelium but generally lacks the deep rete pegs seen in the vagina. The lowermost layer of cells adjacent to the basal lamina is referred to as the *stratum germinativum* or *basal zone.* The next layer, the *parabasal zone* or *stratum spinosum,* is also mitotically active and consists of polyhedral cells attached to one another by prominent intercellular bridges. There is beginning glycogenation. The two highest layers, the *intermediate* and *superficial* zones, contain a mitotically inactive,[2] maturing cell population rich in glycogen, with small pyknotic nuclei and prominent desmosomes.(H & E stain, × 38.)

Figure 44. *Transmission electron photomicrograph, illustrating the basal cells of the native portio epithelium.* The basal cells are part of the generative compartment of the cervical epithelium and have the fine structural characteristics of an actively dividing cell population.[3–5] There are prominent nuclei (N) and nucleoli, and the cytoplasm contains centrioles and abundant cytoplasmic organelles [free ribosomes (R) and mitochondria (Mi)], which take part in protein synthesis. Mitoses and bundles of peripheral tonofilaments (Tf) converging on the attachment plaques of desmosomes (D) are other characteristic features of cervical epithelial basal cells. A well-defined basal lamina (BL) containing hemidesmosomal attachments (arrow) to the basal cells separates the epithelium from the underlying, supporting, collagenous stroma (S). × 7200. ICS: dilated intercellular space.

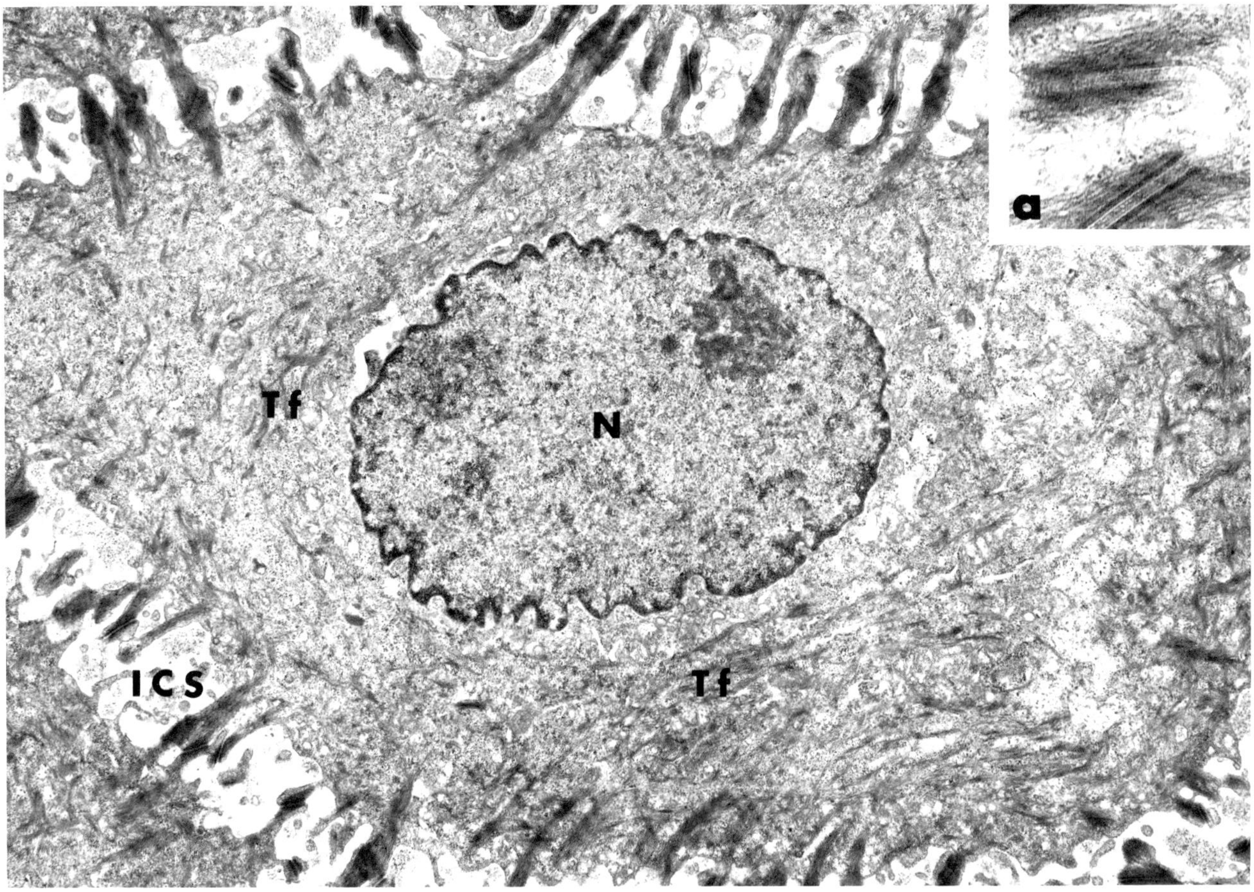

Figure 45. Ultrastructurally, the cells from the *parabasal layer* are similar to the basal cells and contain large, oval nuclei (N) with a slightly convoluted nuclear membrane. The cytoplasmic matrix contains numerous bundles of tonofilaments (Tf), which intermingle with aggregates of glycogen granules, and free ribosomes. Most of the microvillous cytoplasmic projections of adjacent epithelial cells are attached by well-developed tonofilament–desmosome complexes.

Nonepithelial cells are also seen in the cervical mucosa, including emperiopoietic lymphocytes[3] and Langerhans cells.[6] The latter are observed as "clear cells" at the light microscopic level. These nonepithelial components are thought to be related to primary antigen processing within both the epidermis and various mucous membranes.[7,8] × 7200. ICS: dilated intercellular space.

Figure 45a. *Higher magnification* of typical tonofilament–desmosome complexes. In addition to the classical desmosomal plaques there are numerous tight junctional nexuses[9] between adjacent epithelial cells. In these specialized regions the apposed plasma membranes are approximated at a distance of 20 Å and are regarded as low-resistance electrical coupling sites (see **Invasive Epidermoid Carcinoma**). × 11,000.

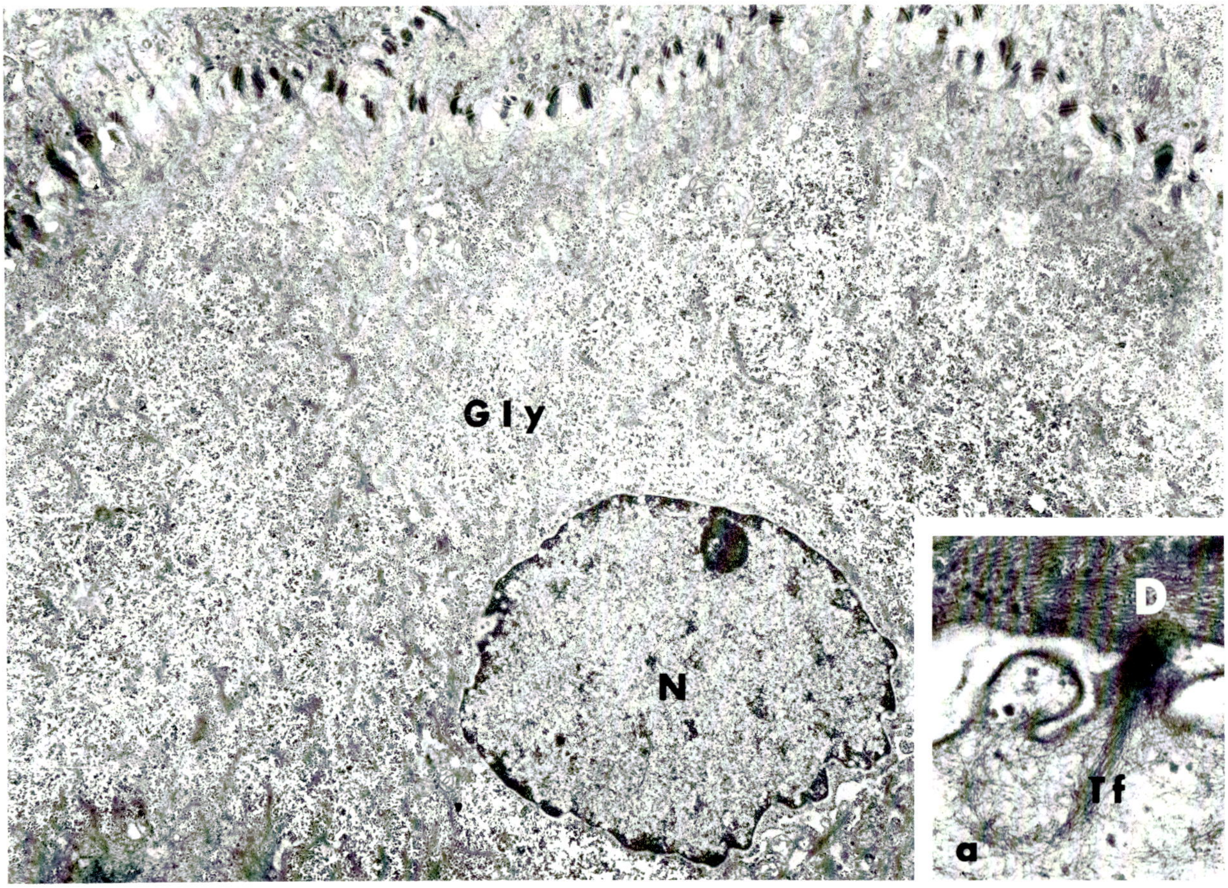

Figure 46. *Native portio. Cells from the upper strata* (intermediate cells) form the differentiated compartment of the cervix and have a conspicuous accumulation of glycogen particles[1,2] (Gly), which are interspersed with numerous bundles of tonofilaments. In keeping with their lack of mitotic or significant metabolic activity, other organelles, such as mitochondria, ribosomes, and endoplasmic reticulum, appear inconspicuous. Note that the nucleo–cytoplasmic ratio is in favor of the cyotplasmic substance. × 6000. N: nucleus.

Figure 46a. *Detailed view,* illustrating the short, stubby intercellular microvilli between cells of the upper strata. × 35,000. D: desmosome; Tf: tonofilaments.

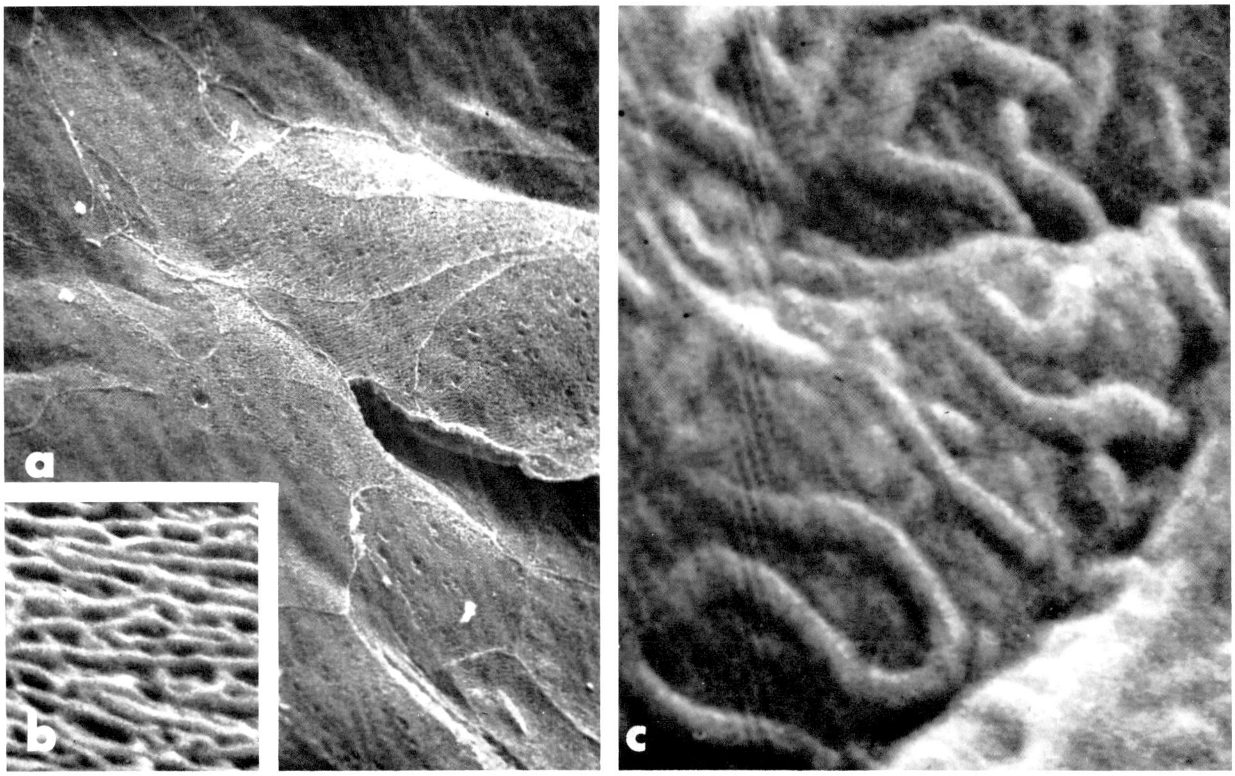

Figure 47a. *Scanning electron micrograph of the most superficial cells of the native portio epithelium.* The cells at the surface of the normal portio epithelium are attached by large numbers of desmosomes. The surfaces of the flattened superficial cells appear to be covered by fine[3] or stubby[2] microvilli at the fine structural level, but these structures are, in reality, a complex network of cytoplasmic microridges,[4-6] the function of which is thought to be related to the "cornified" nature of mature squamous cells, reported to be rich in disulfide keratin precursors.[7] Similar surface specializations are seen in epidermal horny cells. The cells are reinforced by prominent linear, nodular intercellular bridges. × 1000. *From* A. Ferenczy and R. M. Richart. Scanning electron microscopy of the cervical transformation zone. *Am. J. Obstet. Gynecol.* **115:** 151–157 (1973).

Figure 47b. *At a higher magnification,* the surface of the most superficial cells contains an intricate system of interanastomosing microridges. × 10,000. *From* A. Ferenczy and R. M. Richart. Scanning electron microscopy of the cervical transformation zone. *Am. J. Obstet. Gynecol.* **115:** 151–157 (1973).

Figure 47c. *The microridges in the most superficial cells* appear as nodular evaginations of the superficial plasma membrane. × 22,500.

REFERENCES (Figures 46–47c)

1. Jaeger, J. New light and electron microscopic studies on cervical and vaginal epithelium. *Arch. Gynaekol.* **207:** 55 (1969).
2. Luzardo-Baptista, M. J., J. Garcia-Tamayo, and J. T. Nunez-Montiel. Anatomia submicroscopia del exocervix humano normal. *Invest. Clin.* **30:** 23 (1969).
3. Lo Stumbo, F. and P. Buzzoni. Ultrastructure of the normal human uterine cervix. I. The exocervix. *Riv. Ostet. Ginecol.* **22:** (Suppl. 3): 42 (1967).
4. Ferenczy, A. and R. M. Richart. Scanning electron microscopy of the cervical transformation zone. *Am. J. Obstet. Gynecol.* **115:** 151 (1973).
5. Williams, A. E., J. A. Jordan, J. M. Allen, and J. F. Murphy. The surface ultrastructure of normal and metaplastic cervical epithelia and of carcinoma in situ. *Cancer Res.* **33:** 504 (1973).
6. Nasr, M. F., L. D. Lagasse, N. Chang, and J. G. Moore. Scanning electron microscopy of the human cervix. Description of a new method to study the surface anatomy. *Acta Cytol.* **17:** 141 (1973).
7. Ashworth, C. T., F. Luibel, and E. Sanders. Epithelium of normal cervix uteri studied with electron microscopy and histochemistry. *Am. J. Obstet. Gynecol.* **79:** 1149 (1960).

21

Transformation Zone

In most women, mucus-secreting epithelium of the endocervix everts onto the cervical portio during the reproductive period, forming the so-called clinical erosion. This columnar epithelium is subsequently reepithelialized by squamous epithelium, forming the clinical transformation zone, the direction of transformation being centripetal.[1] The eversion and its transformation zone generally occur principally on the anterior and posterior cervical lips.[1,2] The squamocolumnar junction is geographically fluid. The dynamics of its movement and its stability are strongly influenced by the woman's hormonal status, and they change most conspicuously during pregnancy.[3] The squamocolumnar junction is important because virtually all cervical neoplasia begins in the squamous epithelium at this junction;[4] the transformation zone is important because cervical intraepithelial neoplasia spreads on the portio within the transformation zone, and its limits are those of this zone.[4]

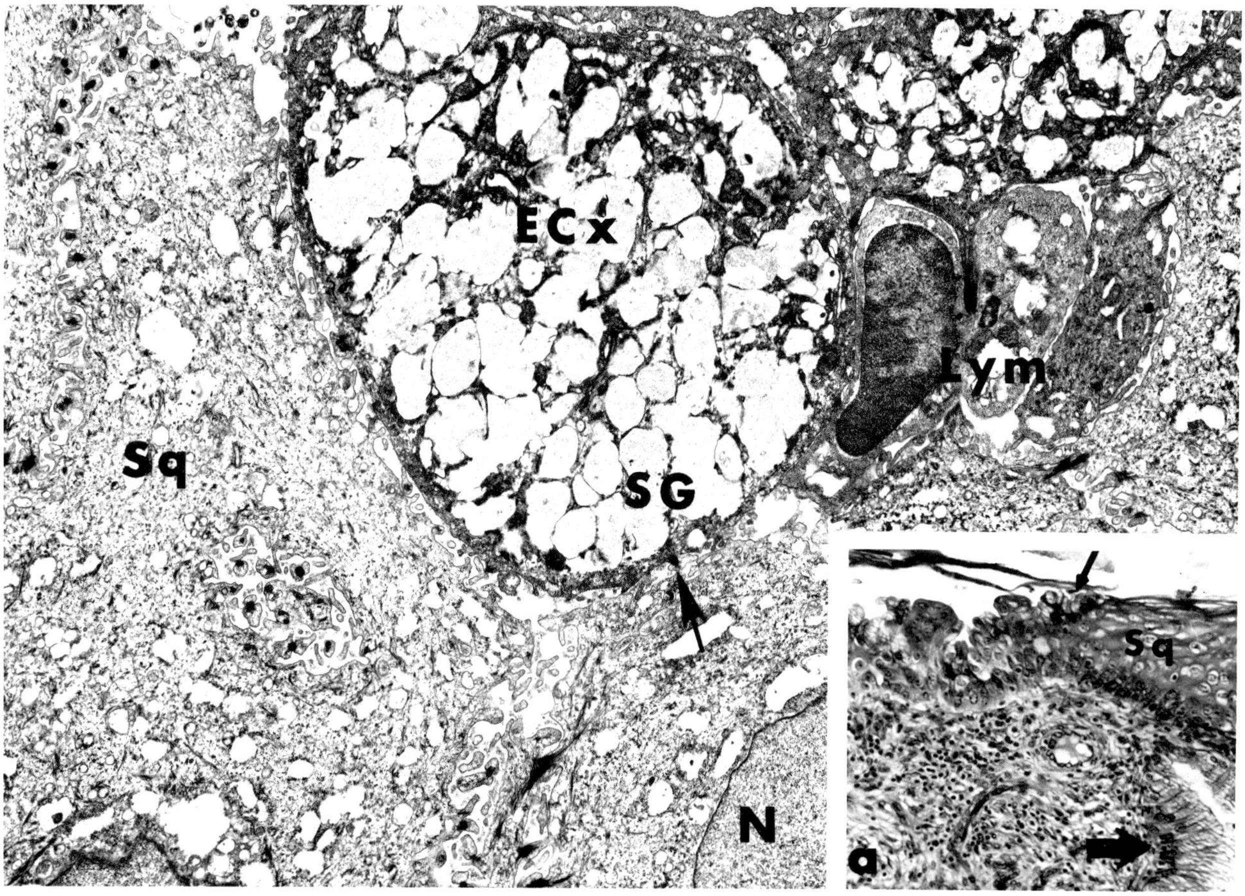

Figure 48a. *Light micrograph of cervical transformation zone.* Masses of stratified squamous epithelium (Sq) grow between the endocervical epithelium and its basal lamina. The cell of origin of this epithelium is controversial, some authors favoring an indirect route via squamous metaplasia,[5] and others suggesting a direct ingrowth from the native portio epithelium.[4] In any event, as the squamous epithelium expands and matures, the endocervical cells are lifted up (small arrow), degenerate, and are shed into the endocervical lumen. The large arrow points to an endocervical gland that has been completely overgrown by the newly formed squamous epithelium of the transformation zone. (H & E stain, × 38.)

Figure 48. *Transmission photomicrograph of cervical transformation zone epithelium* in which degenerating endocervical cells (ECx) are undermined by masses of poorly preserved squamous epithelial cells (Sq). In the process of the formation of the transformation zone, endocervical cells occasionally develop desmosomal attachments with the adjacent squamous epithelial cells (arrow).[6] Several migrating lymphocytes (Lym) are found within the intercellular spaces. × 8000. N: nucleus of squamous epithelial cells; SG: secretory granules.

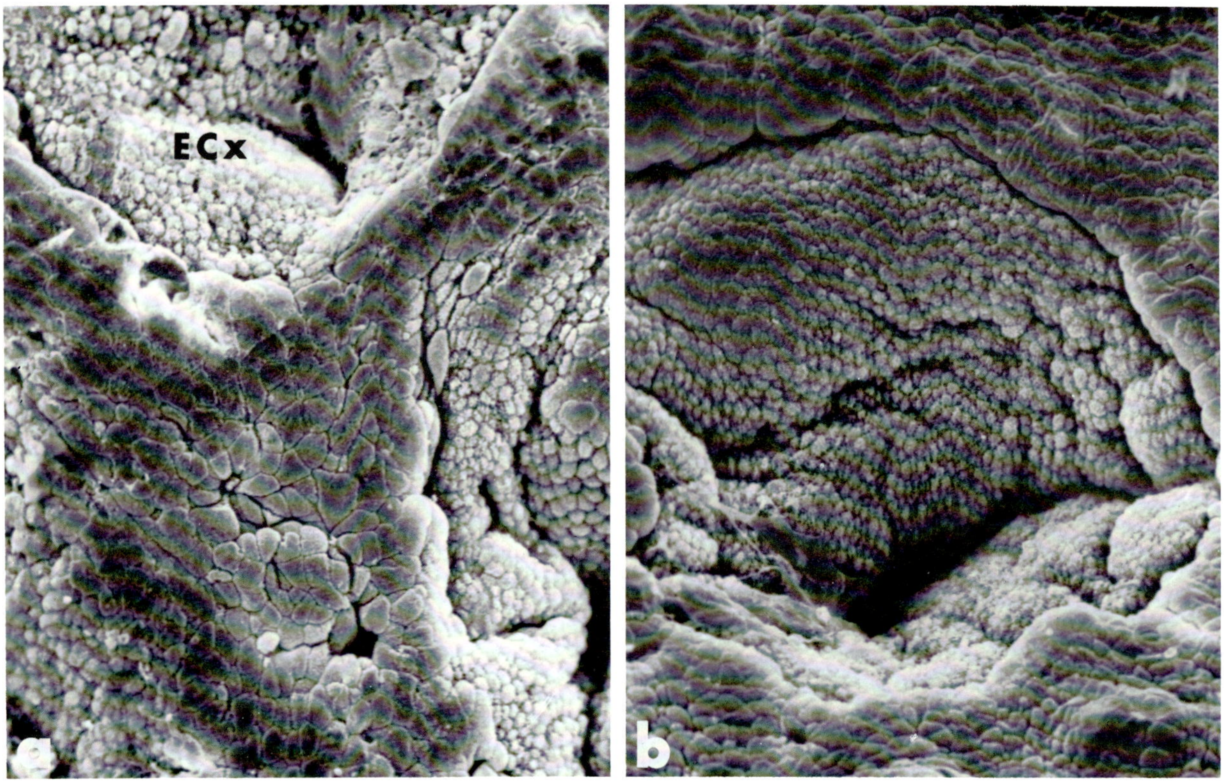

Figure 49a. *Scanning electron microscopic appearance of early transformation zone.* Narrow tongues of squamous epithelium resembling "mosaics" extend onto the cervical mucosa and partially encircle the endocervical gland openings (ECx). Note the sharp demarcation of the two epithelia at the gland mouths, whereas the squamocolumnar junction appears indistinct on the epithelial surface (lower left corner). × 220. Similar observations have been reported by other investigators.[7,8] *From* A. Ferenczy, and R. M. Richart. Scanning electron microscopy of the cervical transformation zone. *Am. J. Obstet. Gynecol.* **115:** 151-157 (1973).

Figure 49b. *Large endocervical opening* completely surrounded by young squamous epithelium. × 220. *From* A. Ferenczy, and R. M. Richart. Scanning electron microscopy of the cervical transformation zone. *Am. J. Obstet. Gynecol.* **115:** 151-157 (1973).

REFERENCES (In most women–Figure 49b)

1. Richart, R. M. Colpomicroscopic studies of the distribution of dysplasia and carcinoma-in-situ on the exposed portion of the human uterine cervix. *Cancer* **18:** 950 (1965).
2. Richart, R. M. Colpomicroscopic studies of cervical intraepithelial neoplasia. *Cancer* **19:** 395 (1966).
3. Wilbanks, G. D. and R. M. Richart. Postpartum cervix and its relation to cervical neoplasia. A colposcopic study. *Cancer* **19:** 273 (1966).
4. Richart, R. M. Natural history of cervical intraepithelial neoplasia. *Clin. Obstet. Gynecol.* **5:** 748 (1968).
5. Coppleson, M., E. Pixley, and B. Reid. *Colposcopy.* Charles C Thomas, Springfield, Ill., 1971.
6. Ferenczy, A. and R. M. Richart. Scanning electron microscopy of the cervical transformation zone. *Am. J. Obstet. Gynecol.* **115:** 151 (1973).
7. Morgenroth, K. and A. Verhagen. The surface structure of the portio ectopia in scanning electron microscopy. *Arch. Gynaekol.* **212:** 423 (1972).
8. Williams, A. E., J. A. Jordan, J. M. Allen, and J. F. Murphy. The surface ultrastructure of normal and metaplastic cervical epithelia and of carcinoma in situ. *Cancer Res.* **33:** 504 (1973).

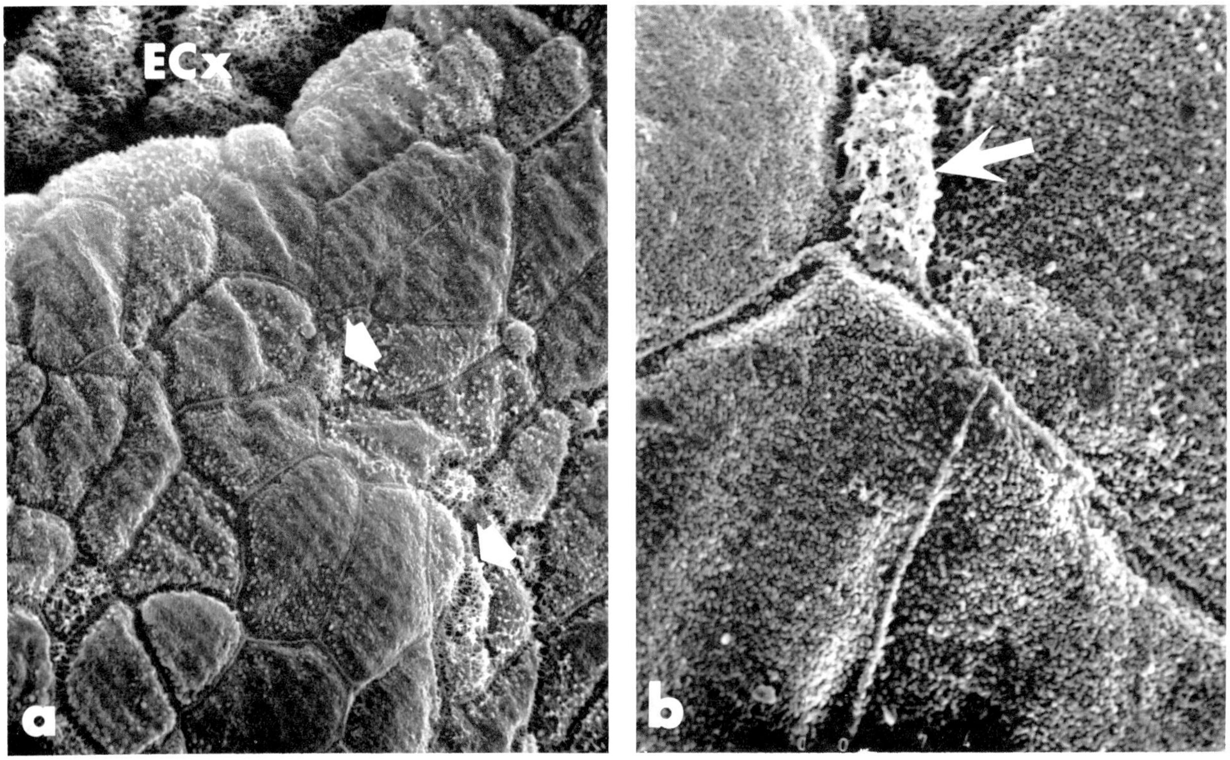

Figure 50a. *Higher magnification of early transformation zone,* containing young squamous epithelium with well-developed intercellular bridges. Among the squamous cells are several individual endocervical cells (arrows). × 885. ECx: endocervical epithelium. *From* A. Ferenczy and R. M. Richart. Scanning electron microscopy of the cervical transformation zone. *Am. J. Obstet. Gynecol.* **115:** 151–157 (1973).

Figure 50b. *A single trapped endocervical cell* (arrow) is apparently interconnected with the neighboring squamous cells by converging intercellular bridges. × 3000. *From* A. Ferenczy and R. M. Richart. Scanning electron microscopy of the cervical transformation zone. *Am. J. Obstet. Gynecol.* **115:** 151–157 (1973).

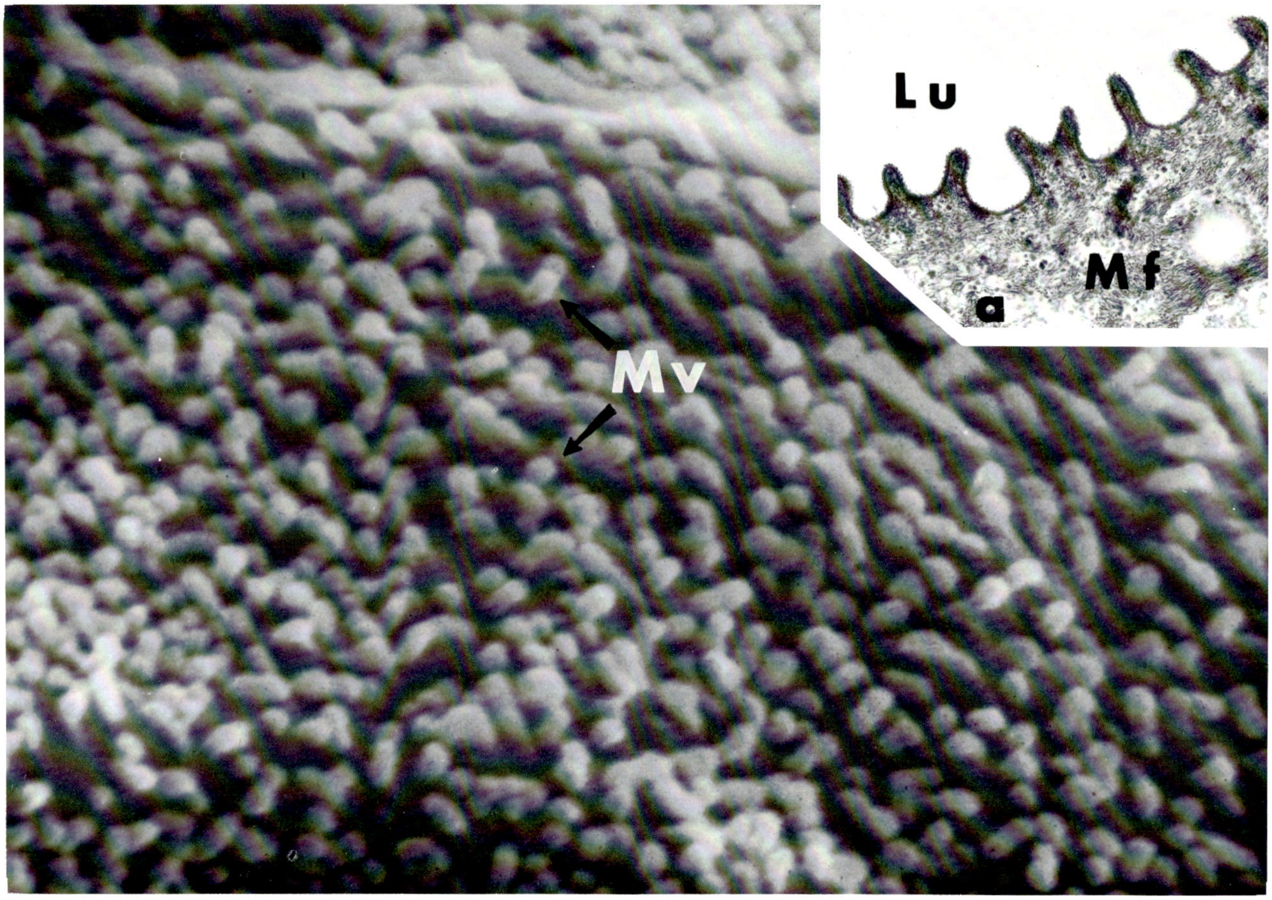

Figure 51. *In contrast to the superficial cells of the mature squamous epithelium,* the superficial cells of the young transformation zone epithelium are covered by numerous well-developed microvillous projections (Mv).[1,2] × 20,000.

Figure 51a. *At the transmission electron microscopic level,* the surface microvilli correspond to the irregular evaginations of the surface plasma membrane. × 25,600. Lu: cervical lumen; Mf: tonofibrils.

REFERENCES (Figures 50a–51a)

1. Ferenczy, A. and R. M. Richart. Scanning electron microscopy of the cervical transformation zone. *Am. J. Obstet. Gynecol.* **115:** 151 (1973).
2. Williams, A. E., J. A. Jordan, J. M. Allen, and J. F. Murphy. The surface ultrastructure of normal and metaplastic cervical epithelia and of carcinoma in situ. *Cancer Res.* **33:** 504 (1973).

22

Endocervical Epithelium

The epithelium of the endocervix, at both the light and the ultrastructural[1-4] level, contains mucus-secreting cells and scattered nonsecretory, ciliated cells. Although cyclic morphologic changes in the endocervical epithelium are inconspicuous, the viscoelastic secretory product, that is, cervical mucus, is subject to profound cyclical alterations. Under estrogenic influence, the endocervical secretions are profuse, watery, and alkaline, facilitating sperm penetration, whereas during the luteal phase they are scant, thick, and acid, contain numerous leukocytes, and are unfavorable for sperm penetration. Biochemical[5] and transmission electron microscopic studies[6,7] have shown that the cervical mucous gel is composed of a heterogeneous micellar network of glycoproteins. The intermicellar space is filled with cervical plasma, rich in sodium chloride and potassium, the ions of which are responsible for the mucous crystallization or fern reaction. During estrogenic stimulation the glycoprotein micelles are arranged parallel to each other at a distance of 5 to 15 mμ,[6] creating a channel system favorable for sperm penetration. Under the influence of endogenous or exogenous progestogens, the micellar channel system is replaced by a dense meshwork composed of numerous intermicellar fiber bridges that preclude sperm penetration.

Ultrastructurally,[1-5] endocervical secretory activity occurs by both the apocrine[2] and the merocrine[1,2] type of expulsion of secretory granules. As in other mucus-secreting units in the body, in the endocervical mucinous cells mucogenesis is initiated in the ribosome–endoplasmic reticulum–Golgi complex.[1,2] The simultaneous occurrence of, and the occasional direct communication[6] between, the light staining secretory granules and granulofibrillar bodies in endocervical cells suggest that the latter store glycoproteins in a granulofilamentous form. Similar fibrillar structures are observed in the mucus-secreting cells of Bartholin's glands (see **Bartholin's Duct, Glands, and Duct Cyst**).

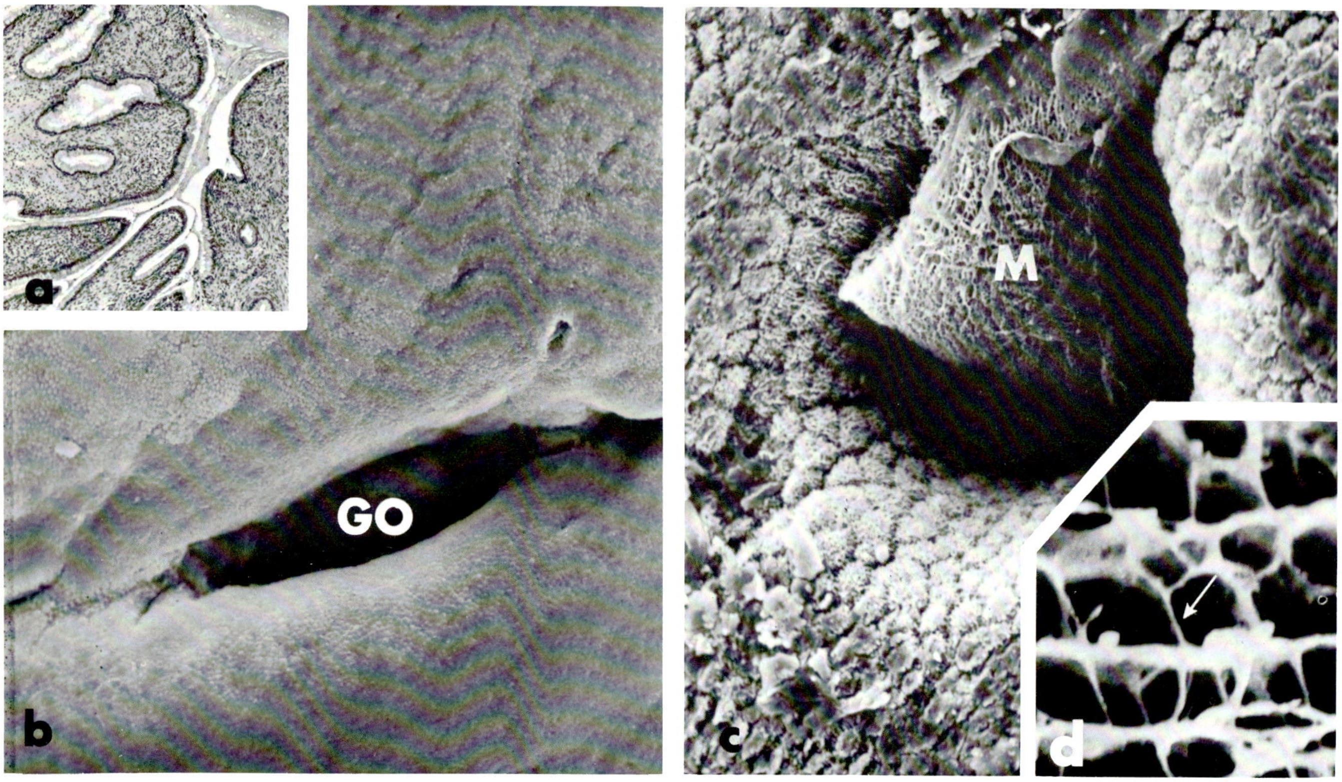

Figure 52a. *Histologically, the endocervix* consists of deeply penetrating tunnels and clefts lined by a single layer of mucus-secreting, columnar epithelium. The columnar epithelial cells characteristically have basally placed nuclei surrounded by a column of mucus, which is also found intraluminally and changes its histological appearance with the stage of the cycle, appearing more dense in the progestational phase. The glands tend to become dilated during pregnancy. There is frequently an abundant metaplastic reaction, which is most pronounced during the reproductive years. (H & E stain, × 12.)

Figure 52b. *Scanning electron microscopic appearance of* endocervical glandular mouth (GO). Note the polygonal cellular contour and the fine microvillous covering of the surface plasma membrane. × 160.

Figure 52c. *Higher magnification of an endocervical opening* with conspicuous mucus secretion (M). × 800.

Figure 52d. *Scanning electron microscopic appearance of* glutaraldehyde-fixed, unpurified cervical mucus in the luteal phase of the menstrual cycle. The mucoid material has a complex meshwork configuration and is composed of long, thick filamentous structures (micelles), interconnected by thin filaments (arrow) that are distributed at regular intervals. This network pattern of the endocervical mucus is unfavorable for sperm penetration. × 3200.

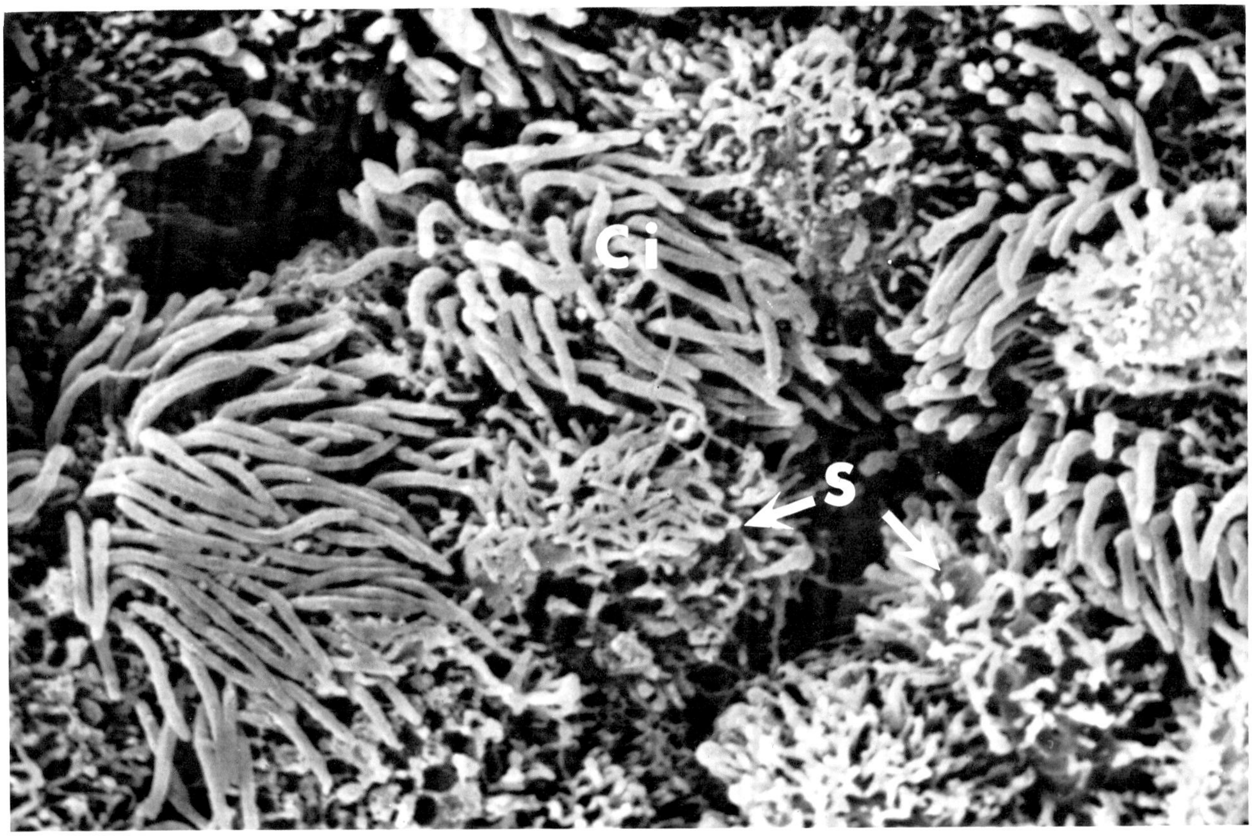

Figure 53. *High-power scanning electron micrograph* of the endocervical epithelium, which is composed of ciliated (Ci) and nonciliated secretory cells (S), the latter being covered by numerous well-developed microvilli. × 4800.

REFERENCES (The epithelium of the endocervix –Figure 53)

1. Nilsson, O. and A. Westman. The ultrastructure of the epithelial cells of the endocervix during the menstrual cycle. *Acta Obstet. Gynecol. Scand.* **40:** 223 (1961).
2. Overbeck, L. and E. Philipp. Die Ultrastruktur des Zervixepithels. *Z. Geburtsh. Gynaekol.* **171:** 159 (1969).
3. Ferenczy, A. and R. M. Richart. Scanning electron microscopy of the cervical transformation zone. *Am. J. Obstet. Gynecol.* **115:** 151 (1973).
4. Williams, A. E., J. A. Jordan, J. M. Allen, and J. F. Murphy. The surface ultrastructure of normal and metaplastic epithelia and of carcinoma in situ. *Cancer Res.* **33:** 504 (1973).
5. Schumacher, G. F. Biochemistry of cervical mucus. *Fertil. Steril.* **21:** 697 (1970).
6. Singer, A. and B. L. Reid. The ultrastructure of cervical mucus. *J. Reprod. Fertil.* **21:** 377 (1970).
7. Van Bruggen, E. F. J. and J. Kremer. Electron microscopy of bovine and human cervical mucus. *Int. J. Fertil.* **15:** 50 (1970).

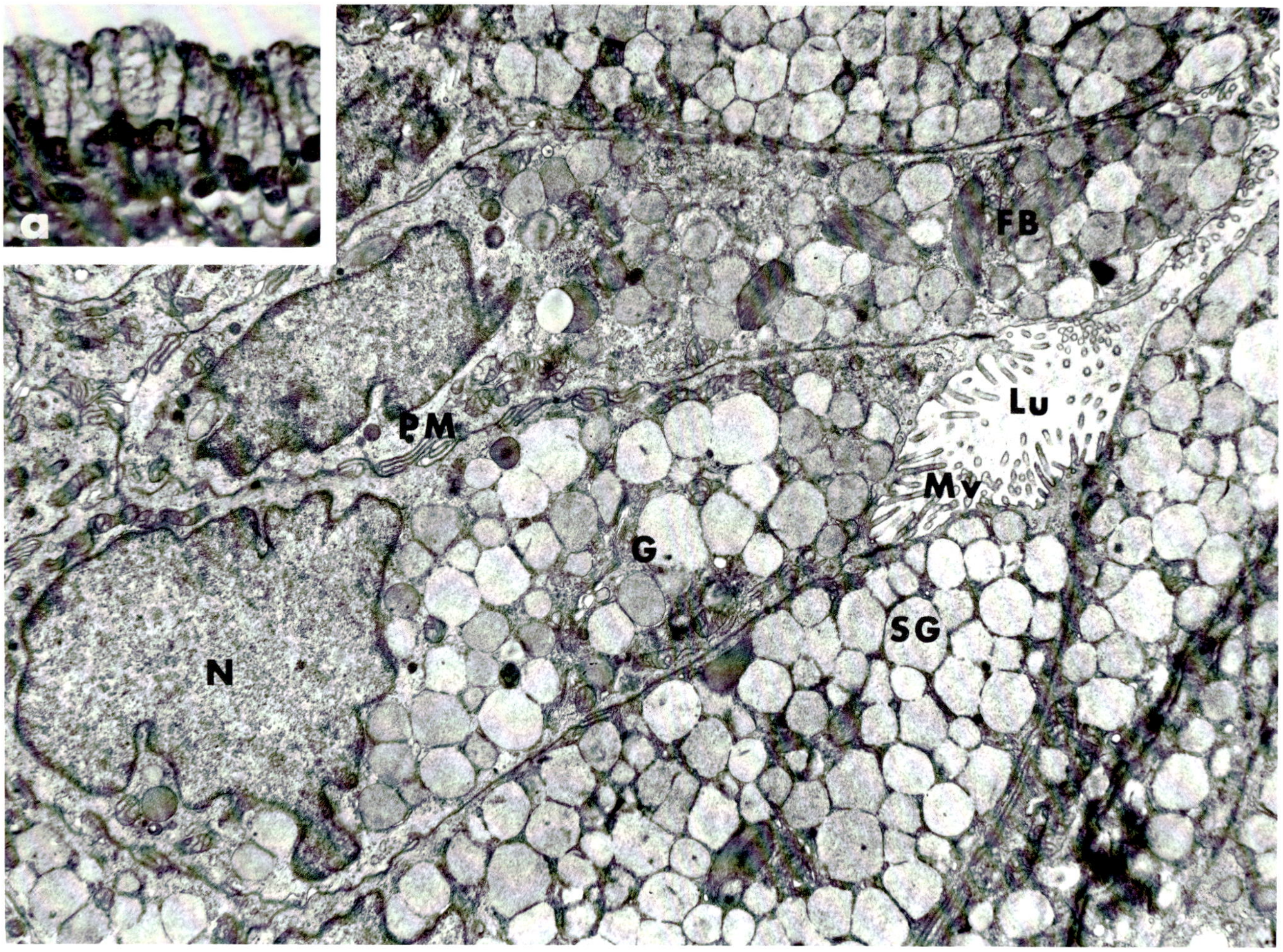

Figure 54a. *Histologic appearance of endocervical epithelium,* which consists of tightly packed mucus-secreting columnar cells (picket fence) in which the nuclei are characteristically located near the basal lamina and the abundant cytoplasmic substance contains granular mucus. (H & E stain, × 64.)

Figure 54. *Endocervix, 12th day of the menstrual cycle.* The typical mucus-secreting endocervical cells have numerous tightly packed, supranuclear (N) secretory granules (SG), fibrillar bodies (FB), and well-developed Golgi apparatuses (G). The luminal plasma membrane contains numerous well-developed and occasionally branching microvilli (Mv). × 9500. Lu: lumen; PM: plasma membrane. *From* L. Overbeck, and E. Philipp. Die Ultrastruktur des Zervixepithels. *Z. Geburtsh. Gynaekol.* **171:** 159–171 (1969).

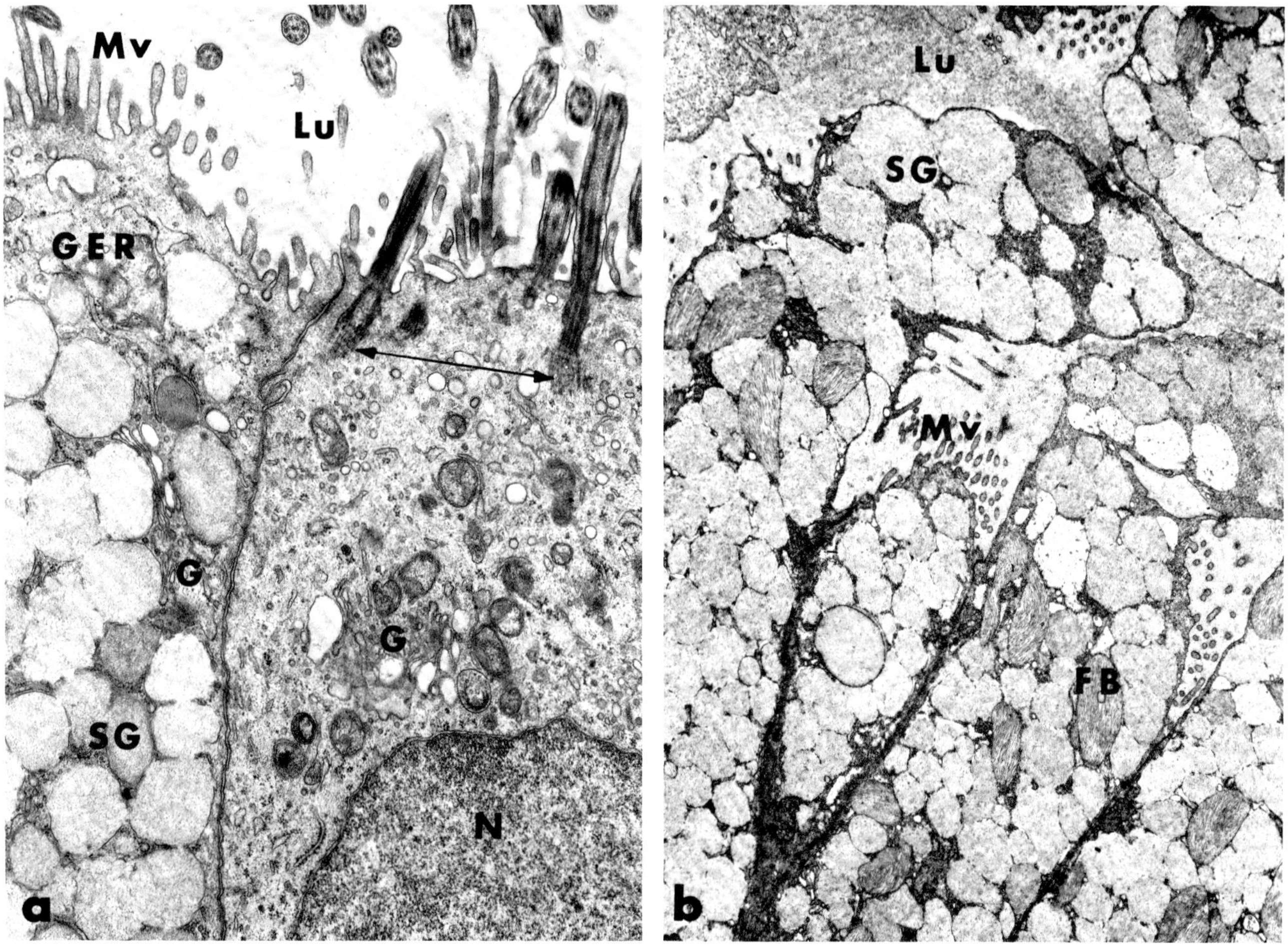

Figure 55a. *Endocervix, 20th day of the menstrual cycle.* The ciliated endocervical epithelial cell contains several well-developed cilia composed of ciliary shafts, basal bodies, and cross-striated rootlets (double-headed arrow). In a supranuclear (N) location are several mitochondria associated with the Golgi (G) and granular, as well as agranular, endoplasmic reticulum. The adjacent secretory cell has numerous microvilli (Mv) and tightly packed secretory granules (SG). The secretory granules are in close association with the Golgi and parallel membranes of granular endoplasmic reticulum (GER). × 18,400. Lu: lumen. *From* L. Overbeck and E. Philipp. Die Ultrastruktur des Zervixepithels. *Z. Geburtsh. Gynaekol.* **171:** 159–171 (1969).

Figure 55b. *Endocervix, 12th day of the menstrual cycle.* Mucus secretion is of the apocrine type, as indicated by the intraluminal (Lu) bulging of the apical cytoplasmic substance packed with secretory granules (SG). Numerous fibrillar bodies (FB) and luminal microvilli (Mv) are seen. × 8000. *From* L. Overbeck and E. Philipp. Die Ultrastruktur des Zervixepithels. *Z. Geburtsh. Gynaekol.* **171:** 159–171 (1969).

REFERENCES (Ultrastructurally, endocervical secretory activity–Figure 55b)

1. Nilsson, O. and A. Westman. The ultrastructure of the epithelial cells of the endocervix during the menstrual cycle. *Acta Obstet. Gynecol. Scand.* **40:** 223 (1961).
2. Overbeck, L. and E. Philipp. Die Ultrastruktur des Zervixepithels. *Z. Geburtsh. Gynaekol.* **171:** 159 (1969).
3. Lo Stumbo, F. and P. Buzzoni. Ultrastructure of the normal human uterine cervix. II. The endocervix. *Riv. Ostet. Ginecol.* **22:** (Suppl.): 43 (1967).
4. Stegner, H. E. and R. Beltermann. The electron microscopy of epithelial cells of cervical glands and of so-called reserve cells. *Arch. Gynaekol.* **207:** 480 (1969).
5. Bonilla-Musoles, F. Electron-microscopical examinations of the cervix uteri. *Gynaekol.-Rundsch.* **8:** 197 (1969).
6. Philipp, E. On the granulo-filamentary transformation of secretory granules in the mucus producing epithelium of the human endocervix. *Z. Zellforsch.* **134:** 555 (1972).

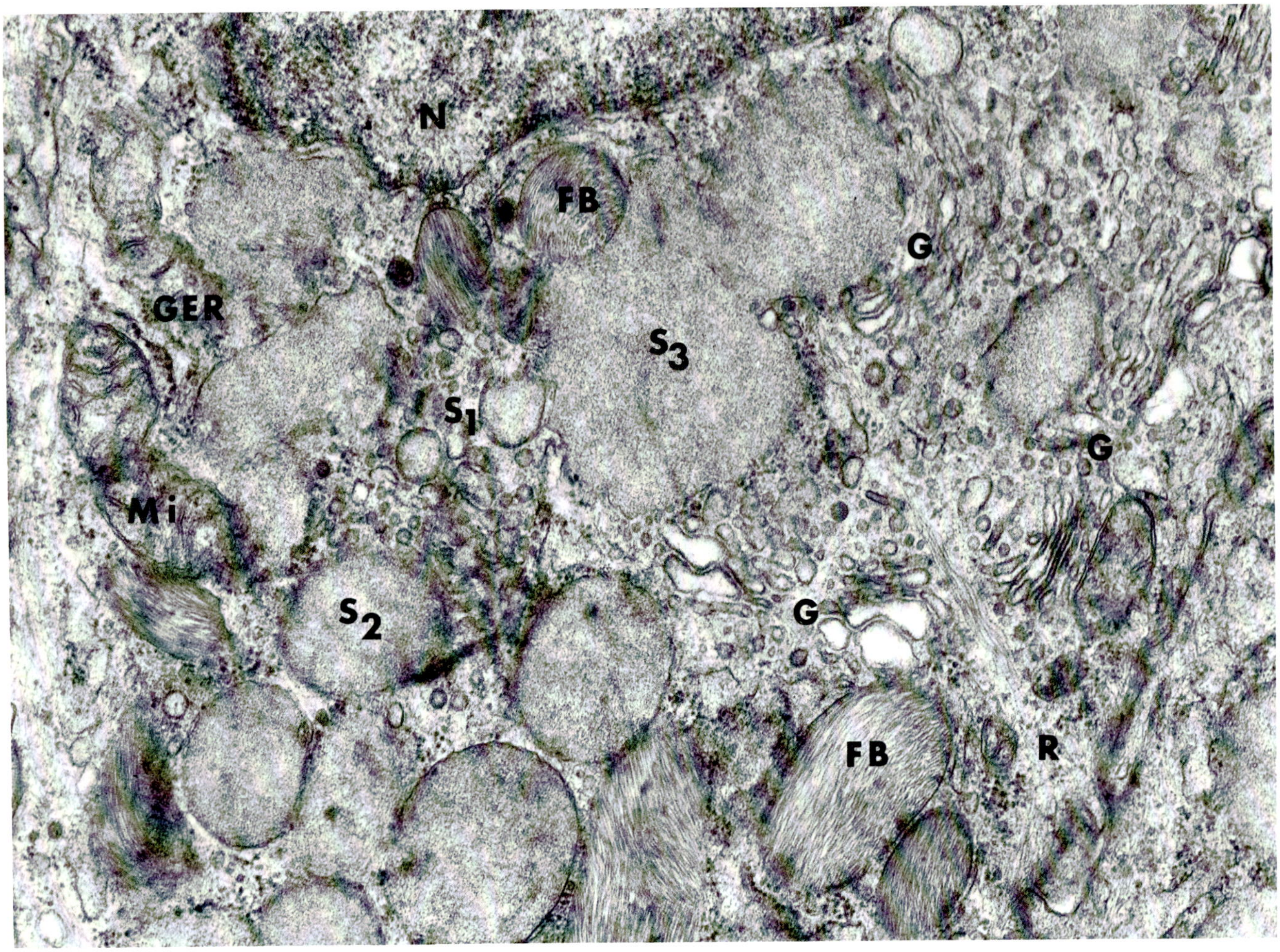

Figure 56. *Endocervix, 12th day of the menstrual cycle.* Detail of endocervical mucinogenesis: the formation of secretory granules is initiated near the perinuclear (N) Golgi zone (G), apparently by coalescence of peripheral Golgi vesicles (S_1); these are transformed into larger secretory granules (S_2), which in turn form by further coalescence prominent secretory granules with granular content (S_3). The Golgi are associated with abundant free ribosomes (R), mitochondria (Mi), and granular endoplasmic reticulum (GER), providing the essential proteins and energy for mucoprotein synthesis. The close association of fibrillar bodies (FB) and secretory vacuoles suggests that the former represent a peculiar filamentous form of glycoprotein storage. × 37,600. *From* L. Overbeck and E. Philipp. Die Ultrastruktur des Zervixepithels. *Z. Geburtsh. Gynaekol.* **171:** 159–171 (1969).

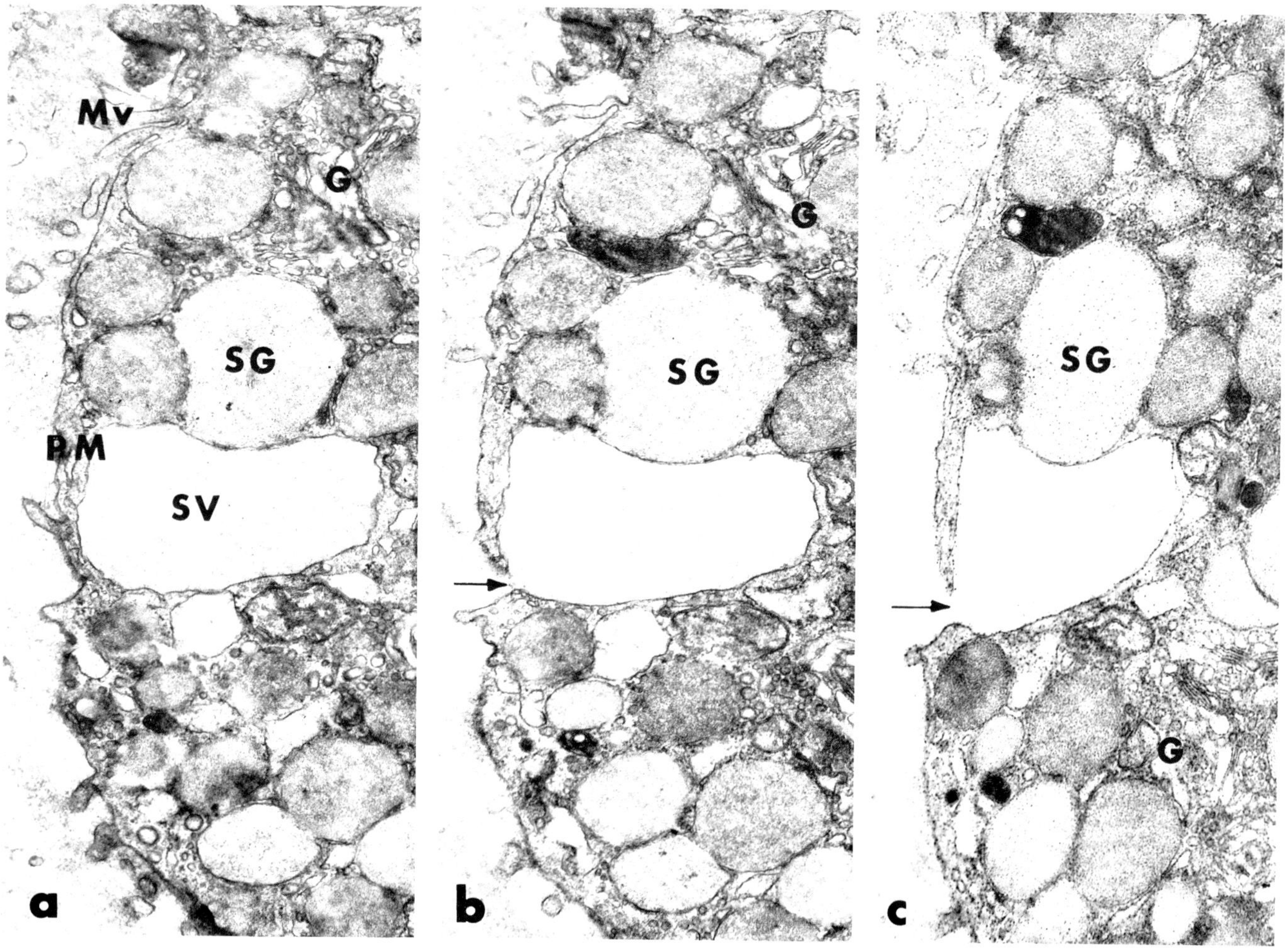

Figures 57a, b, and c. *Serial sections of endocervical epithelium, 15th day of the menstrual cycle.* In addition to apocrine secretion, granules (SG) may be discharged from the cytoplasmic substance by focal, porelike openings (arrows in Figures *b* and *c*) of the surface plasma membrane (PM). In Figure *c*, secretory granules (SG) protrude into the empty vacuole (SV), left behind by the previously expelled secretory products. × 25,600. G: Golgi; Mv: microvilli. *From* L. Overbeck and E. Philipp. Die Ultrastruktur des Zervixepithels. *Z. Geburtsh. Gynaekol.* **171:** 159–171 (1969).

23

Normal Exfoliative Cytology

The microscopic examination of exfoliated vaginal and cervical squamous cells was introduced by George Papanicolaou in 1943. With improved techniques of sampling, the "Pap smear" has proved to be of great value in the detection of cervical neoplasia and various other pathologic conditions of the female genital tract. In addition, because of the close relationship between cellular growth and morphology and ovarian steroid hormones, examination of exfoliated cells is valuable in assessing endocrine function, and cytological "hormonal evaluations" are commonly used.

Under the influence of estrogens, the cells of the superficial zone of the squamous epithelium are stimulated to mature and desquamate. During the proliferative phase of the menstrual cycle, up to 90% of the exfoliated cells are of the mature superficial type. The postovulatory period is dominated by progesterone, and because of its inhibiting effect on the maturation process cells of intermediate type are more commonly shed than those of superficial type. The elevated levels of progesterone that occur during pregnancy accentuate the normal luteal phase pattern, and, in addition, the intermediate cells become heavily glycogenated. In the postpartum and postmenopausal periods parabasal cells predominate because of a relative lack of hormonal stimulation.

The high resolving power of the scanning electron microscope is useful in the study of exfoliated squamous epithelial cells.[1] In our laboratory, the technique employed to obtain acceptable specimens is identical to that used for obtaining routine Papanicolaou smears. The exposed portion of the cervix is cleaned with isotonic saline solution and scraped with a wooden spatula. The specimens obtained are transferred onto glass slides or coverslips and fixed immediately with an isopropyl alcohol-based spray. After fixation, the smears are air-dried, dehydrated, and stained by the Papanicolaou method. They are then examined by light microscopy, and appropriate cell-containing areas approximately 5 mm square are cut from the slide, cleaned in 100% xylene, cemented onto specimen holders, coated with a 150-Å-thick film of gold-palladium, and examined in the scanning electron microscope. The advantages of this method include the ability to examine and process a large number of specimens rapidly, a reliable means of cell identification, and better cellular preservation than is obtained with the previously described techniques.[2]

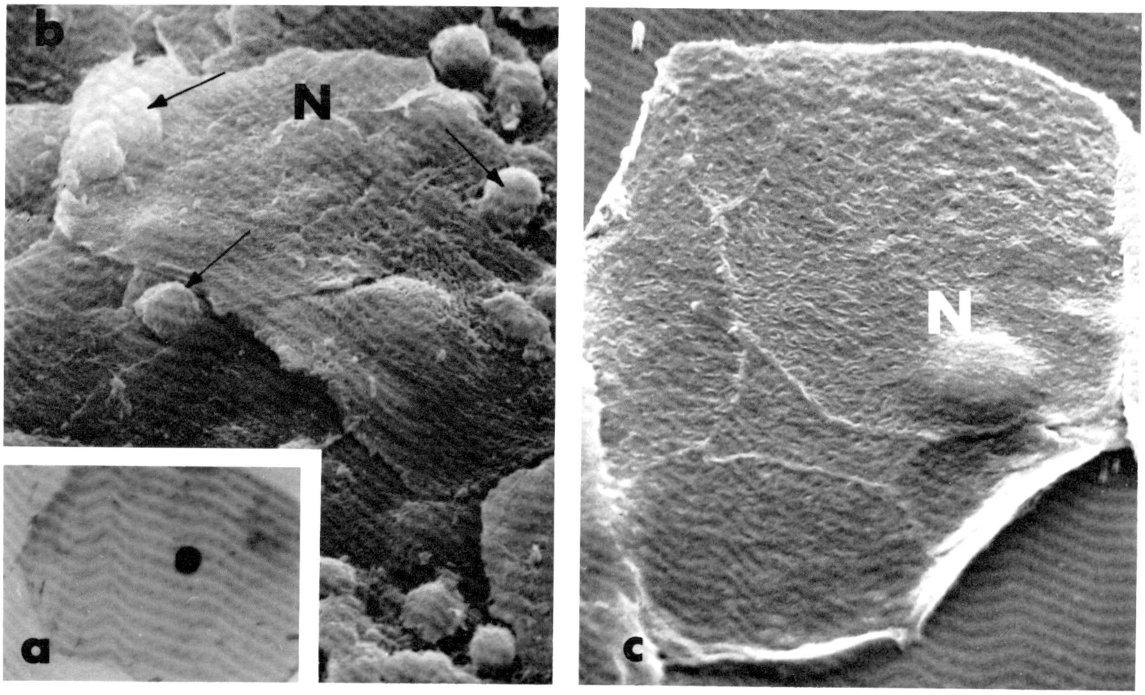

Figure 58a. *Light micrograph of normal superficial, exfoliated cervical squamous cells.* The cytoplasm is abundant (40 to 50μ in diameter), and there is a small, central, pyknotic nucleus. (Papanicolaou stain, × 120.)

Figure 58b. *Scanning electron microscopic appearance* of previously stained (Papanicolaou stain) exfoliated, normal superficial cells. The cells overlap each other, have central bulging nuclei (N), and are covered with leukoctyes (arrows). × 1000.

Figure 58c. *Higher-power view of a superficial cell* with curled edges and a centrally located nucleus (N). The abundant cytoplasm is covered by smooth, shallow, interdigitating microridges. These microridges are distinctive features of both exfoliated[1] and nondesquamated superficial squamous cells of the cervical[3-5] and vaginal squamous mucous membranes and are thought to play a role in surface adhesiveness.[1] Their formation is presumably related to the "cornified" nature of the most superficial and mature squamous cells, which are known to contain disulfide-rich keratin precursors.[6] This contention is further supported by the findings of similar plasma membrane microridges in keratin-containing, epidermal horny cells. In immature squamous epithelium, including the young cervical transformation zone, such surface specializations are not observed.[3,4] × 1400. *From* A. Llanes, C. Farre, A. Ferenczy, and R. M. Richart. Scanning electron microscopy of normal exfoliated squamous cervical cells. *Acta Cytol.* **17:** 507–509 (1973).

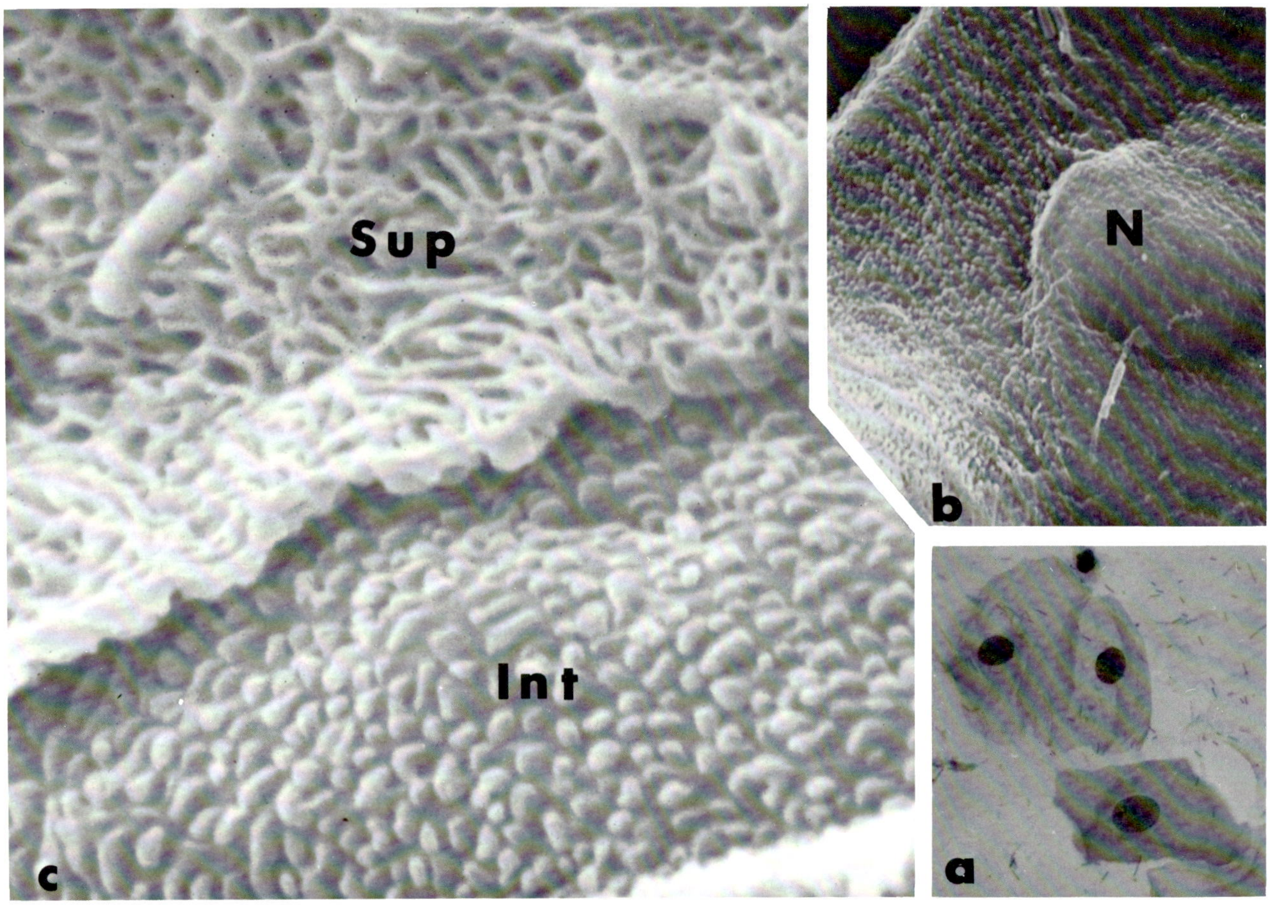

Figure 59a. *Light micrograph of several intermediate cells* (navicular cells) in which the nuclei are large as compared to superficial cells and the peripheral portion of the cytoplasm is often folded. (Papanicolaou stain, × 150.)

Figure 59b. *Scanning electron microscopy of a normal intermediate cell,* demonstrating the presence of numerous microvilli. The cytoplasmic projections are more numerous and prominent along the periphery and tend to flatten out in the region of the nucleus (N). × 2000. *From* A. Llanes, C. Farre, A. Ferenczy, and R. M. Richart. Scanning electron microscopy of normal exfoliated squamous cervical cells. *Acta Cytol.* **17:** 507–509 (1973).

Figure 59c. *Higher magnification of an intermediate cell* (Int). The microvilli appear as projecting, globular extensions with a broad base. The overlying superficial cell (Sup) contains an intricate network of microridges. × 20,000. *From* A. Llanes, C. Farre, A. Ferenczy, and R. M. Richart. Scanning electron microscopy of normal exfoliated squamous cervical cells. *Acta Cytol.* **17:** 507–509 (1973).

REFERENCES (The microscopic examination—Figure 59c)

1. Llanes, A., C. Farre, A. Ferenczy, and R. M. Richart. Scanning electron microscopy of normal exfoliated squamous cervical cells. *Acta Cytol.* **17:** 507 (1973).
2. Friedlander, S. A new method for detecting changes in the surfaces of human exfoliated cervical cells with the scanning electron microscope. *Acta Cytol.* **13:** 288 (1969).
3. Ferenczy, A. and R. M. Richart. Scanning electron microscopy of the cervical transformation zone. *Am. J. Obstet. Gynecol.* **115:** 151 (1973).
4. Williams, A. E., J. A. Jordan, J. M. Allen, and J. F. Murphy. The surface ultrastructure of normal and metaplastic epithelia and of carcinoma in situ. *Cancer Res.* **33:** 504 (1973).
5. Nasr, M. F., L. D. Lagasse, N. Chang, and J. G. Moore. Scanning electron microscopy of the human cervix: description of a new method to study the surface anatomy. *Acta Cytol.* **17:** 141 (1973).
6. Ashworth, C. T., F. Luibel, and E. Sanders. Epithelium of normal cervix uteri studied with electron microscopy and histochemistry. *Am. J. Obstet. Gynecol.* **79:** 1149 (1960).

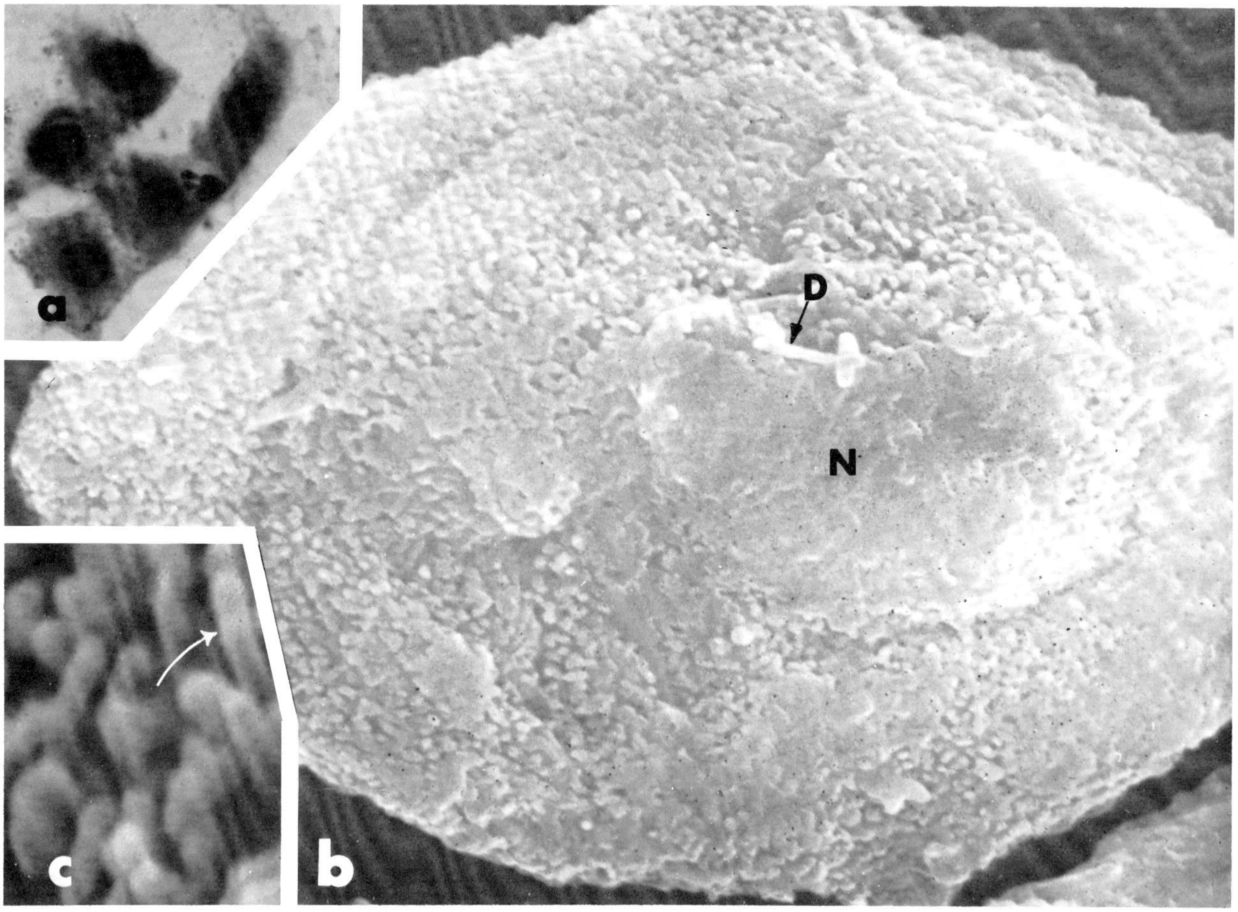

Figure 60a. *Light micrograph of normal parabasal cells* in which the nucleo–cytoplasmic ratio is reduced as compared to normal intermediate cells. (Papanicolaou stain, × 190.)

Figure 60b. *Scanning electron microscopy* of a normal, oval, parabasal cell covered by numerous stubby microvilli. The nucleus (N) is recognized as a protuberant bulge, and scattered Doderlein bacilli (D) are seen. × 2400. *From* A. Llanes, C. Farre, A. Ferenczy, and R. M. Richart. Scanning electron microscopy of normal exfoliated squamous cervical cells. *Acta Cytol.* **17:** 507–509 (1973).

Figure 60c. *Higher magnification,* illustrating the microvilli of a parabasal cell (arrow). × 22,400.

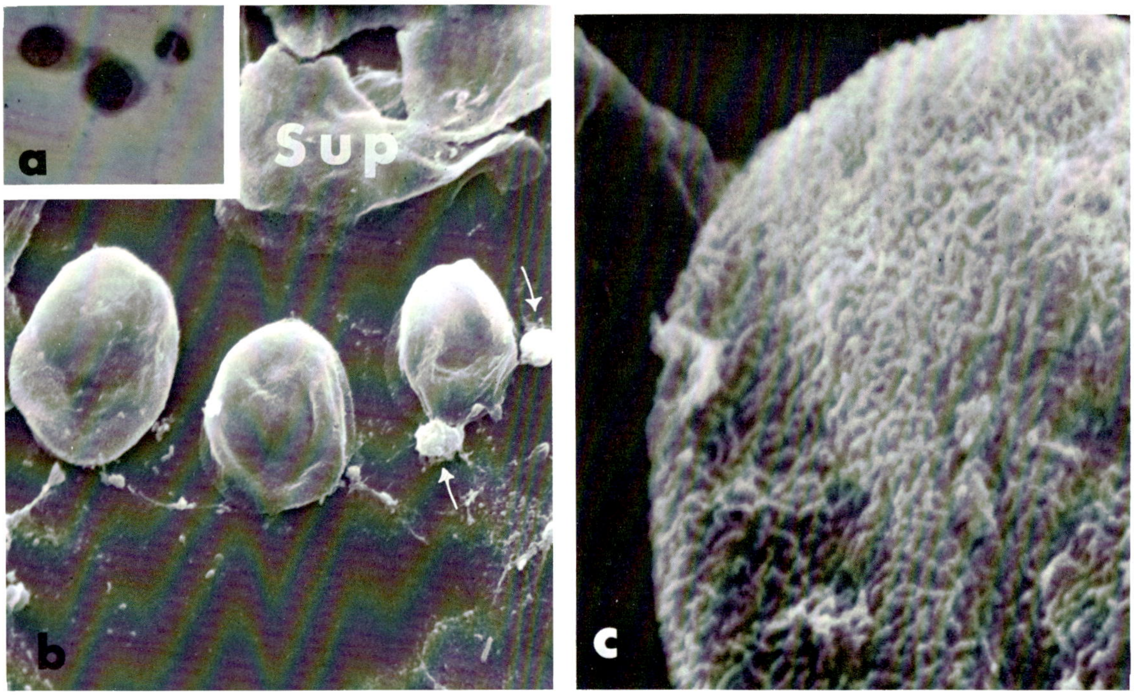

Figure 61a. *Light micrograph of a normal basal cell* recovered from a postmenopausal woman. The nucleo–cytoplasmic ratio is in favor of the nucleus. (Papanicolaou stain, × 190.)

Figure 61b. *Survey photomicrograph,* illustrating the comparative sizes and shapes of normal exfoliated cervical cells. Three basal cells are seen in the center of the photomicrograph, and in the upper right corner there is a superficial cell (Sup). Mucus, bacteria, and a few lymphocytes (arrows) are scattered around the basal cells. × 700. *From* A. Llanes, C. Farre, A. Ferenczy, and R. M. Richart. Scanning electron microscopy of normal exfoliated squamous cervical cells. *Acta Cytol.* **17:** 507–509 (1973).

Figure 61c. *Higher magnification* of the well-developed intricate pattern of the microvilli in a basal cell. The microvilli are more numerous and slender than those covering the parabasal or intermediate cells. The presence of abundant microvillous specialization in immature squamous cells, including the intermediate, parabasal, and basal cells, is thought to increase the overall cell surface, thereby enhancing various surface metabolic functions such as secretion, absorption, and transport of water and electrolytes. × 7000. *From* A. Llanes, C. Farre, A. Ferenczy, and R. M. Richart. Scanning electron microscopy of normal exfoliated squamous cervical cells. *Acta Cytol.* **17:** 507–509 (1973).

24

Cervical Intraepithelial Neoplasia

The precursors to invasive squamous cell carcinoma of the cervix are among the most extensively studied neoplasms occurring in women. They form a continuum of decreasing differentiation that begins with mild dysplasia and ends with carcinoma in situ. It has been suggested that the continuous nature of the process be acknowledged by the use of a generic term, cervical intraepithelial neoplasia, since a compound name (dysplasia-carcinoma in situ) implies a two-disease system.[1] It has been amply demonstrated that detection and treatment of the precursor states prevent the development of invasive carcinoma both in the individual[2] and in the aggregate.[3]

Fine structurally,[4-6] the lesional continuum comprising cervical intraepithelial neoplasia shows qualitative changes that are constant across the disease spectrum but vary quantitatively, depending on the state of epithelial differentiation. The nucleus becomes larger both in absolute terms and in relation to the cytoplasm, and the nuclear membrane becomes complex. The nuclear chromatin has an altered distribution. These changes are correlated with the abnormal nuclear DNA content, which is a constant feature of cervical neoplasia.[7] Changes in cytoplasmic constituents are also prominent and include a relative increase in mitochondria, free ribosomes, and endoplasmic reticulum and a decrease in specialized cell products such as glycogen. There is a decrease in cell contact inhibition and in cellular adhesion,[8,9] which is reflected in fewer and poorly formed desmosomes and tonofilaments.

The surface ultrastructure of the cervix cancer precursors also differs strikingly from the normal architecture,[10,11] the most characteristic feature being the absence of the surface microridges of the normal superficial cell and the presence of abundant microvilli. The microridges have been shown[12] to interdigitate in apposed superficial cell surfaces and presumably help to maintain epithelial integrity. Their absence may account in part for the lack of adhesion between the cells of carcinoma in situ.

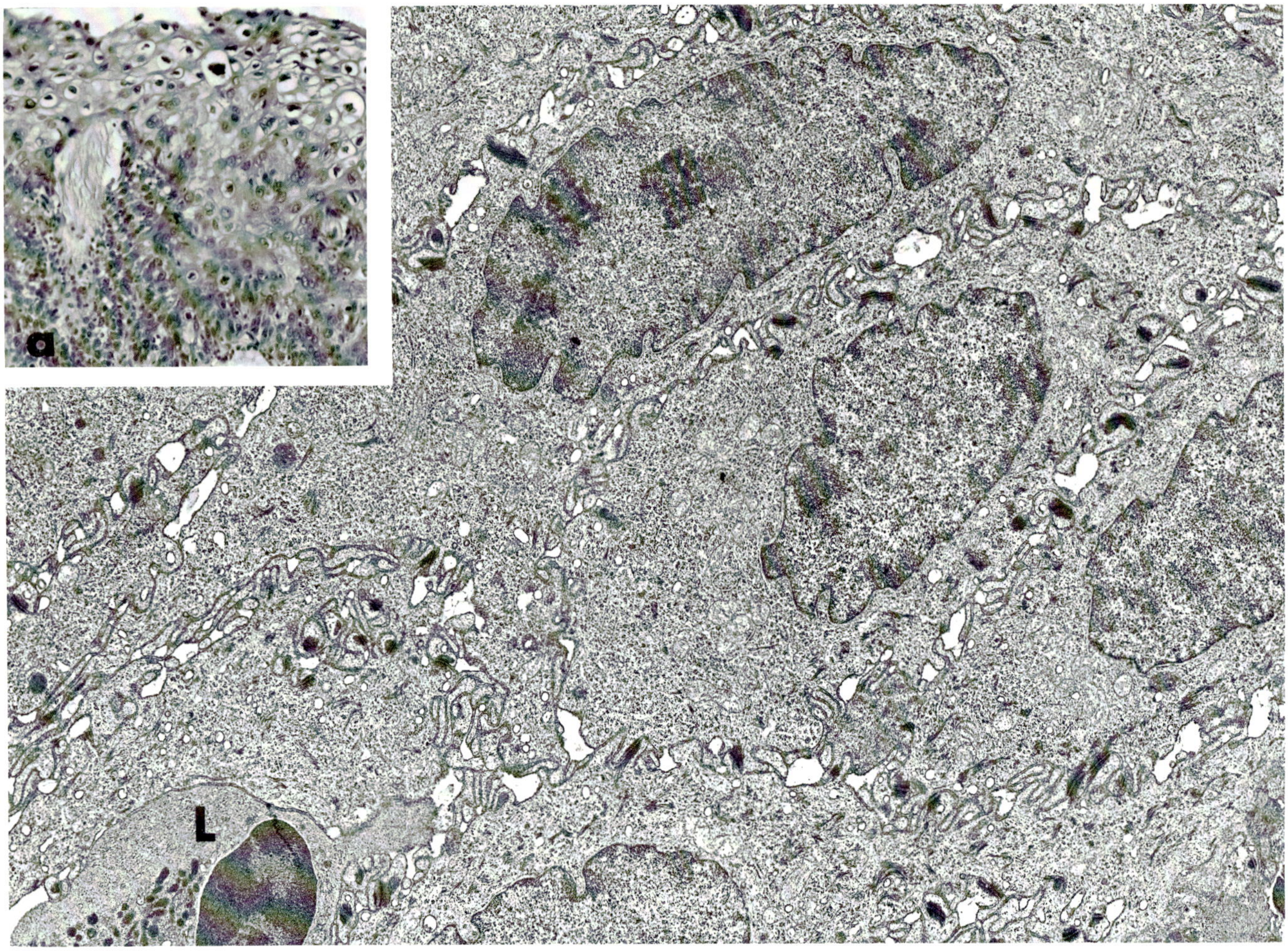

Figure 62a. *Mild dysplasia. Histologically,* the full thickness of the epithelium is replaced by neoplastic cells, with neoplastic basal cells occupying the lowest third of the section. There are several mitotic figures in the lowest third of the epithelium. Loss of cellular orientation and cohesion and disturbed maturation also occur, as shown by the presence of several large squamous cells with irregular prominent nuclei in the upper layer. Characteristically, glycogen-rich cells are few in number and are located mainly in the upper layers of the epithelium. H & E stain, × 30.)

Figure 62. *Mild dysplasia.* The neoplastic cells from the middle third of the epithelium contain enlarged nuclei with irregular contours and several prominent nucleoli. The cytoplasm has numerous mitochondria, free ribosomes, and granular endoplasmic reticulum. The lateral plasma membranes are markedly convoluted, and the intercellular space contains several interdigitating microvilli, some of which are interconnected by tonofilament–desmosome complexes. These are reduced, however, as compared to the normal cervical squamous epithelium. In the left lower corner is an intercellular leukocyte (L) with a well-developed pseudopod. × 6000. *From* H. M. Shingleton. The University of Alabama in Birmingham, Medical Center, 1919 Seventh Avenue South, Birmingham, Ala. 35233.

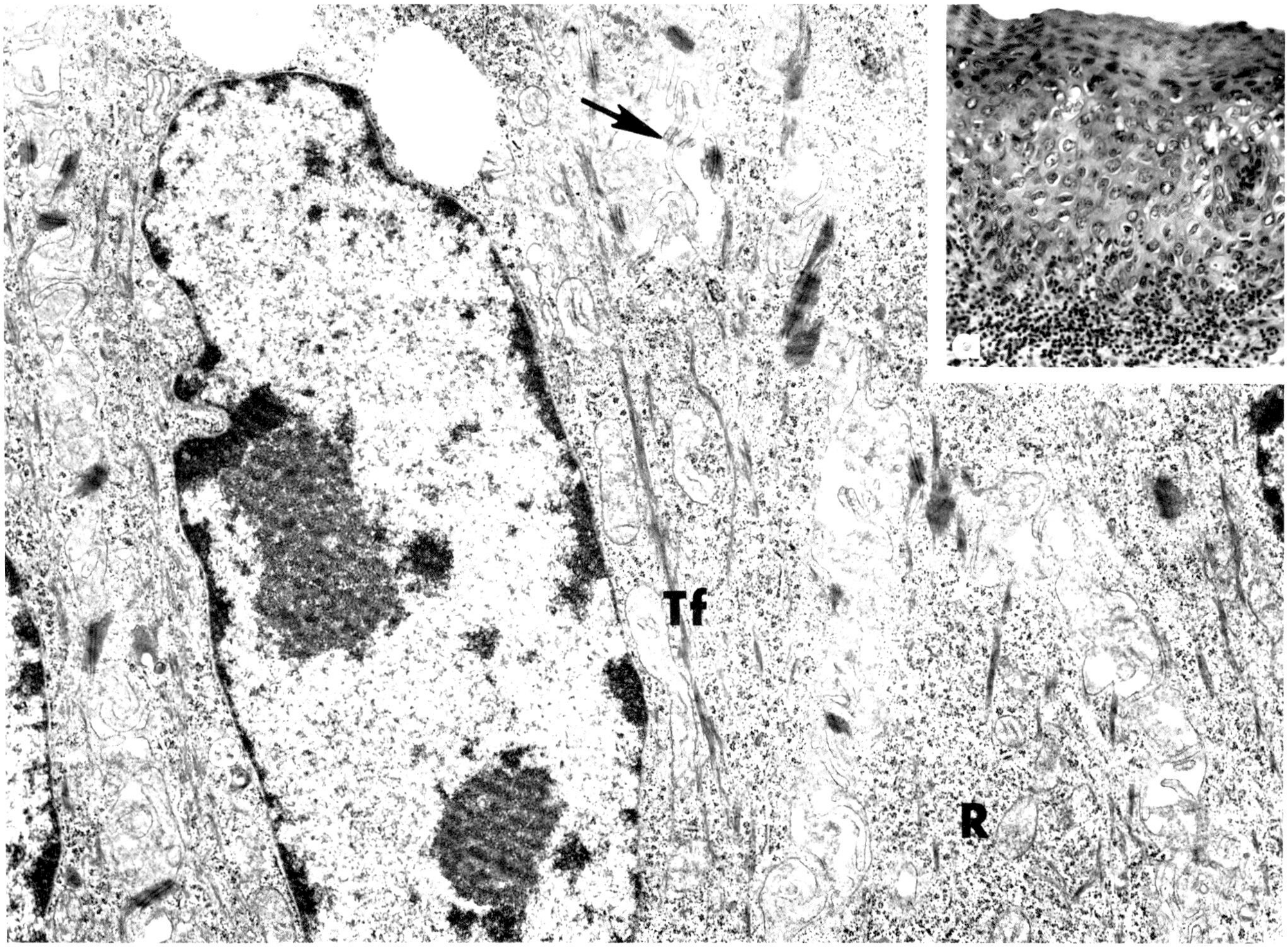

Figure 63a. *Moderate dysplasia* is similar to mild dysplasia, but the neoplastic basal cells may replace more than one half of the epithelium. Characteristically, there is an absence of cellular maturation and intracytoplasmic glycogen. The underlying connective tissue contains aggregates of chronic inflammatory cells. (H & E stain, × 38.)

Figure 63. *Moderate dysplasia.* Ultrastructurally, the cells have abundant intracytoplasmic free ribosomes (R), poorly developed tonofilaments (Tf), and mitochondria. There is a further decrease in the number of desmosomal attachments between neoplastic cells, and most of the microvilli (arrow) project freely into the intercellular spaces. There is a considerable nuclear enlargement with peripheral concentration of the heterochromatin, and the nucleoli are prominent. × 9500. *From* H. M. Shingleton. The University of Alabama in Birmingham, Medical Center, 1919 Seventh Avenue South, Birmingham, Ala. 35233.

REFERENCES (The precursors—Figure 63)

1. Richart, R. M. Natural history of cervical intraepithelial neoplasia. *Clin. Obstet. Gynecol.* **5:** 748 (1968).
2. Stern, E. Rate, stage, and patient age in cervical cancer. An analysis of age specific discovery rates for atypical hyperplasia, in situ cancer, and invasive cancer in a well population. *Cancer* **12:** 933 (1959).
3. Boyes, D. A. The British Columbia screening program. *Obstet. Gynecol. Surv.* **24:** 1005 (1969).
4. Shingleton, H. M., R. M. Richart, J. Wiener, and D. Spiro. Human cervical intraepithelial neoplasia: fine structure of dysplasia and carcinoma in situ. *Cancer Res.* **28:** 695 (1968).
5. Younes, M. S. Electron microscope observations on carcinoma in situ of the cervix. *Obstet. Gynecol. Surv.* **24:** 768 (1969).
6. Bonilla-Musoles, F. Electron-microscopical examinations of the cervix uteri. *Gynaekol. Rundsch.* **8:** 197 (1969).
7. Wilbanks, G. D., R. M. Richart, and J. Y. Terner. DNA content of cervical intraepithelial neoplasia studied by two-wavelength feulgen cytophotometry. *Am. J. Obstet. Gynecol.* **98:** 792 (1967).
8. Wilbanks, G. D. and R. M. Richart. The in vitro interaction of intraepithelial neoplasia, normal epithelium, and fibroblasts from the adult human uterine cervix. *Cancer Res.* **26:** 1641 (1966).
9. Richart, R. M. and V. Lerch. Time-lapse cinematographic observations of normal human cervical epithelium, dysplasia and carcinoma in situ. *J. Natl. Cancer Inst.* **37:** 317 (1966).
10. Williams, A. E., J. A. Jordan, J. M. Allen, and J. F. Murphy. The surface ultrastructure of normal and metaplastic cervical epithelia and of carcinoma in situ. *Cancer Res.* **33:** 504 (1973).
11. Jordan, J. A. and A. E. Williams. Scanning electron microscopy in the study of cervical neoplasia. *J. Obstet. Gynaecol. Brit. Commonw.* **78:** 940 (1971).
12. Hackeman, M., C. Grubb, and K. R. Hill. The ultrastructure of normal squamous epithelium of the human cervix uteri. *J. Ultrastruct. Res.* **22:** 443 (1968).

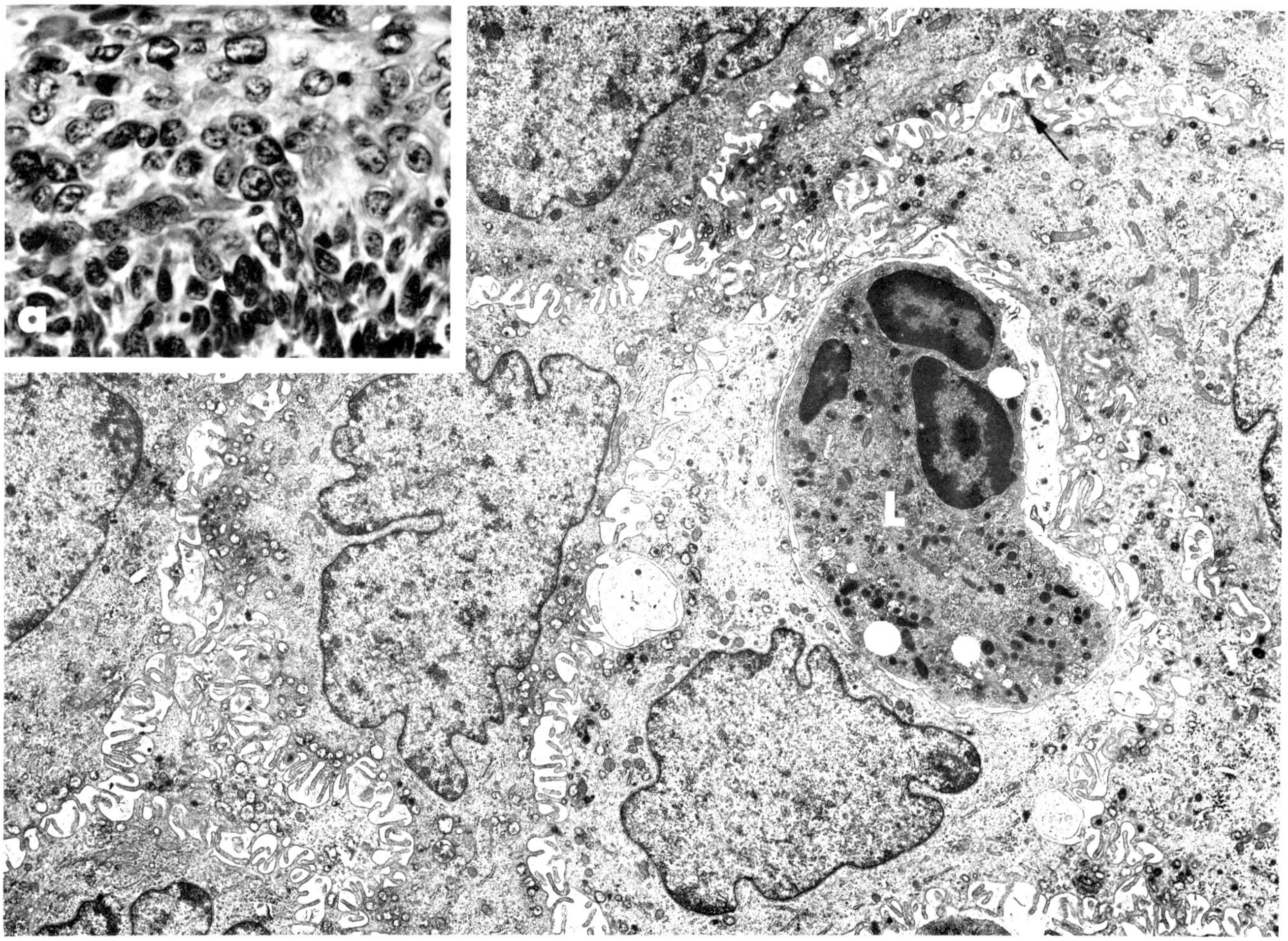

Figure 64a. *In severe dysplasia, neoplastic basal cells* occupy approximately three-fourths of the full thickness of the epithelium. The nucleo–cytoplasmic ratio is in favor of the nucleus, which is enlarged and contains prominent chromatin aggregates. Note the absence of glycogen-rich cells. The cytoplasmic membranes and intercellular attachments are ill defined. (H & E stain, × 96.)

Figure 64. *Severe dysplasia.* Section through the mid-portion of the neoplastic epithelium. The nuclei are enlarged with deeply convoluted membranes. The cytoplasm contains peripherally concentrated mitochondria, granular endoplasmic reticulum, and free ribosomes. Characteristically, tonofilaments are inconspicuous or absent. Note the markedly interdigitating appearance of the intercellular microvilli, which contain rare, poorly developed, desmosomal attachments (arrow). The intercellular space is occasionally distended by migrating intraepithelial leukocytes (L). × 6000. *From* H. M. Shingleton. The University of Alabama in Birmingham, Medical Center, 1919 Seventh Avenue South, Birmingham, Ala. 35233.

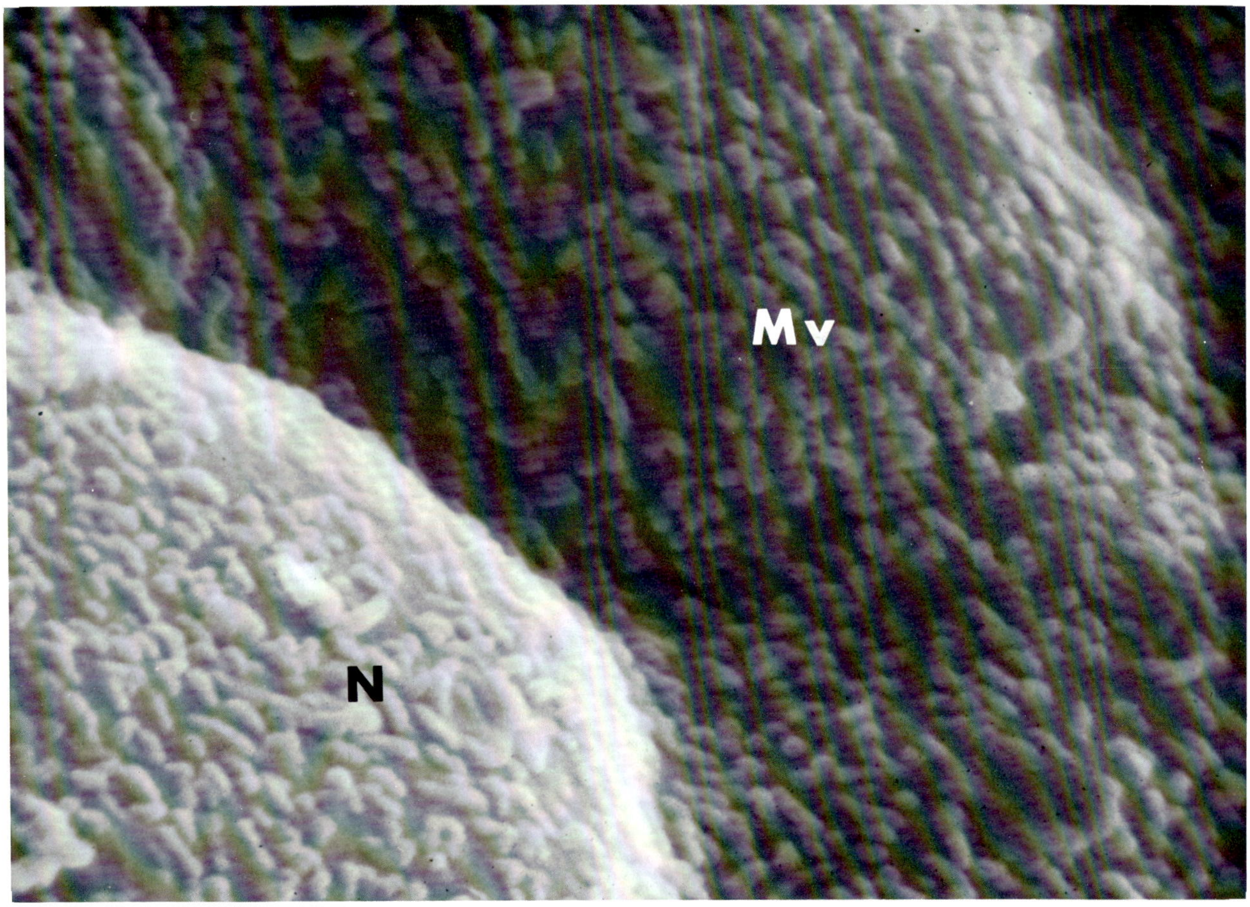

Figure 65. *Severe dysplasia*. Scanning electron microscopic appearance of the most superficial cells in severe dysplasia, which contain numerous stubby microvilli (MV). The topographic appearance of the neoplastic cells provides indirect evidence for loss of maturation, since in mature, superficial squamous cells of normal cervical mucous membrane microridges, rather than microvilli, are found. × 11,200. N: nucleus.

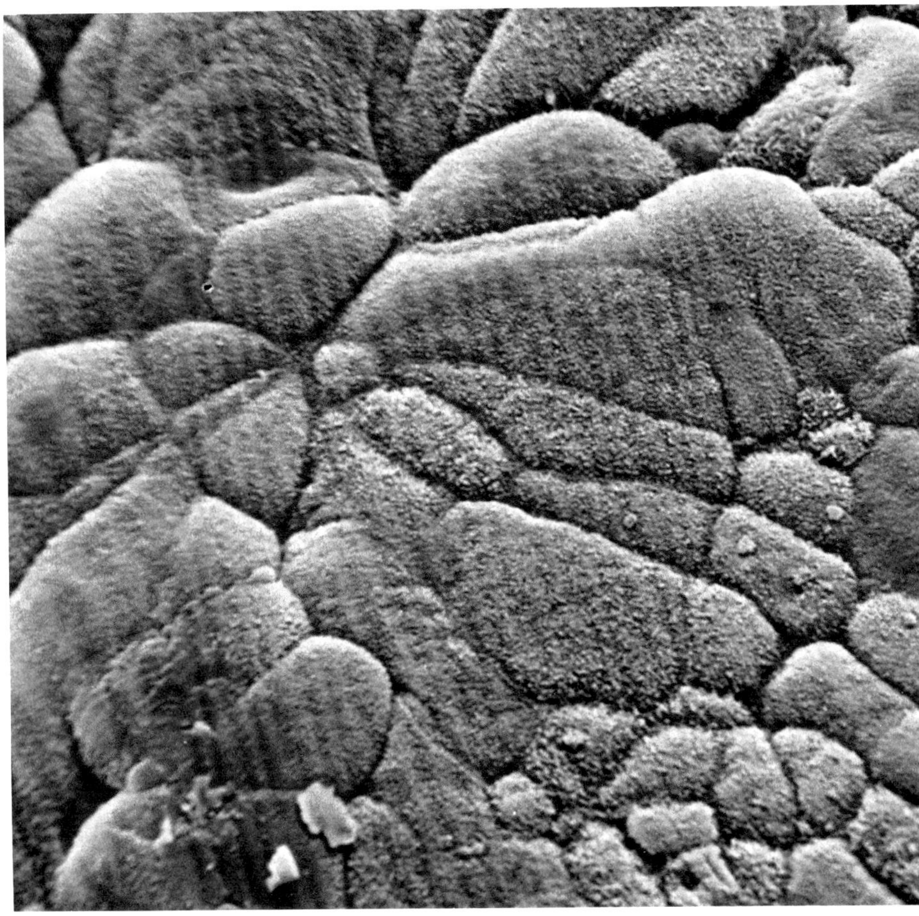

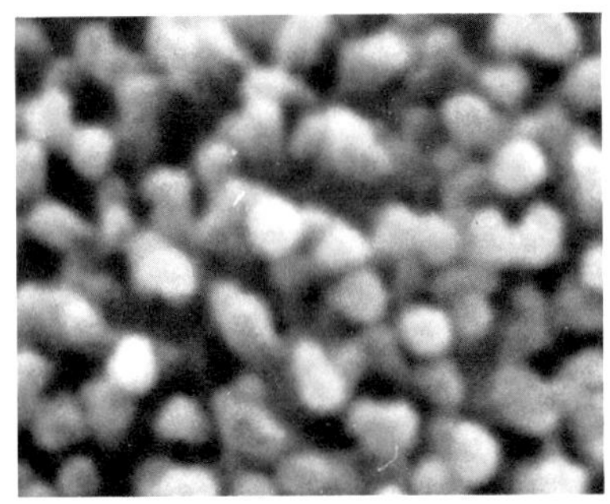

Figure 66. *Scanning electron microscopy of carcinoma in situ.* In contrast to mature squamous epithelium, the most superficial cells in carcinoma in situ are small with an irregular contour and a bulging microvillous cytoplasmic surface membrane. Although the general surface pattern resembles the young squamous epithelium of the transformation zone, the neoplastic cervical cells may be distinguished from the cells that are simply immature, by virtue of their cellular disorganization and lack of well formed intercellular attachments. × 2200. *From* A. E. Williams, J. A. Jordan, J. M. Allen, and J. F. Murphy. The surface ultrastructure of normal and metaplastic cervical epithelia and of carcinoma in situ, *Cancer Res.* **33:** 504–513 (1973).

Figure 66a. *Higher magnification* of tightly packed, blunt ended microvilli. × 26,500. *From* A. E. Williams, J. A. Jordan, J. M. Allen, and J. F. Murphy. The surface ultrastrutcure of normal and metaplastic cervical epithelia and of carcinoma in situ. *Cancer Res.* **33:** 504–513 (1973).

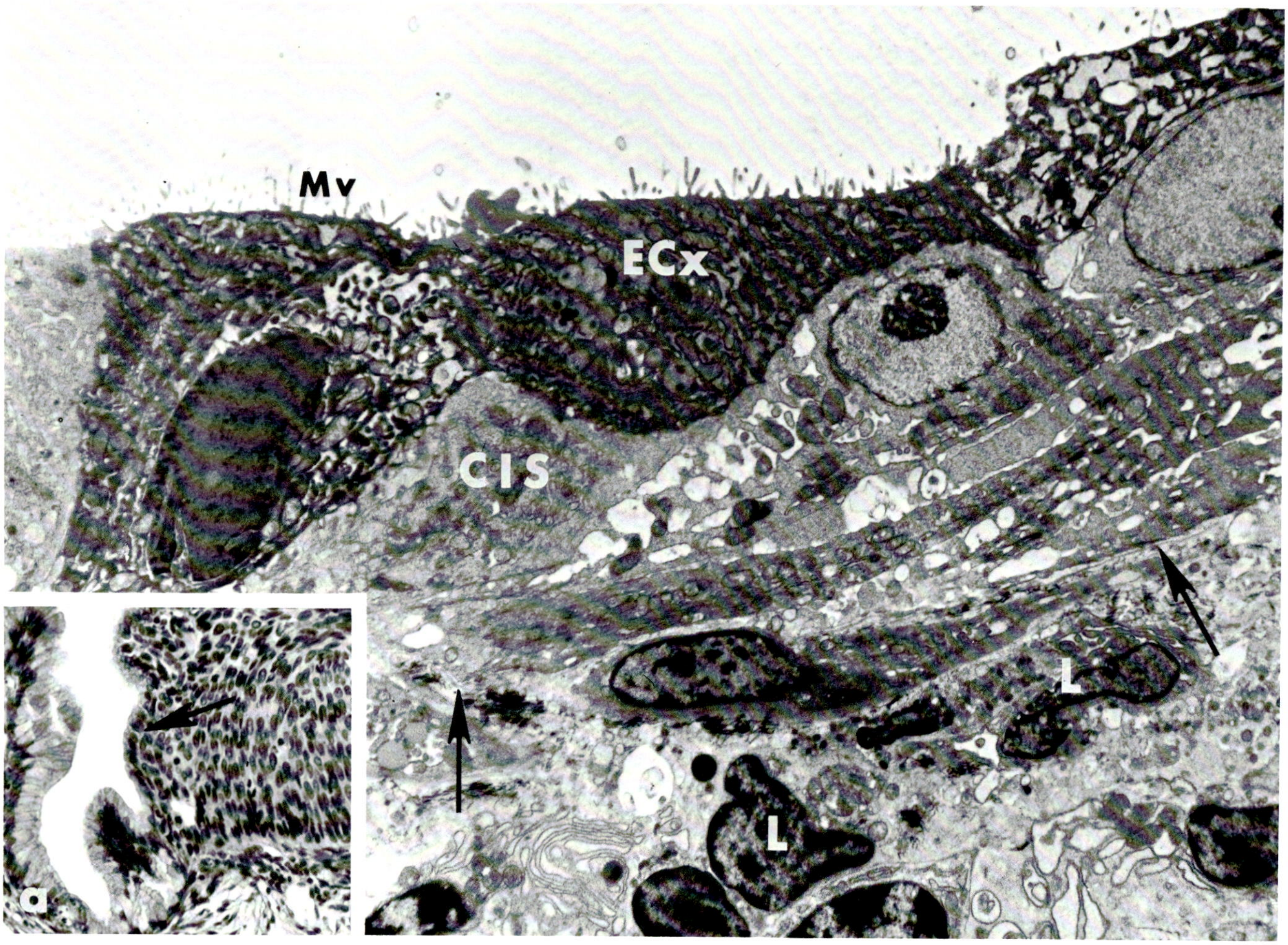

Figure 67a. *Histologic appearance of carcinoma in situ with gland involvement.* Masses of undifferentiated neoplastic cells involving the entire thickness of the epithelium extend along the basal membrane of an endocervical gland by lifting up the endocervical epithelium (arrow). (H & E stain, × 48.)

Figure 67. *At the transmission electron microscopic level* tongues of neoplastic cells (CIS) are seen between the basal lamina (arrows) and the overlying endocervical epithelium (ECx). Because the endocervical epithelium is separated by the neoplastic cells from its supporting tissue, it degenerates, as indicated by the electron-dense cytoplasmic matrix and swelling of the endoplasmic reticulum. × 4200. Mv: microvilli; L: stromal leukocytes. *From* H. M. Shingleton. The University of Alabama in Birmingham, Medical Center, 1919 Seventh Avenue South, Birmingham, Ala. 35233.

25

Invasive Epidermoid Carcinoma

Invasive epidermoid carcinoma of the cervix represents one of the most common malignancies of the female genital tract and is responsible for about 10,000 cancer deaths each year among American women. It occurs in multiparous women in the late reproductive period and is generally preceded by preinvasive cervical neoplasia.

Epidemiologically,[1] cervix cancer is closely related to a number of environmental covariables which have as their common basis sexual intercourse, and evidence is accumulating to suggest that carcinoma of the cervix is a venereal disease with a long latency period. Serological studies have shown that a higher proportion of cervix cancer patients have antibodies to herpesvirus type II than occurs in matched controls,[2] and herpesvirus has been isolated from cervical cancer cells grown in tissue culture.[3] Although these associations do not establish the virus as an oncogen, it is a prime suspect.

Ultrastructurally, the neoplastic cells of invasive epidermoid carcinoma of the cervix[4,5] show organellar alterations, such as an increase in polyribosomes, dilatation, and fragmentation of the granular endoplasmic reticulum and aggregation of the tonofilaments. In the lesser differentiated lesions desmosomal plates are few and are incompletely[6] or poorly developed. Loss of desmosomal attachments and gap junction nexuses,[6] together with separation of tonofilament–desmosome complexes, presumably leads to loss of cellular cohesion. Essentially similar submicroscopic features are observed in invasive epidermoid carcinoma[7-10] of the squamous mucous membranes and epidermis of extragenital sites.

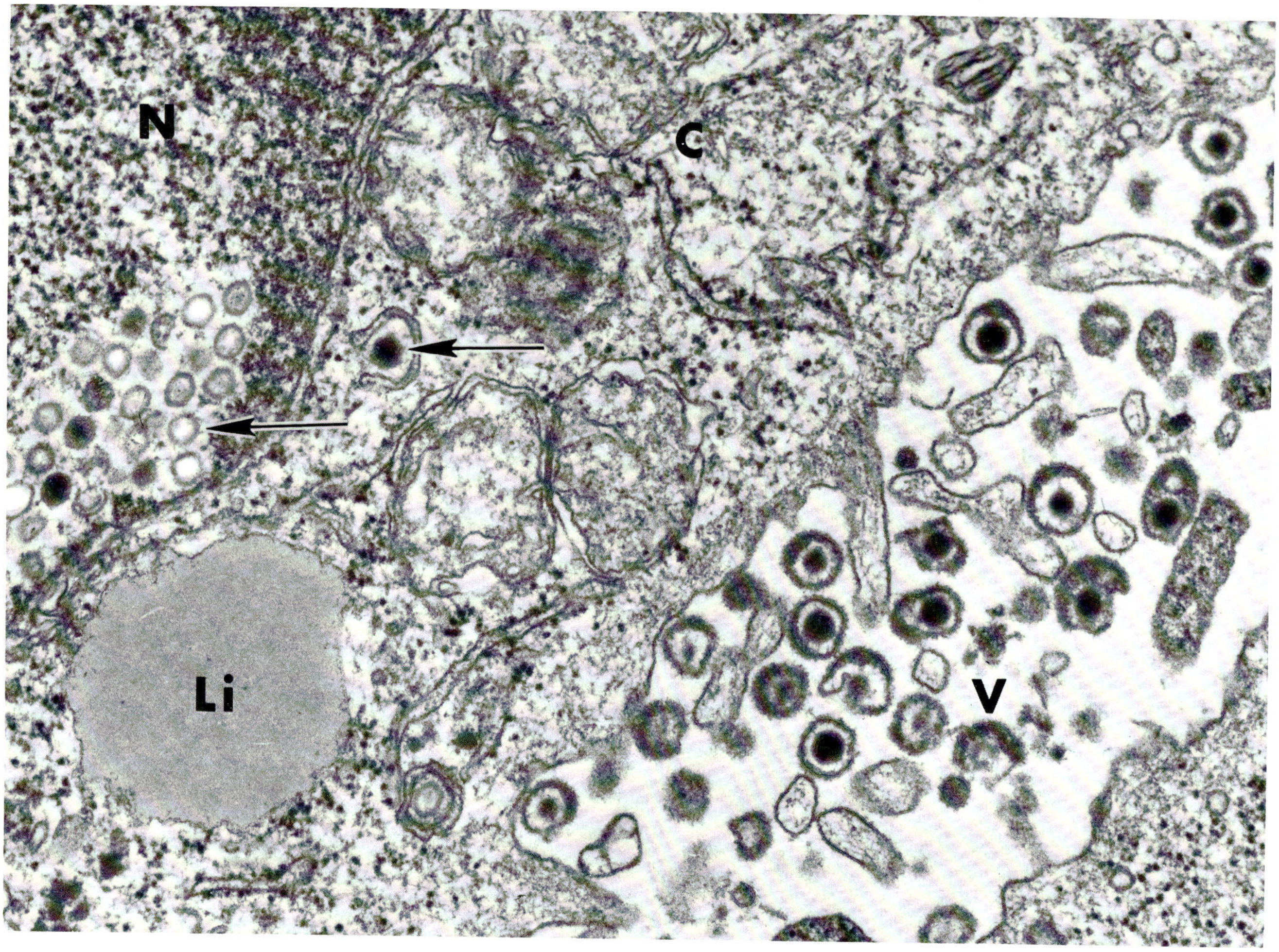

Figure 68. *Electron micrograph of HEp-2 cell infected with herpes simplex virus type II, isolated from a tissue culture line of cervical tumor cells.* Unenveloped nucleocapsids (arrows) are clustered at the periphery of the nucleus (N) and are also found in the cytoplasm (C). Mature enveloped virions (V) can be seen in the intercellular space. × 58,000. Li: large cytoplasmic lipid droplets. *From* L. Aurelian, and J. D. Strandberg. Division of Laboratory Animal Medicine, The Johns Hopkins University School of Medicine, Baltimore, Md.

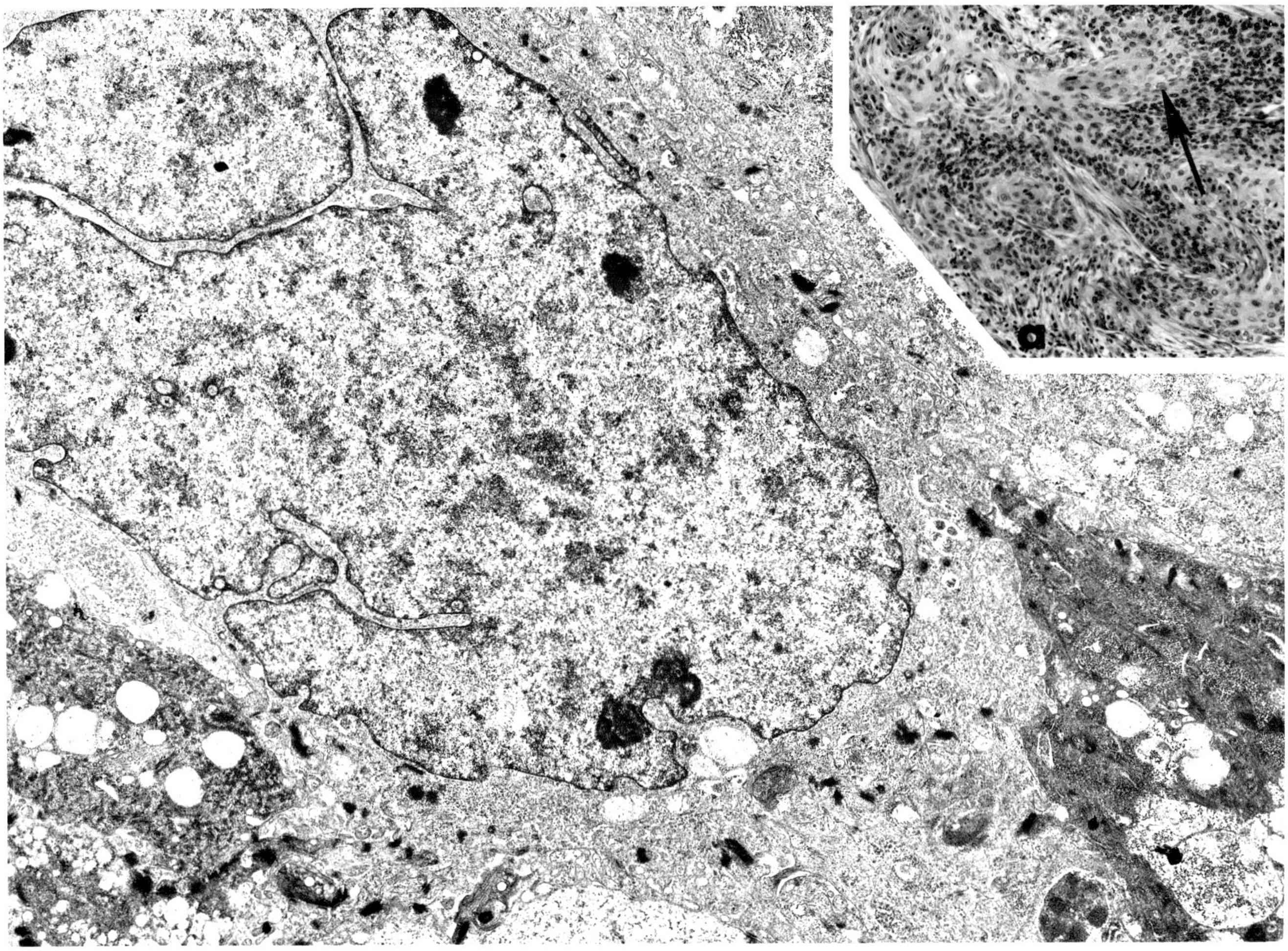

Figure 69a. *Histologic appearance of a moderately well-differentiated invasive epidermoid carcinoma of the cervix.* Large tongues of neoplastic squamous cells (arrow) invade the chronically inflamed cervical stroma. (H & E stain, × 30.)

Figure 69. *Transmission electron microscopic appearance* of cells from invasive epidermoid carcinoma containing markedly enlarged nuclei with deep nuclear infoldings. Several small nucleoli are seen within the nuclear substance. The cytoplasm is reduced and contains abundant free ribosomes and occasional desmosomal attachments with the adjacent neoplastic cells. In the right lower corner a portion of a degenerated neoplastic cell is seen. × 6000.

REFERENCES (Invasive epidermoid carcinoma—Figure 69)

1. Barron, B. and R. M. Richart. An epidemiologic study of cervical neoplastic disease, based on a self-selected sample of 7,000 women in Barbados, West Indies. *Cancer* **27:** 978 (1971).
2. Rawls, W. E., H. L. Gardner, and R. L. Kaufman. Antibodies to genital herpesvirus in patients with carcinoma of the cervix. *Am. J. Obstet. Gynecol.* **107:** 710 (1970).
3. Aurelian, L., J. D. Strandberg, L. V. Melendez, and L. A. Johnson. Herpesvirus type 2 isolated from cervical tumor cells grown in tissue culture. *Science* **174:** 704 (1971).
4. Ashworth, C. T., V. Stembridge, and F. Luibel. Symposium on probable or possible malignant cervical lesions—carcinoma in situ. I. Histology of carcinoma in situ and invasive carcinoma of uterine cervix utilizing electron microscopy and histochemical methods. *Acta Cytol.* **5:** 369 (1961).
5. Bhowmick, D. K. and A. Mitra. Ultrastructural morphology of squamous carcinoma of human exocervix. *Indian J. Med. Res.* **56:** 282 (1968).
6. McNutt, N. S. and R. S. Weinstein. Carcinoma of the cervix: deficiency of nexus intercellular junctions. *Science* **165:** 597 (1969).
7. Barocci, C. and B. Birabell. Aspetti ultrastrutturali del carcinoma di epithelio pavimentoso della laringe. *Otorinolaringol. Ital.* **32:** 121 (1963).
8. Sugar, J. An electron study of early microscopic invasive growth in human skin tumors and laryngeal carcinoma. *Eur. J. Cancer* **4:** 33 (1968).
9. Hirone, T. and Y. Eryu. Fine structure of squamous cell carcinoma. *Skin Res. (Osaka)* **12:** 352 (1970).
10. Klehr, H. U. and G. Klingmuller. Different forms of the endoplasmic reticulum in neoplastic keratinocytes. Investigations on the squamous cell carcinoma. *Arch. Dermatol. Forsch.* **242:** 111 (1972).

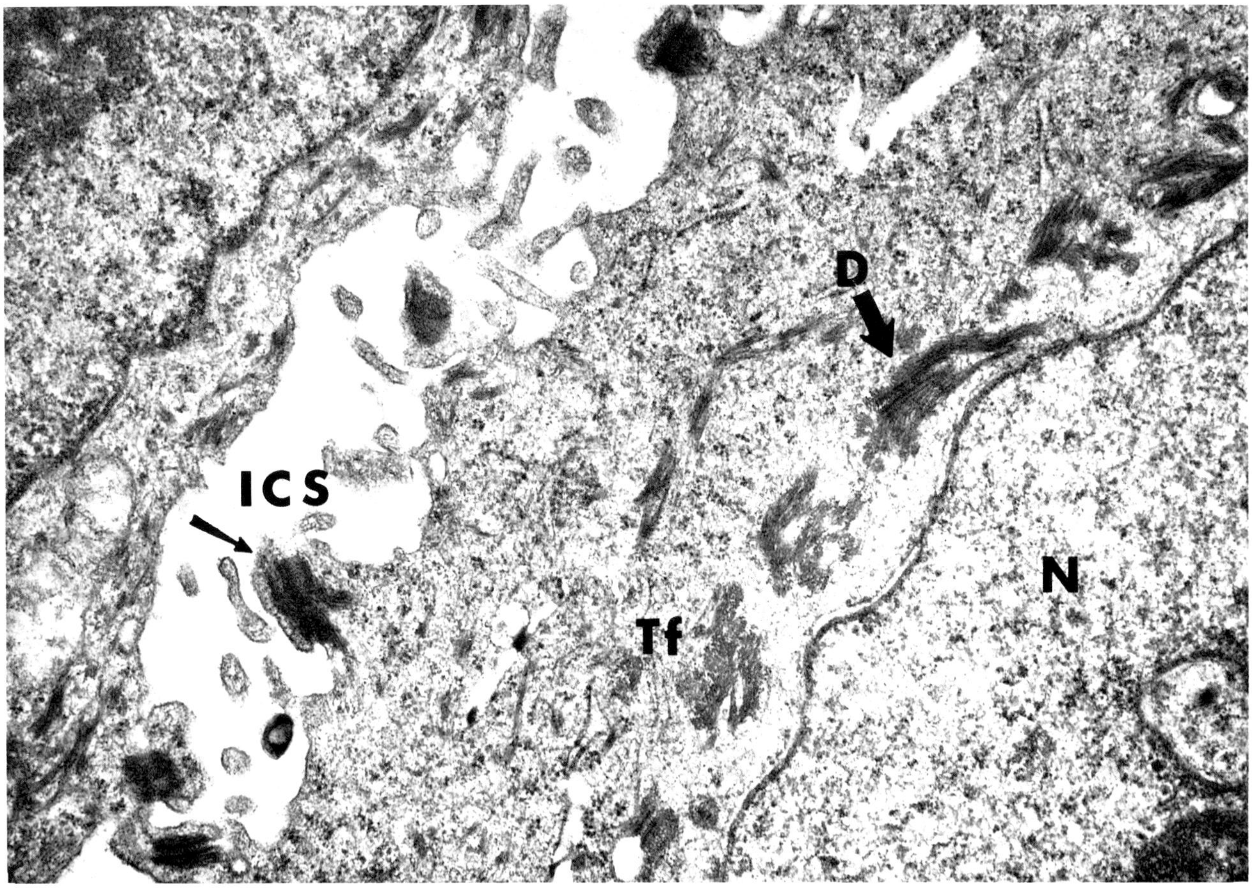

Figure 70. *High-power view of invasive epidermoid carcinoma cells.* There are several short bundles of tonofilaments (Tf) and retracted desmosome–tonofilament complexes (D) in a perinuclear location. The plasma membrane contains several microvilli projecting into dilated intercellular spaces (ICS), and retracted tonofilament–desmosome complexes are occasionally seen (arrow). × 34,010.

REFERENCES (Figures 70–71)

1. McNutt, N. S. and R. S. Weinstein. Carcinoma of the cervix: deficiency of nexus intercellular junctions. *Science* **165:** 597 (1969).
2. Revel, J. P., A. G. Yee, and A. J. Hudspeth. Gap junctions between electronically coupled cells in tissue culture and in brown fat. *Proc. Natl. Acad. Sci. U.S.* **68:** 2924 (1971).
3. Steere, R. L. and J. R. Sommer. Stereo ultrastructure of nexus faces exposed by freeze-fracturing. *J. Microsc.* **15:** 205 (1972).
4. Jamakosmanovic, A. and W. R. Loewenstein. Intercellular communication and tissue growth. 3. Thyroid cancer. *J. Cell Biol.* **38:** 556 (1968).

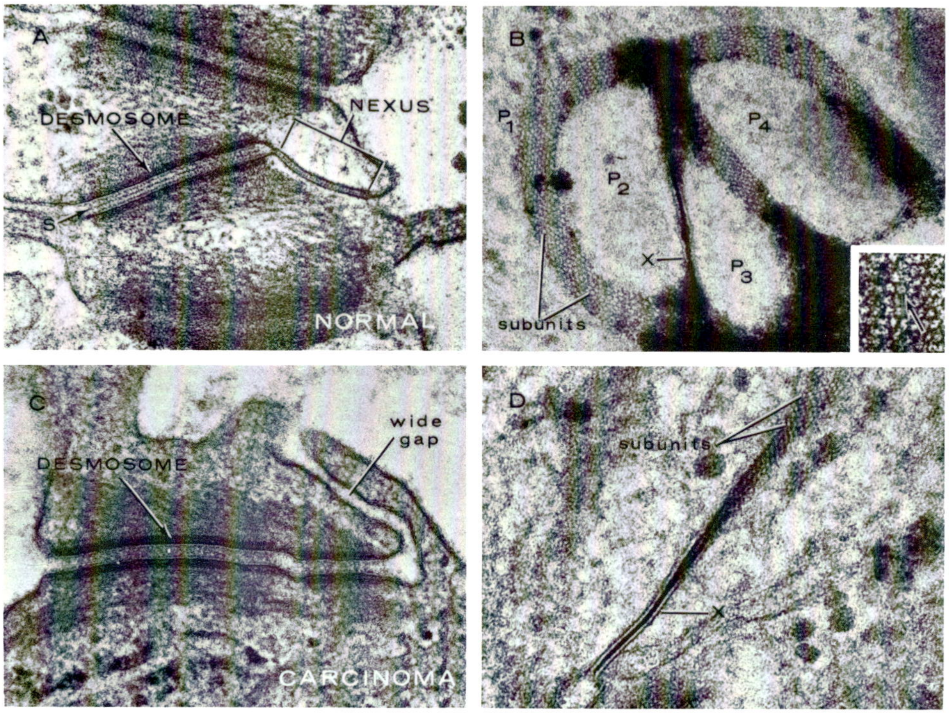

Figure 71. *Electron micrographs of regions of contact between adjacent cervical epithelial cells. From* N. S. McNutt and R. S. Weinstein. Carcinoma of the cervix: deficiency of nexus intercellular junctions. *Science* **165:** 597–599, Fig. 1 (1969).

(A) Normal cervical epithelium. Intermediate layer cells are connected to each other by attachment of their surface processes with desmosomes and nexuses. At a nexus, the cell membranes are very closely apposed and the intercellular space is reduced to 20 Å. At a desmosome, the membranes are attached by dense proteinaceous material, often showing a distinct central stratum (S). × 51,000.

(B) Normal cervical epithelium. Four thin-cell processes (P_{1-4}) are attached at the nexuses. Opaque lanthanum hydroxide fills the thin channels of the extracellular space around the subunits, extending between the nexus membranes. Nexuses viewed *en face* show that the lanthanum-outlined subunits are in a closely packed array with 100-Å center-to-center spacing. In cross section, the subunit pattern is obscured because of section thickness, and only a dark, central 70-Å line is seen (X). × 71,000. *Inset:* High magnification of a subunit array *en face* shows individual subunits (arrow) outlined by the lanthanum. Stereomicroscopic observations of replicas of freeze-etched[2] and freeze-fractured nexuses have demonstrated the subunits to be composed of hollow hexagonal tubules arranged in a honeycomb pattern[3] and forming an open channel system between adjacent cells, through which electrolytes[1] and molecules of 60,000 daltons can traverse.[3] It has also been suggested that intercellular nexuses may play a role in cell contact inhibition and in the formation of low-resistance electrical coupling sites between normal cells.[2,4] A deficiency of nexuses in invasive cervical carcinoma[1] may therefore be responsible for the loss of contact inhibition and the lack of electrical coupling[1] in neoplastic cells, and perhaps for the invasive character of malignant neoplasms.[1] × 168,000.

(C) Invasive squamous carcinoma of the cervix. Processes of adjacent cells may be attached at desmosomes but nexuses are infrequent, since the plasma membranes rarely approach each other at a distance less than 100 Å. Some tumor desmosomes lack a central dense stratum. This possibly represents a stage in desmosome formation, since many tumor desmosomes have a normal laminar substructure. × 54,000.

(D) Invasive squamous carcinoma of the cervix. A rare nexus connects two tumor cells and has trapped the lanthanum, revealing the characteristic cross section (X), as well as a closely packed subunit array with a center-to-center spacing of 100 to 110 Å. × 87,000.

26
Adenocarcinoma

Adenocarcinoma of the cervix originates in the epithelium of the endocervix and comprises 3 to 5% of all cervical malignancies. In contrast to squamous cell carcinoma of the cervix, adenocarcinoma is not believed to be associated with venereal etiologic factors. Histologically, adenocarcinomas vary from extremely well-differentiated in-situ carcinomas, in which most of the general characteristics of endocervical epithelium are retained, to poorly differentiated adenocarcinoma without an obvious glandular pattern. Ultrastructural observations[1,2] confirm the light microscopic and histochemical findings of a gradual decrease and an eventual loss of mucogenesis in increasingly dedifferentiated neoplasms of the endocervix. In addition to common adenocarcinoma and adenocarcinoma with squamous metaplasia (adenoacanthoma), other endocervical neoplasms have been examined by electron microscopy, including clear cell adenocarcinoma,[1] mesonephric carcinoma of Gartner's duct (Wolffian duct) origin,[2,3] and adenoid cystic carcinoma (cylindroma).[4]

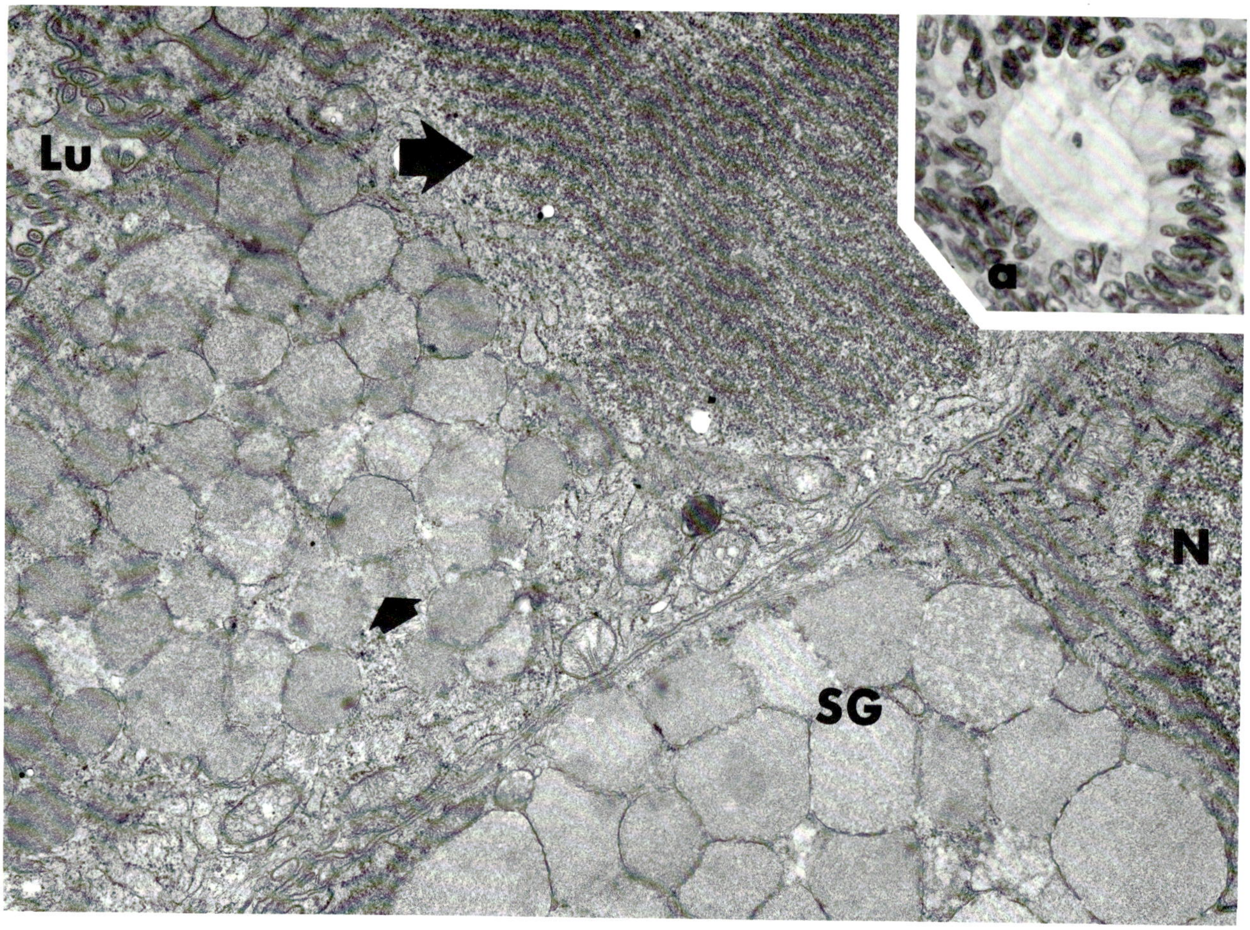

Figure 72a. *Invasive adenocarcinoma of the cervix.* This is a moderately well-differentiated, mucus-secreting adenocarcinoma in which the glandular lining epithelium contains several mucus-filled, signet-ring cells. The glandular lumen is also rich in mucous secretions. (H & E stain, × 150.)

Figure 72. *Ultrastructurally,* the neoplastic signet-ring cells contain large collections of supranuclear (N), membrane-bound secretory granules (SG) with finely granular content, in all respects identical with that of gastrointestinal or ovarian origin (see **Mucinous Cystadenocarcinomas** of ovary). Many of the secretory granules are fused together by intercoalescence (short arrow). Membranes of granular endoplasmic reticulum, as well as mitochondria, are displaced at the periphery of the cytoplasm. The cell in the upper portion of the micrograph is presumably in mitosis (long arrow). Several small microvilli project into the glandular lumen (Lu). × 15,000.

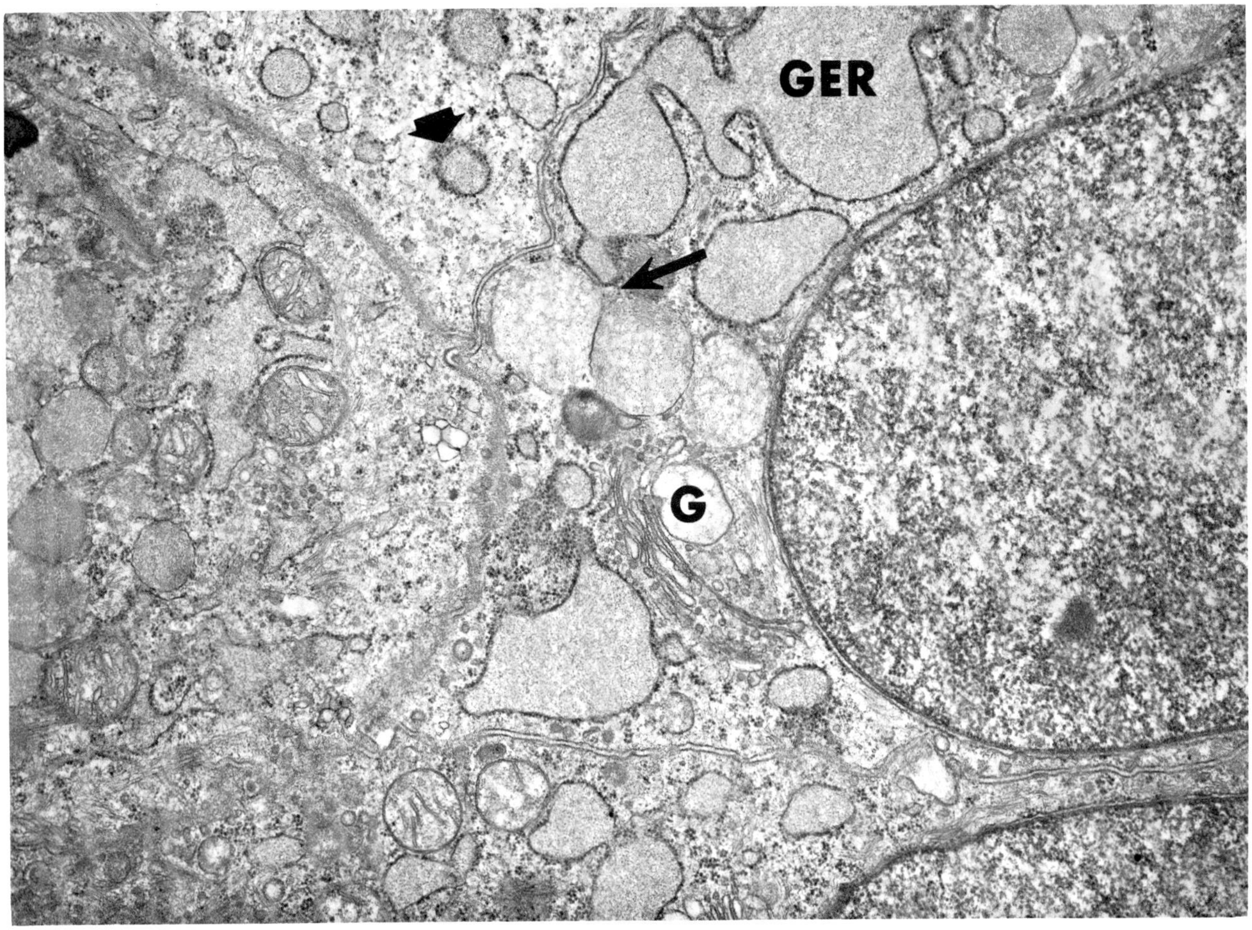

Figure 73. *Detail of mucogenesis in neoplastic glandular cells.* As in normal endocervical cells, the formation of mucus-containing secretory granules (long arrow) is initiated in the perinuclear ribosome–granular endoplasmic reticulum (GER)–Golgi (G) complex. Unlike the normal endocervical epithelium, however, the neoplastic cells have markedly distended endoplasmic reticulum filled with fine, granular material, indicating metabolic alterations in mucoprotein synthesis. In addition to several coated vesicles (short arrow), there are abundant mitochondria providing the necessary energy for mucogenesis. × 17,000.

REFERENCES (Adenocarcinoma–Figure 73)

1. Woyke, S., W. Damagala, and W. Olszewski. Mesonephroma of the uterine cervix. Submicroscopical study and comparison with fine structure of endocervical adenocarcinoma. *Virchows. Arch. Abt. Pathol. Anat.* **355:** 29 (1972).
2. Bonilla-Musoles, F. Electron-microscopical examinations of the cervix uteri. *Gynaekol. Rundsch.* **8:** 197 (1969).
3. Changus, G. W., J. E. Towne, C. J. Smith, and T. N. Yonan. Fine structure of the so-called mesonephric carcinoma (abstract). *Lab. Invest.* **20:** 579 (1969).
4. Gordon, H. W., N. J. McMahon, C. M. Agliozzo, P. R. Rao, and J. Rogers. Adenoid cystic (cylindromatous) carcinoma of the uterine cervix: report of two cases. *Am. J. Clin. Pathol.* **58:** 51 (1972).

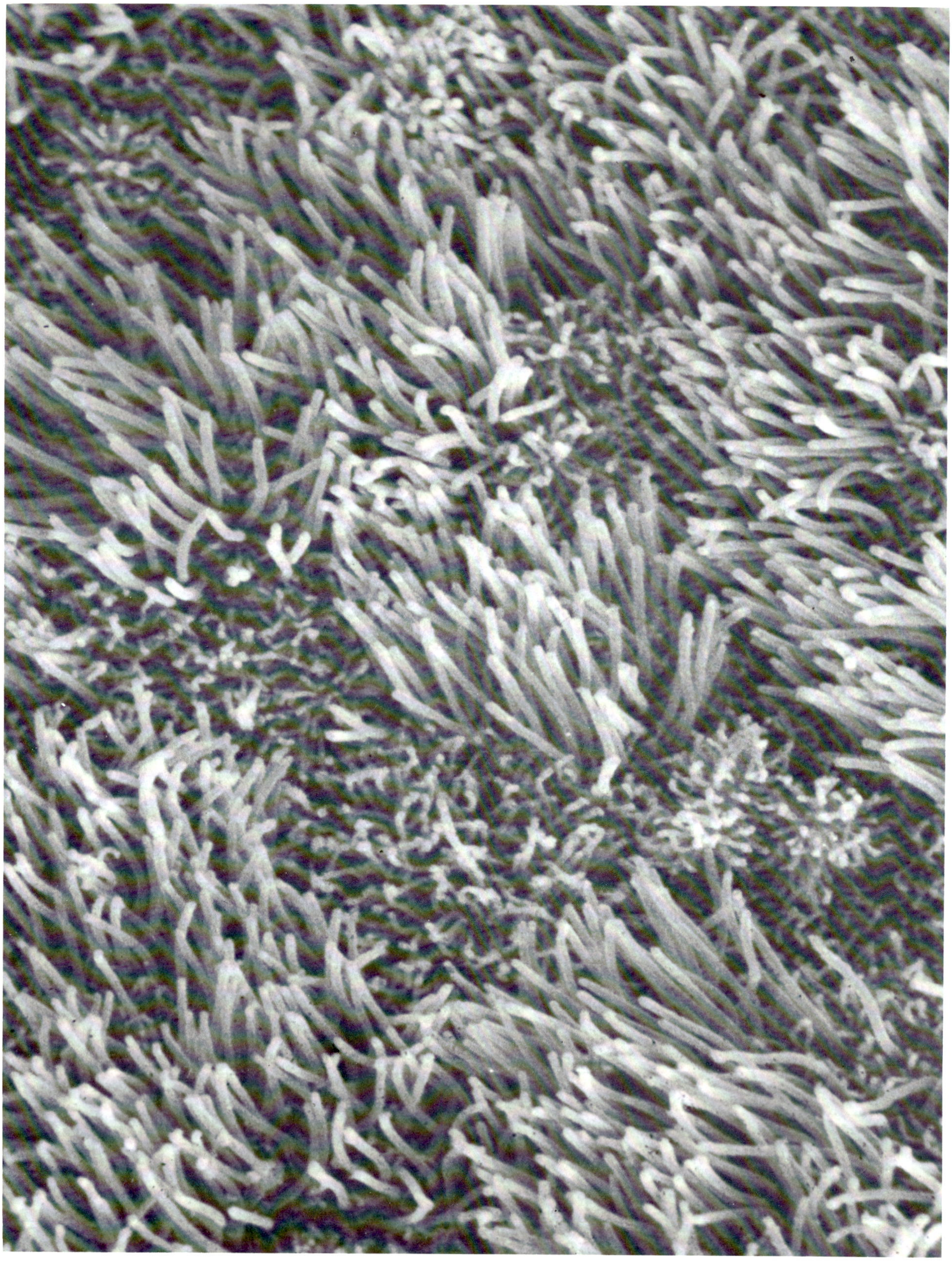

Scanning electron micrograph of the endometrial surface epithelium during the late proliferative phase of the menstrual cycle. Clusters of ciliated cells intermingle with noncilated microvillous cells. $\times$ 7500.

ENDOMETRIUM

The endometrial mucosa consists of two segments: the inactive basalis and the overlying functionalis (spongiosa and compacta). The endometrial glands open on the epithelial surface and are supported in their course through the endometrium by endometrial stromal cells. The endometrium is richly supplied by blood vessels that have a spiral course from the basalis to the surface. The menstrual cycle, mediated by the ovarian hormones, affects the glands, the stroma, and the endometrial vasculature. During the proliferative phase the synthesis of new cells predominates, whereas in the secretory phase cell organization is programmed for the elaboration and expulsion of secretory products and the development of predecidua.

The ultrastructural and histochemical observations on the human cyclical endometrium are in concordance with the biochemical, autoradiographic, and cell fractionation studies of the mechanism of action of estrogen that suggest that its major effect is to stimulate rapid cell growth by accelerating DNA-dependent RNA synthesis[1] (probably by influencing the transcription phase), glycogen and phospholipid metabolism, the synthesis of alkaline and acid phosphatase,[2] and mitotic activity. The effect of progesterone on the endometrial glandular cell is to produce a further accumulation and secretion of glycogen, mucopolysaccharides, lipids, and hydrolytic enzyme activity.[2] On a morphologic basis, endometrial secretory activity involves the ergastoplasm (proteins), glycogen, mitochondria (phosphorylation), and Golgi, resulting in the formation of secretory vesicles with acid mucopolysaccharide contents.

REFERENCES

1. O'Malley, B. W. Mechanisms of action of steroid hormones. *New Engl. J. Med.* **284:** 370 (1971).
2. Henzl, M. R., R. E. Smith, G. Boost, and E. T. Tyler. Lysosomal concept of menstrual bleeding in human. *J. Clin. Endocrinol. Metab.* **34:** 360 (1972).

27

Normal Menstrual Cycle

GLANDULAR EPITHELIUM

The glands, as well as the surface epithelium, are lined by a single layer of columnar epithelium, composed of secretory and ciliated cells. Degenerating peg cells have also been noted, especially in the surface epithelium. The existence of reserve cells has not been unequivocally demonstrated.

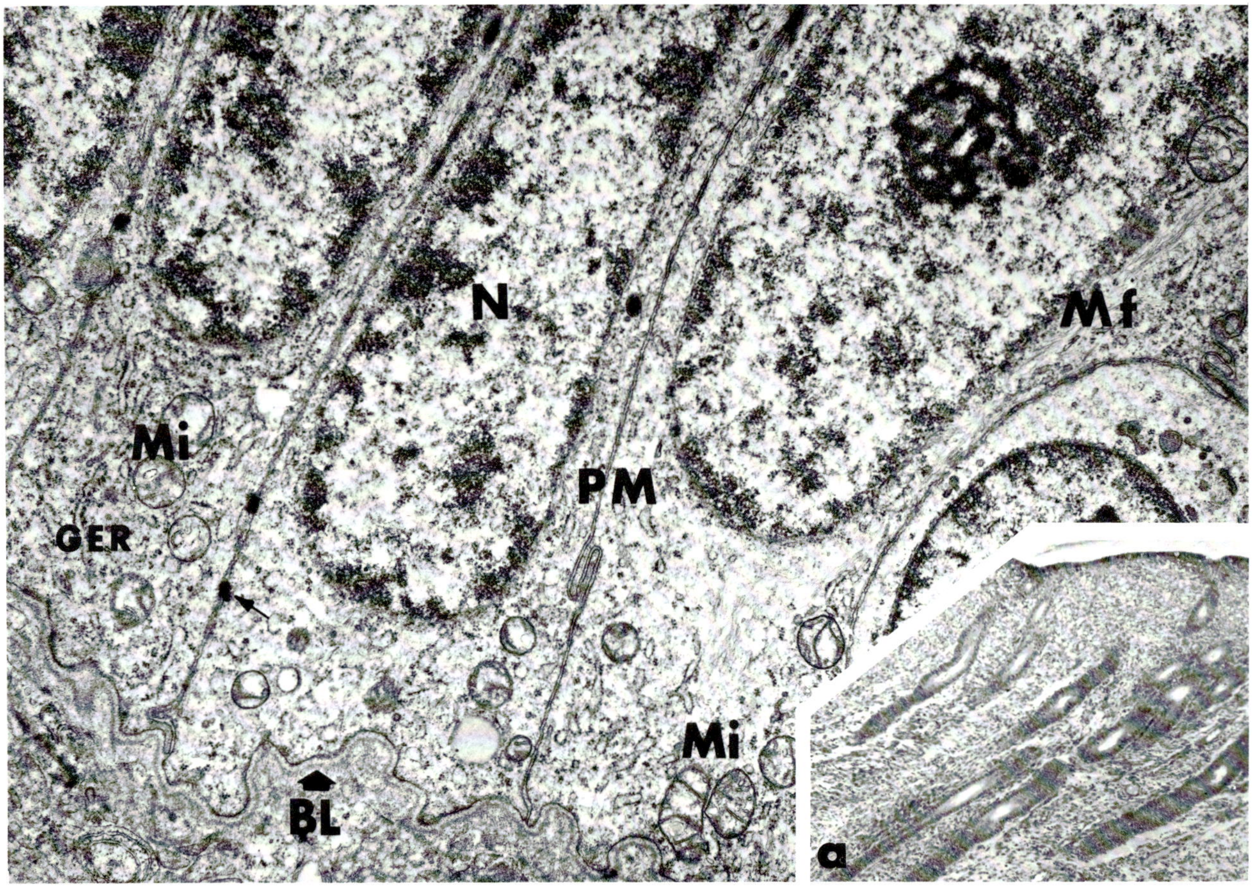

In the mid-proliferative phase (8–10th days) mitotic activity is at its peak,[1] accompanied by nucleolar enlargement and an increase in RNA synthesis. These changes are associated with high 6,7-^{3}H-estradiol-17-β uptake,[2] as well as with elevated estradiol competitive binding capacity[3] in uteri, removed during the first half of the menstrual cycle.

Figure 74a. *During the early proliferative phase (4–7th days* of a 28-day cycle), narrow, straight glands are generated from the underlying basalis. (H & E stain, × 12.)

Figure 74. *At the ultrastructural level,* the epithelial surface contains ATP-ase[1,2] and alkaline phosphatase-positive microvilli,[1,3,4] which become shorter in the luteal phase. The cytoplasmic organelles involved in protein synthesis, such as free ribosomes, granular endoplasmic reticulum (GER), and mitochondria (Mi), are poorly developed, and the nuclei (N) are elongated with compact chromatin. The tightly apposed lateral plasma membranes (PM) are reinforced by a few desmosomes (arrow). × 18,400. MF: microfilaments; BL: basal lamina.

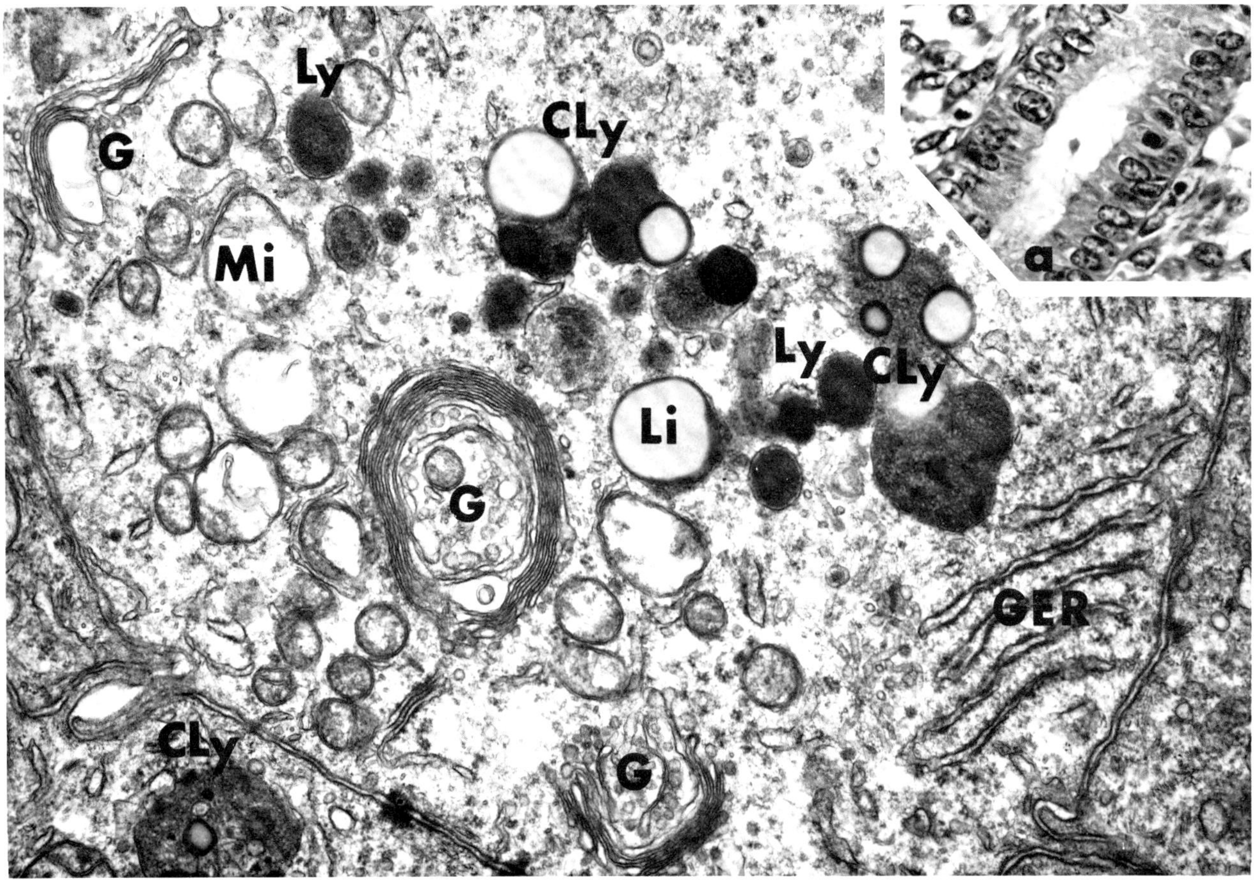

Figure 75a. *Higher magnification* of an endometrial gland in the proliferative phase, lined by low columnar (6 μ) epithelium and a few ciliated cells. Mitoses, under the control of preovulatory estrogens, are common. (H & E stain, × 120).

Figure 75. *Endometrial glands in the early proliferative phase* are rich in acid phosphatase-positive cytolysosomes (CLy) and lysosomes (Ly) near the Golgi (G),[1,3,5] and lipid droplets (Li) are numerous. × 29,200. Mi: mitochondria; GER: granular endoplasmic reticulum.

REFERENCES (Figures 74–75)

1. Colville, E. A. The ultrastructure of the human endometrium. *J. Obstet. Gynaecol. Brit. Commonw.* **75:** 342 (1968).
2. Sirtori, C. Some ultrastructural aspects of human uterine physiopathology: cyclosenility, senility, antisenile and antitumoral therapies, and contraceptive drugs. In *Proceedings of International Symposium on Obstetrics and Gynaecology,* J. A. Chalmers, R. Merger, and G. B. Candiani (Eds.). Carlo Erba Foundation, Milan, 1969, pp. 129–154.
3. Nilsson, O. Electron microscopy of the glandular epithelium in the human uterus. I. Follicular phase. *J. Ultrastruct. Res.* **6:** 413 (1962).
4. Sawaragi, I. and R. M. Wynn. Ultrastructural localization of metabolic enzymes during the human endometrial cycle. *Obstet. Gynecol.* **34:** 50 (1969).
5. Cavazos, F., J. A. Green, D. G. Hall, and F. V. Lucas. Ultrastructure of the human endometrial glandular cell during the menstrual cycle. *Am. J. Obstet. Gynecol.* **99:** 833 (1967).

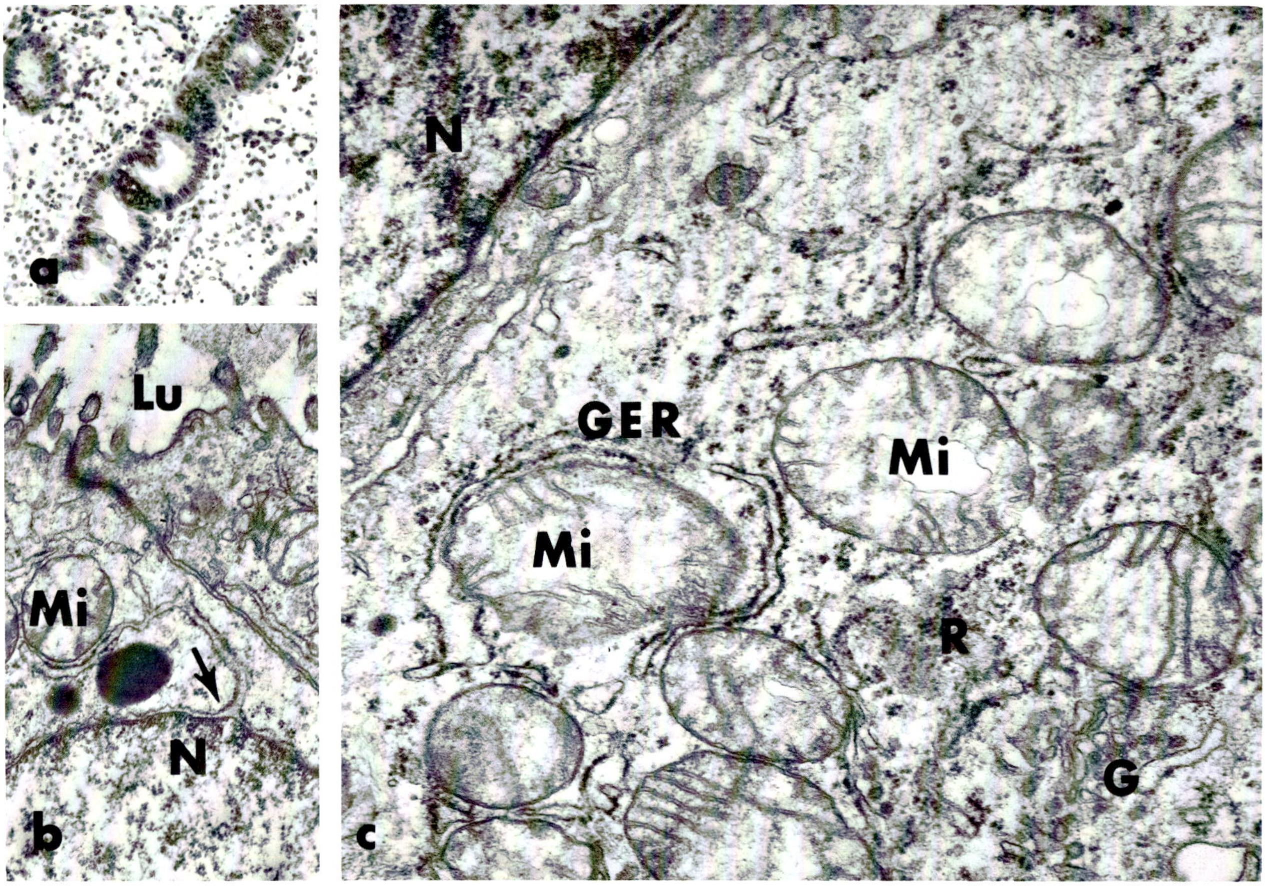

Figure 76a. *In the mid-proliferative phase,* still under the influence of preovulatory estrogens, the glands become longer with segmental tortuosity. (H & E stain, × 30.)

Figure 76b. *Ultrastructurally,* a considerable increase in RNA synthesis is noted, reflected in the abundance of free ribosomes and granular endoplasmic reticulum in a subnuclear (N) location. The latter is often seen in connection with the nuclear membrane (arrow) and mitochondria (Mi). The appearance of annulate lamellae[4] and bundles of microfilaments[5,6] is an additional characteristic of this stage of the cycle. × 23,040. Lu: glandular lumen.

Figure 76c. *Note the close spatial relationship* between the mitochondria (Mi), parallel membranes of granular endoplasmic reticulum (GER), Golgi (G), and free ribosomes (R). × 41,200. N: nucleus.

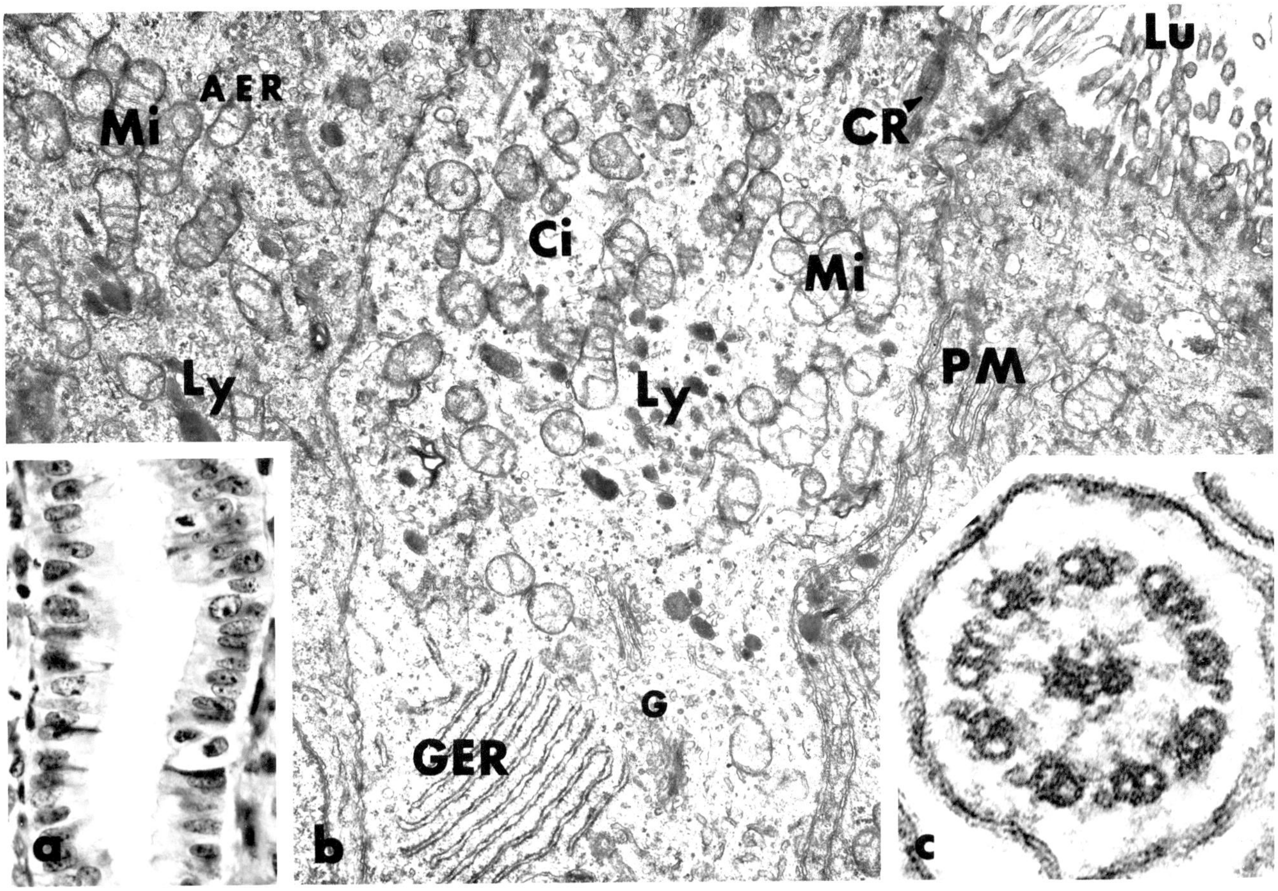

Figure 77a. *Mid-proliferative endometrium.* The lining epithelium becomes tall columnar and contains numerous mitoses and ciliated cells. (H & E stain, × 120.)

Figure 77b. *The endometrial ciliated cells* (Ci) are indistinguishable from tubal ciliated cells[7,8] in their cytoplasmic organization and the formation of ciliary apparatuses. Their clear appearance with the light microscope is due to the relatively clear cytoplasmic matrix. In the postovulatory period, a considerable decrease in ciliated cells is observed,[9-13] suggesting that ciliogenesis is estrogen dependent. Mitoses are not found in ciliated cells, and they are thought to be derived from precursor, clear cells, located near the basal lamina.[8] Loss of cilia during the cycle occurs by the shedding of individual ciliary shafts and their apical cytoplasmic fragments.[14] The cytoplasmic ciliary bodies invariably remain, however, providing for ciliary regeneration. The primary function of ciliated cells in the endometrial gland is probably related to the distribution of glandular secretions. The significance of the frequent finding of anomalous ciliary shafts in endometrial ciliated cells is not apparent.[15,16] × 15,600. CR: ciliary rootlets, Ly: lysosomes; Mi: mitochondria; G: Golgi; PM: plasma membranes; GER: granular endoplasmic reticulum; AER: agranular endoplasmic reticulum; Lu: glandular lumen.

Figure 77c. *Higher-power view of cross-sectioned ciliary shaft* containing nine double peripheral tubules and a pair of central tubules. × 84,275.

REFERENCES (In the mid-proliferative phase—Figure 77c)

1. Wagner, D., R. M. Richart, and J. Y. Terner. DNA content of human endometrial gland cells during the menstrual cycle. *Am. J. Obstet. Gynecol.* **100:** 90 (1968).
2. Brush, M. G., R. W. Taylor, and R. J. L. King. The uptake of (6,7-^{3}H) oestradiol by the normal human female reproductive tract. *J. Endocrinol.* **39:** 599 (1967).
3. Henderson, S. R. and D. S. Schalch. Estrogen receptors in the human uterus. *Am. J. Obstet. Gynecol.* **112:** 762 (1972).
4. Ancla, M. and J. de Brux. Occurrence of intranuclear tubular structures in the human endometrium during the secretory phase, and of annulate lamellae in hyperestrogenic states. *Obstet. Gynecol.* **26:** 23 (1965).
5. Cavazos, F., J. A. Green, D. G. Hall, and F. V. Lucas. Ultrastructure of the human endometrial glandular cell during the menstrual cycle. *Am. J. Obstet. Gynecol.* **99:** 833 (1967).

6. Cavazos, F., J. A. Green, D. G. Hall, and F. V. Lucas. The microtubular system in the cytoplasm of the human endometrial glandular cell during the menstrual cycle. *Am. J. Obstet. Gynecol.* **94:** 824 (1966).
7. Ferenczy, A., R. M. Richart, J. F. Agate, Jr., M. L. Purkerson, and E. W. Dempsey. Scanning electron microscopy of the human endometrial surface epithelium. *Fertil. Steril.* **23:** 515 (1972).
8. Ferenczy, A. and R. M. Richart. Scanning and transmission electron microscopy of the human endometrial surface epithelium. *J. Clin. Endocrinol. Metab.* **36:** 183 (1973).
9. Nilsson, O. Electron microscopy of the glandular epithelium in the human uterus. I. Follicular phase. *J. Ultrastruct. Res.* **6:** 413 (1962).
10. Nilsson, O. Electron microscopy of the glandular epithelium in the human uterus. II. Early and late luteal phase. *J. Ultrastruct. Res.* **6:** 422 (1962).
11. Gompel, C. The ultrastructure of the human endometrial cell studied by electron microscopy. *Am. J. Obstet. Gynecol.* **84:** 1000 (1962).
12. Wynn, R. M. and J. A. Harris. Ultrastructural cyclic changes in the human endometrium. I. Normal preovulatory phase. *Fertil. Steril.* **18:** 632 (1967).
13. Terzakis, J. A. The nucleolar channel system of human endometrium. *J. Cell Biol.* **27:** 293 (1965).
14. Hamperl, H.: Uber die "hellen" Flimmerepithelzellen dermenschlichen Uterusschleimhaut. *Virchows. Arch. Pathol. Anat.* **319:** 265 (1950).
15. Hando, T., D. M. Okada, and L. Zamboni. Atypical cilia in human endometrium. *J. Cell Biol.* **39:** 475 (1968).
16. Sengel, A. and P. Stoebner. Ultrastructure of the normal human endometrium. II. The glandular cells. *Z. Zellforsch.* **109:** 260 (1970).

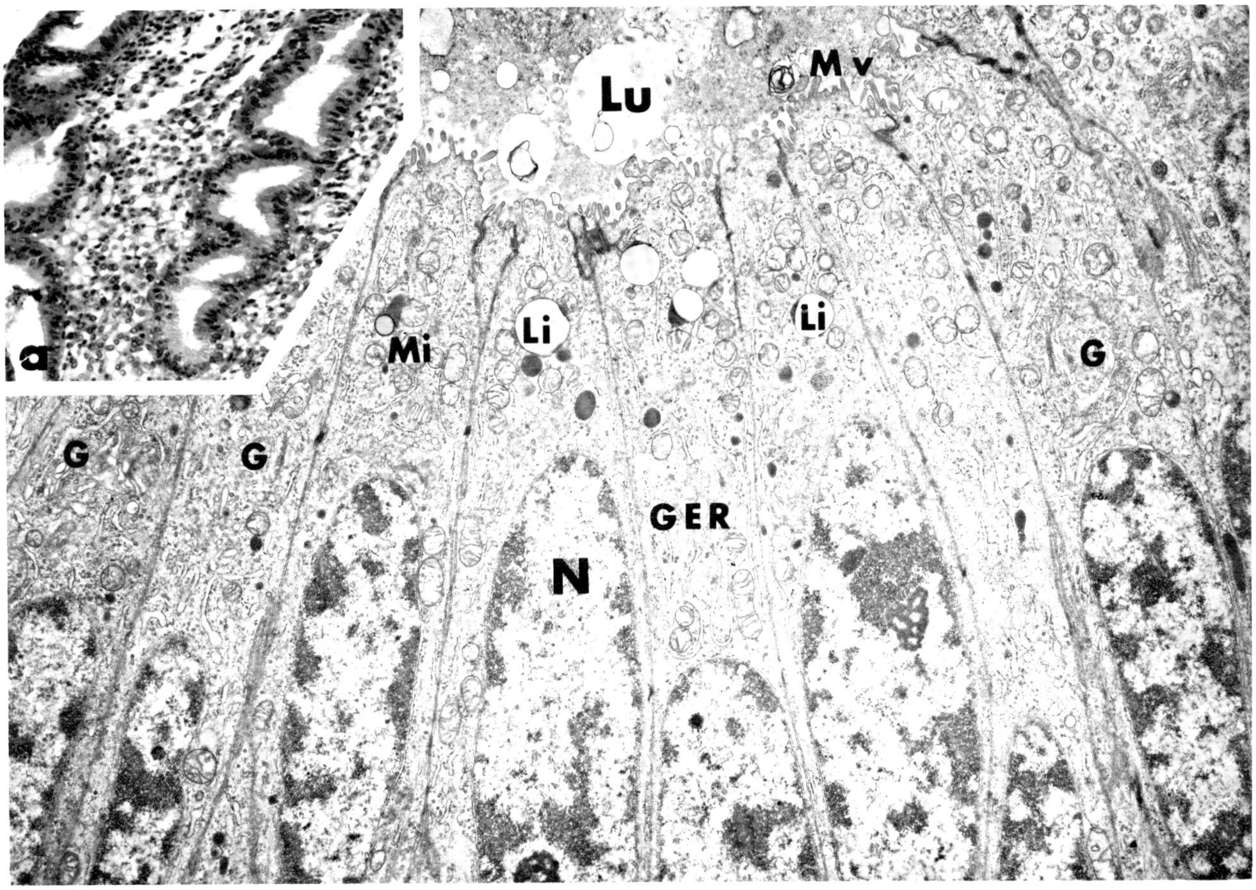

Figure 78a. *The late proliferative phase (11-14th days)* is characterized by increased tortuosity of the glands. (H & E stain, × 38.)

Figure 78. *Fine structurally,* the cells have abundant supranuclear RNA synthesis and well-developed Golgi (G), associated with numerous secretory vesicles,[1-3] annulate lamellae,[4] and lipid droplets (Li). The lateral plasma membranes are still straight and numerous, and well-developed microvilli (Mv) project into the glandular lumen (Lu). The nuclei (N) of the late proliferative and the early secretory phase contain one or more compact nucleoli. × 5600. GER: granular endoplasmic reticulum.

REFERENCES (Figures 78–79)

1. Nilsson, O. Electron microscopy of the glandular epithelium in the human uterus. I. Follicular phase. *J. Ultrastruct. Res.* **6:** 413 (1962).
2. Nilsson, O. Electron microscopy of the glandular epithelium in the human uterus. II. Early and late luteal phase. *J. Ultrastruct. Res.* **6:** 422 (1962).
3. Sengel, A. and Stoebner, P.: Ultrastructure of the normal human endometrium. II. The glandular cells. *Z. Zellforsch.* **109:** 260, 1970.
4. Cavazos, F., J. A. Green, D. G. Hall, and F. V. Lucas. Ultrastructure of the human endometrial glandular cell during the menstrual cycle. *Am. J. Obstet. Gynecol.* **99:** 833 (1967).

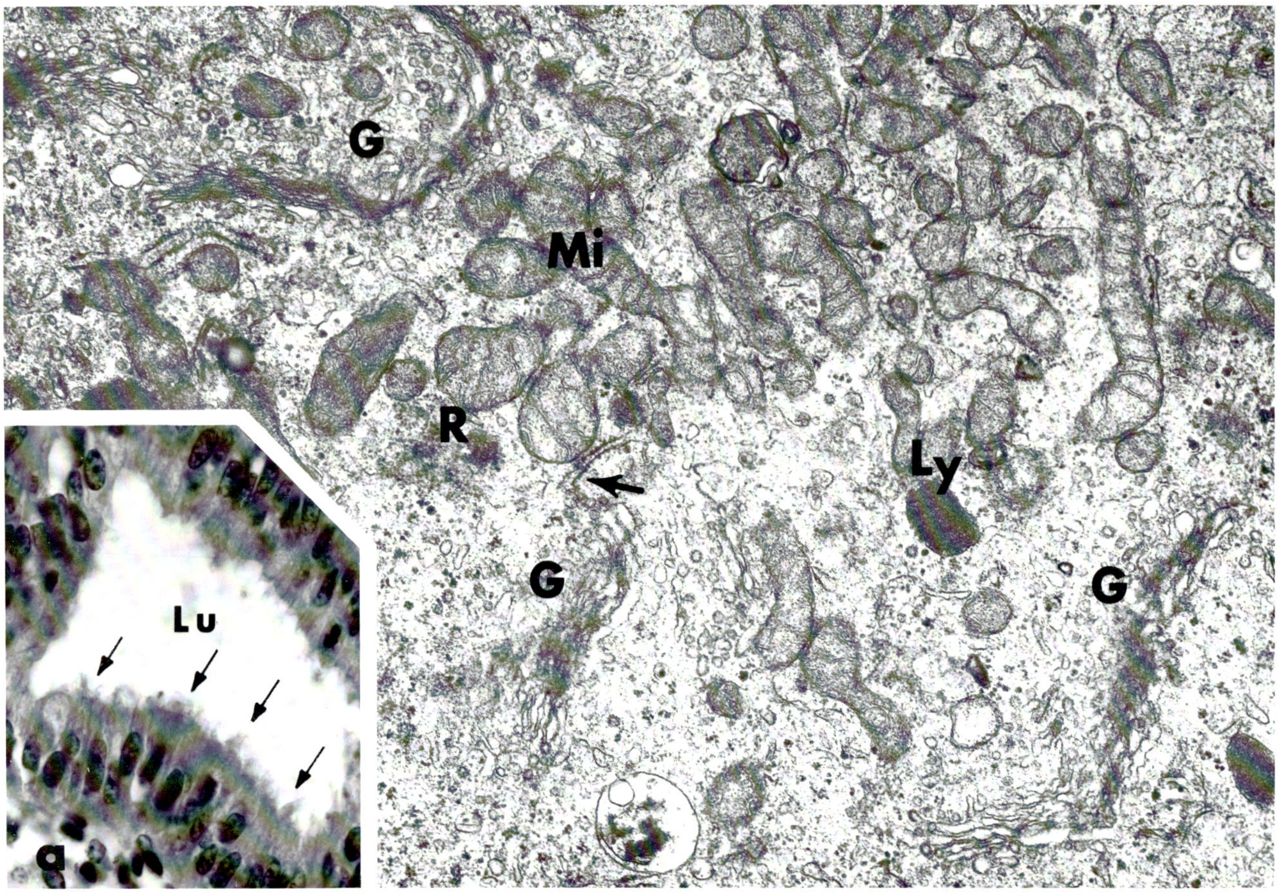

Figure 79a. *Late proliferative endometrium.* The glands are lined by tall, piled-up, columnar epithelium, resulting in pseudostratification. Apical alkaline phosphatase and mitotic activity, as well as ciliated cells (arrows), are abundant. (H & E stain, × 153.) Lu: glandular lumen.

Figure 79. *Large subnuclear aggregates* of mitochondria (Mi) are associated with well-developed Golgi (G) and granular endoplasmic reticulum (arrow). Free ribosomes (R) are dispersed throughout the cytoplasm. × 25,600. Ly: lysosome.

Between the 14th and 16th days of the cycle, under the combined influence of estrogen and progesterone, aggregates of glycogen appear in the basal portions of the glandular cells.[1-5]

Figure 80a. *In the early postovulatory phase (16th day),* the glands are extremely tortuous and the still pseudostratified epithelium contains irregular, small, subnuclear vacuoles corresponding to deposits of glycogen particles. (H & E stain, × 150.) Lu: glandular lumen.

Figure 80. *The 16th day of the menstrual cycle.* Concomitantly to subnuclear accumulation of glycogen particles (Gly), the neighboring mitochondria (Mi) began to increase in size and number, reflecting greater metabolic activity and enzymatic secretions,[3,5,6-8] and the granular endoplasmic reticulum is associated with glucose-6 phosphatase activity.[9] During the ovulatory period and in the following days, groups of subnuclear mitochondria in close association with granular endoplasmic reticulum (GER) and free ribosomes (R) are interconnected by undulating bundles of perinuclear microfilaments (Mf) to supranuclear Golgi and are thought to play a role in the transport of glycogen particles to the Golgi apparatus.[2,6] The arrow indicates the close relationship between bundles of microfilaments and glycogen particles. In the early postovulatory phase the lateral plasma membranes (PM) contain focal areas of convolutions, and microvillous projections (MvP) appear near the basal lamina (BL). × 20,300.

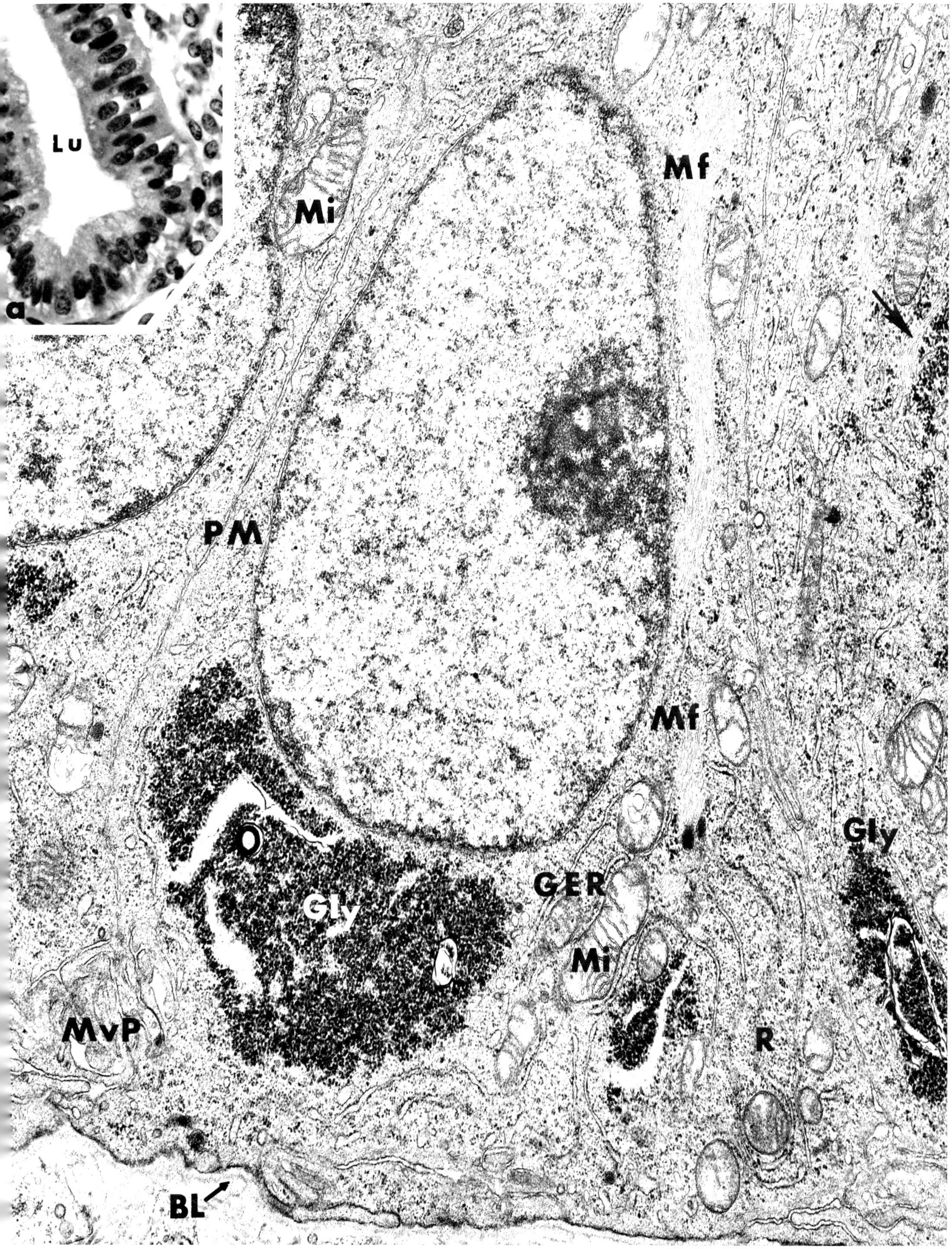

Lu
a
Mi
Mf
PM
Mf
Gly
GER
Gly
Mi
MvP
R
BL

REFERENCES (Between the 14th and 16th days—Figure 80)

1. Colville, E. A. The ultrastructure of the human endometrium. *J. Obstet. Gynaecol. Brit. Commonw.* **75:** 342 (1968).
2. Ancla, M. and J. de Brux. Occurrence of intranuclear tubular structures in the human endometrium during the secretory phase, and of annulate lamellae in hyperestrogenic states. *Obstet. Gynecol.* **26:** 23 (1965).
3. Gompel, C. The ultrastructure of the human endometrial cell studied by electron microscopy. *Am. J. Obstet. Gynecol.* **84:** 1000 (1962).
4. Wynn, R. M. and J. A. Harris. Ultrastructural cyclic changes in the human endometrium. I. Normal preovulatory phase. *Fertil. Steril.* **18:** 632 (1967).
5. Sengel, A. and P. Stoebner. Ultrastructure of the normal human endometrium. II. The glandular cells. *Z. Zellforsch.* **109:** 260 (1970).
6. Cavazos, F., J. A. Green, D. G. Hall, and F. V. Lucas. Ultrastructure of the human endometrial glandular cell during the menstrual cycle. *Am. J. Obstet. Gynecol.* **99:** 833 (1967).
7. Nilsson, O. Electron microscopy of the glandular epithelium in the human uterus. II. Early and late luteal phase. *J. Ultrastruct. Res.* **6:** 422 (1962).
8. Merker, H. J., R. Herbst, and K. Kloss. An electron-microscopical study of the mitochondria of the human uterine epithelium during the secretory phase. *Z. Zellforsch.* **89:** 139 (1968).
9. Sawaragi, I. and R. M. Wynn. Ultrastructural localization of metabolic enzymes during the human endometrial cycle. *Obstet. Gynecol.* **34:** 50 (1969).

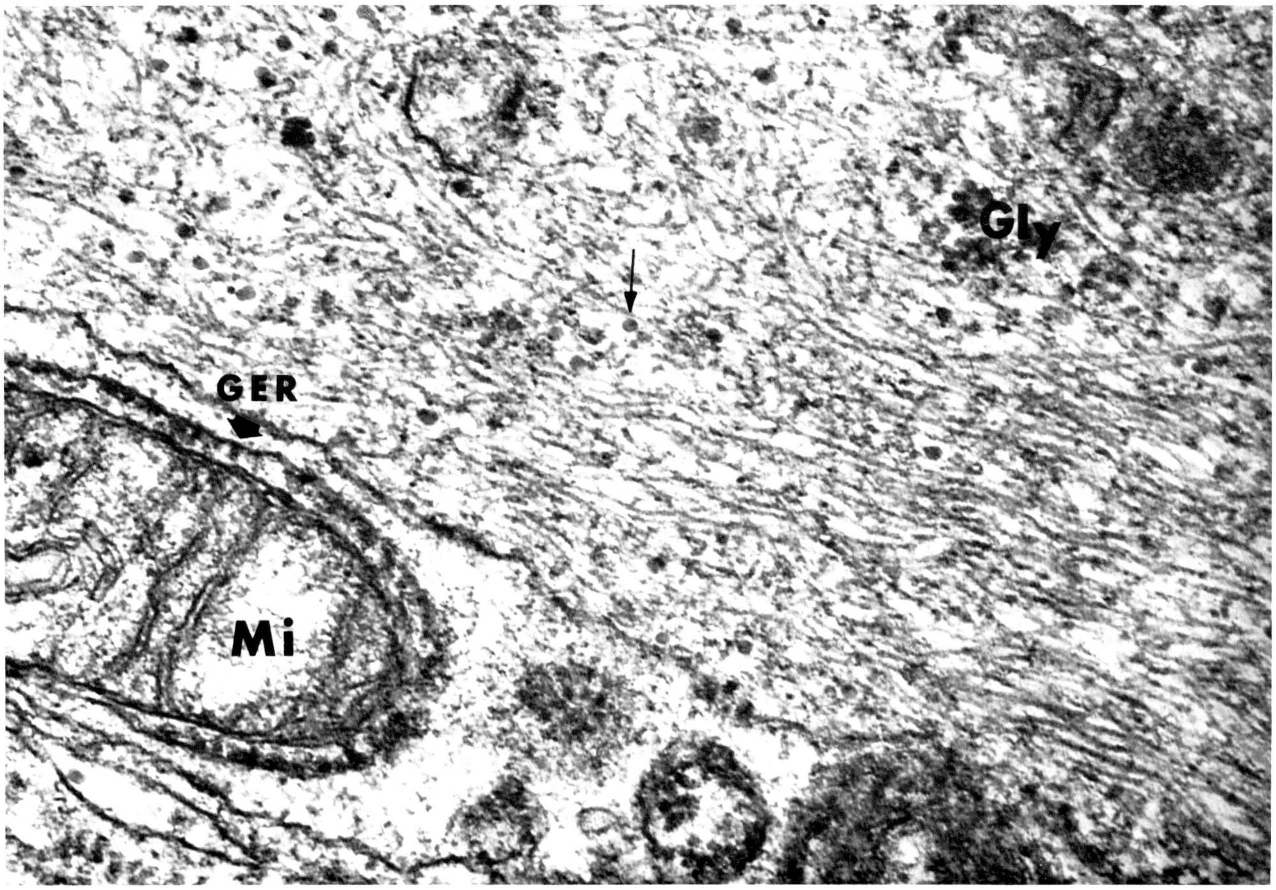

Figure 81. *The 16th day of the cycle.* High-power view of perinuclear microfilaments, each measuring approximately 100 Å in width. In the interfilamentous space are several glycogen granules (Gly), some in a monoparticulate form (arrow), and the adjacent mitochondrion (Mi) is enveloped by membranes of granular endoplasmic reticulum (GER). Note that the inner side of the membrane that faces the mitochondrion contains numerous ribosomes, whereas the outer membrane is virtually devoid of such granularity. × 67,000.

REFERENCES (Figure 81 and 82)

1. Sirtori, C. Some ultrastructural aspects of human uterine physiopathology: cyclosenility, senility, antisenile and antitumoral therapies, and contraceptive drugs. In *Proceedings of International Symposium on Obstetrics and Gynaecology,* J. A. Chalmers, R. Merger, and G. B. Candiani (Eds.). Carlo Erba Foundation, Milan, 1969, pp. 129–154.
2. Nilsson, O. Electron microscopy of the glandular epithelium in the human uterus. II. Early and late luteal phase. *J. Ultrastruct. Res.* **6:** 422 (1962).
3. Sengel, A. and P. Stoebner. Ultrastructure of the normal human endometrium. II. The glandular cells. *Z. Zellforsch.* **109:** 260 (1970).
4. Wynn, R. M. and R. S. Woolley. Ultrastructural cyclic changes in the human endometrium. II. Normal postovulatory phase. *Fertil. Steril.* **18:** 721 (1967).

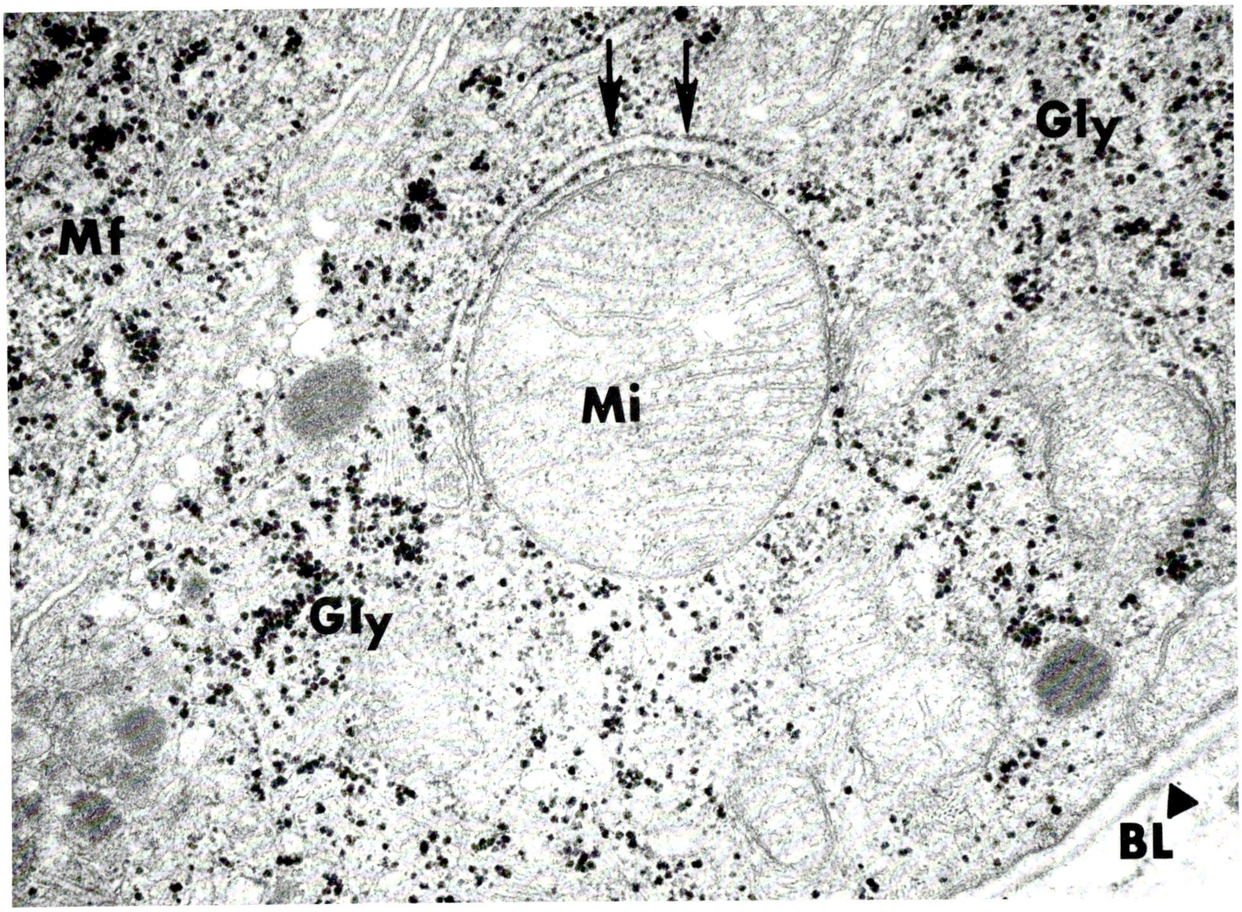

Figure 82. *The 16th day of the cycle.* The subnuclear accumulation of glycogen (Gly) is accompanied by an increase in mitochondrial size (Mi: giant mitochondria), and numerous secretory vesicles become concentrated around the Golgi and mitochondria.[1-4] The enlargement of subnuclear mitochondria suggests that they are related to glycogen synthesis.[2,3] The giant mitochondrion is partly covered by parallel membranes of granular endoplasmic reticulum (arrows), and microfilaments (Mf) are in close association. $\times$ 41,000. BL: basal lamina.

On the 17th day of the cycle, at the ultrastructural level, ovulation is followed by the appearance of an intranucleolar channel system (NCS).[1] These structures, first described by Dubrauszky and Pohlmann in 1960,[2] are apparently unique to human endometrial nucleoli and can be seen as early as the 16th day of the cycle. They reach a maximum on the 21st day and presumably represent a response to rising progesterone levels.[3-6]

The NCS measures up to 1.5 μ in diameter and is composed of a series of anastomosing spherical channels, lined by a triple-layered limiting membrane.[1] When the canaliculi (400–600 Å in diameter) are cut transversally, they form a honeycomb pattern. The NCS is usually found at the periphery of the nucleoli and is often located near the nuclear membrane. On occasion, continuity between the NCS and the cytoplasmic matrix and granular endoplasmic reticulum, through either the perinuclear space or nuclear openings (not the nuclear pores), has been demonstrated.[1] The exact significance of the NCS is obscure. Despite the finding of intracanalicular particles, structurally similar to nucleolar ribonuclease-positive material,[1] the NCS is unlikely to play a role in the transport or metabolism of cytoplasmic RNA, for RNA synthesis is considerably decreased when the NCS is at its maximum.

The exclusive presence of the NCS in the postovulatory period suggests that these unique structures are formed under the combined stimulus of estrogen and progesterone. This is further supported by their absence under abnormal hormonal conditions, such as prolonged administration of progestins or luteal insufficiency.[3,7] The need for progestational agents in the development of NCS is also suggested by organ culture studies of proliferative endometrium. In these experiments, the administration of progesterone, specifically those progestational steroids that contain an acyl group in the 17-beta position,[8] provoked secretory activity and the appearance of NCS, but both were invariably absent in the control proliferative endometria treated with estrogen alone, with cortisol,[9] or with 19-nortestosterone compounds lacking the acyl group in the 17-beta position.[8,9]

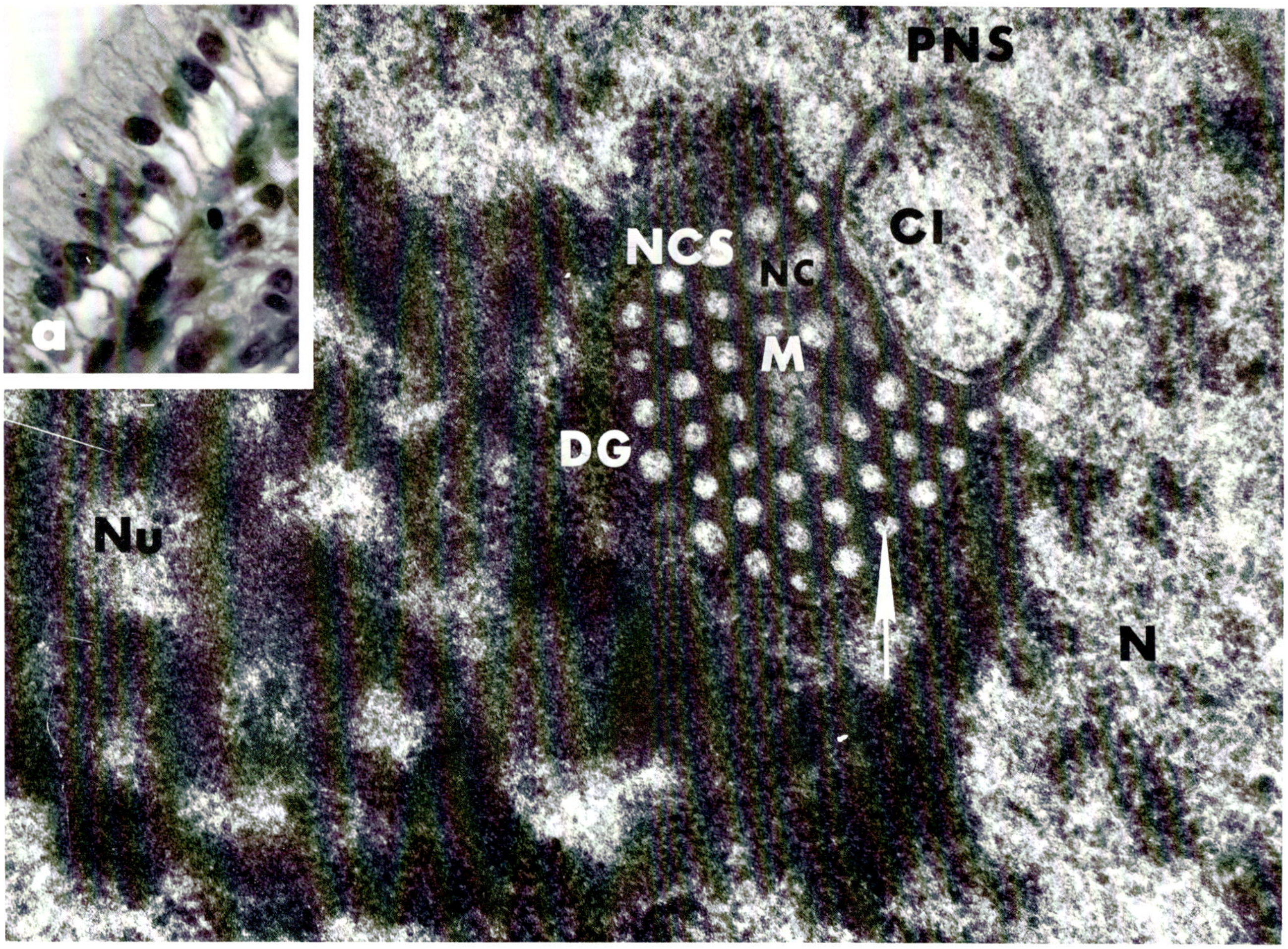

Figure 83a. *On the 17th day of the cycle* the subnuclear vacuoles become uniform and prominent and occupy the lowest one-third of the cell, elevating the nuclei. These morphological features provide the first reliable histologic evidence that ovulation has occurred. (H & E stain, × 190.)

Figure 83. *A portion of an endometrial secretory cell nucleus (N) and nucleolus (NU).* Note that the nucleolar channel system (NCS) is located at the periphery of the nucleus. Note also that a cytoplasmic arm (Cl) has pushed its way into the nucleus. The nucleolar channel system is cross sectioned, showing a large number of channels (NC) in circular profile about 500 to 600 Å in diameter. Within the channels are amorphous material of low density and small granules. One granule (arrow) has a hollow central portion, giving it a ring-shaped appearance. The channels are embedded in a rather dense, amorphous matrix material (M). Just peripheral to the matrix is a row of very densely staining, 150-Å granules (DG). Note the difference in staining between these granules and those in the rest of the nucleolus. × 79,000. PNS: perinuclear space. *From* J. A. Terzakis. The nucleolar channel system of human endometrium. *J. Cell Biol.* **27**: 293–304 (1965).

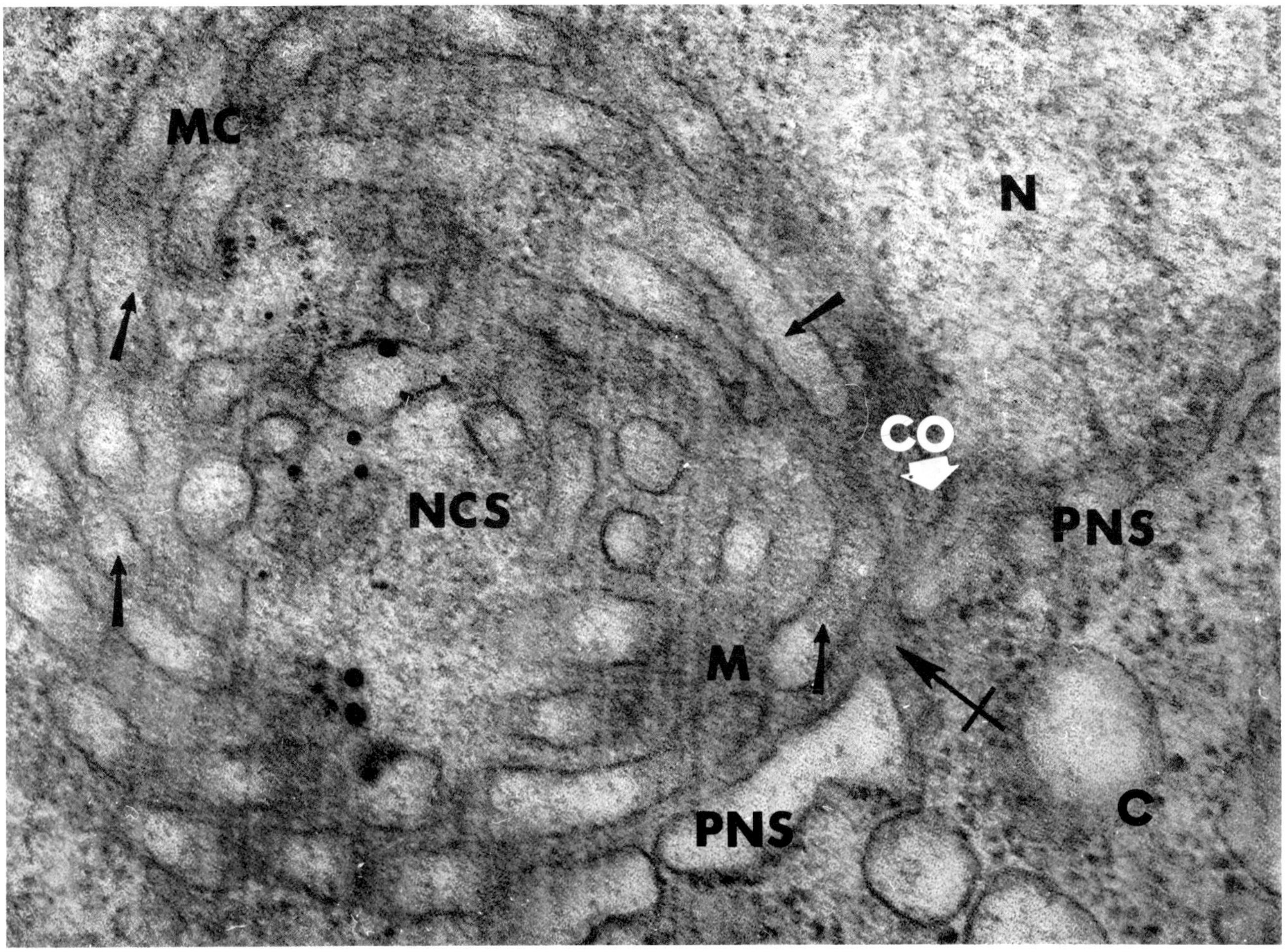

Figure 84. *This high-power view of an endometrial cell nucleus (N) and cytoplasm (C)* shows the nucleolar channel system (NCS) on the periphery of the nucleus. The individual channels have a triple-layered membrane 50 to 70 Å wide (MC), consisting of two dense lines 17 to 25 Å wide, between which is a less dense area 15 to 20 Å wide; 50- to 75-Å fibrils (⟵) are seen in the interior of the channels. There is a communication (CO) between a channel and the perinuclear space (PNS). Just adjacent to this is an open gap (⟻) in the nuclear membrane, not bridged by a diaphragm, which puts the cytoplasm in direct communication with the matrix (M) of the nucleolar channel system. × 112,000. *From* J. A. Terzakis. The nucleolar channel system of human endometrium. *J. Cell Biol.* **27:** 293–304 (1965).

REFERENCES (On the 17th day—Figure 84)

1. Terzakis, J. A. The nucleolar channel system of human endometrium. *J. Cell Biol.* **27:** 293 (1965).
2. Dubrauszky, V. and G. Pohlmann. Strukturveranderungen am Nukleolus von Korpusendometriumzellen während der Sekretionsphase. *Naturwissenschaften,* **47:** 523 (1960).
3. Ancla, M. and J. de Brux. Occurrence of intranuclear tubular structures in the human endometrium during the secretory phase, and of annulate lamellae in hyperestrogenic states. *Obstet. Gynecol.* **26:** 23 (1965).
4. Clyman, M. J. A new structure observed in the nucleolus of the human endometrial epithelial cell. *Am. J. Obstet. Gynecol.* **86:** 430 (1963).
5. Ancla, M., J. de Brux, and J. Belaisch. Influence of the estrogen-progesterone balance on the ultrastructure of the human endometrium. I. Morphology and development of the intranuclear corpuscles present in the glandular cells of the endometrium under the effect of noresthérone and in essential sterility. *Gynécol. Obstét (Paris)* **63:** 239 (1964).
6. Moricard, R. and F. Moricard. Modifications cytoplasmiques et nucléaires ultrastructurales utérines au cours de l'état follicolutéinique à glycogène massif. *Gynécol. Obstét. (Paris)* **63:** 203 (1964).
7. Clyman, M. Electron-microscopic changes produced in the human endometrium by norethindrone acetate with ethinyl estradiol. *Fertil. Steril.* **14:** 352 (1963).
8. Kohorn, E. I., S. I. Rice, S. Hemperly, and M. Gordon. The relation of the structure of progestational steroids to nucleolar differentiation in human endometrium. *J. Clin. Endocrinol. Metab.* **34:** 257 (1972).
9. Kohorn, E. I., S. I. Rice, and M. Gordon. In vitro production of nucleolar channel system by progesterone in human endometrium. *Nature (London)* **228:** 671 (1970).

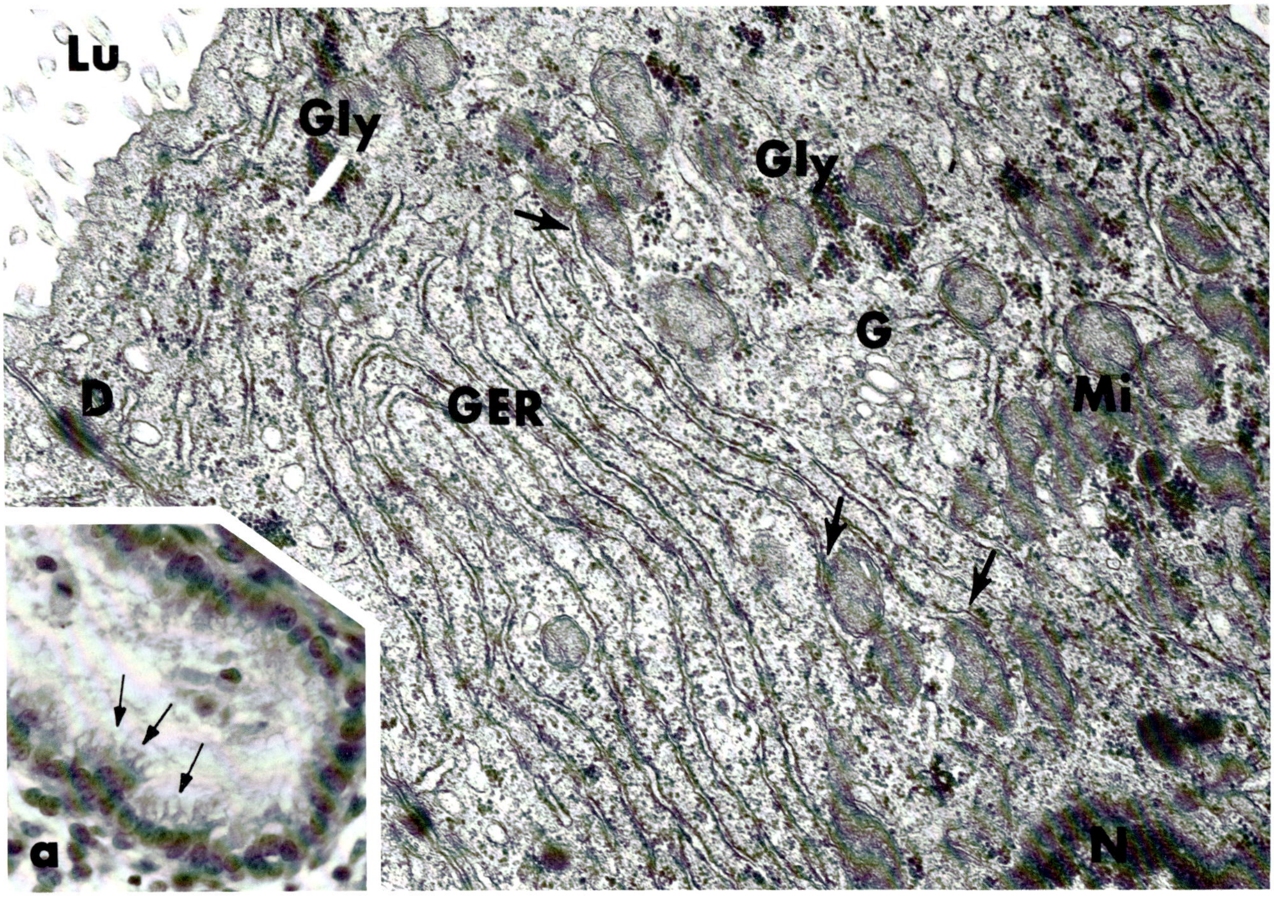

Figure 85a. *On the 19th day,* most of the secretions (arrows) have been expelled and the epithelium becomes flattened. (H & E stain, × 120.)

Figure 85. *At the ultrastructural level,* secretory activity is preceded by the appearance of numerous small vesicles, originating from prominent Golgi (G),[1] and glycogen (Gly), both of which accumulate beneath the surface plasma membrane.[2-4] During this period, the mitochondria (Mi) and Golgi are at their maximum,[1,2] glycogen particles occur throughout the cytoplasm, and bundles of microfilaments are formed and become intermingled with the glycogen and Golgi and attached to the desmosomes.[2] Prominent stalks of granular endoplasmic reticulum (GER) are in close association (arrows) with supranuclear mitochondria (Mi). × 23,060. N: nucleus; Lu: glandular lumen; D: desmosome.

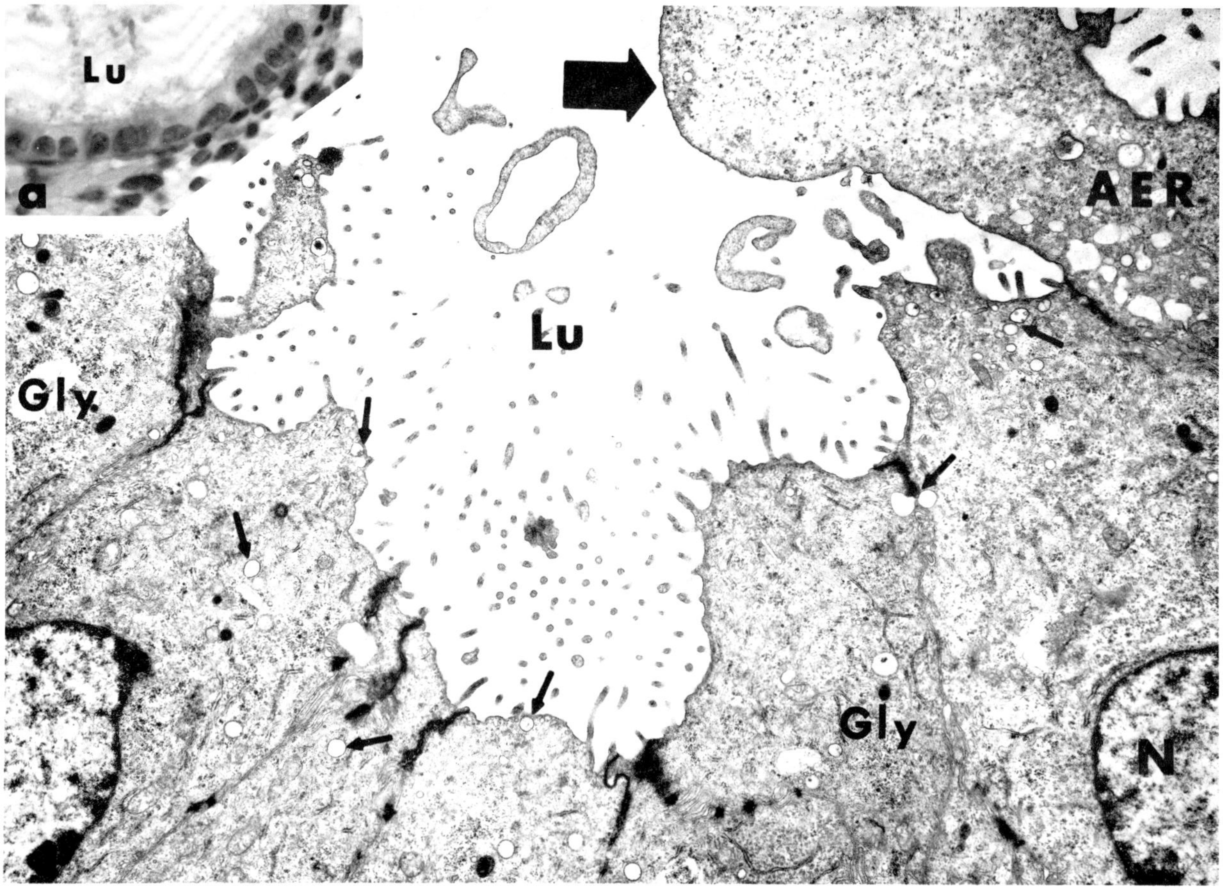

Figure 86a. *On the 20th day*, several glands exhibit secretory "exhaustion." (H & E stain, × 120.) Lu: glandular lumen.

Figure 86. *The apical accumulations of large aggregates of glycogen* (Gly) and various organelles cause large portions of the cytoplasm to protrude (large arrow) and eventually rupture into the glandular lumen (Lu). This apocrine type of secretion[5-7] reaches its maximum activity between the *19th and 21st days of the cycle*. Note the tightly apposed but convoluted lateral plasma membranes, especially near the glandular lumen. × 5600. AER: dilated agranular endoplasmic reticulum; arrows: membrane-coated vesicles.

REFERENCES (Figures 85–86a)

1. Sengel, A. and P. Stoebner. Ultrastructure of the normal human endometrium. II. The glandular cells. *Z. Zellforsch.* **109:** 260 (1970).
2. Cavazos, F., J. A. Green, D. G. Hall, and F. V. Lucas. Ultrastructure of the human endometrial glandular cell during the menstrual cycle. *Am. J. Obstet. Gynecol.* **99:** 833 (1967).
3. Nilsson, O. Electron microscopy of the glandular epithelium in the human uterus. II. Early and late luteal phase. *J. Ultrastruct. Res.* **6:** 422 (1962).
4. Gompel, C. The ultrastructure of the human endometrial cell studied by electron microscopy. *Am. J. Obstet. Gynecol.* **84:** 1000 (1962).
5. Wynn, R. M. and R. S. Woolley. Ultrastructural cyclic changes in the human endometrium. I. Normal postovulatory phase. *Fertil. Steril.* **18:** 721 (1967).
6. Wetzstein, R. and H. Wagner. Elektronenmikroskopische Untersuchungen am menschlichen Endometrium. *Anat. Anz.* **108:** 362 (1960).
7. Svajger, A. Die apokrine Extrusion. *Anat. Anz.* **123:** 137 (1968).

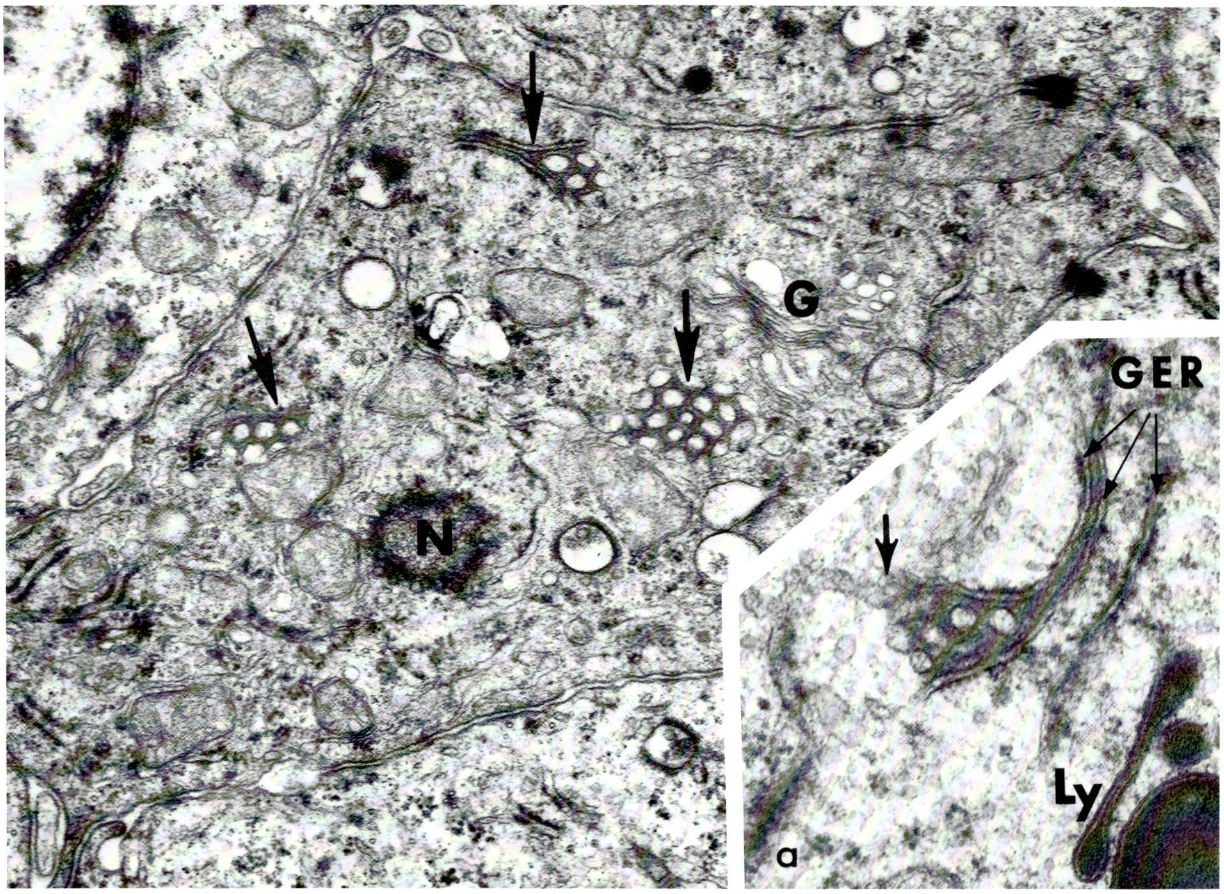

Figure 87. *On the 23rd day of the cycle,* several cells contain "alveolate" structures (arrows), composed of agranular vesicles surrounded by an electron-dense amorphous matrix. These structures are in close relationship with membranes of granular endoplasmic reticulum and Golgi (G). × 35,1000. N: portion of tangentionally sectioned nucleus with nuclear pores.

Figure 87a. *Detailed view of "alveolate" structures.* Vesicles of uniform size and the surrounding dark matrix are partly enveloped by parallel membranes of granular endoplasmic reticulum (GER). Several smaller vesicles (arrow) and lysosomes (Ly) are seen in the immediate neighborhood. × 54,000.

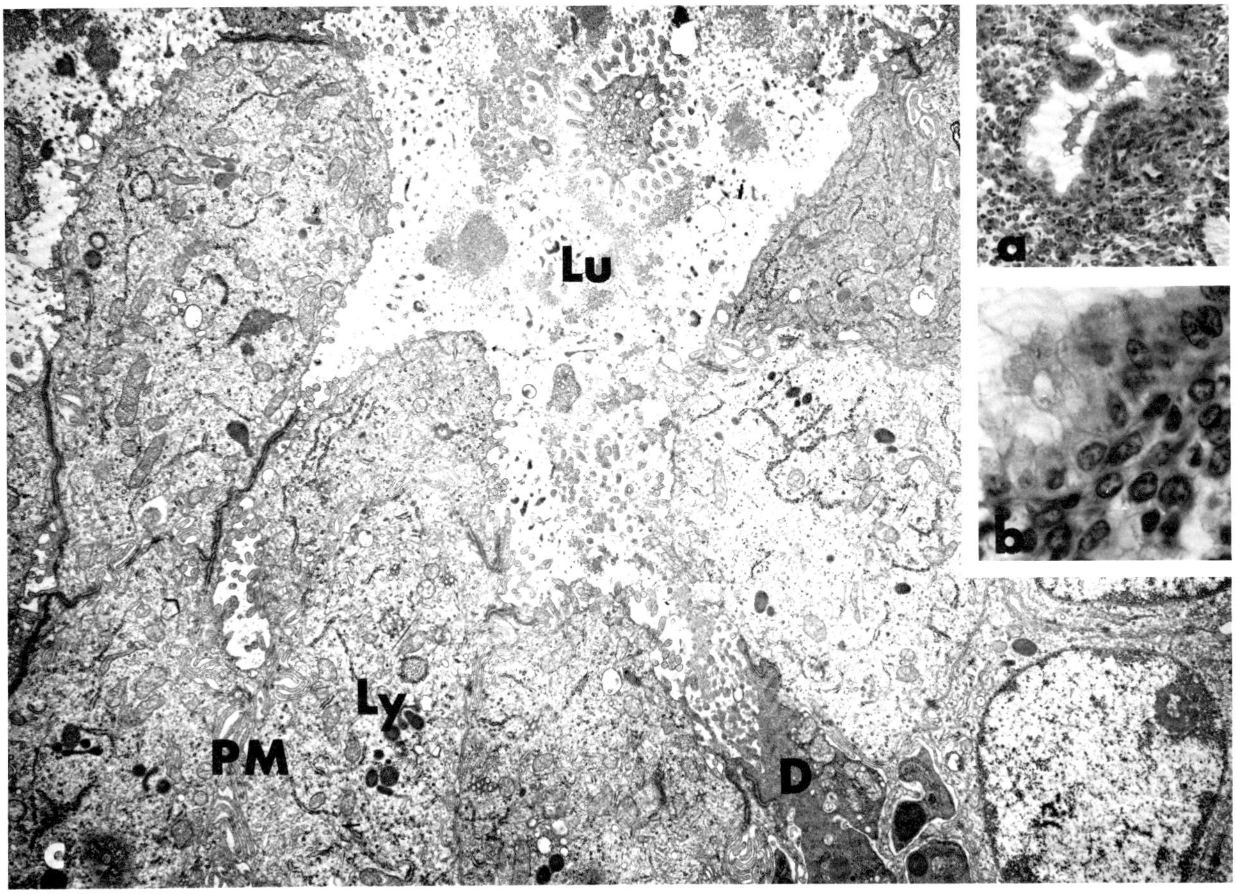

Figure 88a. *The accumulated intraluminal secretions,* a prominent feature of *the 24th day of the cycle,* contain glycogen, acid and neutral mucopolysaccharides, lipids, and various enzymes, including acid phosphatase.[1] Note the well-developed periarteriolar predecidua in the center of the photomicrograph. (H & E stain, × 30.)

Figure 88b. *Higher-power view* of the glandular lining epithelium containing prominent bulging of the apical cytoplasmic substance. (H & E stain,× 150.)

Figure 88c. *The glandular cells themselves contain the submicroscopic features* of involuting secretory activity, as indicated by regression of the Golgi with a decrease in the number of vesicles and ribosomes[2,3] and by the presence of several electron-dense degenerating cells (D). Clusters of membrane-bound lysosomes (Ly) appear. Large portions of the apical cytoplasm protrude into the glandular lumen (Lu), and the luminal microvilli appear short and scant. The lumen contains detached fragments of cytoplasm and finely granular material. The lateral plasma membranes (PM) are extremely convoluted, and the intercellular space has numerous interdigitating microvilli. × 5600.

REFERENCES (Figures 87–88c)

1. Henzl, M. R., R. E. Smith, G. Boost, and E. T. Tyler. Lysosomal concept of menstrual bleeding in humans. *J. Clin. Endocrinol. Metab.* **34:** 360 (1972).
2. Cavazos, F., J. A. Green, D. G. Hall, and F. V. Lucas. Ultrastructure of the human endometrial glandular cell during the menstrual cycle. *Am. J. Obstet. Gynecol.* **99:** 833 (1967).
3. Sengel, A. and P. Stoebner. Ultrastructure of the normal human endometrium. II. The glandular cells. *Z. Zellforsch.* **109:** 260 (1970).

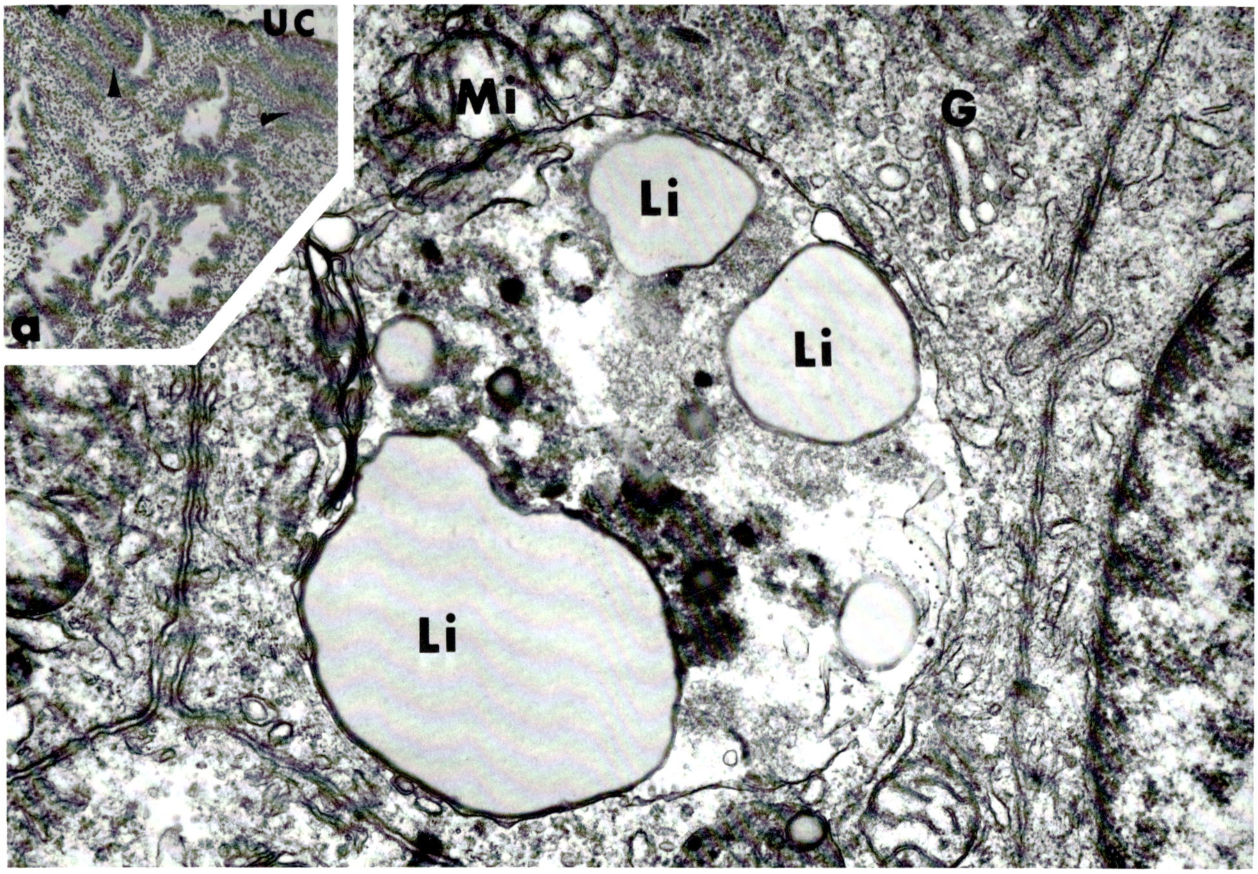

From *the 25th day,* most of the cells lack glycogen and microfilamentous systems. Acid phosphatase-containing lysosomes and Golgi [1-3] become abundant and pleomorphic,[4-6] corresponding to the high acid phosphatase levels found by earlier investigators.[7] In the late luteal phase, hydrolytic enzyme secretion involves the lateral plasma membranes, desmosomes, and basal lamina.[6] The elevated levels of acid phosphatase are thought to be the result of the increased permeability of the lysosomal membranes due to the effect of progesterone in the luteal phase.[6] The increase in lysosomal activity (autocytolysosomes) is believed to be associated with focal cytoplasmic membranes due to the effect of progesterone in the luteal phase.[6] The increase in lysosomal activity (autocytolysosomes) is believed to be associated with focal cytoplasmic degeneration[6] and perhaps with autoregulation of excess secretory material.[1,5] Focal (and eventually total) cell degeneration with expulsion of the cellular debris into the lumen occurs increasingly as the cycle approaches the menstrual period.[5]

Figure 89a. *Histologically, the 25th day of the cycle* is characterized by the development of subsurface (UC) predecidua (arrow heads), and the glands have numerous intraluminal projections, resulting in the so-called saw-tooth pattern. (H & E stain, × 30.)

Figure 89. *The 25th day of the cycle.* Electron photomicrograph of a prominent autocytolysosome containing lipid droplets (Li) and fragments of ingested cytoplasmic debris. × 25,600. G: Golgi; Mi: mitochondria.

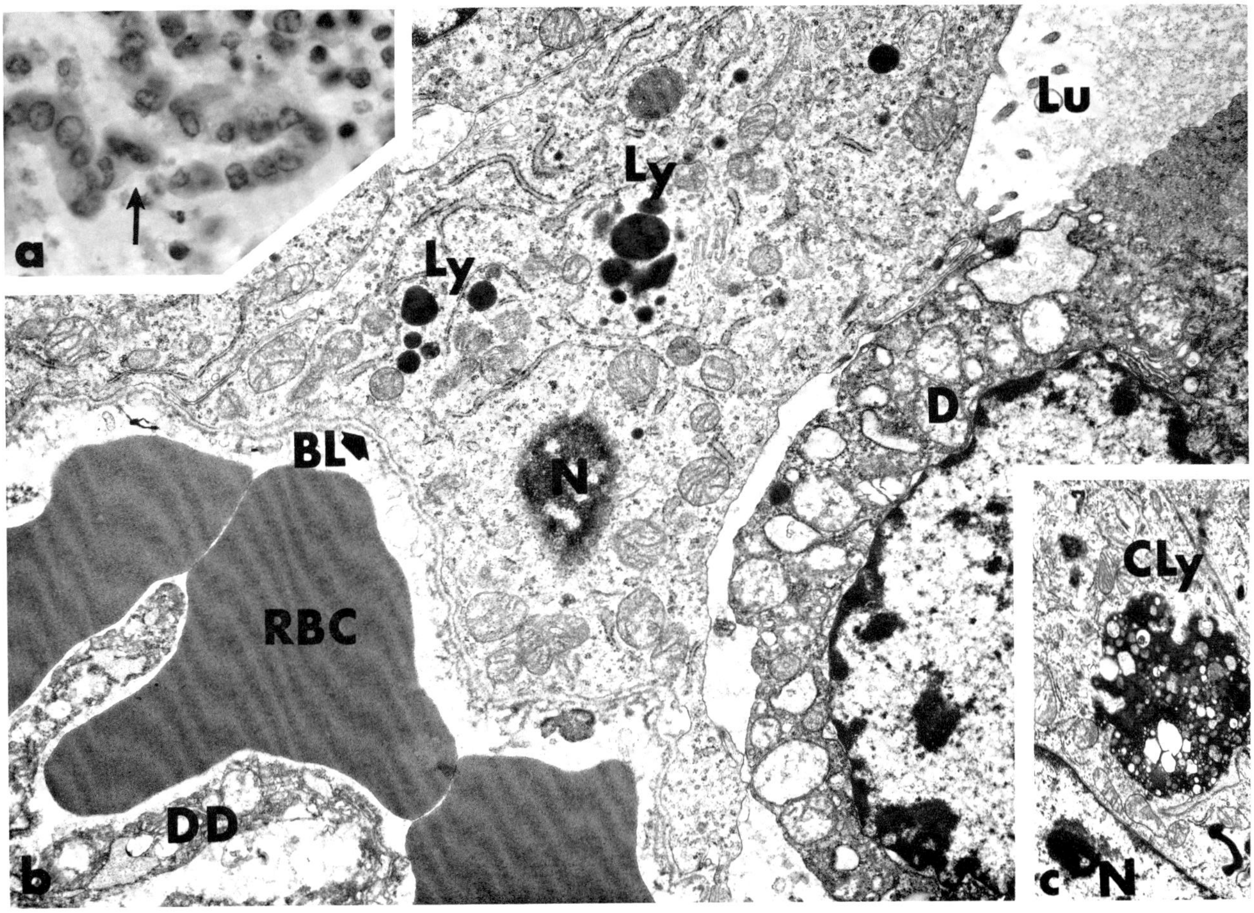

Figure 90a. *Histologically, the early menstrual endometrium* has focal areas of subepithelial stromal degeneration, with or without extravasated red blood cells. Many of the glands are collapsed (arrow), and there are numerous intraluminal and intraepithelial leukocytes and cellular debris. From the second menstrual day, there is a massive collapse of the entire endometrium, resulting in an intermixture of stromal and glandular elements with leukoerythrocytic debris.

Figure 90b. *Ultrastructurally,* many of the glandular cells are degenerated (D) with vacuolated organelles and widened intercellular spaces with loss of desmosomal attachments, leading to cellular collapse.[6] The adjacent, apparently intact, glandular cells contain aggregates of lysosomes (Ly), and the stroma contains extravasated red blood cells (RBC) and degenerated predecidual elements (DD). × 6400. Lu: glandular lumen; N: portion of nucleus; BL: basal lamina.

Figure 90c. *On the 2nd and 3rd menstrual days,* rupture of the basal lamina with disruption of the glandular cells, cytolysosomes (CLy), and heterolysosomes is noted.[5,6] × 5600. N: nucleus.

REFERENCES (From the 25th day–Figure 90c)

1. Sirtori, C. Some ultrastructural aspects of human uterine physiopathology: cyclosenility, senility, antisenile and antitumoral therapies, and contraceptive drugs. In *Proceedings of International Symposium on Obstetrics and Gynaecology,* J. A. Chalmers, R. Merger, and G. B. Candiani (Eds.). Carlo Erba Foundation, Milan, 1969, pp. 129–154.
2. Sawaragi, I. and R. M. Wynn. Ultrastructural localization of metabolic enzymes during the human endometrial cycle. *Obstet. Gynecol.* **34:** 50 (1969).
3. Bitensky, L. and S. Cohen. The variation of endometrial acid phosphatase activity with the menstrual cycle. *J. Obstet. Gynaecol. Brit. Commonw.* **72:** 769 (1965).
4. Cavazos, F., J. A. Green, D. G. Hall, and F. V. Lucas. Ultrastructure of the human endometrial glandular cell during the menstrual cycle. *Am. J. Obstet. Gynecol.* **99:** 833 (1967).
5. Sengel, A. and P. Stoebner. Ultrastructure of the normal human endometrium. II. The glandular cells. *Z. Zellforsch.* **109:** 260 (1970).
6. Henzl, M. R., R. E. Smith, G. Boost, and E. T. Tyler. Lysosomal concept of menstrual bleeding in humans. *J. Clin. Endocrinol Metab.* **34:** 360 (1972).
7. McKay, D. B., A. T. Hertig, W. A. Bardawil, and J. T. Velardo. Histochemical observations on the endometrium. I. Normal endometrium. *Obstet. Gynecol.* **8:** 22 (1956).

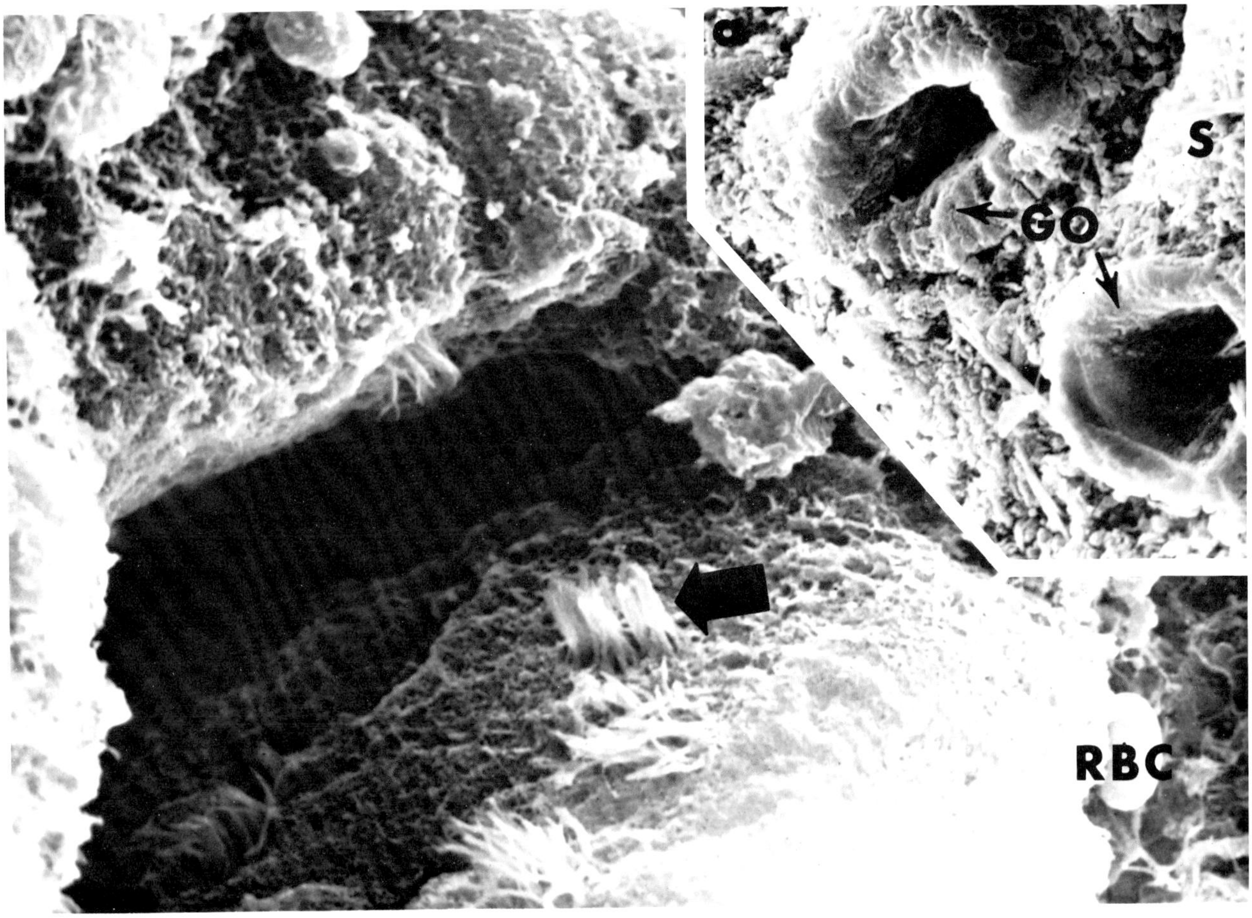

Figure 91a. *Scanning electron microscopic appearance of the glands in the zona basalis during the 2nd to 3rd days of menstruation.* The glands have prominent openings (GO), and the stroma (S) is covered by cellular debris. × 160.

Figure 91. *Higher magnification of a glandular opening of the 2nd to 3rd menstrual days.* The presence of well-developed ciliated cells (arrow) in this period suggests that endometrial ciliogenesis may begin as early as the 2nd or 3rd day of the menstrual period.[1] × 1920. RBC: red blood cells. *From* A. Ferenczy and R. M. Richart. Scanning and transmission electron microscopy of the human endometrial surface epithelium. *J. Clin. Endocrinol. Metab.* **36:** 999–1008 (1973).

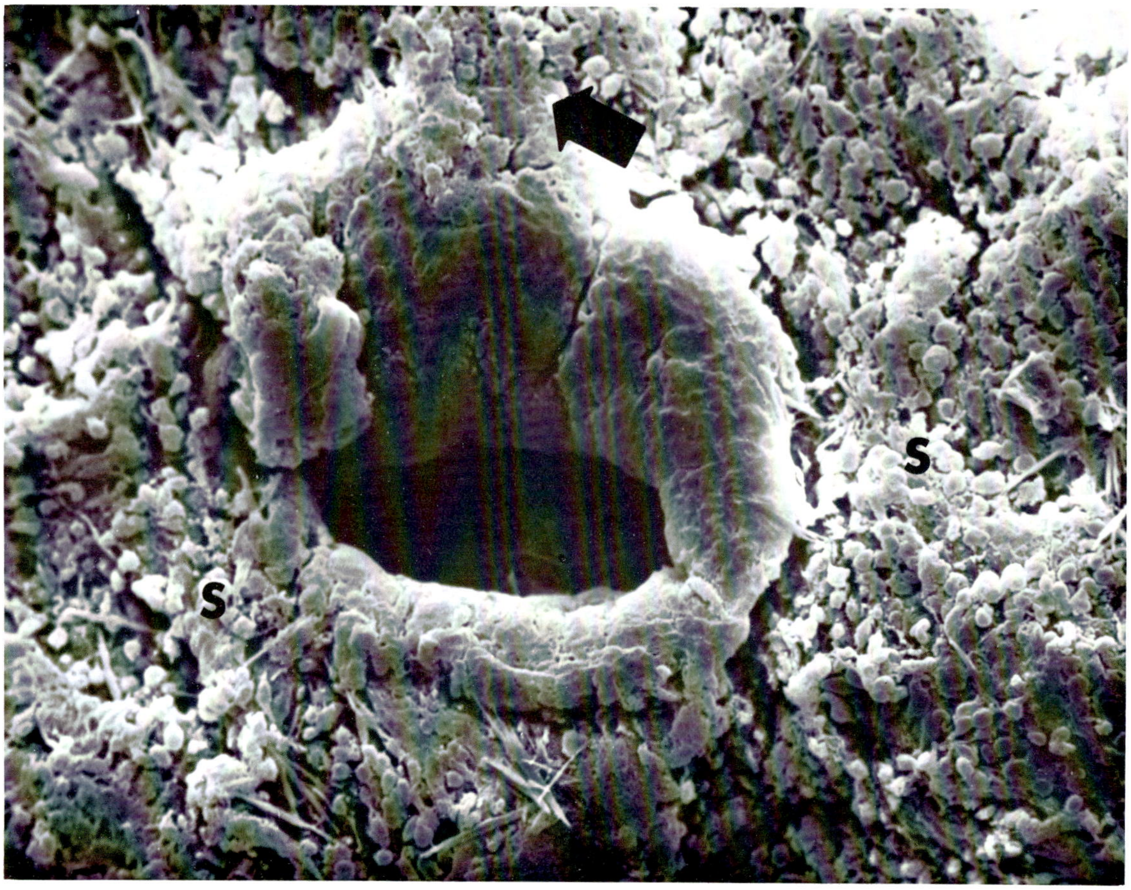

Figure 92. *On the 2nd to 3rd days of menstruation,*[1,2] several glands in the remaining basalis are greatly dilated with epithelial extensions (arrow) onto the surrounding stroma (S), suggesting early reepithelialization. × 600. *From* A. Ferenczy, R. M. Richart, F. J. Agate, Jr., M. L. Purkerson, and E. W. Dempsey. Scanning electron microscopy of the human endometrial surface epithelium. *Fertil. Steril.* **23:** 515–521 (1972).

REFERENCES (Figures 91–92)

1. Ferenczy, A. and R. M. Richart. Scanning and transmission electron microscopy of the human endometrial surface epithelium. *J. Clin. Endocrinol. Metab.* **36:** 999 (1973).
2. Ferenczy, A., R. M. Richart, F. J. Agate, Jr., M. L. Purkerson, and E. W. Dempsey. Scanning electron microscopy of the human endometrial surface epithelium. *Fertil. Steril.* **23:** 515 (1972).

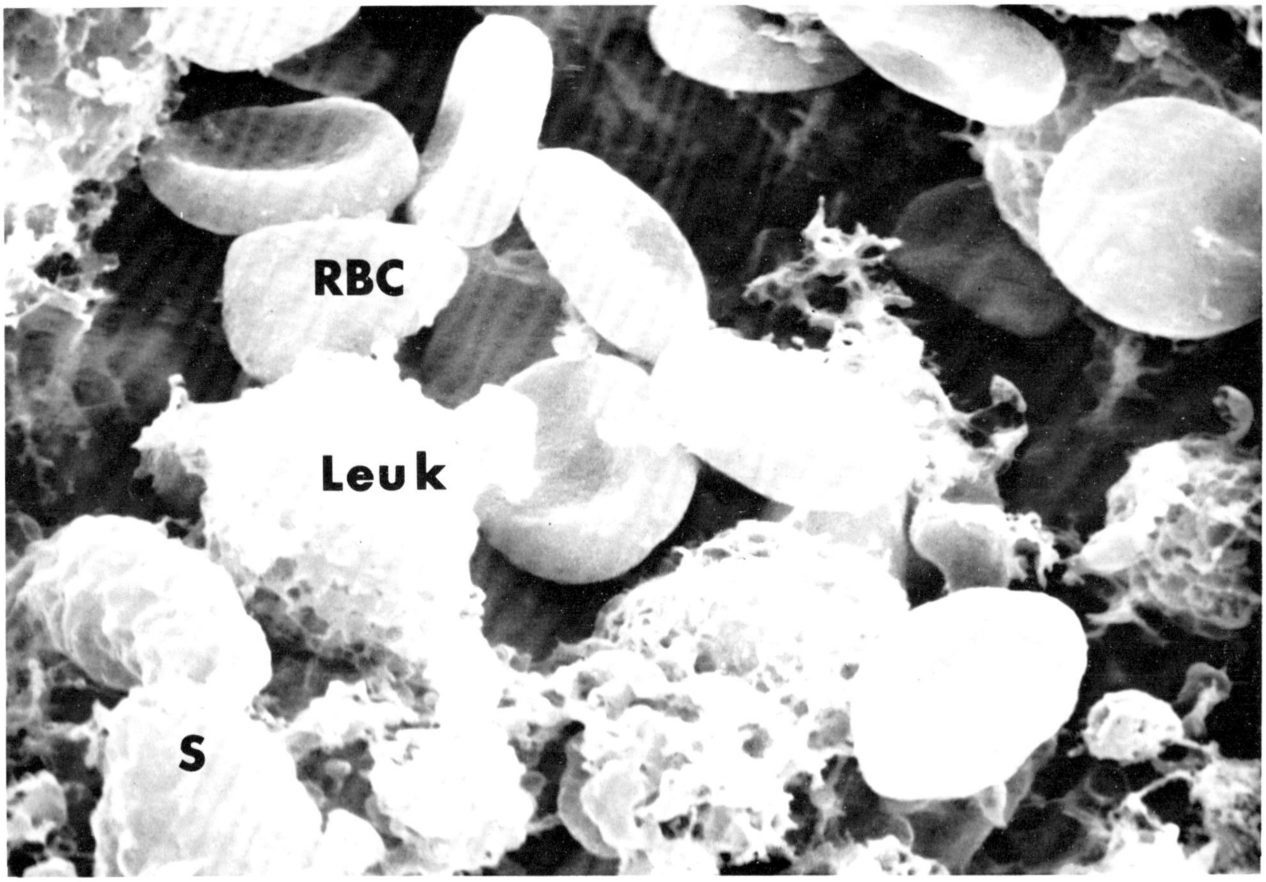

Figure 93. *Scanning electron microscopy of menstrual blood.* Well-preserved red blood cells (RBC) devoid of fibrin network intermingle freely with leukocytes (Leuk) and degenerated stromal cells (S). × 4800.

MENSTRUAL BLOOD

Both scanning and transmission electron microscopic examinations of the menstrual endometrium and blood confirm the premise[1] that menstrual blood does not clot,[2] presumably because the high fibrinolytic activity[3] inhibits the formation of fibrin polymers.

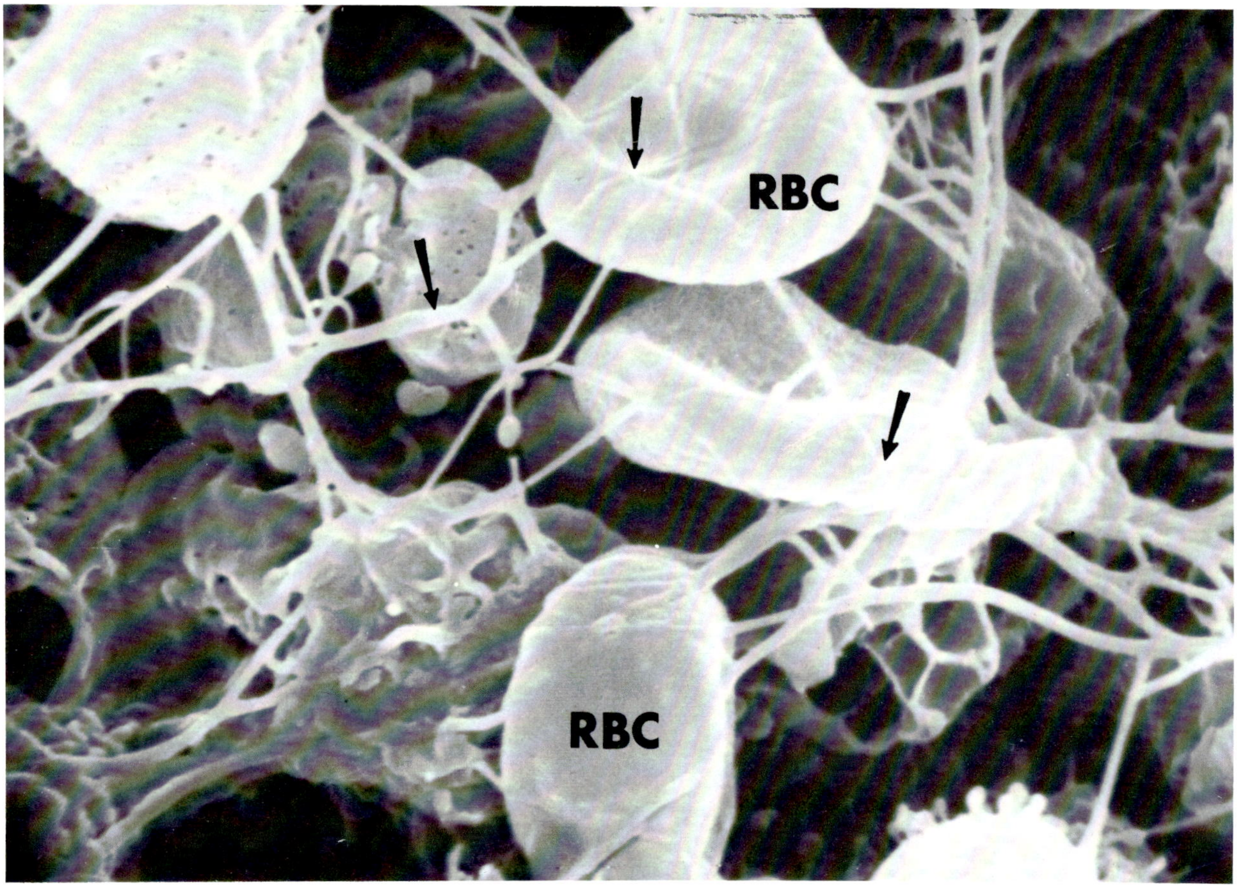

Figure 94. *Scanning electron micrograph of normal blood clot.* In contrast to menstrual blood, coagulated blood contains red blood cells (RBC) that are enmeshed in a delicate fibrin network (arrows). × 6400.

REFERENCES (Both scanning and transmission—Figure 94)

1. Beller, F. K. Observations on the clotting of menstrual blood and clot formation. *Am. J. Obstet. Gynecol.* **111:** 535 (1971).
2. Ferenczy, A. and R. M. Richart. Scanning and transmission electron microscopy of the human endometrial surface epithelium. *J. Clin. Endocrinol. Metab.* **36:** 183 (1973).
3. Schmidt-Matthiesen, H. Die fibrinolytische Aktivität von Endometrium und Myometrium, Dezidua und Plazenta, Kollum- und Korpuskarzinomen. Physiologic, Pathologie und klinisch-therapeutische Konsequenzen. *Fortschr. Geburtsch. Gynaekol.* **31:** 1 (1967).

SURFACE EPITHELIUM

The uterine surface epithelium, at the light, histochemical,[1] transmission,[2-6] and scanning[7-11] electron microscopic levels, is dissimilar[7,8] to its glandular counterpart during the second half of the menstrual cycle. Specific dissimilarities include a greater number of ciliated cells,[7,8] the earlier appearance and longer persistence of intracytoplasmic glycogen, and a constant rate of RNA synthesis.[1]

The uterine lining epithelium does not undergo major morphologic cellular alterations in response to the cyclic hormonal stimuli, and in this regard it bears a close resemblance to the tubal mucosa, in which secretory activity and ciliogenesis experience minimal cyclic changes.[12] Since cellular modifications in the endometrium are hormone dependent, it is possible that the surface epithelium has a different sensitivity to hormonal stimuli from that of the glandular epithelium, reflecting different cellular functions which, in both the uterine and the tubal lining epithelium, are related to the mobility, nutrition, and reception of sperm and blastocysts.[7,8,13]

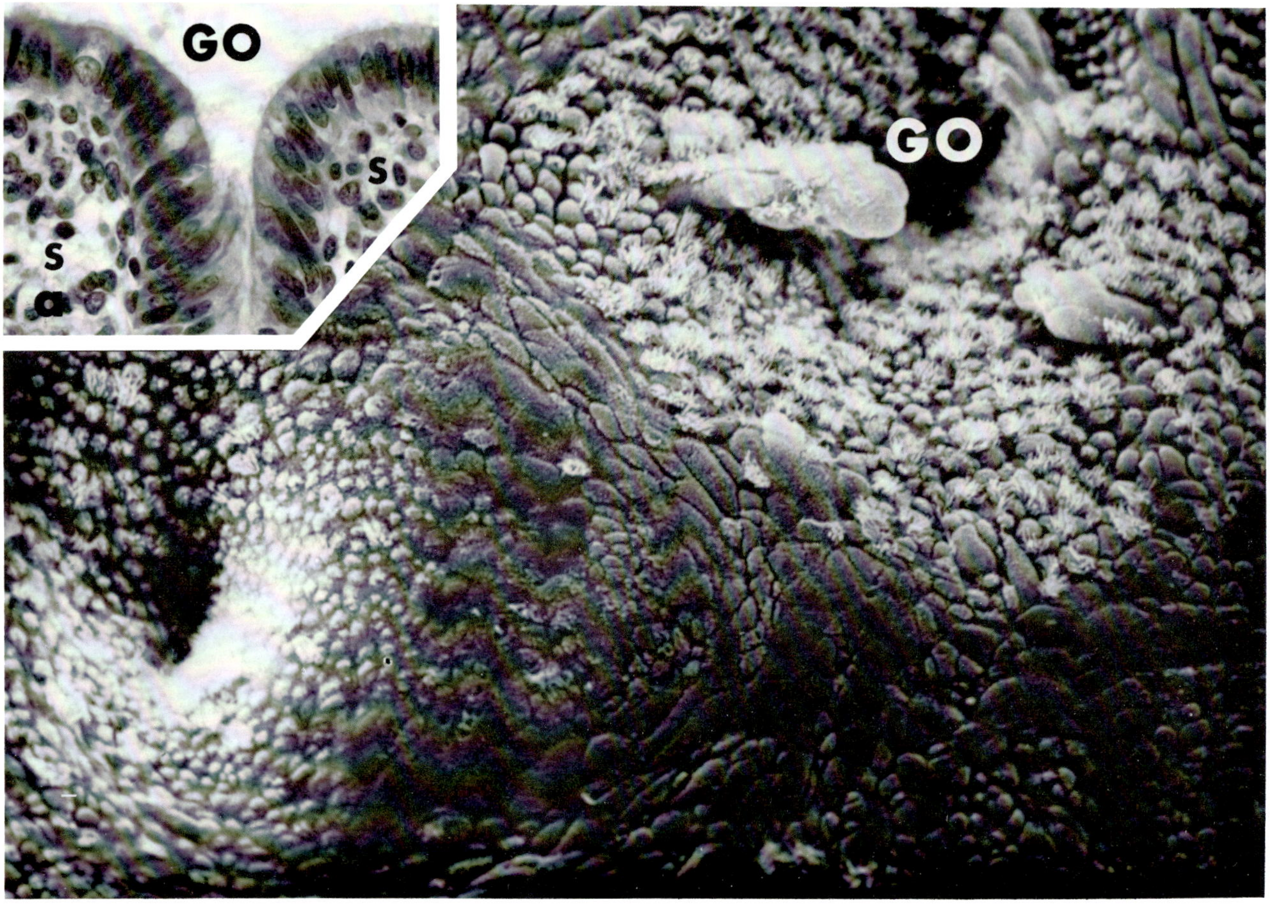

Figure 95a. *Microscopically, during the early proliferative phase (4–7th days) of the cycle,* the epithelium forming the glandular opening (GO) has numerous ciliated cells. (H & E stain, × 120.) S: subepithelial stroma.

Figure 95. *Early proliferative endometrium.* The surface contains two circular openings (GO), characteristically surrounded by numerous ciliated cells. × 800. *From* A. Ferenczy and R. M. Richart. Scanning and transmission electron microscopy of the human endometrial surface epithelium. *J. Clin. Endocrinol. Metab.* **36:** 999–1008 (1973).

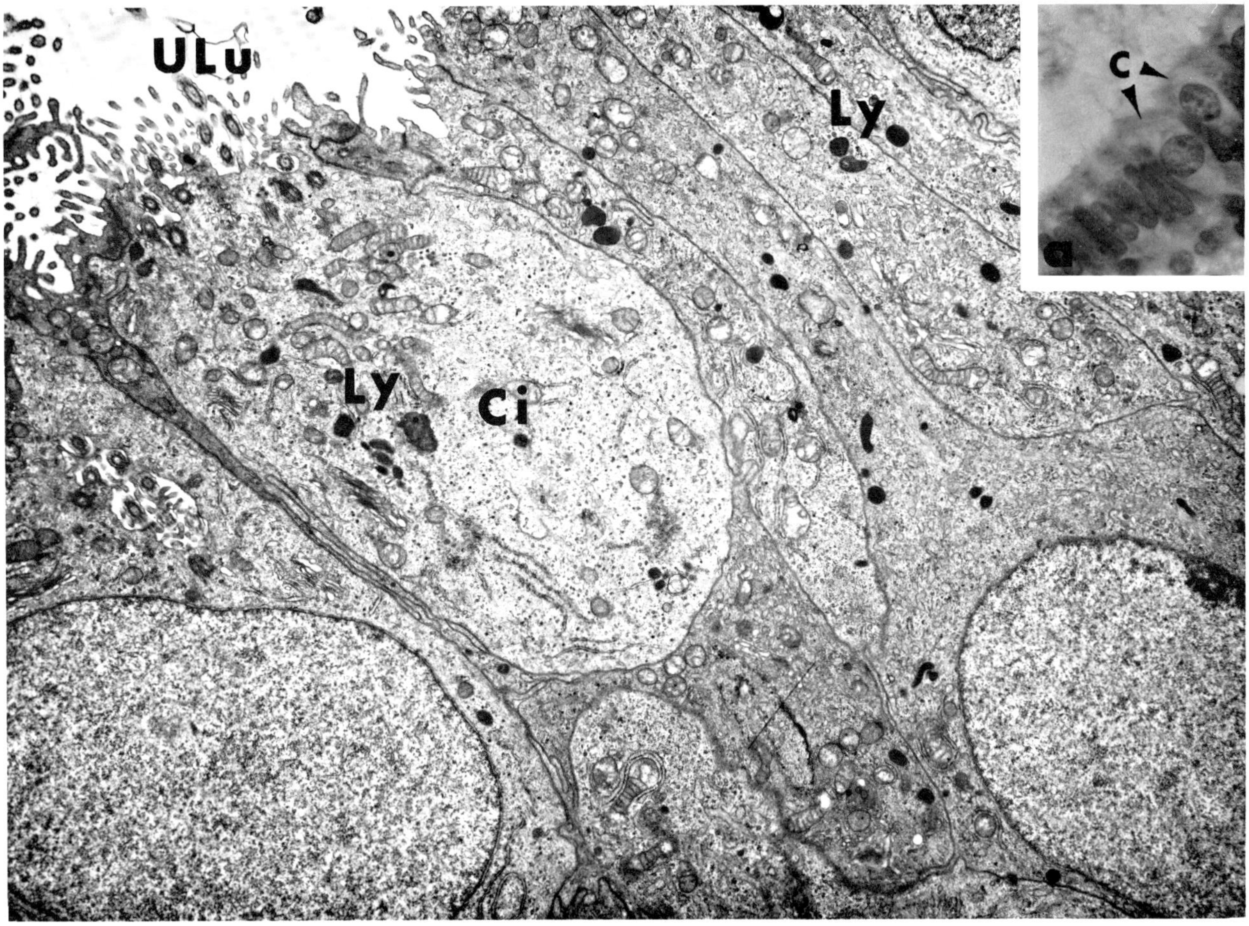

Figure 96a. *Early proliferative phase of the cycle.* High-power view of the endometrial surface epithelium, containing tall columnar, ciliated cells (C) with pale cytoplasm and centrally located round nuclei. (H & E stain, × 120.)

Figure 96. *Early proliferative endometrium.* Slightly oblique section of the surface epithelium, containing two light-ciliated (Ci) and narrow, columnar, nonciliated cells (right) with numerous membrane-bound dense bodies (Ly) and relatively few organelles. Short bundles of microfilaments are seen in the nonciliated cells. × 3600. ULu: uterine lumen. *From* A. Ferenczy and R. M. Richart. Scanning and transmission electron microscopy of the human endometrial surface epithelium. *J. Clin. Endocrinol. Metab.* **36:** 999–1008 (1973).

REFERENCES (The uterine surface epithelium—Figure 96)

1. Dallenbach-Hellweg, G. *Histopathology of the Endometrium.* Springer-Verlag, New York, 1971.
2. Wynn, R. M. and J. A. Harris. Ultrastructural cyclic changes in the human endometrium. I. Normal preovulatory phase. *Fertil. Steril.* **18:** 632 (1967).
3. Wetzstein, R. and H. Wagner. Elektronenmikroskopische Untersuchungen am menschlichen Endometrium. *Anat. Anz.* **108:** 362 (1960).
4. Bitensky, L. and S. Cohen. The variation of endometrial acid phosphatase activity with the menstrual cycle. *J. Obstet. Gynaecol. Brit. Commonw.* **72:** 769 (1965).
5. Fisher, W. Neuere Forschungsergebnisse am Endometrium. *Dtsch. Gesund. Wochenschr. Gesamt. Med.* **40:** 1714 (1963).
6. Komae, Y. Electron microscopic studies of the endometrium of the human uterus. *J. Jap. Obstet. Gynec. Soc.* **20:** 741 (1968).
7. Ferenczy, A., R. M. Richart, F. J. Agate, Jr., M. L. Purkerson, and E. W. Dempsey. Scanning electron microscopy of the human endometrial surface epithelium. *Fertil. Steril.* **23:** 515 (1972).
8. Ferenczy, A. and R. M. Richart. Scanning and transmission electron microscopy of the human endometrial surface epithelium. *J. Clin. Endocrinol Metab.* **36:** 999 (1973).
9. Nilsson, O. and K. G. Nygren. Scanning electron microscopy of human endometrium. *Upsala J. Med. Sci.* **77:** 3 (1972).
10. Morgenroth, K. and A. Verhagen. Submicroscopic surface structure of the endometrium. *Arch. Gynaekol.* **212:** 30 (1972).
11. Johannisson, E. and L. Nilsson. Scanning electron microscopic study of the human endometrium. *Fertil. Steril.* **23:** 613 (1972).
12. Ferenczy, A., R. M. Richart, F. J. Agate, Jr., M. L. Purkerson, and E. W. Dempsey. Scanning electron microscopy of the human Fallopian tube. *Science* **175:** 783 (1972).
13. Ferenczy, A. and R. M. Richart. Scanning electron microscopy of the human female genital tract. *N.Y. State J. Med.* (in press).

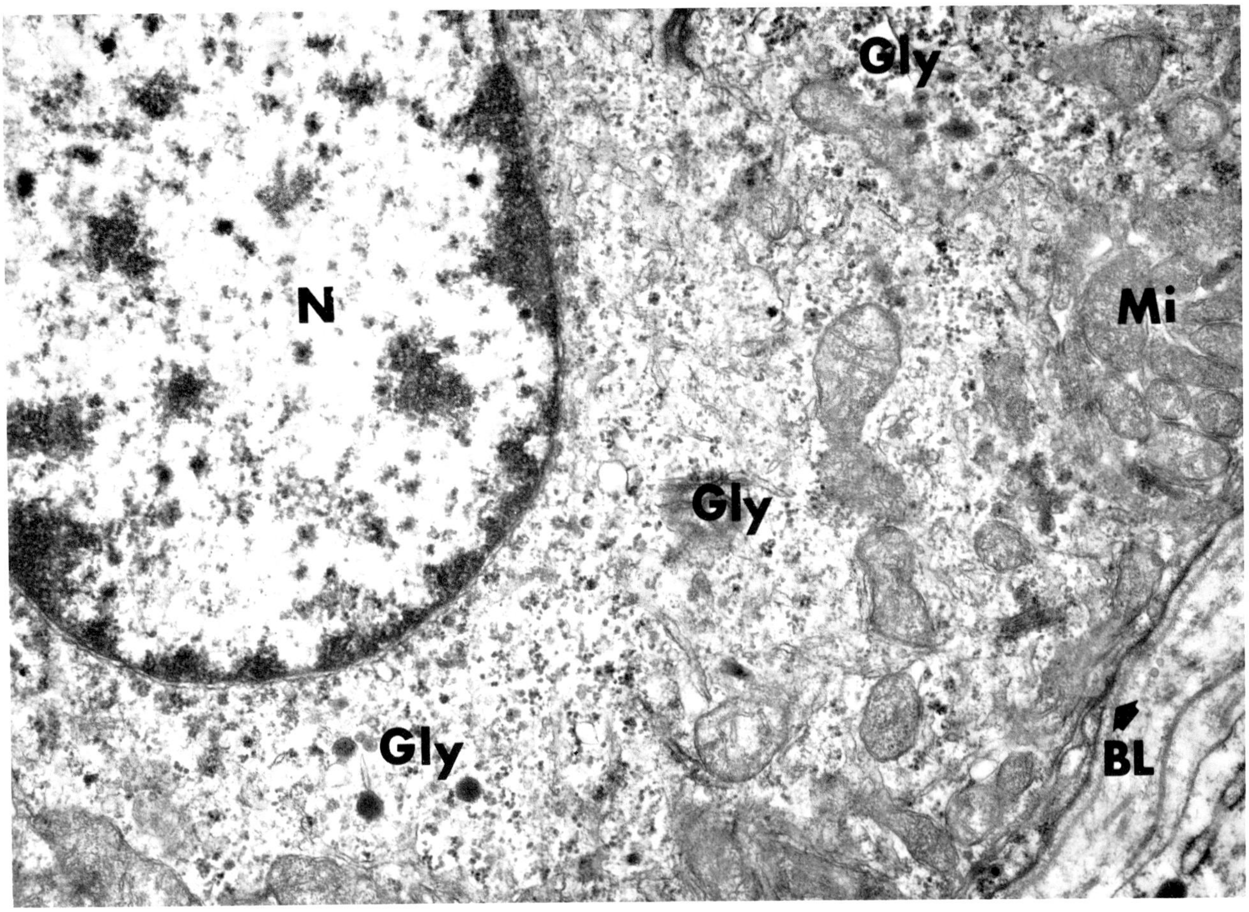

Figure 97. *Mid-proliferative endometrium.* About the 12th day of the cycle, subnuclear (N) crowding of mitochondria (Mi) and the precocious appearance of glycogen granules (Gly) are noted. × 11,600. BL: basal lamina. *From* A. Ferenczy and R. M. Richart. Scanning and transmisison electron microscopy of the human endometrial surface epithelium. *J. Clin. Endocrinol. Metab.* **36:** 183–192 (1973).

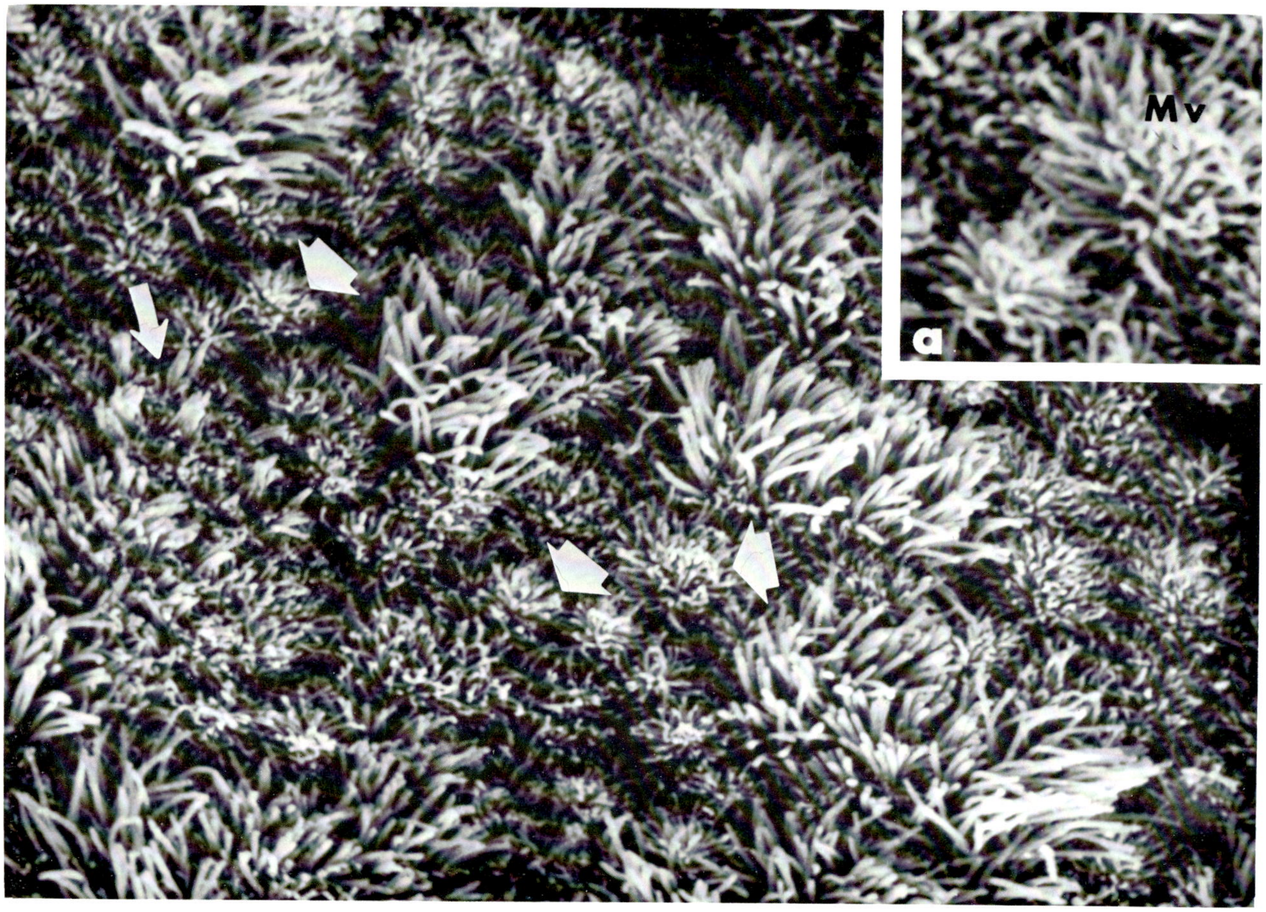

Figure 98. *Late proliferative phase.* In addition to the periosteal concentration of ciliated cells (early proliferative phase), during the mid-proliferative and late proliferative phases numerous ciliated cells are also seen in the interglandular zones of the endometrial surface. Generation of new cilia is observed in several cells (long arrow). The nonciliated cells are covered by abundant and well-developed microvilli, resembling microvillous promontories (short arrows). × 3200.

Figure 98a. *Higher magnification* of a microvillous promontory in which the microvilli (Mv) are slender and occasionally interbranhcing. × 6400.

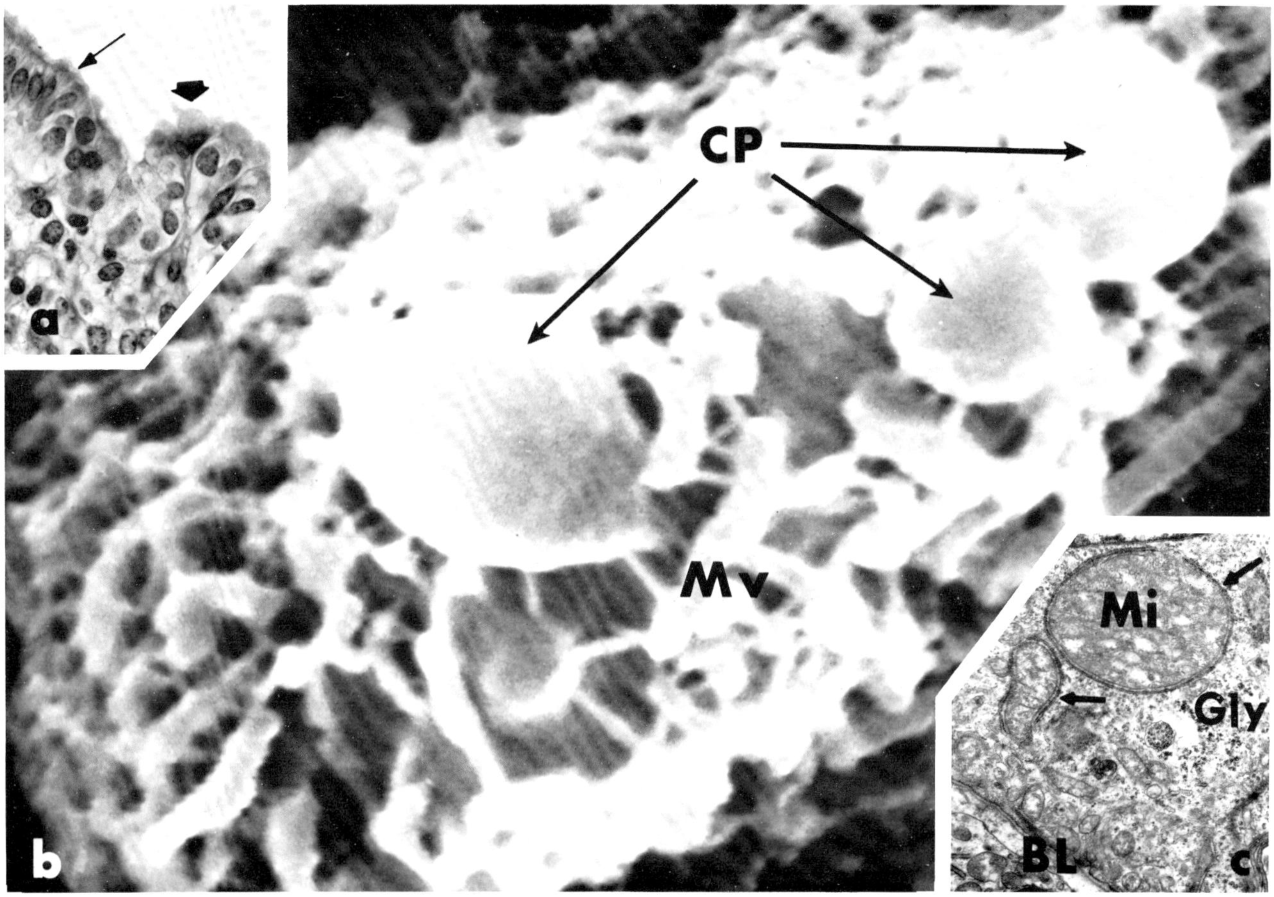

Figure 99a. *On the 22nd day of the menstrual cycle,* the endometrial surface epithelium is tall columnar, with numerous ciliated cells (long arrow) and other cell types having prominent apical cytoplasmic protrusions (short arrow) that denote an apocrine secretion. (H & E stain, × 120.)

Figure 99b. *Scanning electron microscopic appearance* of apocrine secretions which occurs on the endometrial surface between the 20th and 24th days.[1,2] A secretory cell on the 22nd day of the cycle contains three apical cytoplasmic protuberances (CP) that are rich in glycogen, acid mucopolysaccharides, and several enzymes, providing an optimal environment for sperm and blastocysts. The microvilli (Mv) are shorter and fewer than those in the proliferative phase of the cycle. × 25,600.

Figure 99c. *On the 21st day of the menstrual cycle,* subnuclear giant mitochondria (Mi), in close association with membranes of granular endoplasmic reticulum (arrows) and glycogen particles (Gly), are observed. These subcellular modifications in both the surface and the glandular endometrial cells reflect the effect of progesterone. × 6200. BL: basal lamina. *From* A. Ferenczy and R. M. Richart. Scanning and transmission electron microscopy of the human endometrial surface epithelium. *J. Clin. Endocrinol. Metab.* **36:** 999–1008 (1973).

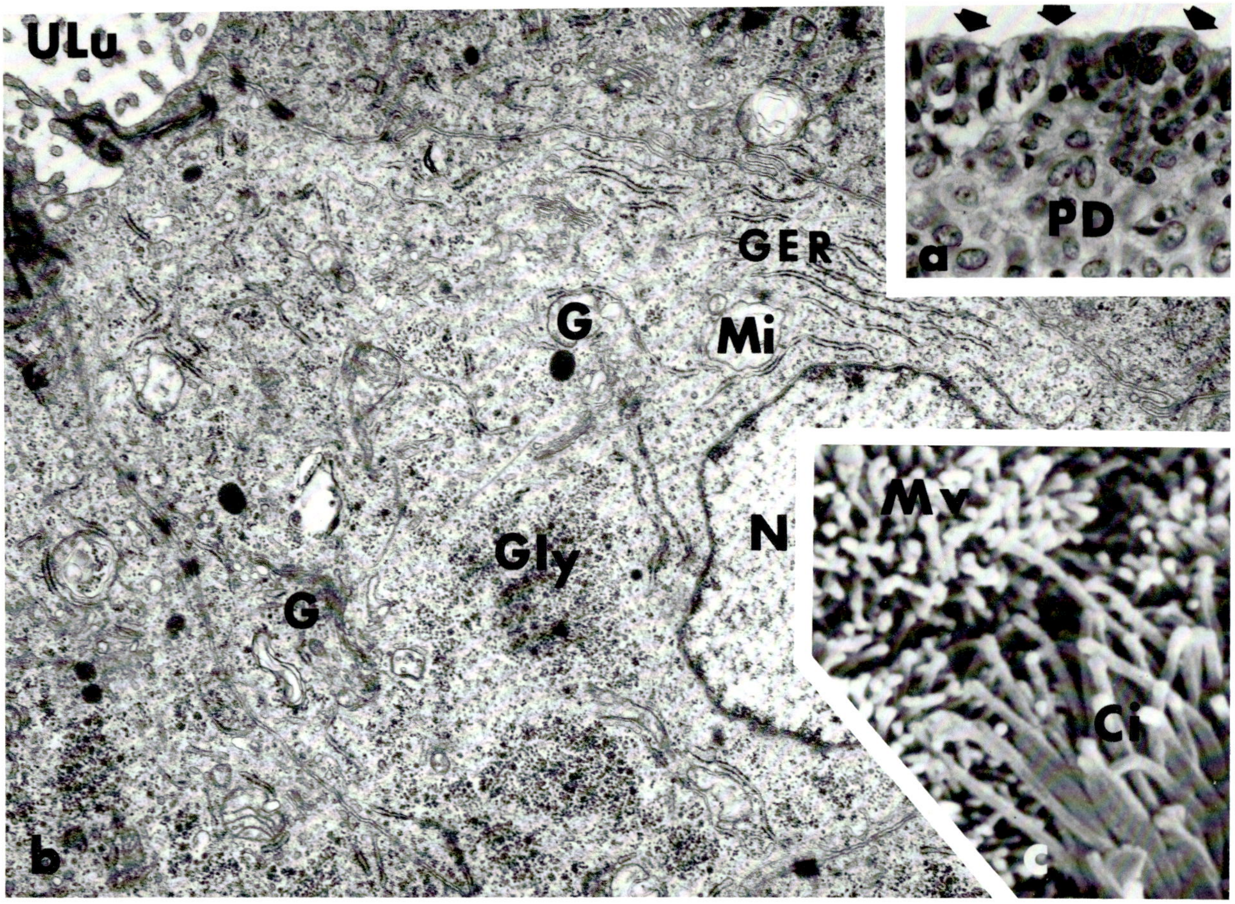

Figure 100a. *On the 26th day of the menstrual cycle,* the endometrial surface epithelium remains tall columnar with numerous ciliated cells (arrows). (H & E stain, × 120.) PD: subepithelial predecidua.

Figure 100b. *The 26th day secretory endometrium.* Collections of supranuclear (N) glycogen granules (Gly) are associated with granular endoplasmic reticulum (GER) and Golgi (G). × 16,900. ULu: uterine lumen; Mi: mitochondria. *From* A. Ferenczy and R. M. Richart. Scanning and transmission electron microscopy of the human endometrial surface epithelium. *J. Clin. Endocrinol. Metab.* **36:** 999 (1972).

Figure 100c. *The 27th day of the menstrual cycle.* Note the persistent presence of ciliated cells (Ci) with well-developed ciliary shafts and the adjacent secretory cells with well-preserved, but shorter and less branching, microvillous projections (Mv), as compared to the microvilli of the preovulatory period. × 8000.

REFERENCES (Figures 99a–100c)

1. Ferenczy, A., R. M. Richart, F. J. Agate, Jr., M. L. Purkerson, and E. W. Dempsey. Scanning electron microscopy of the human endometrial surface epithelium. *Fertil. Steril.* **23:** 515 (1972).
2. Ferenczy, A. and R. M. Richart. Scanning and transmission electron microscopy of the human endometrial surface epithelium. *J. Clin. Endocrinol. Metab.* **36:** 999 (1973).

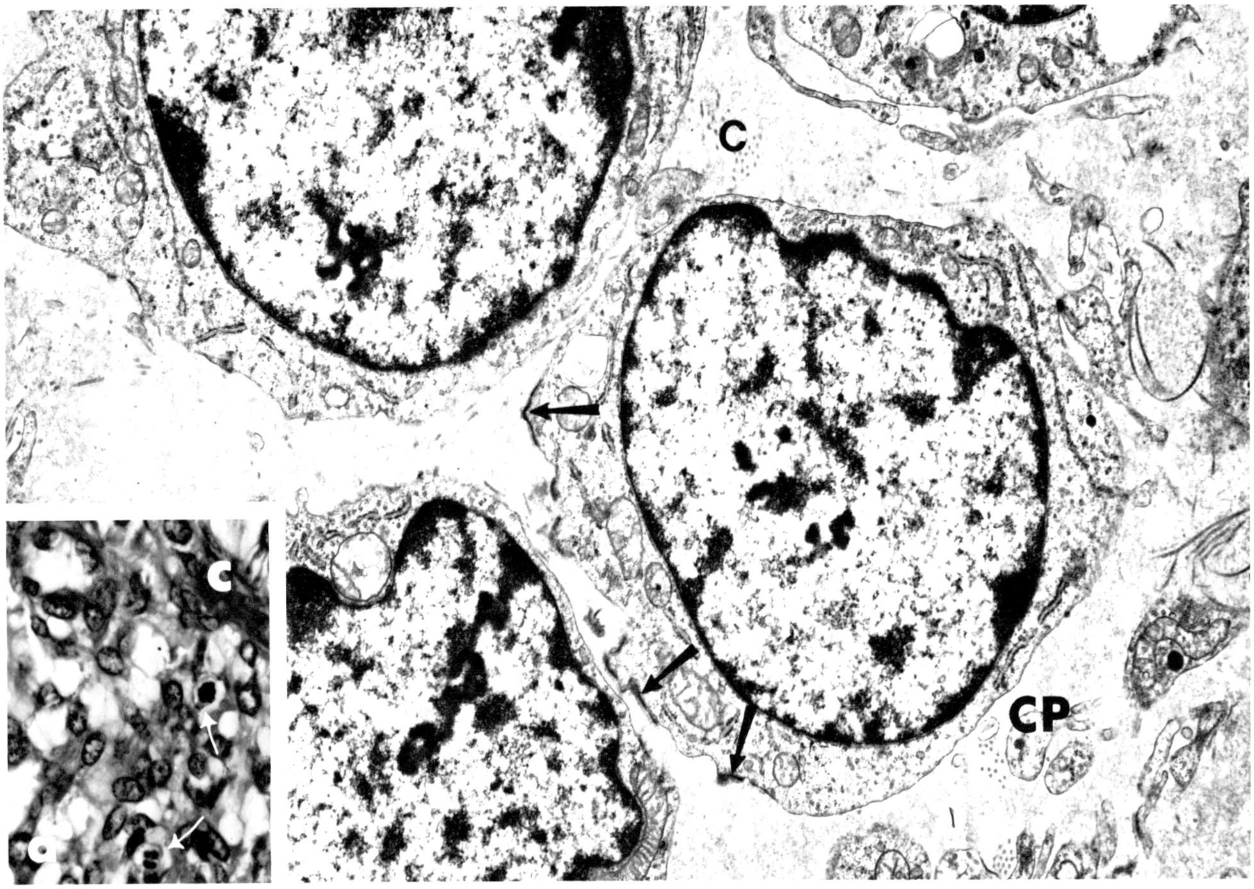

ENDOMETRIAL STROMA

The endometrial mesenchymal cells and vasculature undergo hormonally stimulated cyclical variations, characterized by proliferation, differentiation, and maturation.[1]

Figure 101a. *In the early proliferative phase,* the stromal cells have an immature, spindle-shaped appearance with stellate cytoplasmic processes. The cytoplasm is scant, and nuclear DNA synthesis is the dominant feature. The intercellular stroma is loose and myxoid. (H & E stain, × 120.) C: intercellular collagen.

Figure 101. *Transverse section of stromal cells in the immediately postmenstrual period.* The nuclei are prominent with peripheral condensation of the nuclear heterochromatin. The scant cytoplasmic substance contains few organelles, and the plasma membrane has occasional dense bodies (arrows). A basal lamina is absent from endometrial stromal cells. × 11,200. CP: cross-sectioned cytoplasmic processes; C: intercellular collagen.

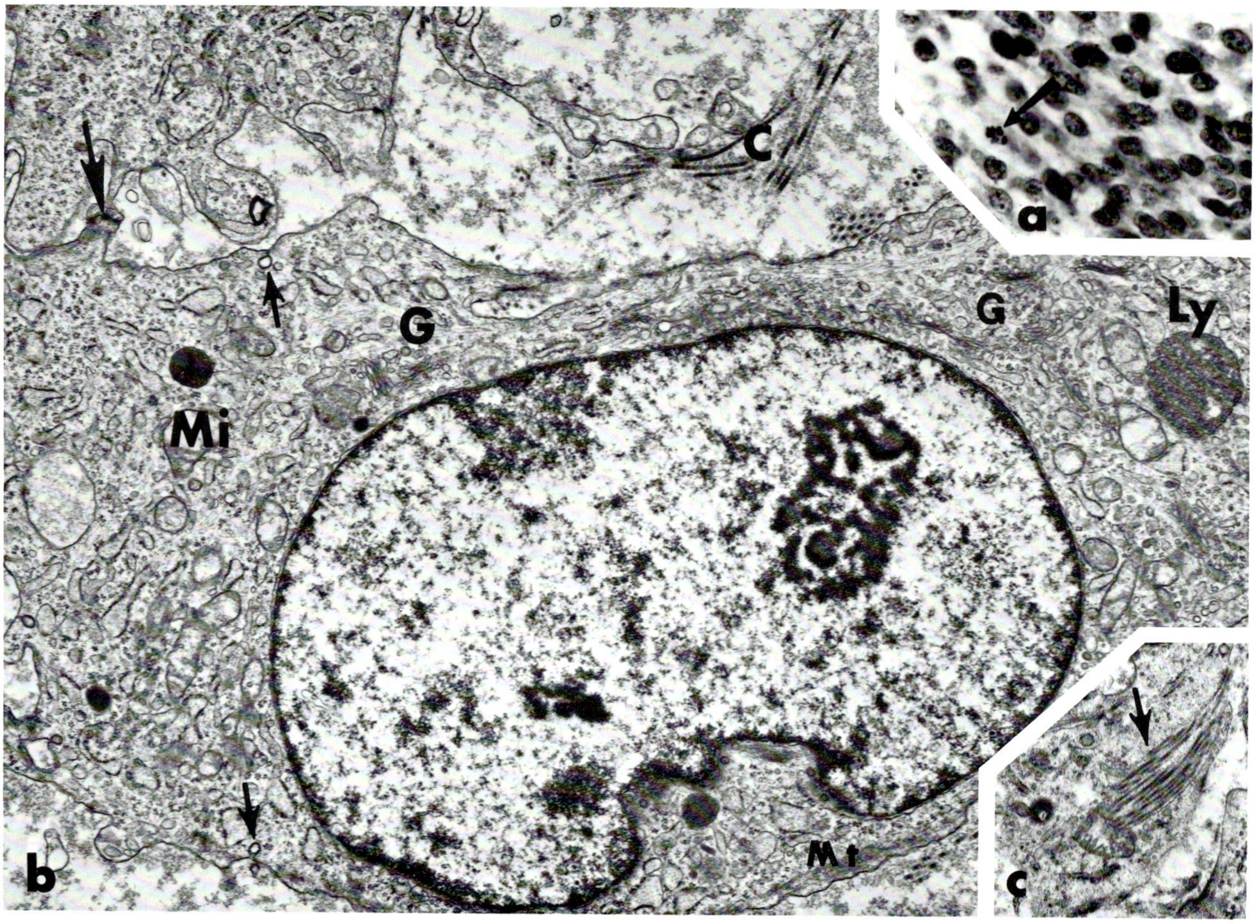

Figure 102a. *In the mid-proliferative phase,* the rapid development of cytoplasmic RNA synthesis begins and there is increased mitotic activity (arrow). (H & E stain, × 120.)

Figure 102b. *Ultrastructurally,* the stromal cells resemble mature fibroblasts, as indicated by the striking increase in mitochondria (Mi), granular endoplasmic reticulum, Golgi (G), and free ribosomes and the appearance of both intracytoplasmic tropocollagen (Mf) and pericellular collagen fibers (C).[1-6] The production of collagen is considered to be the primary function of the endometrial stromal cells, which thus provide supporting tissue for the endometrial glands.[1] × 12,600. Ly: lysosome; small arrows: pinocytic vesicles; large arrows: intercellular attachment complex.

Figure 102c. *Mid-proliferative phase.* Collagen fibers (arrow) are often formed within deep intracytoplasmic recesses in direct contact with the cytoplasmic matrix. × 6800.

REFERENCES (The endometrial mesenchymal cells—Figure 102c)

1. Wienke, E. C., F. Cavazos, D. G. Hall, and F. V. Lucas. Ultrastructure of the human endometrial stroma cell during the menstrual cycle. *Am. J. Obstet. Gynecol.* **102:** 65 (1968).
2. Wetzstein, R. and H. Wagner. Elektronenmikroskopische Untersuchungen am menschlichen Endometrium. *Anat. Anz.* **108:** 362 (1960).
3. Dubrauszky, V. and G. Pohlmann. Die Ultrastruktur des Korpus endometriums wahren des Cyclus. *Arch. Gynaekol.* **196:** 180 (1961).
4. Hoffmeister, H. and H. Schulz. Lichtopische und elektronenoptische Befunde am Endometrium den geschlechtsreifen Frau wahrend der Proliferations und Sekretionsphase unter besonderer Berucksichtigung der Faserstrukturen. *Beitr. Pathol. Anat.* **124:** 415 (1961).
5. Wynn, R. M. and R. S. Woolley. Ultrastructural cyclic changes in the human endometrium. II. Normal postovulatory phase. *Fertil. Steril.* **18:** 721 (1967).
6. Sengel, A. and P. Stoebner. Ultrastructure of the normal human endometrium. I. The stroma. *Z. Zellforsch.* **109:** 245 (1970).

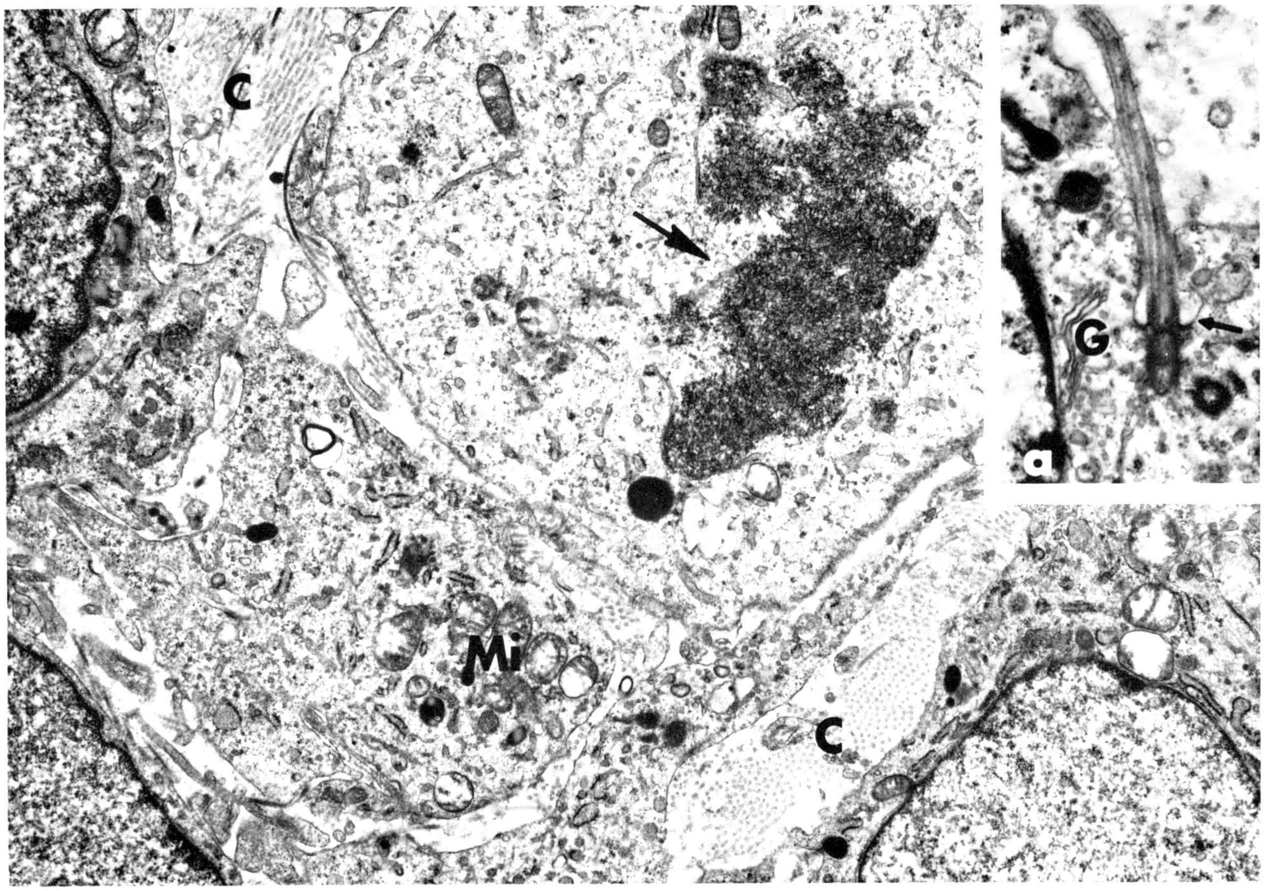

Figure 103. *Late proliferative phase.* A stromal cell is in mitotic prophase (arrow), whereas the adjacent cells have numerous mitochondria (Mi), bound and free ribosomes, and few membrane-bound dense bodies (lysosomes). The intercellular stroma contains abundant collagen fibers (C). × 12,600.

Figure 103a. *Occasional stromal cells* have well-developed, single cilia in a perinuclear location. The ciliary body is associated with a centriole, Golgi (G), and centriolar vesicles (arrow). The ciliary shaft projects into the intercellular space. The precise significance of single cilia in endometrial stromal cells is unknown. × 20,600.

In the early secretory phase no striking cellular modifications are observed; by the 20th day of the cycle, however, additional maturation is noted, and there are abundant cytoplasmic RNA, ergastoplasm, and Golgi vesicles,[1] as well as intracytoplasmic glycogen and lipid droplets.[2] The appearance of lipid droplets is related to estrogenic stimulation, and the occasional finding of large, lipid-laden stromal cells in proliferative and, more frequently, in hyperplastic and neoplastic endometria is thought to be a reflection of hyperestrogenism.[3] On the next 2 days (days 21 and 22), conspicuous stromal edema develops because of the local liberation of histamine, coincident with the highest estrogen levels found during the luteal phase.

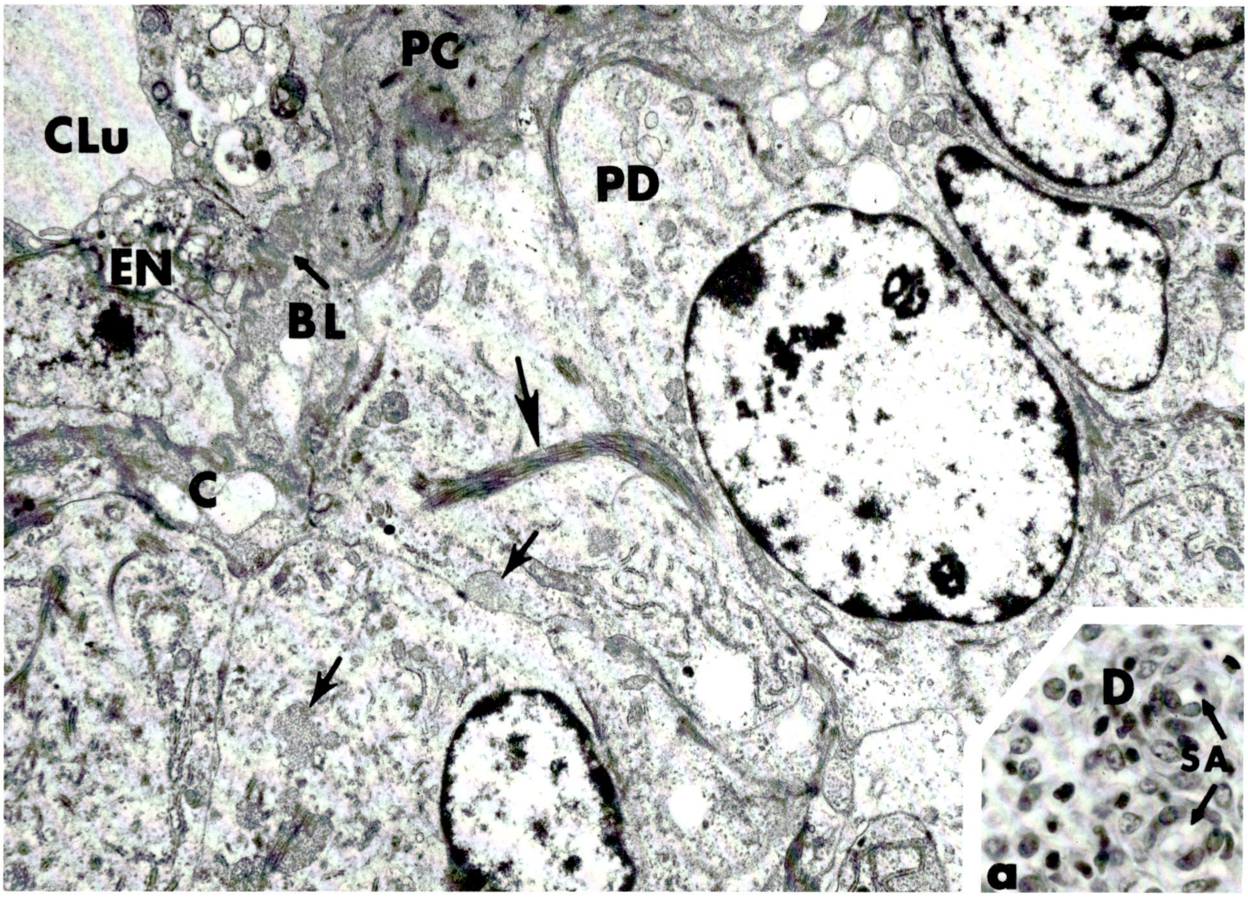

Figure 104a. *On the 23rd day, spiral arterioles* (SA) become prominent and the surrounding stromal cells enlarge, resulting in perivascular predecidualization (D). (H & E stain, × 120.)

Figure 104. *Predecidual cells* (PD) have voluminous round nuclei and well-developed Golgi, granular endoplasmic reticulum, mitochondria, and free ribosomes. There is a concomitant increase in protein synthesis. These changes are under the primary control of progesterone, which is thought to stimulate stromal DNA-dependent RNA synthesis.[4] Collagen synthesis is inconspicuous,[2] and numerous acid phosphatase-rich[5] lysosomes contain fragments of partly digested collagen fibers[1,2,5,6] (short arrows). Large bundles of undigested collagen fibers (long arrow) are occasionally seen free within the cytoplasmic matrix. Perivascular predecidual cells are separated from the endothelial cells (EN) by a narrow zone of collagenous stroma (C). Coincidentally with the formation of predecidua, the endothelium enlarges and perithelial cells (PC) with abundant myofilaments become conspicuous. × 5600. CLu: capillary lumen; BL: capillary basal lamina.

REFERENCES (Figures 103–104)

1. Sengel, A. and P. Stoebner. Ultrastructure of the normal human endometrium. I. The stroma. *Z. Zellforsch.* **109:** 245 (1970).
2. Wienke, E. C., F. Cavazos, D. G. Hall, and F. V. Lucas. Ultrastructure of the human endometrial stroma cell during the menstrual cycle. *Am. J. Obstet. Gynecol.* **102:** 65 (1968).
3. Dallenbach-Hellweg, G. *Histopathology of the Endometrium.* Springer-Verlag, New York, 1971.
4. O'Malley, B. W. Mechanisms of action of steroid hormones. *New Engl. J. Med.* **284:** 370 (1971).
5. Henzl, M. R., R. E. Smith, G. Boost, and E. T. Tyler. Lysosomal concept of menstrual bleeding in humans. *J. Clin. Endocrinol. Metab.* **34:** 360 (1972).
6. Wynn, R. M. and R. S. Woolley. Ultrastructural cyclic changes in the human endometrium. II. Normal post-ovulatory phase. *Fertil. Steril.* **18:** 721 (1967).

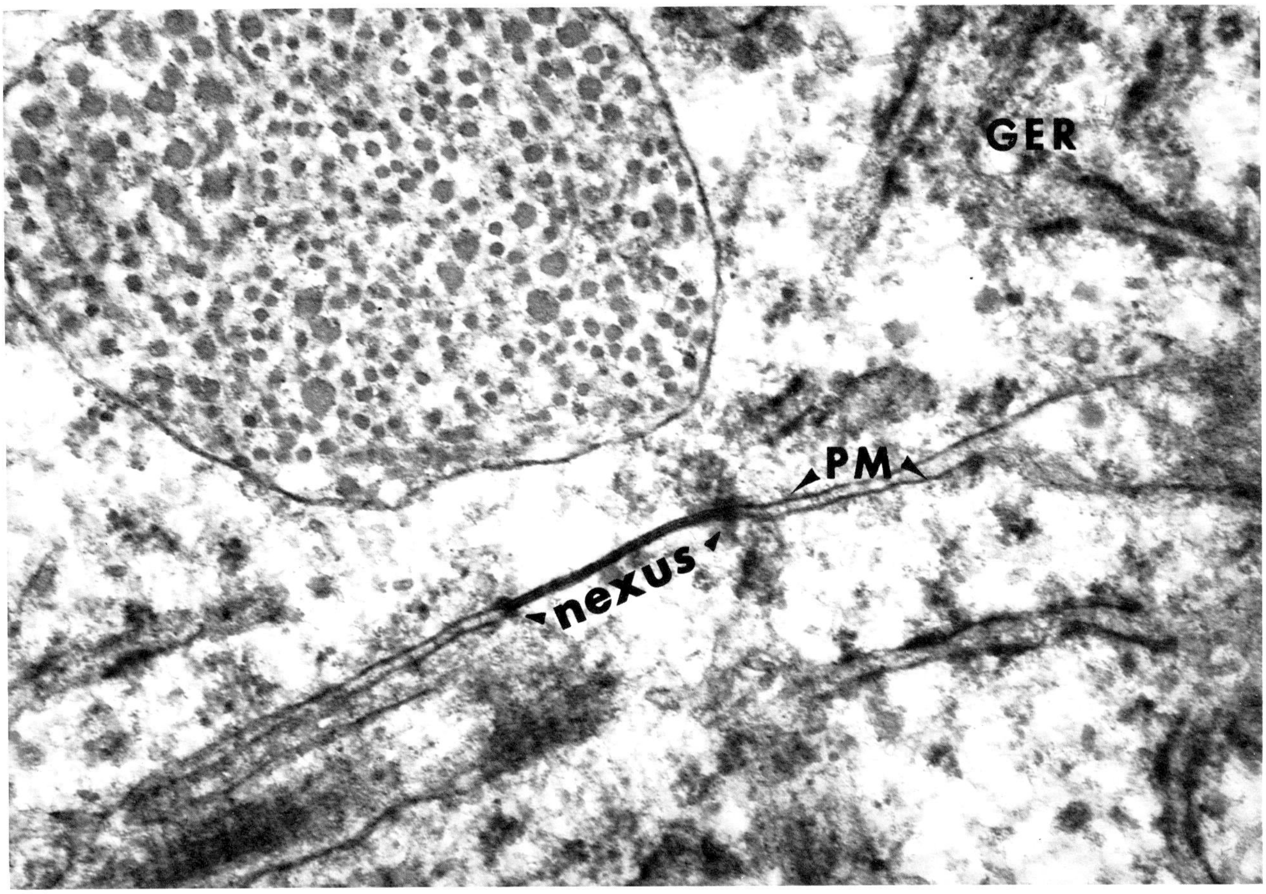

Figure 105. *The characteristic honeycomb pattern* of the predecidual cells is due to the frequent intercellular boundaries in the form of tight gap junctions[1] or pentalaminar nexuses (nexus). A large vacuole contains fragments of partly digested collagen fibers. × 75,000. PM: plasma membranes of two adjacent predecidual cells; GER: granular endoplasmic reticulum.

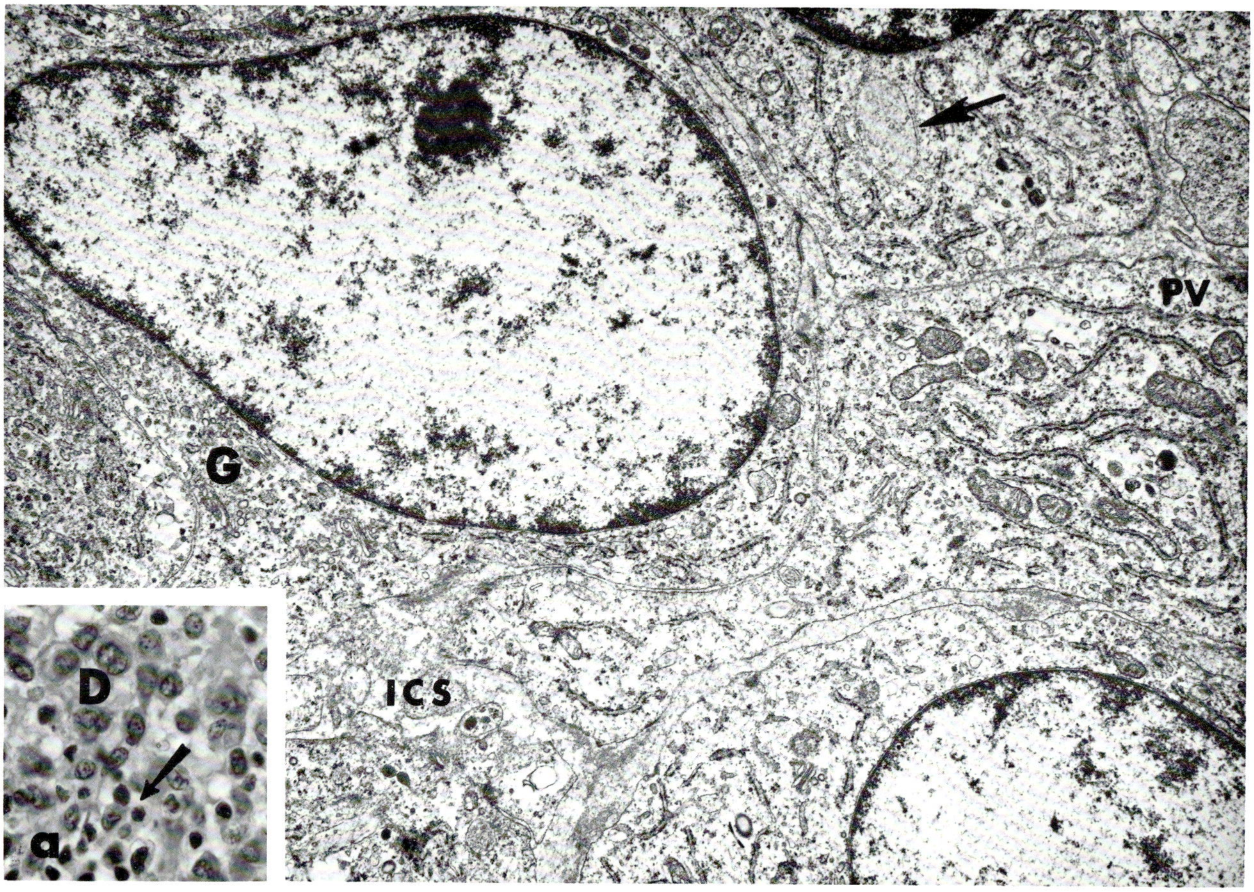

Further predecidualization continues centrifugally from the spiral arterioles, and *on the 25th day* the superficial compacta contains a large subepithelial band of predecidual cells, rich in organelles.[1]

Figure 106. *The 26th day of the cycle.* This substructurally well-equipped population of predecidual cells is capable of biosynthetic and secretory activity,[1] in addition to its supportive function, and it has been suggested that these cells also participate in the nutrition of the implanting blastocyst.[2] × 12,600. G: Golgi; PV: pinocytotic vesicle; arrow: vacuole with collagen fibers; ICS: intercellular space.

Figure 106a. *From the 26th day,* the entire compacta and a large portion of the spongiosa become predecidualized (D) and the number of inflammatory cells (arrow) progressively increases. (H & E stain, × 120.)

REFERENCES (Figures 105–106)

1. Lawn, A. M., E. W. Wilson, and C. A. Finn. The ultrastructure of human decidual and predecidual cells. *J. Reprod. Fertil.* **26:** 85 (1971).
2. McKay, D. G., A. T. Hertig, W. A. Bardawil, and J. T. Velardo. Histochemical observations on the endometrium. I. Normal endometrium. *Obstet. Gynecol.* **80:** 22 (1956).

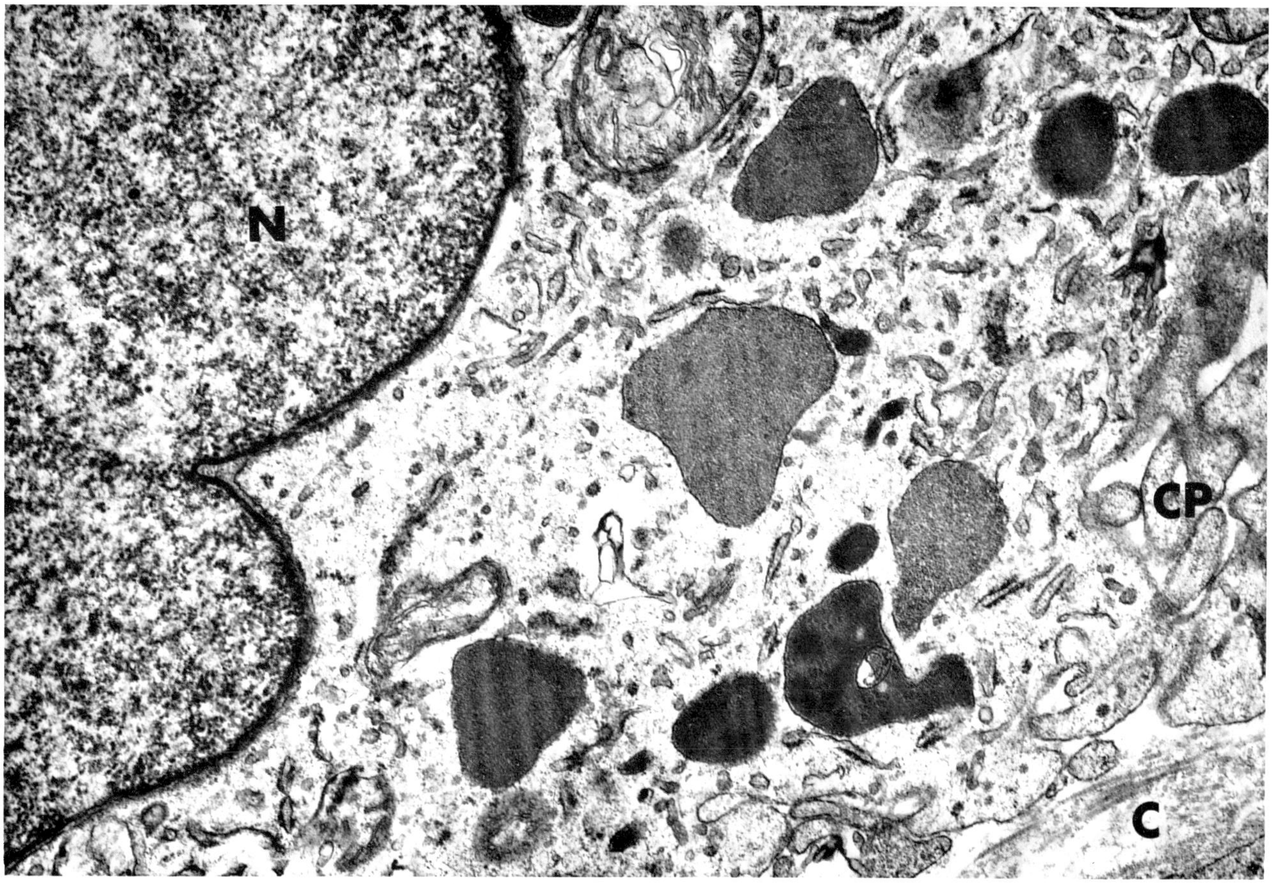

In addition to the stroma cells, other cell types occur in the nonglandular portion of the endometrium, including lymphocytes (which form occasional lymphoid aggregates), histiocytes, eosinophiles, mast cells, and the so-called *endometrial granulocytes*.[1,2] The endometrial granulocytes, thought to differentiate from native stromal cells during the second half of the menstrual cycle, are also present during pregnancy. They are small, mononuclear cells with phloxinophilic granules and are thought to contain relaxin, presumably bound to lysosomes. The liberation of relaxin, upon the action of progesterone, would contribute to the dissolution of the premenstrual stromal reticulin skeleton and, presumably, would aid in nidation.[1]

Figure 107. *Endometrial granulocyte.* The cytoplasm contains several membrane-bound granules of differing size, shape, and content, scattered with vesicular endoplasmic reticulum. × 29,000. CP: cytoplasmic processes; C: intercellular collagen; N: nucleus.

REFERENCES (In addition to the stroma cells—Figure 108)

1. Dallenbach-Hellweg, G. *Histopathology of the Endometrium.* Springer-Verlag, New York, 1971.
2. Jaeger, J. and G. Dallenbach-Hellweg. Elektronenmikroskopische Befunde an den endometrialen Körnchenzellen des Menschen. *Gynaecologia (Basel)* **168:** 117 (1969).
3. Henzl, M. R., R. E. Smith, G. Boost, and E. T. Tyler. Lysosomal concept of menstrual bleeding in humans. *J. Clin. Endocrinol. Metab.* **34:** 360 (1972).

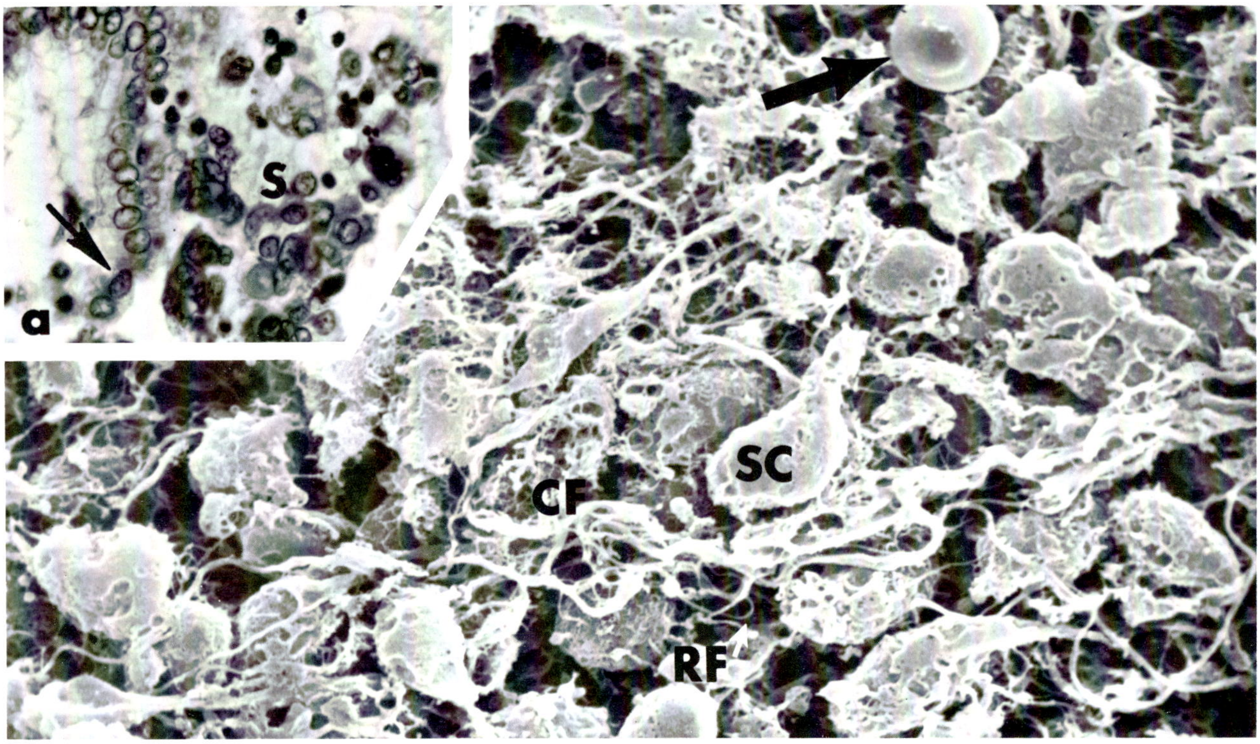

In the absence of pregnancy, there is a decrease in estrogen and progesterone, involution of the predecidua occurs, and acid phosphatase activity increases[3] leading to the disruption, degradation, and collapse of the reticulin network of the functional zone.

Figure 108. *Scanning electron microscopy of menstrual stroma.* Degenerated stromal cells (SC) are invested in haphazardly arranged bundles of collagen (CF) and reticulum fibers (RF). A well-preserved red blood cell (arrow) is seen. × 1600.

Figure 108a. *Menstrual endometrium (2nd menstrual day).* Secondarily to the collapse of the supportive fibrous network of the endometrium, stromal cells (S) aggregate in clusters, intermingling with acute and chronic inflammatory cells. Concomitantly with the stromal changes, the glands undergo a gradual degenerative process (arrow), rupture, and eventual dissolution. × 120.

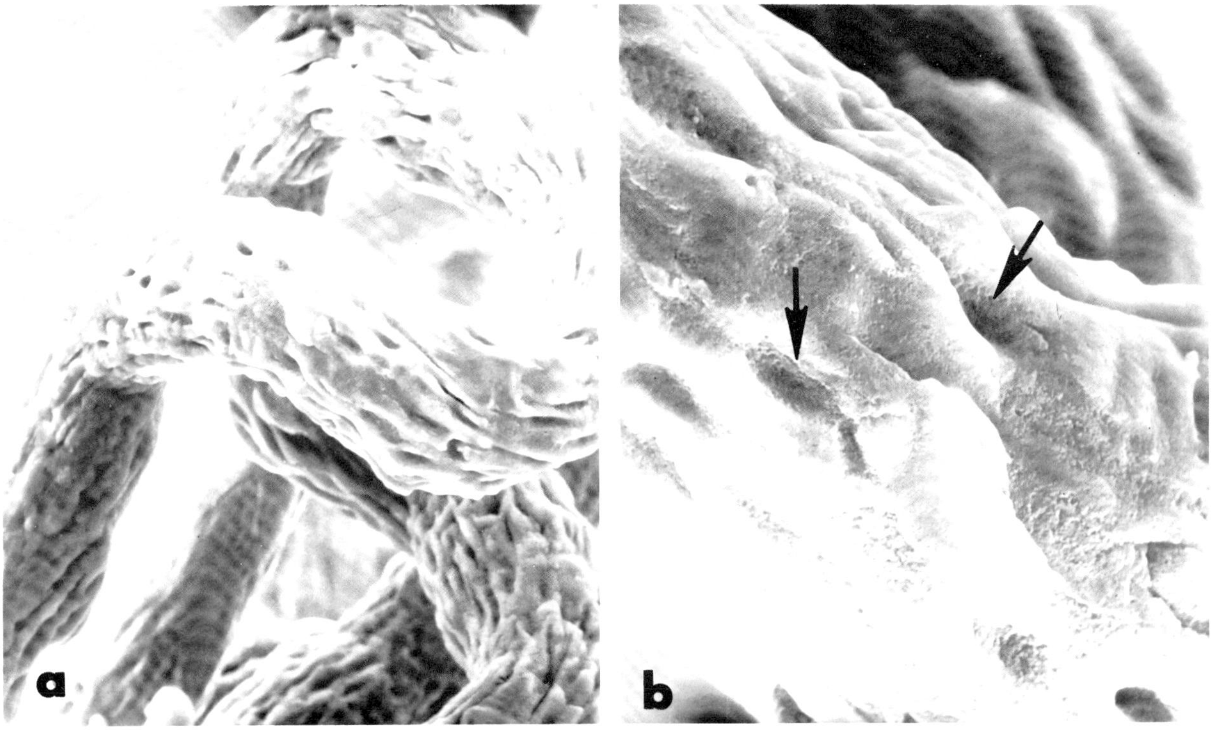

Figure 109a. *Rhesus monkey (Macaca mulatta), 23rd day of the menstrual cycle.* Corrosion cast of endometrial spiral artery, located near the endomyometrial junction. Note the counterclockwise coiling pattern, a characteristic feature of uterine and ovarian vessels. × 160.

Figure 109b. *Rhesus monkey, 23rd day of the menstrual cycle.* Detail of Figure 109*a*, illustrating the spindle-shaped depressions (arrows), which presumably correspond to the endothelial nuclear imprints. × 1600.

ENDOMETRIAL VASCULATURE

The endothelial lining of the circulatory system in the functional zone is sensitive to cyclical hormonal stimuli. During the first half of the cycle, the growth and development of a new capillary bed, originating from the basal spiral arteries, predominates.[1] From typical flattened cells during the early proliferative phase, a progressive development of the Golgi, ergastoplasm, RNA, mitochondria, and pinocytic vesicles occurs, and these organelles become prominent by the end of the follicular phase.[2,3]

During the luteal phase, the spiral arteries become longer and more tortuous and extend into the spongiosa. The endothelial cells increase in size and number, and numerous mitotic figures are seen. Simultaneously, the capillaries in the compacta acquire a well-developed, smooth muscle layer. In the mid-secretory phase, further development of the ergastoplasm–Golgi complex is noted. In the premenstrual phase the arterial capillaries contain prominent hydrolytic enzyme activity and intraluminal endothelial cells, perhaps contributing to capillary breakdown[4] and to the ischemic phenomenon[2] brought about by the contraction of the endomyometrial radial arteries[5] at the onset of menses.

The configuration of the convoluted vessels at different segments of the endometrium is especially well demonstrated by latex perfusion and corrosion techniques. Ordinary household latex (for painting purposes) is diluted with isotonic saline in a ratio of 75 cc latex to 25 cc saline and, after exsanguination, is intravascularly, (artery or vein) injected under controlled pressure (according to the normal values of the blood pressure of the animal studied). When vascular filling has been completed, the intravascular latex is allowed to dry for a minimum of 2 hours, after which the injected organ is digested by caustic agents (HCl). The resulting vascular cast is washed, air dried, coated with a 150-Å-thick film of gold-palladium, and examined with the SEM.

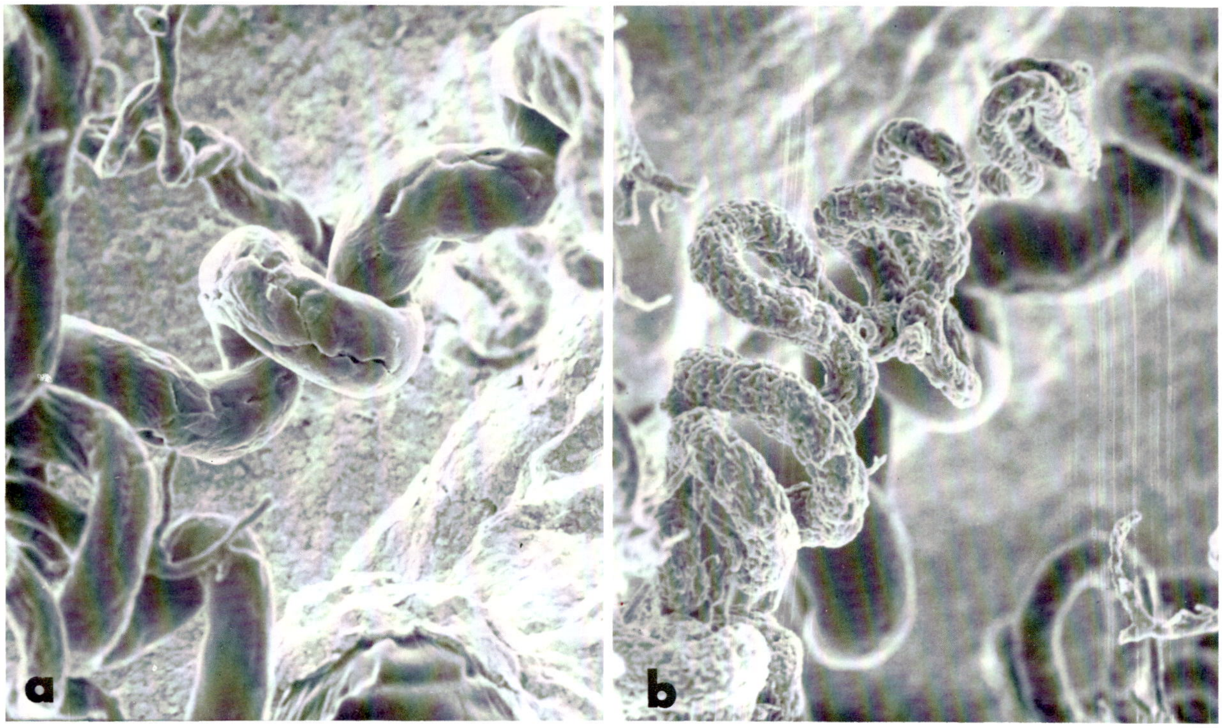

Figure 110a. *Rhesus monkey, 24th day of the menstrual cycle.* Corrosion cast of a markedly convoluted endometrial spiral arteriole of the upper spongiosa, which has several spirals with the characteristic counterclockwise rotation. × 480.

Figure 110b. *Rhesus monkey, 25th day of the menstrual cycle.* Corrosion cast of complexly branching endometrial capillary network of the upper compact layer. × 400.

REFERENCES (The endothelial lining–Figure 110b)

1. Ramsey, E. M. Vascular anatomy of the uterus. In *Cellular Biology of the Uterus,* R. M. Wynn (Ed.). Appleton-Century-Crofts, New York, 1967.
2. Sengel, A. and P. Stoebner. Ultrastructure of the normal human endometrium. I. The stroma. *Z. Zellforsch.* **109:** 245 (1970).
3. Ancla, M. and J. de Brux. Etude au microscope électronique des artérioles spiralées de l'endomètre humain. *Ann. Anat. Pathol. (Paris)* **9:** 209 (1964).
4. Henzl, M. R., R. E. Smith, G. Boost, and E. T. Tyler. Lysosomal concept of menstrual bleeding in humans. *J. Clinol. Endocrin. Metab.* **34:** 360 (1972).
5. Bartelmez, G. W. The form and the functions of the uterine blood vessels in the Rhesus monkey. *Contrib. Embryol. Carnegie Inst. Wash.* **36:** 153 (1957).

28

Endometrium of Gestation (Arias-Stella Reaction)

At the time of implantation, on about the 21st day of the cycle, there is a striking increase in endometrial glandular secretions, accompanied by stromal edema, decidualization and vascular engorgement, and proliferation. The proliferation is thought to occur in response to a glycoprotein that has been termed the angiogenesis factor.[1] This factor is apparently secreted only by the trophoblast,[1] although a similar substance, called the tumor angiogenesis factor (TAF),[1] is elaborated by neoplasms and stimulates the capillary endothelium to form new vessels, providing the blood supply to support tumor growth. Although electron microscopic observations of the human uterine surface at the time of implatation have not been reported, scanning[2,3] and transmission[4] microscopy of the rat endometrial surface has been carried out, and it has been reported that the microvilli become flattened during the preattachment period. The significance of this observation is obscure. Similar topographic observations have been made in the human endometrial lining during the mid-luteal phase of the cycle.[5,6]

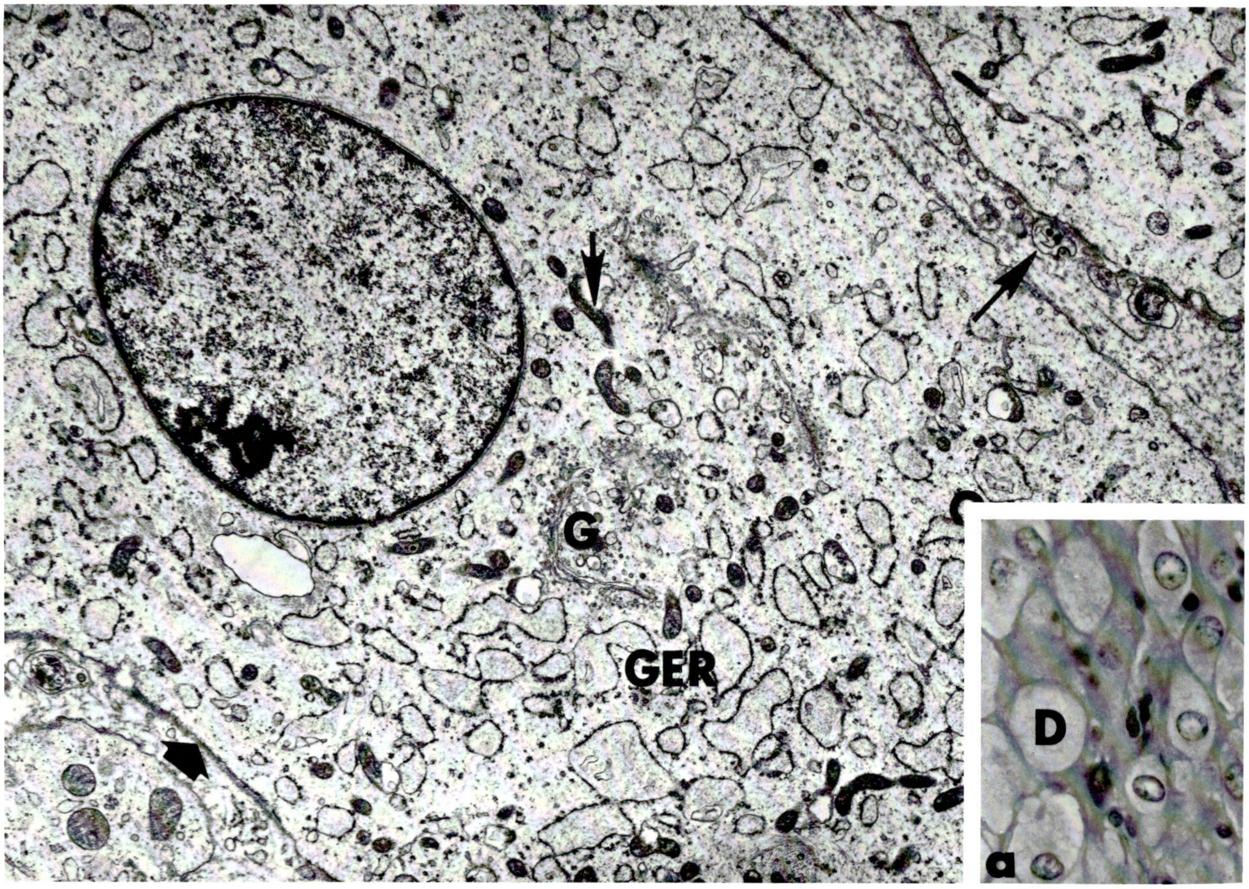

Figure 111a. *On the 2nd day after blastocyst penetration,* the decidual response is well developed and the decidualized stroma (D) is composed of well-differentiated, plump cells with increased RNA synthesis, glycogen, and an increase in various enzymes, most notably carbonic anhydrase.[7] (H & E stain, × 120.)

Figure 111. *The gestational decidual cells* have prominent, dilated, granular endoplasmic reticulum (GER) filled with a fine granular material, Golgi (G), and distinctly small mitochondria (short arrow). The decidual cells also form basal lamina[8] (thick arrow) and elaborate cytoplasmic processes (long arrow), which contain inclusion bodies and collagen fibers,[9] possibly endocytotic in nature. × 6800. C: stroma with scant collagen fibers.

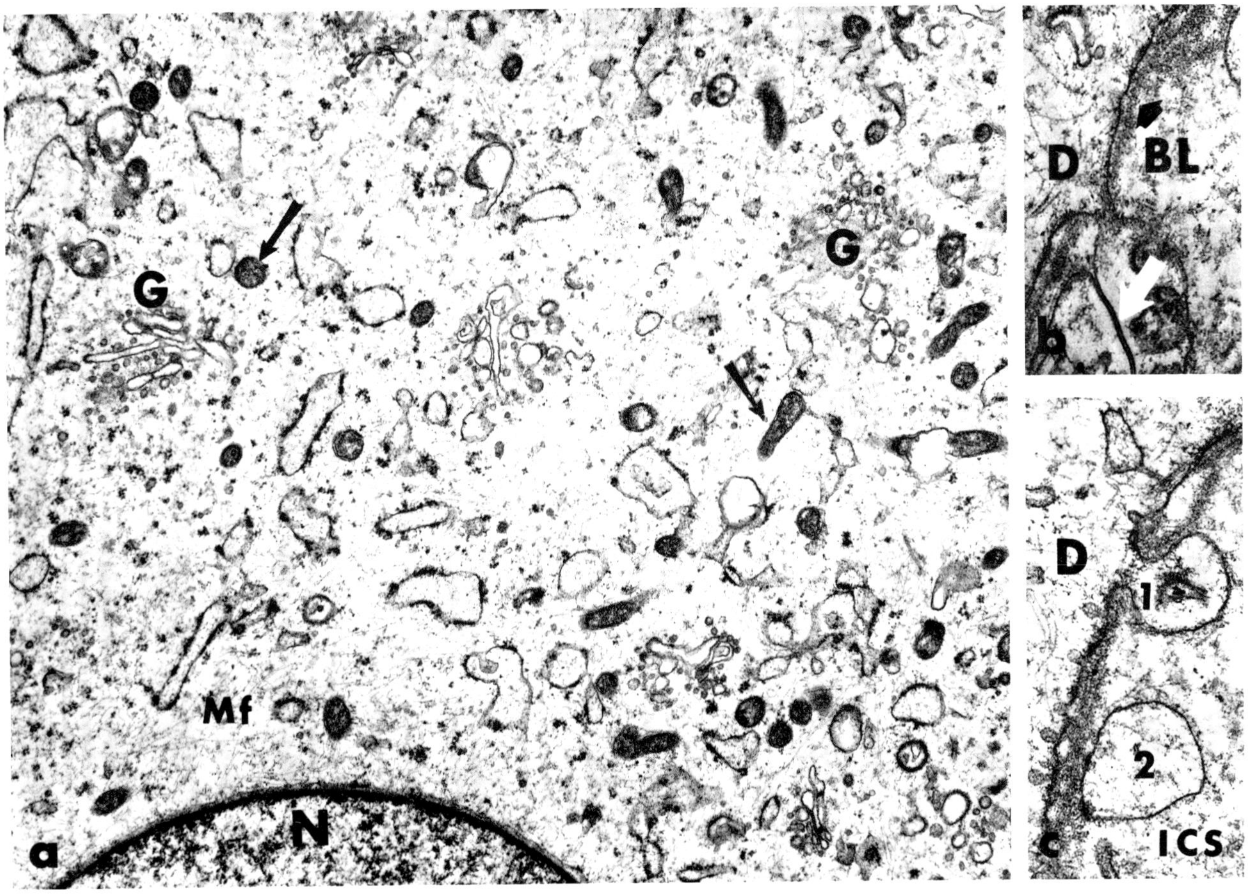

Figure 112a. *Higher-power view of gestational decidual cell.* The cytoplasmic matrix is pale and contains scattered, fine microfilaments (Mf), Golgi (G), granular endoplasmic vesicles, and cigar-shaped mitochondria (arrows). × 20,600. N: nucleus.

Figure 112b. Although *predecidual cells* are occasionally interconnected by gap junctions (nexuses), *in the decidua vera* similar attachments are seen only between cytoplasmic processes of the same cell[8] (arrow). × 35,000. D: decidual cell; BL: basal lamina of decidual cell.

Figure 112c. *Gestational decidual cell (D).* The plasma membrane contains rows of micropinocytotic vesicles and prominent evaginations (1) into the intercellular space (ICS), which are often detached (2) from the cell. × 35,000.

REFERENCES (At the time of implantation—Figure 112c)

1. Folkman, J. Tumor angiogenesis: therapeutic implications. *New Engl. J. Med.* **285:** 1182 (1971).
2. Psychoyos, A. and P. Mandon. Scanning electron microscopy of the surface of the rat uterine epithelium during delayed implantation. *J. Reprod. Fertil.* **26:** 137 (1971).
3. Bergstrom, S. Scanning electron microscopy of ovoimplantation. *Arch. Gynaekol.* **212:** 285 (1972).
4. Nilsson, O. Some ultrastructural aspects of ovo-implantation. In *Ovo-Implantation, Human Gonadotropins and Prolactin,* P. O. Hubinont, F. Leroy, C. Robyn, and P. LeLeux (Eds.). S. Karger, Basel, 1970, pp. 52–72.
5. Nilsson, O. and K. G. Nygren. Scanning electron microscopy of human endometrium. *Upsala J. Med. Sci.* **77:** 3 (1972).
6. Ferenczy, A. and R. M. Richart. Scanning and transmission electron microscopy of the human endometrial surface epithelium. *J. Clin. Endocrinol. Metab.* **36:** 999 (1972).
7. Dallenbach-Hellweg, G. *Histopathology of the Endometrium.* Springer-Verlag, New York, 1971.
8. Lawn, A. M., E. W. Wilson, and C. A. Finn. The ultrastructure of human decidual and predecidual cells. *J. Reprod. Fertil.* **26:** 85 (1971).
9. Wessel, W. Die Menschlichen Decidua-zellen und ihre "Kollagen einschlüsse" im Elektronenmikroscop. *Virchows Arch. Pathol. Anat.* **332:** 224 (1959).

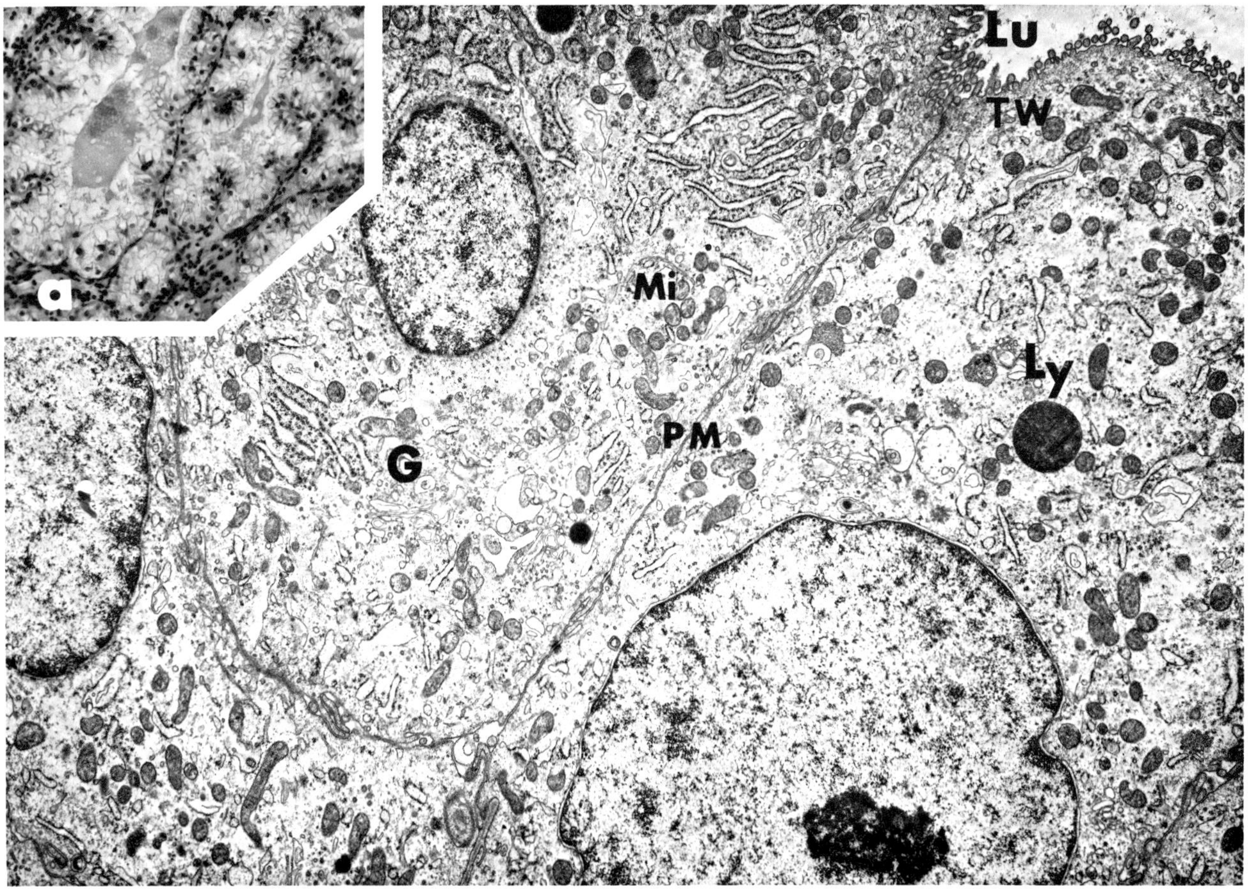

Figure 113a. *In early and late pregnancy, islands of packed hypersecretory glands are noted.* Their lining epithelium contains prominent clear cells with hyperchromatic and pleomorphic nuclei. These nuclear alterations, commonly known as the *Arias-Stella reaction* (ASR), are a result of nuclear polyploidy.[1] They are produced by glandular hyperstimulation with estrogens, progesterone, and chorionic gonadotropin and occur during normal or ectopic pregnancy, as well as in association with trophoblastic disease or after the administration of ovulating agents to nonpregnant women. (H & E stain, × 73.)

Figure 113. *At the ultrastructural level,*[2-4] Arias-Stella cells have a complex cytoplasmic organization reflecting the increased metabolic activity in the glands of ASR. The absence of giant mitochondria (Mi) and the paucity of glycogen granules suggest that gestational progesterone may not play an important role in the development of ASR, and that the accentuated organelles, such as free and bound ribosomes and Golgi (G), are related to protein, rather than mucopolysaccharide, synthesis. The increased, but uniform, pattern of the nuclear chromatin in ASR cells is consistent with the polyploid DNA values discussed previously.[1] × 23,00. PM: plasma membranes; Ly: lysosome; TW: filamentous terminal webb; Lu: glandular lumen.

In early gestation the endometrial glands undergo intense secretory activity and glycogen production, both of which become inconspicuous after the first trimester. With advancing pregnancy, "glandular exhaustion" occurs; ultrastructurally, the organelles, especially the mitochondria, are diminished, and lipid gradually accumulates.

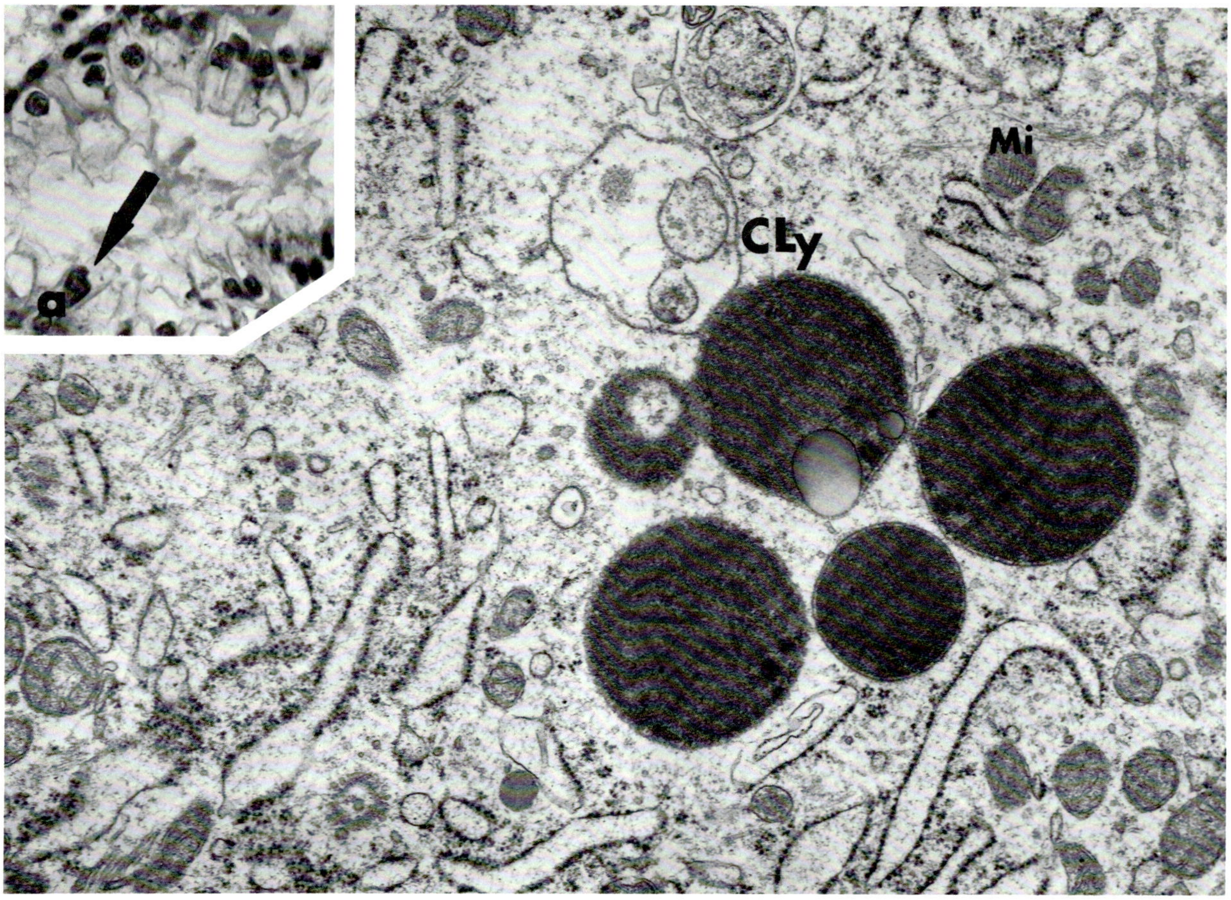

Figure 114a. *High-power light micrograph of ASR.* The glandular cells have voluminous clear cytoplasm and prominent nuclei with irregular nuclear membranes (arrow). (H & E stain, × 120.)

Figure 114. *Detailed view of the cytoplasmic content of Arias-Stella cells.* Clusters of membrane-bound cytolysosomes (CLy) with lipid droplets and needle-shaped dense bodies are surrounded by membranes of granular endoplasmic reticulum and small mitochondria (Mi). × 29,200.

REFERENCES (Figures 113–114)

1. Wagner, D. and R. M. Richart. Polyploidy in the human endometrium with the Arias-Stella reaction. *Arch. Pathol.* **85:** 475 (1968).
2. de Brux, J. and M. Ancla. Arias-Stella endometrial atypias. Case study with the electron microscope. *Am. J. Obstet. Gynecol.* **89:** 661 (1964).
3. Wynn, R. M. and J. A. Harris. Ultrastructure of trophoblast and endometrium in invasive hydatidiform mole (chorioadenoma destruens). *Am. J. Obstet. Gynecol.* **99:** 1125 (1967).
4. Thrasher, T. V. and R. M. Richart. Ultrastructure of the Arias-Stella reaction. *Am. J. Obstet. Gynecol.* **112:** 113 (1972).

29

Inactive and Atrophic Endometrium

INACTIVE ENDOMETRIUM

The inactive (resting) endometrium is most common in the few years preceding and following the clinical menopause, or climacterium. Because of the cessation of ovarian steroidogenesis, the endometrium becomes thinned and contains glands resembling those seen in the first half of the proliferative phase. The lining epithelium, however, differs from the proliferative epithelium by the absence of mitotic activity and glycogen.

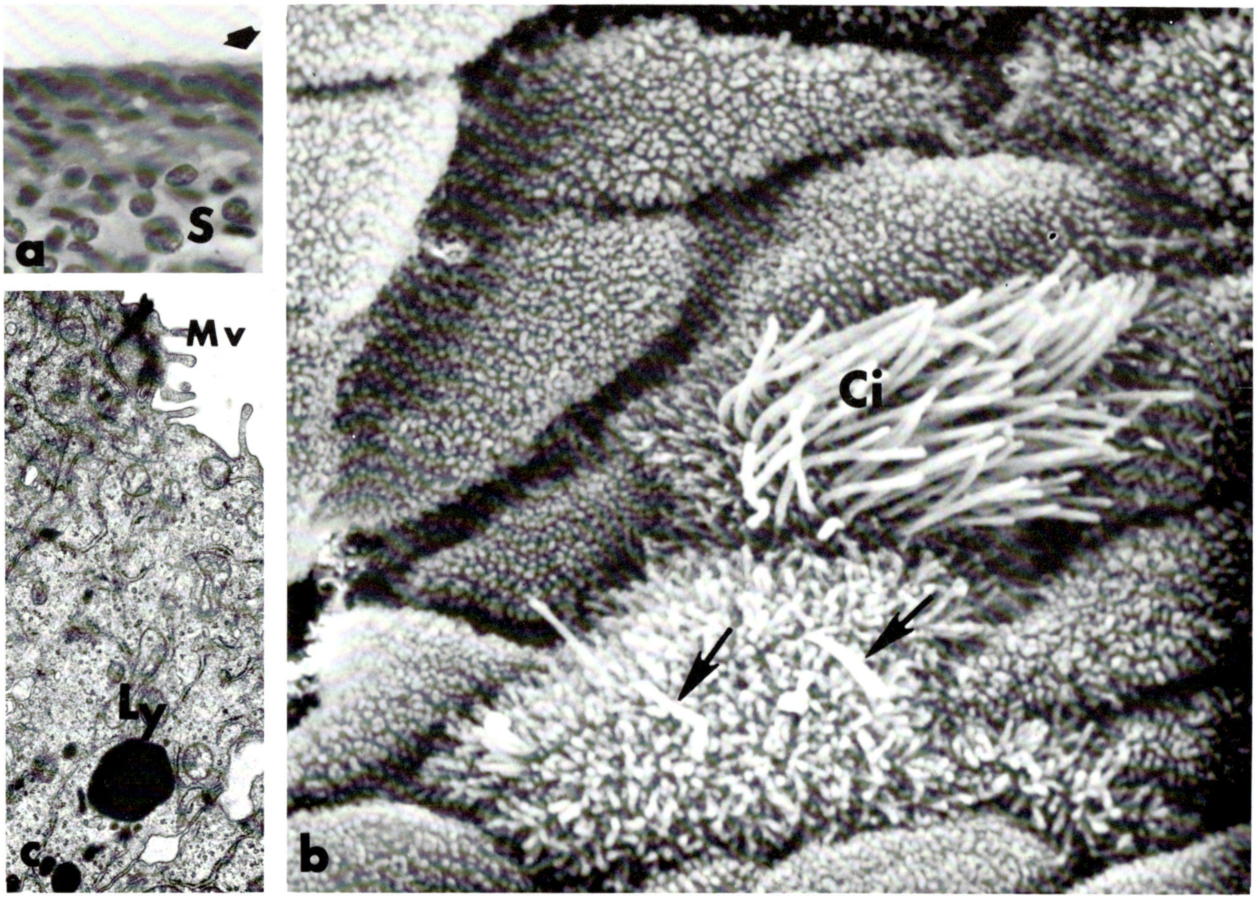

Figure 115a. *Inactive endometrium.* The endometrial surface epithelium appears low cuboidal, and there are scattered ciliated cells (arrow). The stroma (S) varies from dense to loose, is frequently myxoid, and contains narrow, spindle-shaped cells, with ultrastructural evidence of decreased RNA synthesis. (H & E stain, × 120.)

Figure 115b. *At the scanning electron microscopic level,* the uterus lining cells are flattened and are covered by abundant, but short, microvilli. Well-developed ciliated cells (Ci) are infrequent; others have few and short ciliary shafts (arrows). × 4800.

Figure 115c. *Inactive endometrium.* In comparison to the endometrium found in women in the reproductive period, there is, in addition, a relative decrease in the ergastoplasm[1] and in the height of microvilli (Mv) of the lining,[2] confirming the histochemical findings of low levels of cytoplasmic RNA and apical alkaline phosphatase.[3] × 20,600. Ly: lysosome with electron-dense amorphous content.

ATROPHIC (SENILE) ENDOMETRIUM

The atrophic (senile) endometrium is very thin and is composed of a narrow zone of basalis, containing scattered atrophic glands that are surrounded by a dense fibrocellular stroma. These changes are a consequence of the physiological cessation of ovarian hormone production.

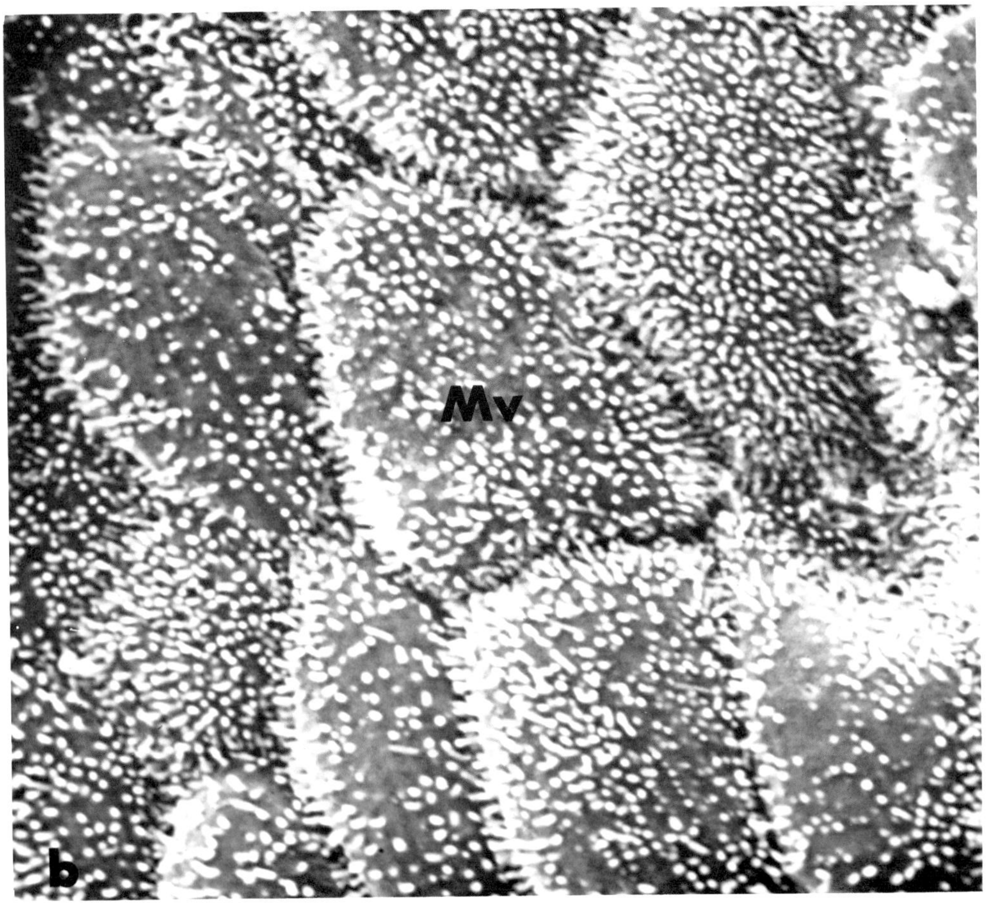

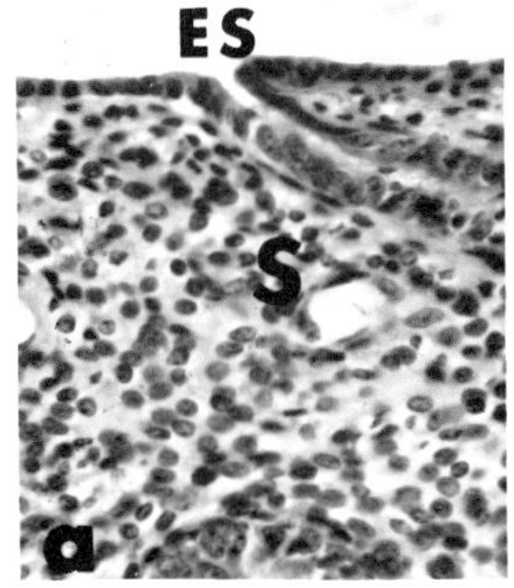

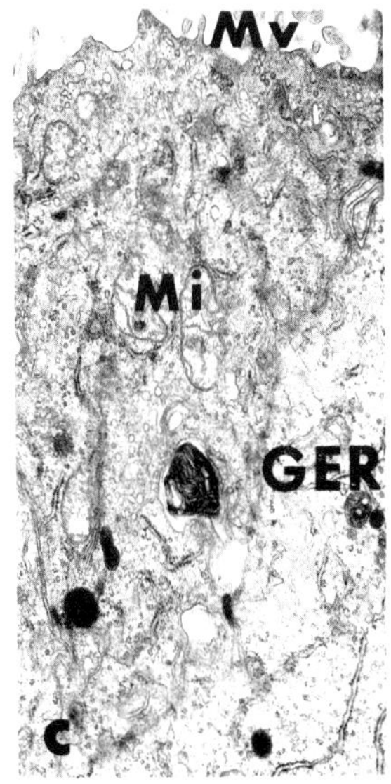

Figure 116a. *Atrophic (senile) endometrium.* Most of the cells lining the endometrial surface (ES) and glands are low cuboidal with scant cytoplasm and are uniformly devoid of ciliary shafts. The stromal cells (S) have the appearance of indifferent, spindle-shaped cells with scant cytoplasmic substance and RNA. The relative lack of collagen production results in a loosely arranged, intracellular matrix. Similar histologic and histochemical findings are observed in the atrophic endometrium of premenarche or castration.[3] (H & E stain, × 75.)

Figure 116b. *Atrophic (senile) endometrium.* Although some reports describe the occurrence of ciliated cells in the senile endometrium,[4] they are extremely rare and, when present, have a smaller number of short ciliary shafts. They are uniformly absent in the advanced climacterium.[2] There is also a significant decrease in the number and height of the surface microvilli (Mv) in the superficial senile epithelium. × 4800. *From* A. Ferenczy and R. M. Richart. Scanning electron microscopy of hyperplastic and neoplastic endometria. In *Scanning Electron Microscopy/1973* Part III. *Proceedings of the Workshop on Scanning Electron Microscopy in Pathology*, O. Johari (Ed.). IIT Research Institute, Chicago, 1973, pp. 613–620.

Figure 116c. *Atrophic (senile) endometrium.* The low cuboidal epithelium lining either the uterine surface or small, involuted, or cystic glands is poor in cytoplasmic organelles, and a loss of progesterone[5] and estradiol[5] binding capacity has been reported. × 7200. GER: granular endoplasmic reticulum; Mi: mitochondria; Mv: surface microvilli.

REFERENCES (Figures 115a–116c)

1. Borell, U., O. Nilsson, and A. Westman. The cyclical changes occurring in the epithelium lining the endometrial glands. An electron microscopical study in the human being. *Acta Obstet. Gynecol. Scand.* **38:** 364 (1959).
2. Ferenczy, A. and R. M. Richart. Scanning electron microscopy of the human female genital tract. *N.Y. State J. Med.* (in press).
3. Dallenbach-Hellweg, G. *Histopathology of the Endometrium.* Springer-Verlag, New York, 1971.
4. Sirtori, C. and E. Morano. The senile endometrium examined by means of the electron microscope. In *Cancer of the Uterus, from Gross Appearance to Ultrastructure,* 2nd ed. C. Sirtori and E. Morano (Eds.). Charles C Thomas, Springfield, Ill., 1963, pp. 321–329.
5. Haukkamaa, M., O. Karjalainen, and T. Luukkainen. In vitro binding of progesterone by the human endometrium during the menstrual cycle and by hyperplastic, atrophic and carcinomatous endometrium. *Am. J. Obstet. Gynecol.* **111:** 205 (1971).
6. Henderson, S. R. and D. S. Schalch. Estrogen receptors in the human uterus. *Am. J. Obstet. Gynecol.* **112:** 762 (1972).

30

Endometrium Associated with Hyperestrogenic States

Hyperestrogenic, anovulatory cycles are associated with persistent proliferative endometrium, which resembles, both histologically and ultrastructurally, normal proliferative (early, mid-, or late) endometrium, including the presence of annulate lamellae[1] and bundles of microfilaments in association with scattered glycogen particles. When the estrogen levels decrease, the endometrium is no longer hormonally supported and withdrawal bleeding occurs. The ultrastructures of the glandular uterine lining, ciliated, and microvillous secretory cells are morphologically and distributionally similar to those seen in normal proliferative endometrium.

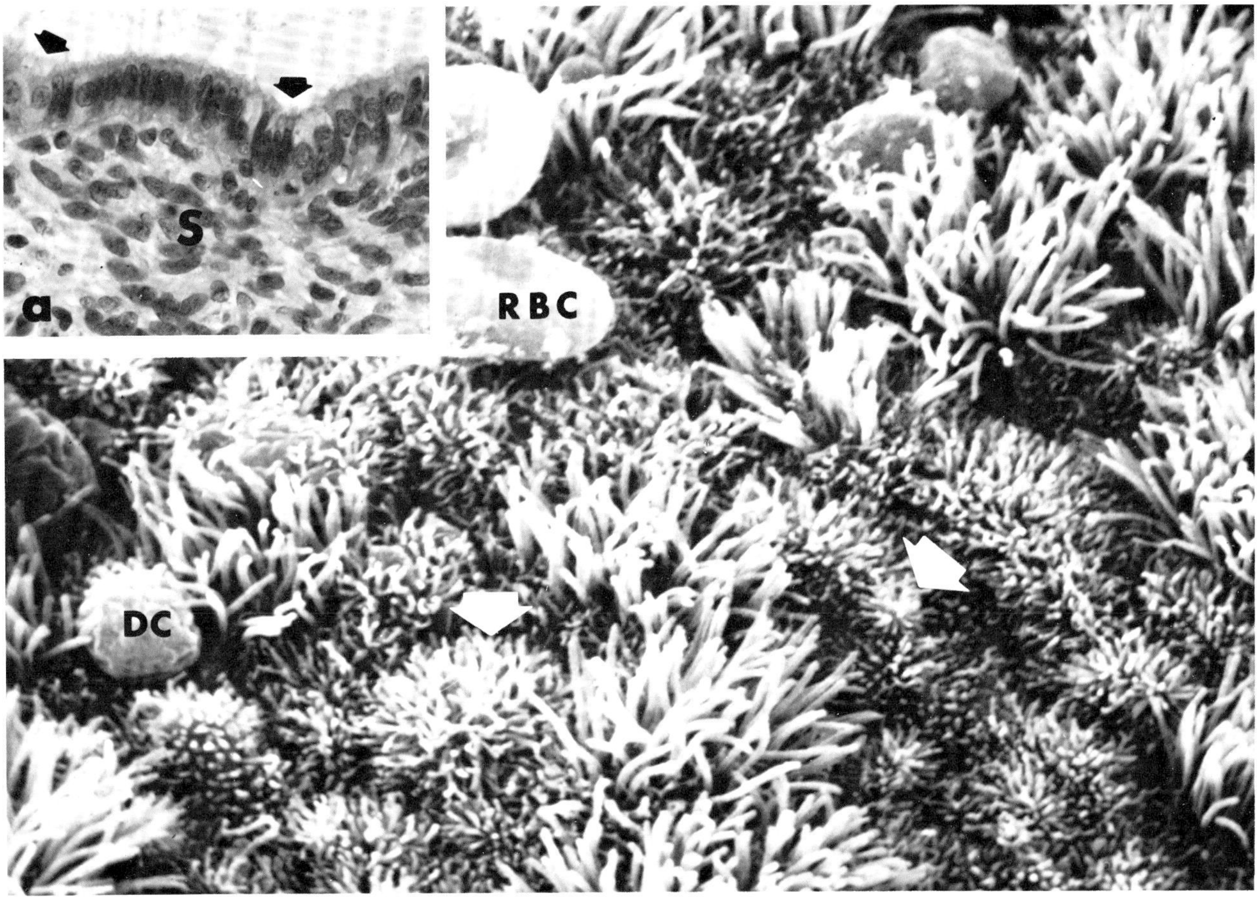

Figure 117a. *Endometrial surface epithelium in anovulatory cycles.* The lining cells are tall columnar with elongated, spindle-shaped nuclei, interspersed with numerous ciliated cells (arrows) with pale cytoplasmic substance. (H & E stain, × 120.) S: subepithelial stroma.

Figure 117. *In the persistent proliferative endometrium,* the surface contains numerous well-developed ciliated cells occurring in clusters. The adjacent nonciliated cells have abundant microvilli with occasional microvillous promontories (arrows). Several nonciliated cells exhibit wrinkled cytoplasmic protrusions devoid of microvilli (DC) that represent degenerated "peg" cells. Note the close resemblance of this epithelium to that often seen during the late proliferative phase of the normal menstrual cycle. × 6200. RBC: well-preserved red blood cell.

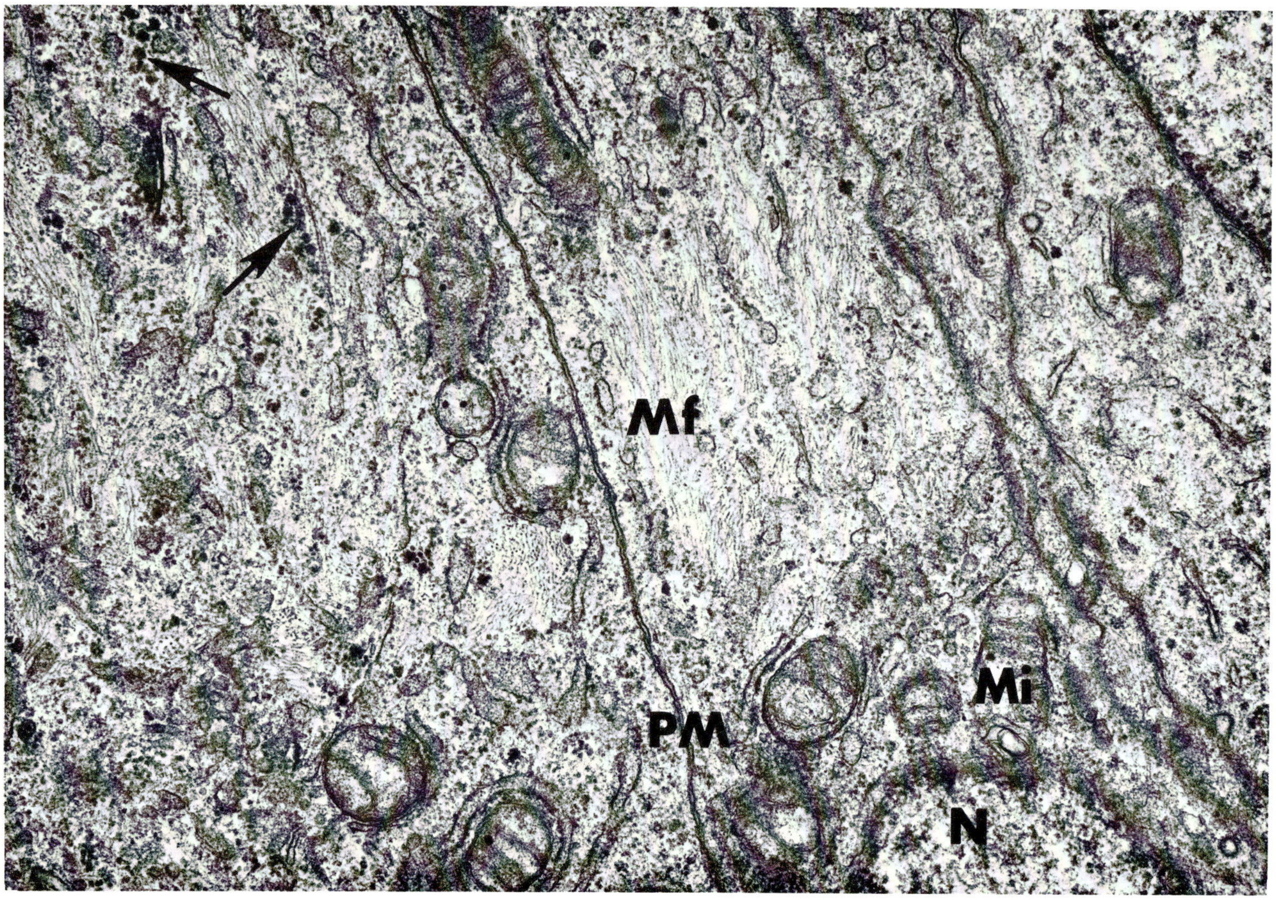

Figure 118. *Ultrastructurally,* the persistent proliferative uterine lining cells have numerous sub- and supranuclear (N) granular endoplasmic reticula in close relationship with mitochondria (Mi) and abundant bundles of microfilaments (Mf) oriented parallel to the lateral plasma membranes (PM). In addition to scattered free ribosomes, there are a few aggregates of glycogen granules (arrows), the presence of which suggests that progesterone is produced, although in inadequate quantities. Many of the anovulatory cycles associated with "unopposed estrogens" should be regarded as relative, rather than absolute, hyperestrogenic conditions × 7500.

REFERENCE (Hyperestrogenic, anovulatory cycles–Figure 118)

1. Ancla, M. and J. de Brux. Occurrence of intranucleolar tubular structures in the human endometrium during the secretory phase, and of annulate lamellae in hyperestrogenic states. *Obstet. Gynecol.* **26:** 23 (1965).

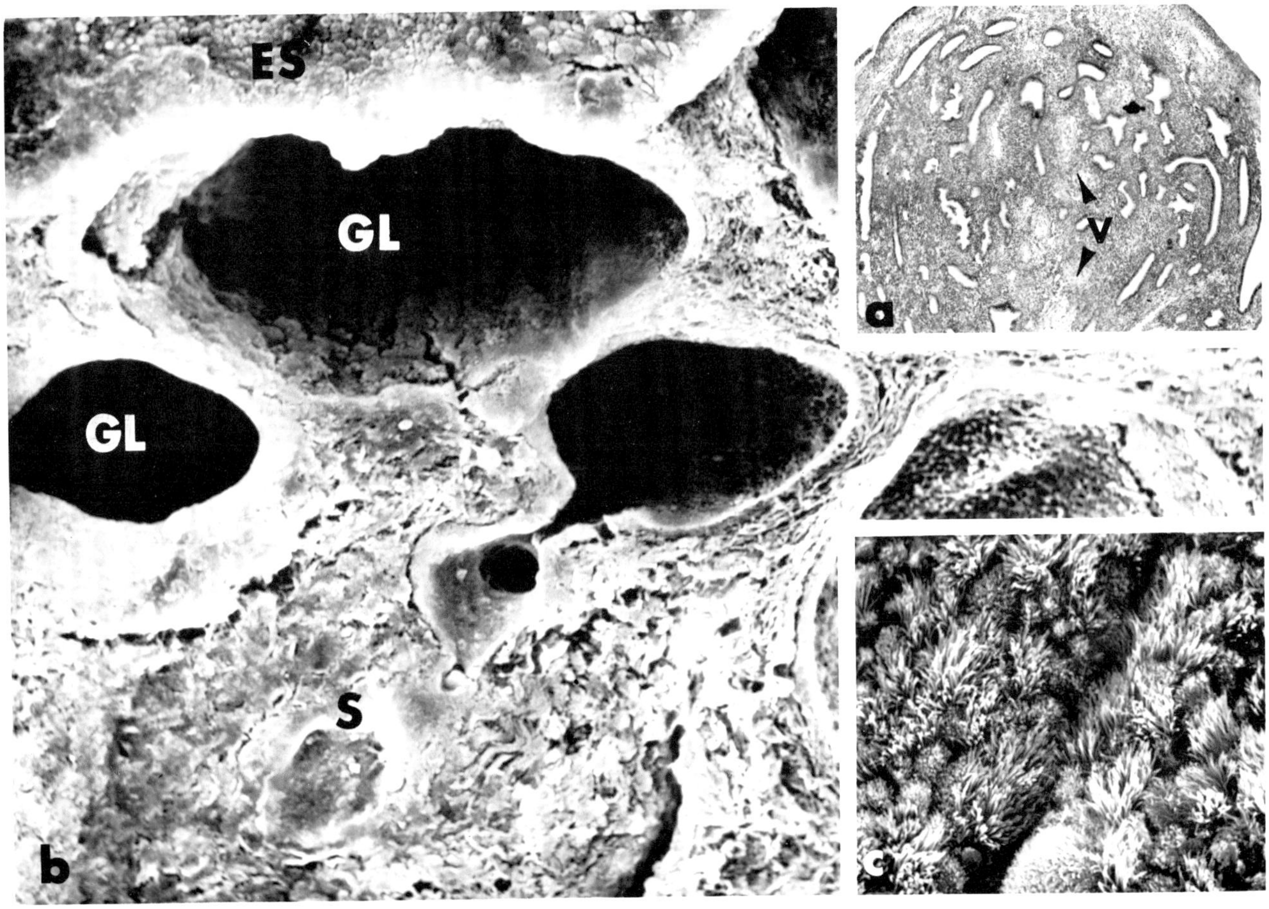

POLYPS

Endometrial polyps are not true neoplasms, but focal, polyploid overgrowths originating from the basalis.

Figure 119a. *Histologically,* the stroma is dense and fibrocellular and contains glands oriented in all directions. In most instances, the glandular epithelium is of the proliferative type, but it may also contain inactive epithelium or foci of cystic glandular, or adenomatous, hyperplasia. (H & E stain, × 10). V: feeding vessels of endometrial polyp.

Figure 119b. *Scanning electron microscopy* of a cross-sectioned endometrial polyp with focal cystic glandular hyperplasia. Beneath the endometrial surface (ES) are several cystically dilated glands (GL) embedded in a fibrocellular stroma (S). × 160.

Figure 119c. *Higher magnification* of the endometrial epithelium covering the polyp. Numerous ciliated cells intermingle with dome-shaped microvillous cells. The submicroscopic characteristics of the various epithelia seen in endometrial polyps are identical with those of their nonpolyp counterparts, including cystic or adenomatous hyperplasia and adenocarcinoma. × 1000.

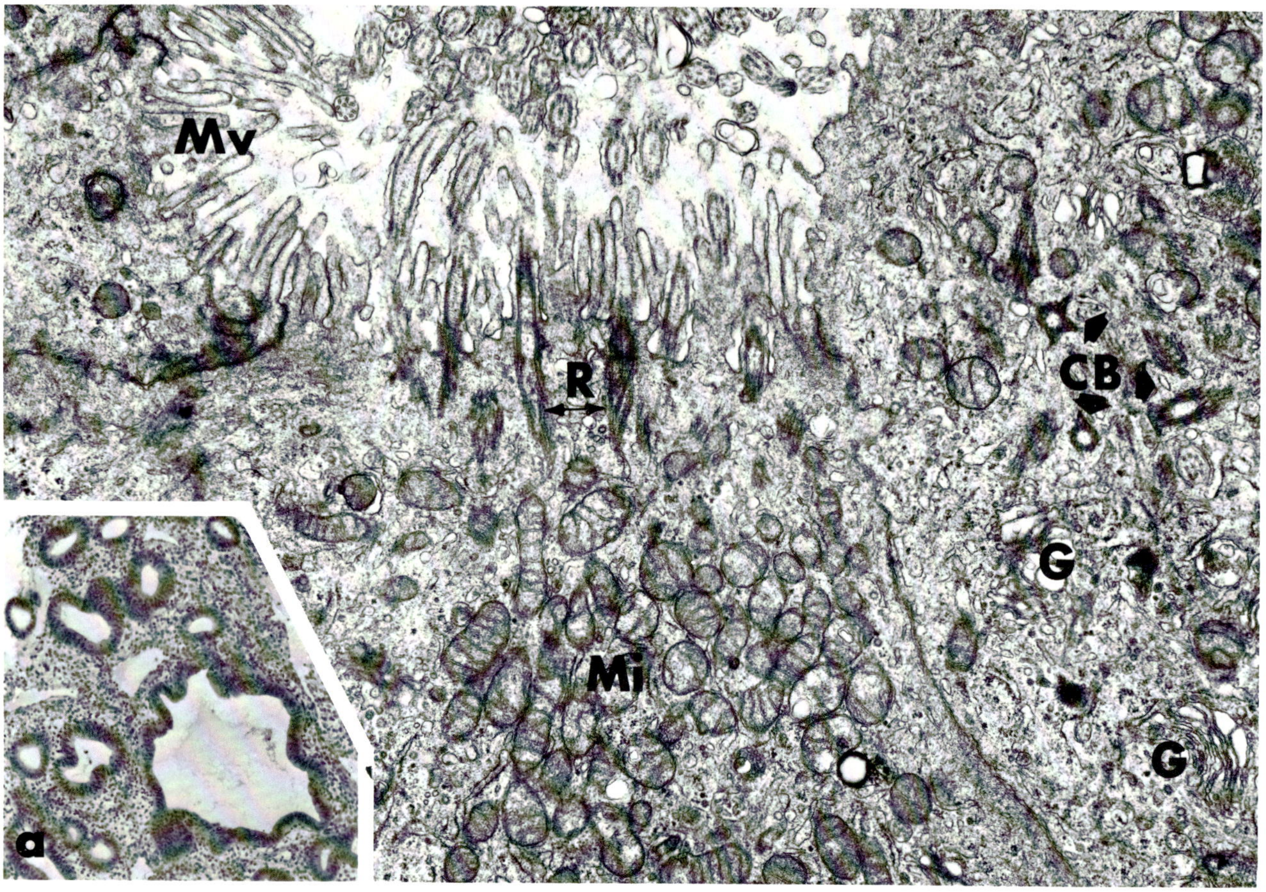

REFERENCES (Figures 119a–120)

1. Terenius, L., A. Lindell, and B. H. Persson. Binding of estradiol-17-β to human cancer tissue of the female genital tract. *Cancer Res.* **31:** 1895 (1971).
2. Wessel, W. Die glandular-cystische Hyperplasie des menschlichen Endometriums in elektronenmikroskopischen Bild. *Virchows Arch. Pathol. Anat.* **334:** 181 (1961).
3. Fasske, E., K. Morgenroth, H. Themann, and A. Verhagen. Vergleischende elektronenmikrosckopische Untersuchengen von Proliferationsphase, glandular-cystischer Hyperplasie und Adenocarcinom der Schleimhaut des Corpus Uteri. *Arch. Gynaekol.* **200:** 473 (1965).

CYSTIC GLANDULAR HYPERPLASIA

Cystic glandular hyperplasia is generally seen in long-standing hyperestrogenic states associated with abnormally high estrone levels or exogenous estrogen administration.

Figure 120a. *Histologically,* the lesion may be focal or diffuse, and in most instances both the glands and the stroma are hyperplastic. The glands are numerous and tortuous, and many of them are cystically dilated ("Swiss cheese pattern"). The lining epithelium is tall and columnar, often pseudostratified, and contains numerous mitoses and ciliated cells. Estrogenic hyperstimulation results in an increase in cytoplasmic RNA synthesis and apical alkaline phosphatase activity, and a high 17-β-estradiol binding receptor content is found.[1] (H & E stain, × 20.)

Figure 120. *At the ultrastructural level,* the extensive organellar development associated with mucopolysaccharide synthesis is noted and abundant lipid droplets are observed.[2,3] Characteristically there are parallel membranes of granular endoplasmic reticulum in close association with mitochondria (Mi), the former occasionally occurring in a concentric arrangement. Bundles of microfilaments, in both supra- and subnuclear locations, are a prominent feature. The luminal microvillous processes (Mv) are well developed, and ciliary bodies have cone-shaped, cross-striated rootlets (R-double-headed arrow). × 15,600. G: Golgi; CB: tangentially sectioned ciliary bodies with satellite processes.

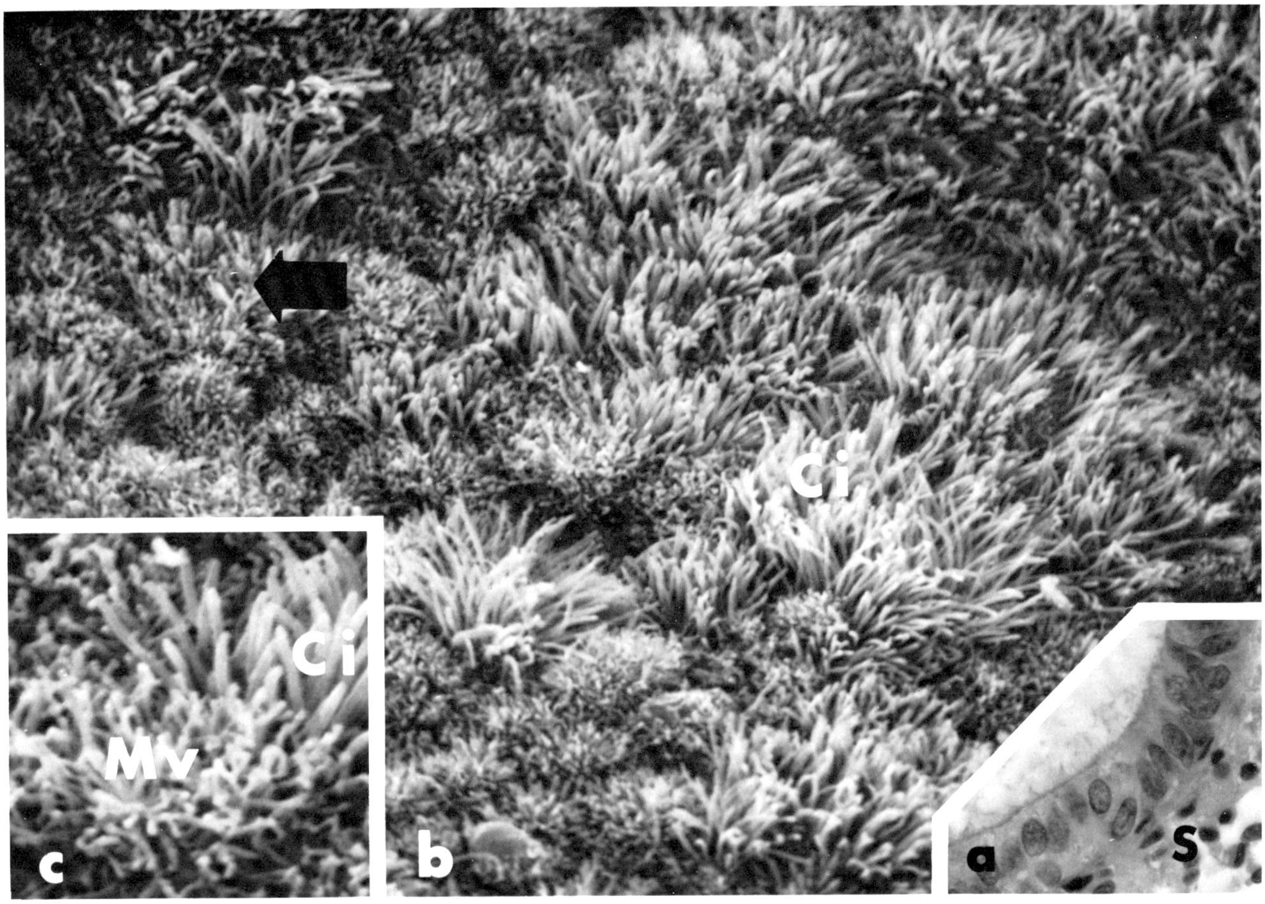

Figure 121a. *Cystic glandular hyperplasia.* The uterine lining has numerous ciliated cells. The hyperplastic stroma (S) contains tightly packed, spindle-shaped cells, ultrastructurally resembling the stromal cells of the late proliferative endometrium. Collagen synthesis is minimal, and the intercellular matrix contains abundant mucopolysaccharides. Mast cells and lipid-laden stromal cells are frequently encountered. The subepithelial sinusoids are often dilated and are frequently filled with hyalin thrombi. (H & E stain, × 150.)

Figure 121b. *Scanning electron microscopy* of the uterine surface epithelium in cystic glandular hyperplasia. There are more ciliated cells (Ci) and microvillous projections than are found in normal proliferative endometria, and these increases are more pronounced in the uterine surface epithelium[1] than in the endometrial glands. The number of ciliated cells and microvillous projections is reduced in the highly dilated cystic glands. Numerous cells generate new ciliary shafts (arrow). × 2400.

Figure 121c. *High magnification* of a microvillous promontory with slender, branching microvilli (Mv). × 6400. Ci: ciliated cell. *From* A. Ferenczy and R. M. Richart. Scanning electron microscopy of hyperplastic and neoplastic endometria. In *Scanning Electron Microscopy/1973.* Part III. *Proceedings of the Workshop on Scanning Electron Microscopy in Pathology,* O. Johari (Ed.). IIT Research Institute, Chicago, 1973, pp. 613–620.

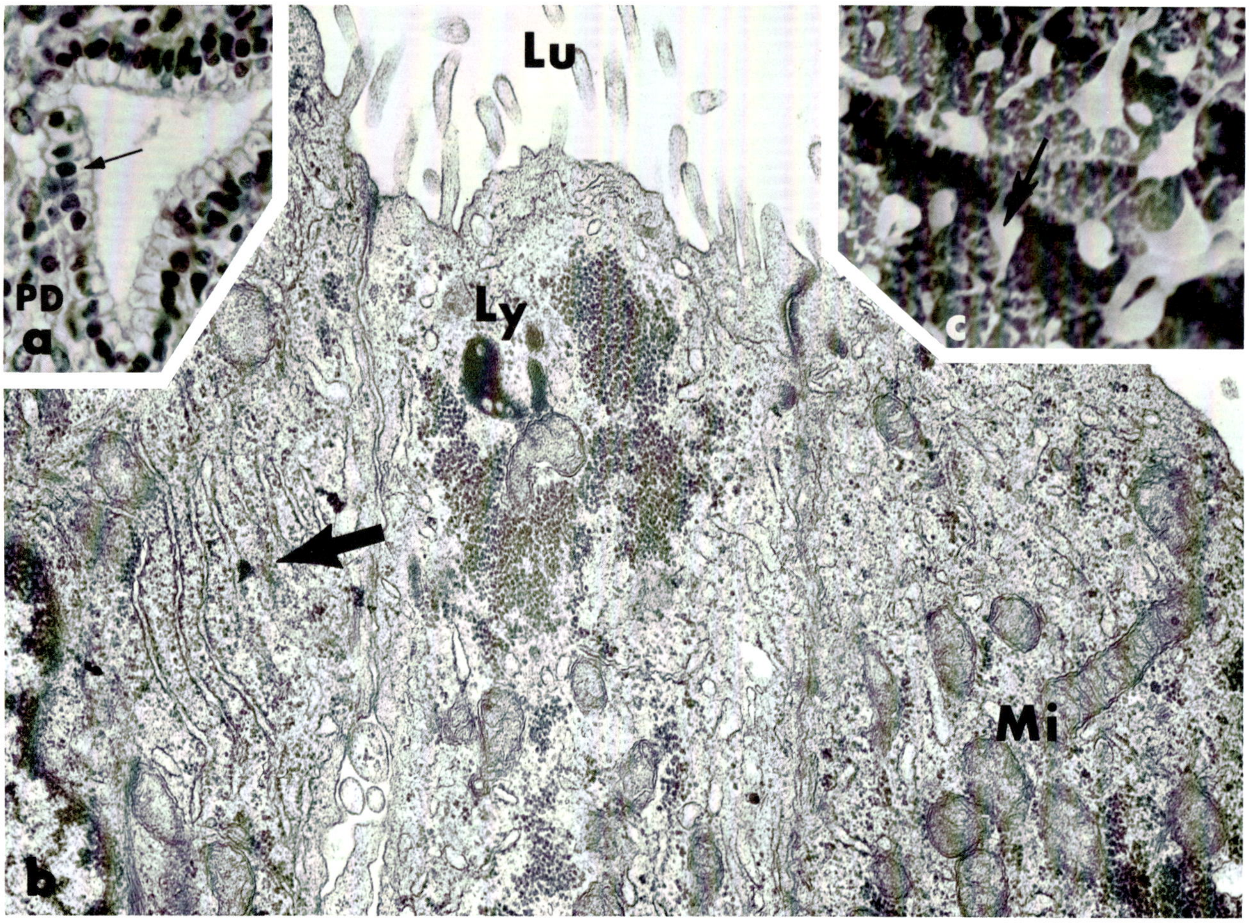

CYSTIC GLANDULAR HYPERPLASIA WITH PROGESTIN EFFECT

Secretory activity in cystic, as well as in adenomatous, glandular hyperplasia may be induced by exogenous progestins. These drugs initiate the accumulation of aggregates of glycogen and a conspicuous intraluminal, acid mucopolysaccharide-rich secretion.[1,2] Glycogen is not produced by estrogen stimulation alone, but estrogens are apparently a prerequisite for progesterone-induced synthesis.[3]

Long-term progestogen administration, such as occurs in the treatment of pelvic endometriosis, leads to complete glandular atrophy and a massive pseudodecidual reaction. In such patients, surface epithelial ciliogenesis and microvilli decrease and secretory activity increases. The dramatic response of hyperplastic endometria to progestogens may be explained by the high progesterone binding capacity found in hyperplastic endometrial tissues.[4]

Figure 122a. *Cystic glandular hyperplasia* treated with large doses of Depo-Provera® (medroxyprogesterone acetate) for 6 months. Note the glandular exhaustion with diffuse supranuclear vacuolization (arrow). The gland is surrounded by well-developed pseudodecidual cells (PD). (H & E stain, × 120.)

Figure 122b. *At the ultrastructural level,* the supranuclear vacuoles correspond to the accumulation of large aggregates of glycogen granules, associated with prominent membranes of granular endoplasmic reticulum (arrow) and mitochondria (Mi). The luminal microvilli appear short and sparse. × 21,000. Lu: glandular lumen; Ly: lysosomal bodies.

Figure 122c. *The surface epithelial cells* contain abundant secretory granules (arrow); short microvilli and ciliated cells are absent. × 2400. From Ferenczy, A. and R. M. Richart. Scanning electron microscopy of hyperplastic and neoplastic endometria. In *Scanning Electron Microscopy/1973.* Part III. *Proceedings of the Workshop on Scanning Electron Microscopy in Pathology,* O. Johari (Ed.). IIT Research Institute, Chicago, 1973, p. 613–620.

REFERENCES (Figures 121a–122c)

1. Ferenczy, A. and R. M. Richart. Scanning electron microscopy of hyperplastic and neoplastic endometria. In *Scanning Electron Microscopy/1973*. Part III. *Proceedings of the Workshop on Scanning Electron Microscopy in Pathology,* O. Johari (Ed.). IIT Research Institute, Chicago, 1973, p. 613.
2. Rorat, E., A. Ferenczy, and R. M. Richart. The ultrastructure of endometrial clear cell adenocarcinoma. *Cancer* (in press).
3. Hackl, H. To the hormonal control of glykogensynthesis in the human endometrium. *Arch. Gynaekol.* **211:** 617 (1971).
4. Haukkamaa, M., O. Karjalainen, and T. Luukkainen. In vitro binding of progesterone by the human endometrium during the menstrual cycle and by hyperplastic, atrophic and carcinomatous endometrium. *Am. J. Obstet. Gynecol.* **111:** 205 (1971).

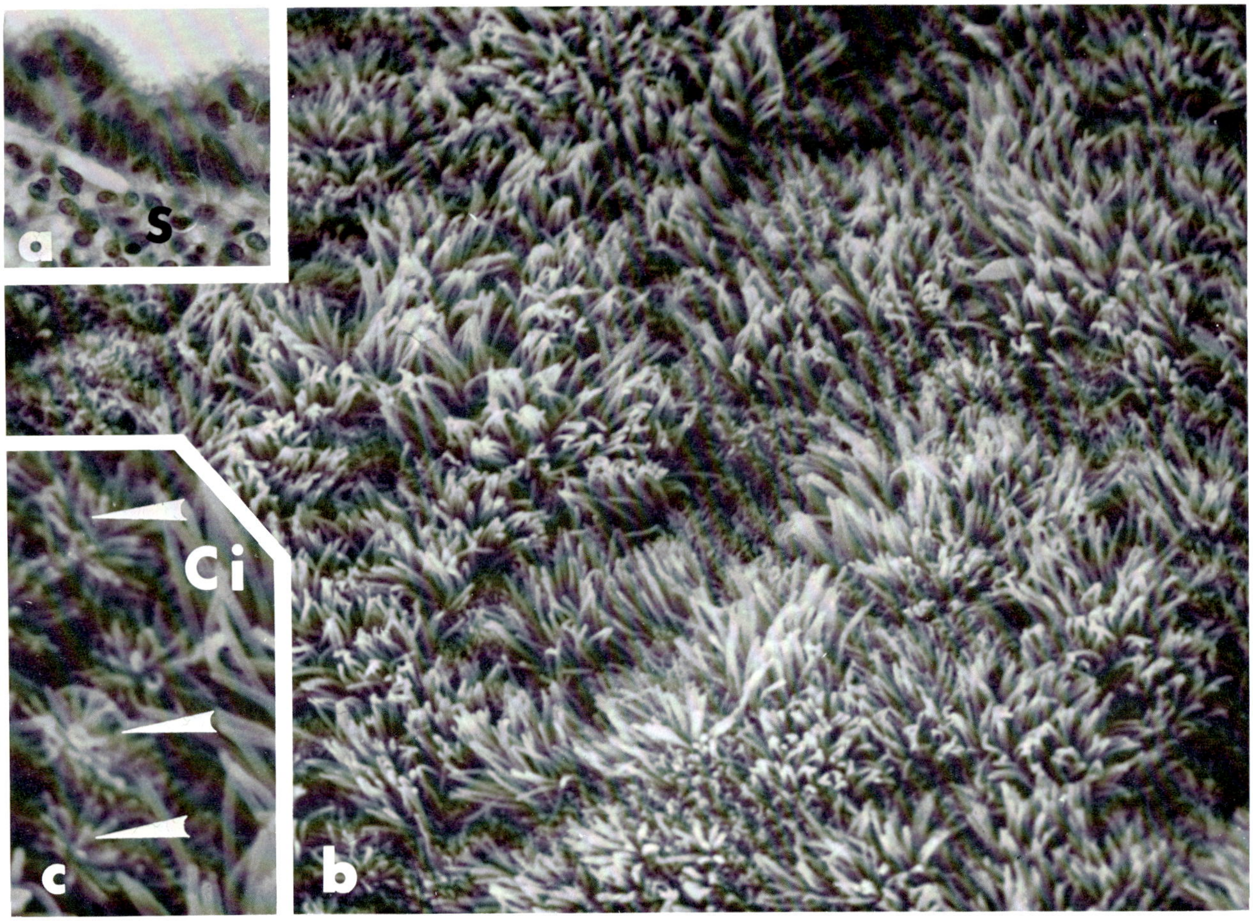

ADENOMATOUS HYPERPLASIA

Adenomatous hyperplasia, like cystic glandular hyperplasia, develops in association with unopposed estrogen stimulation and is most commonly seen in the peri- and postmenopausal period. Although the ovarian stroma is frequently hyperplastic in patients with adenomatous hyperplasia, it has recently been suggested that the postmenopausal estrogens indirectly derive from circulating steroid precursors. Estrone,[1] reported to be the major estrogenic compound found in postmenopausal women, is derived from circulating Δ-4-androstenedione, which is peripherally converted to estrone and estriol, independently of the ovaries or adrenals.[2] Since neither estrone nor estriol has been proved to have a carcinogenic uterine effect, these hormones are unlikely to be directly related to endometrial carcinogenesis.[2]

Adenomatous hyperplasia may occur as a focal or diffuse lesion, may be associated with cystic glandular hyperplasia or adenocarcinoma, or may be confined within an endometrial polyp.

Figure 123a. *The endometrial surface lining* in adenomatous hyperplasia is pseudostratified and contains numerous ciliated cells. (H & E stain, × 120.) S: stromal cells.

Figure 123b. With the *scanning electron microscope,* large areas are seen to be composed principally of cilitated cells; the microvillosity of nonciliated cells is more pronounced than in the normal endometrium or in cystic glandular hyperplasia.[3] × 2400.

Figure 123c. *High magnification* of a nonciliated cell with more than one microvillous promontory (arrow). × 6400. Ci: ciliated cell. *From* A. Ferenczy and R. M. Richart. Scanning electron microscopy of hyperplastic and neoplastic endometria. In *Scanning Electron Microscopy/1973.* Part III. *Proceedings of the Workshop on Scanning Electron Microscopy in Pathology,* O. Johari (Ed.). IIT Research Institute, Chicago, 1973, pp. 613–620.

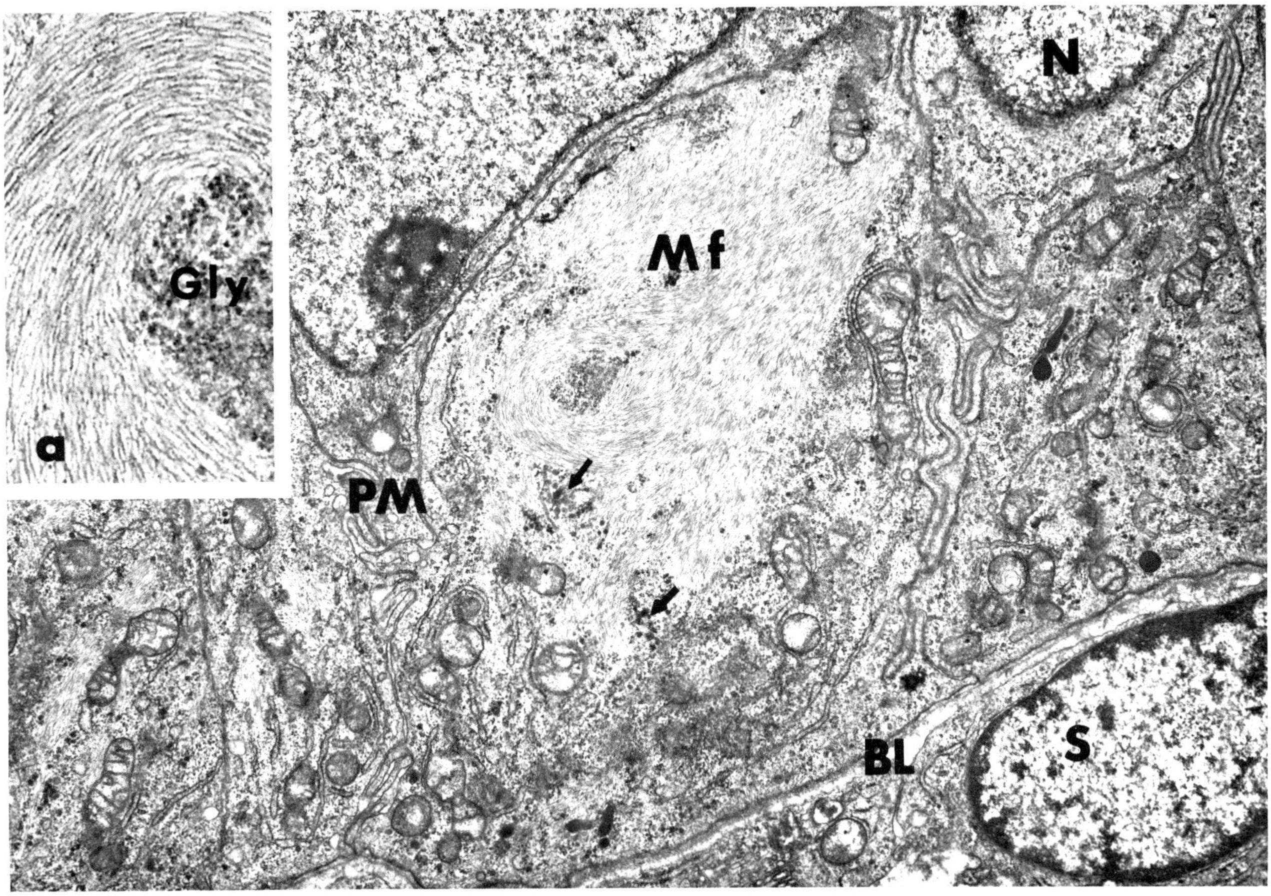

Figure 124. *Ultrastructurally,* the cytoplasmic organelles are more numerous than those found in cystic glandular hyperplasia, and, in addition, the plasma membranes (PM) and endoplasmic reticulum are more convoluted. In contrast to cystic glandular hyperplasia and to normal endometrium, the microfilaments (Mf) in adenomatous hyperplasia are arranged in large masses with a focal, concentric pattern and are invariably located at the basal portion of individual cells. Although a close association between the supranuclear Golgi and the microfilaments is not seen, the latter have an architecture similar to that of the microfilaments found in normal endometrium and occasionally contain scattered glycogen particles (arrows) and ribosomes. × 12,600. N: nucleus; BL: basal lamina; S: stroma cell.

Figure 124a. *Detail of Figure 124,* illustrating the close relationship between bundles of microfilaments (75–100 Å thick) and glycogen particles (Gly). × 48,000.

REFERENCES (Adenomatous hyperplasia—Figure 124a)

1. MacDonald, P. C., J. S. Grodin, and P. K. Siiteri. The utilization of plasma androstenedione for estrone production in women. In *Progress in Endocrinology: Proceedings of the Third International Congress of Endocrinology, Mexico, D.F., June 30 to July 5, 1968.* Excerpta Medica Foundation, Amsterdam, 1969, pp. 770–776.
2. Lemon, H. M., D. M. Miller, and J. F. Foley. Competition between steroids for hormonal receptor. *Natl. Cancer Inst. Monogr.* **34:** 77 (1971).
3. Ferenczy, A. and R. M. Richart. Scanning electron microscopy of hyperplastic and neoplastic endometria. In *Scanning Electron Microscopy/1973.* Part III. *Proceedings of the Workshop on Scanning Electron Microscopy in Pathology,* O. Johari (Ed.). IIT Research Institute, Chicago, p. 613.

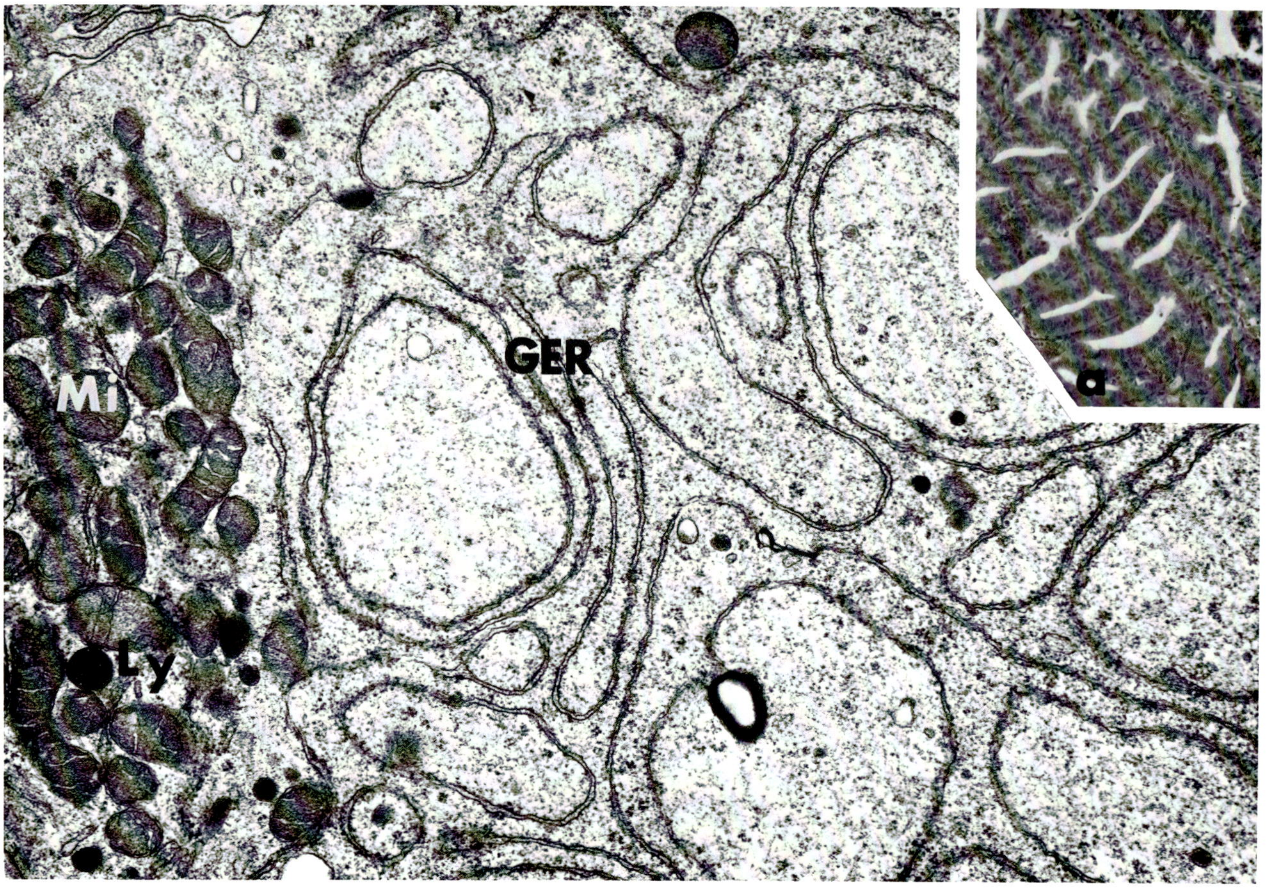

Figure 125a. *Adenomatous hyperplasia.* Histologically, there is extreme glandular crowding with numerous intraluminal papillary projections, and a "gland-in-gland" pattern is frequently observed. Some glands may be in tight apposition ("back to back") and may be separated only by their respective basal lamina. The glands are lined by a florid, often pseudostratified, epithelium with numerous mitoses and ciliated cells. The nuclei, as in cystic glandular hyperplasia, are regular and contain a DNA distribution pattern similar to that in normal endometrium. In approximately 20% of cases of adenomatous hyperplasia, nuclear pleomorphism and an aneuploid nuclear DNA distribution pattern are present.[1] (H & E stain, × 30.)

Figure 125. *Adenomatous hyperplasia.* A striking feature in adenomatous hyperplasia is the marked convolution of the cisternae of granular endoplasmic reticulum (GER). Mitochondria (Mi) are numerous, with an electron-dense, amorphous matrix, often arranged in clusters. As in cystic glandular hyperplasia, cytoplasmic alkaline phosphatase activity and estrogen receptor content[2] are strikingly increased. × 24,400. Ly: lysosome.

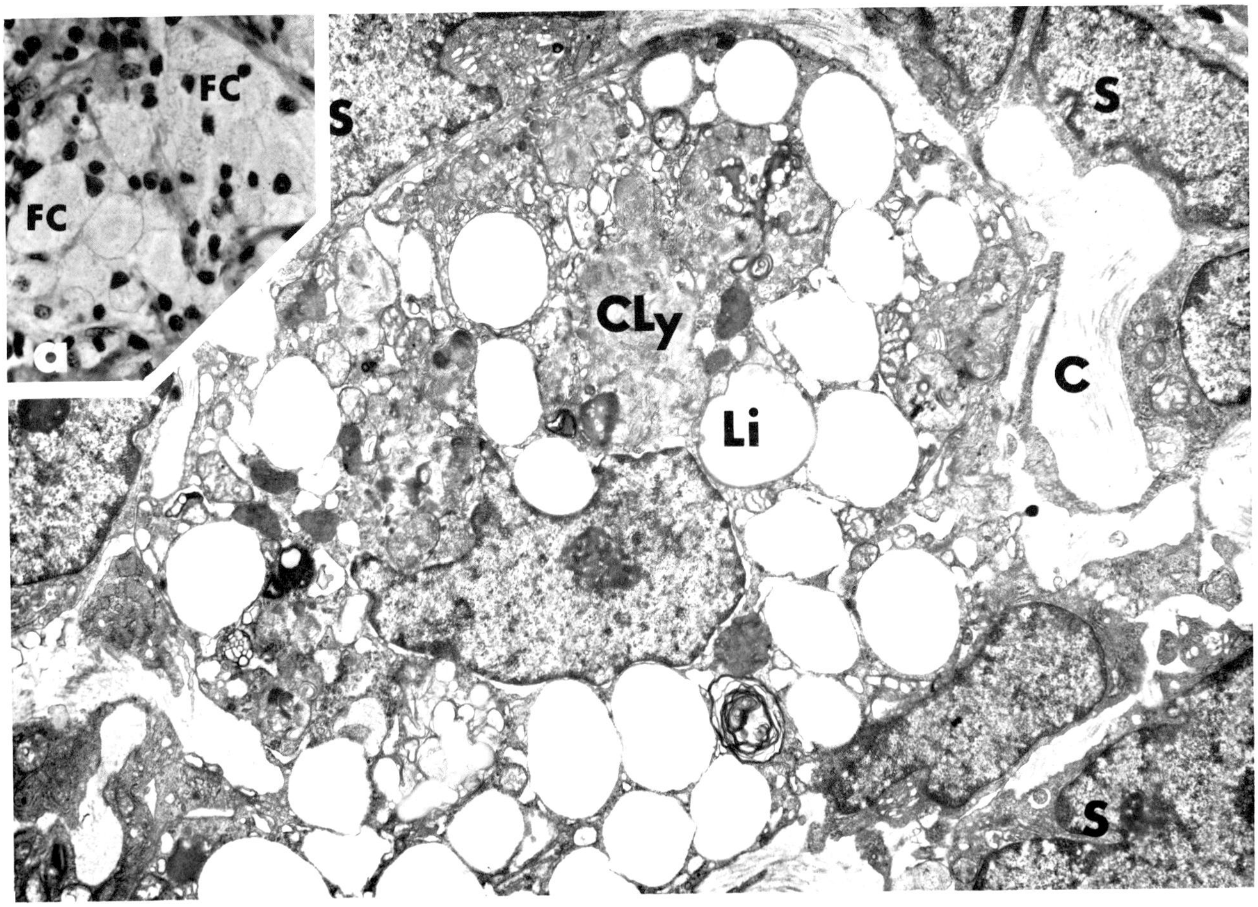

Figure 126a. *The supporting stroma in adenomatous hyperplasia* is hypercellular and frequently contains collections of foam cells (FC), in which autofluorescent lipid droplets, probably cholesterol or estrogen derivatives, can be demonstrated.[3] (H & E stain, × 120.)

Figure 126. *At the electron microscopic level,* foam cells are filled with lipid droplets (Li) (most of which are extracted during preparative procedures), prominent cytolysosomes (CLy), and numerous membrane-bound dense bodies. Foam cells often establish close contact with the adjacent spindle-shaped stromal cells (S) by their respective cytoplasmic processes. Histologically and ultrastructurally, similar lipid-laden macrophages contaning cholesterol are seen in cholesterolosis of the gall bladder, where they accumulate in response to a local disturbance of lipid metabolism.[4] The abundance of lipid-laden macrophages in hyperestrogenic conditions, especially adenomatous hyperplasia, is generally interpreted as a reflection of estrogenic stimulation of the endometrial stromal cells and is thought to be related to increased or disturbed steroid synthesis.[3] × 5600. C: stromal collagen.

REFERENCES (Figures 125–126)

1. Wagner, D., R. M. Richart, and J. Y. Terner. Deoxyribonucleic acid content of presumed precursors of endometrial carcinoma. *Cancer* **20:** 2067 (1967).
2. Terenius, L., A. Lindell, and B. H. Persson. Binding of estradiol-17-beta to human cancer tissue of the female genital tract. *Cancer Res.* **31:** 1895 (1971).
3. Dallenbach-Hellweg, G. *Histopathology of the Endometrium.* Springer-Verlag, New York, 1971.
4. Nevalainen, T. and M. Laitio. Ultrastructure of gall bladder with cholesterolosis. *Virchows Arch. Zellpathol.* **10:** 237 (1972).

31

Endometrium Associated with Hormonal Therapy (Oral Contraceptives)

Most oral contraceptive agents contain 19-nortestosterone or 17-hydroxyprogesterone as progestogen and mestranol or 1,7-α-ethinylestradiol as estrogen. The most commonly used oral contraceptives are combination preparations of estrogens and progestogens in a ratio of approximately 1 to 20. These medications produce varying degrees of glandular atrophy, depending on the duration of the treatment. *Ultrastructurally, under cyclic therapy,* the cytoplasmic organelles are poorly developed,[1-6] protein synthesis is minimal, and lipids are abundant. The nucleolar channel system,[5] a constant ultrastructural feature of the normal postovulatory period, is absent, and the estradiol competitive binding capacity is decreased.[7] The stroma contains foci of spindle-shaped cells, and, if differentiation into predecidualike cells occurs, it does so prematurely. These pseudodecidual cells contain abundant glycogen, Golgi, and endoplasmic reticulum.[8] Characteristically, spiral arterioles fail to develop, but there is a striking endothelial[2] and smooth muscle proliferation of the subepithelial vessels.

Under prolonged administration of progesterone for the treatment of endometriosis, a diffuse glandular atrophy, devoid of secretory activity and stromal decidualization, develops. The glandular epithelium contains decreased ergastoplasm and mitochondria, many of which are poorly formed and contain few cristae. There is an increase in supranuclear lipids.[1,5]

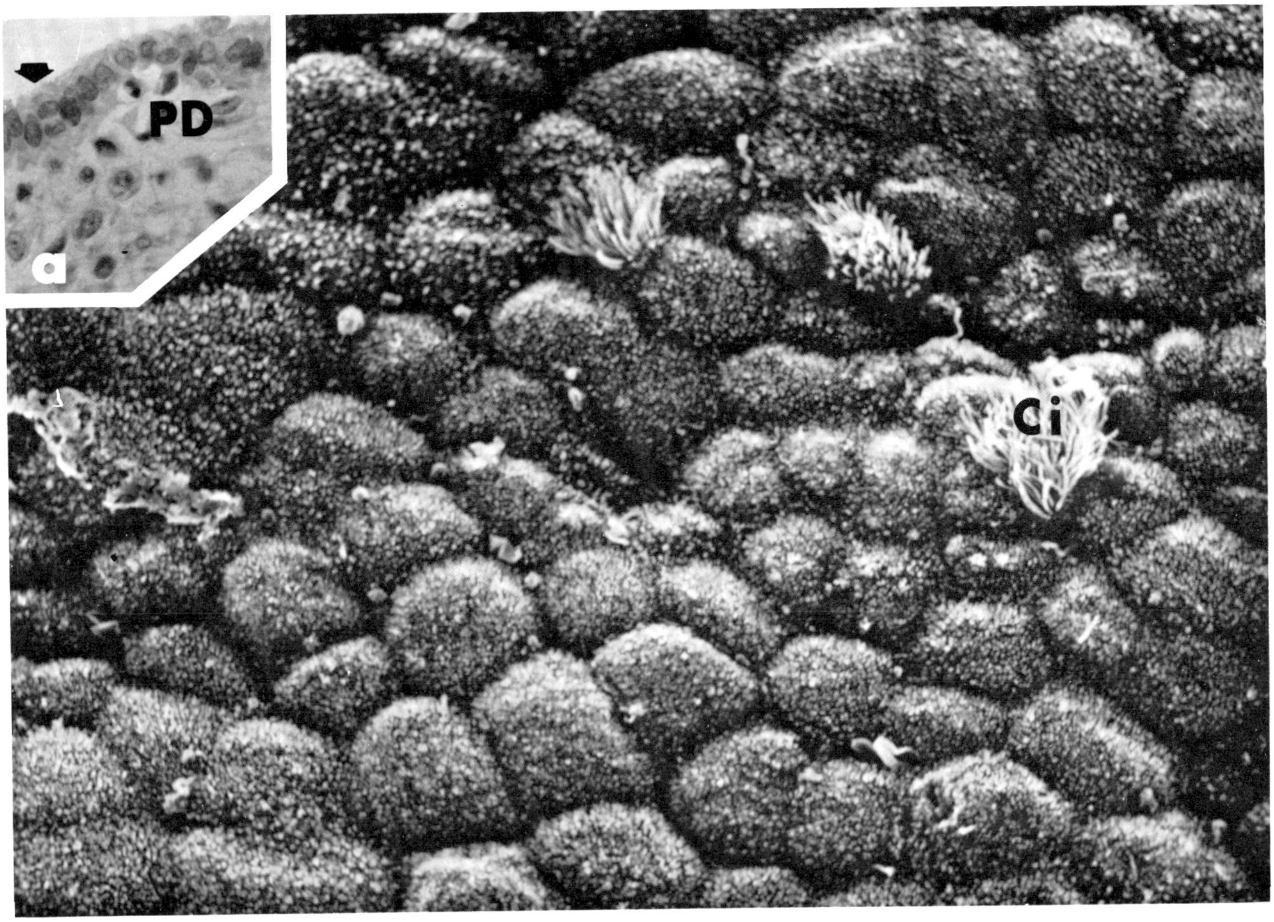

Figure 127a. *The surface epithelium,* although less atrophic than its glandular counterpart, contains low cuboidal cells and few ciliated cells (arrow). The pseudodecidual cells (PD) are indistinguishable from those seen in gestational endometrium, and they are rich in granular endoplasmic reticulum and free ribosomes.[1] (H & E stain, × 120.)

Figure 127. *With the scanning electron microscope the surface epithel cells* have short and sparce microvilli and ciliated cells (Ci) resembling the atrophic epithelium of the late postmenopausal period. × 1,600.

32

Endometrium in the Presence of Copper-Containing Intrauterine Contraceptive Device (Cu-T IUCD)

The recently introduced[9] metal-covered, intrauterine contraceptive devices such as the Cu-T and Cu-7 IUCD produce no significant morphologic alterations of the endometrial mucosa, in respect to its cyclic response to ovarian hormonal stimuli.[10] The antifertility effect of these devices is local and is thought to be related to the metallic copper released into the endometrial secretions, which renders them blastocytotoxic and thereby inhibits nidation.[10,11]

Figure 128a. *Histologic appearance* of the endometrial surface epithelium near the implantation site of a Cu-T IUCD. Foci of degenerating epithelial cells (arrow) alternate with tall columnar, hypertrophic cells (arrow heads). The subjacent stroma (S) contains acute and chronic inflammatory exudate. Aside from the mild to moderate amount of chronic inflammatory reaction, the cyclic morphologic changes in the glandular epithelium are generally not affected. (H & E stain, × 75.)

Figure 128b. *Topographically*, near the implantation site of the device, there are numerous narrow zones of atrophic (A) epithelium alternating with zones of hypertrophic (H) cells with bulging surface plasma membranes and an irregular contour. In these regions, ciliated cells are absent. × 480.

Figure 128c. *Higher magnification*, illustrating a ruptured (arrow) surface epithelial cell. × 1000.

REFERENCES (Most oral contraceptive agents— Figure 128c)

1. Clyman, M. J. Electron microscopic changes produced in the human endometrium by norethindrone acetate with ethinyl estradiol. *Fertil. Steril.* **14:** 352 (1963).
2. Ancla, M., P. Simon, and J. De Brux. Modifications endométriales après administration prolongée de lynéstrénol. Etude au microscope optique et éléctronique. *Gynécol. Obstét. (Paris)* **64:** 231 (1965).
3. Verhagen, A. and H. Theman. Elektronenmikroskopische Endometrium befunde nach Behandlung mit ovulationshemmenden Stoffen. *Arch. Gynaekol.* **202:** 253 (1965).
4. Friedrich, E. R. Effects of contraceptive hormone preparations on the fine structure of the endometrium. *Obstet. Gynecol.* **30:** 201 (1967).
5. Sirtori, C. Some ultrastructural aspects of human uterine physiopatholgy: cyclosenility, senility, antisenile and antitumoral therapies, and contraceptive drugs. In *Proceedings of International Symposium on Obstetrics and Gynaecology,* J. A. Chalmers, R. Merger, and G. B. Candiani (Eds.). Carlo Erba Foundation, Milan, 1969, pp. 129–154.
6. Wynn, R. M. and I. Sawaragi. Effects on intra-uterine and oral contraceptives on the ultrastructure of the human endometrium. *J. Reprod. Fertil.* (Suppl.) **8:** 45 (1969).
7. Henderson, S. R. and D. S. Schalch. Estrogen receptors in the human uterus. *Am. J. Obstet. Gynecol.* **112:** 762 (1972).
8. Wienke, E. C., F. Cavazos, D. G. Hall, and F. V. Lucas. Ultrastructural effects of norethynodral and mestranol on human endometrial stroma cell. *Am. J. Obstet. Gynecol.* **103:** 102 (1969).
9. Zipper, J. A., H. J. Tatum, L. Pastene, M. Medel, and M. Rivera. Metallic copper as an intrauterine contraceptive adjunct to the "T" device. *Am. J. Obstet. Gynecol.* **105:** 1274 (1969).
10. Salaverry, G., M. D. C. Mendez, J. Zipper, and M. Medel. Copper determination and localization in different morphologic components of human endometrium during the menstrual cycle in copper intrauterine contraceptive device wearers. *Am. J. Obstet. Gynecol.* **115:** 163 (1973).
11. Noeslund, G. Blastocystotoxic effect of copper in vitro. *Contraception* **6:** 281 (1972).
12. Hagenfeldt, K., E. Johannisson, and P. Brenner. Intrauterine contraception with the copper-T device. III. Effect upon endometrial morphology. *Contraception* **6:** 207 (1972).

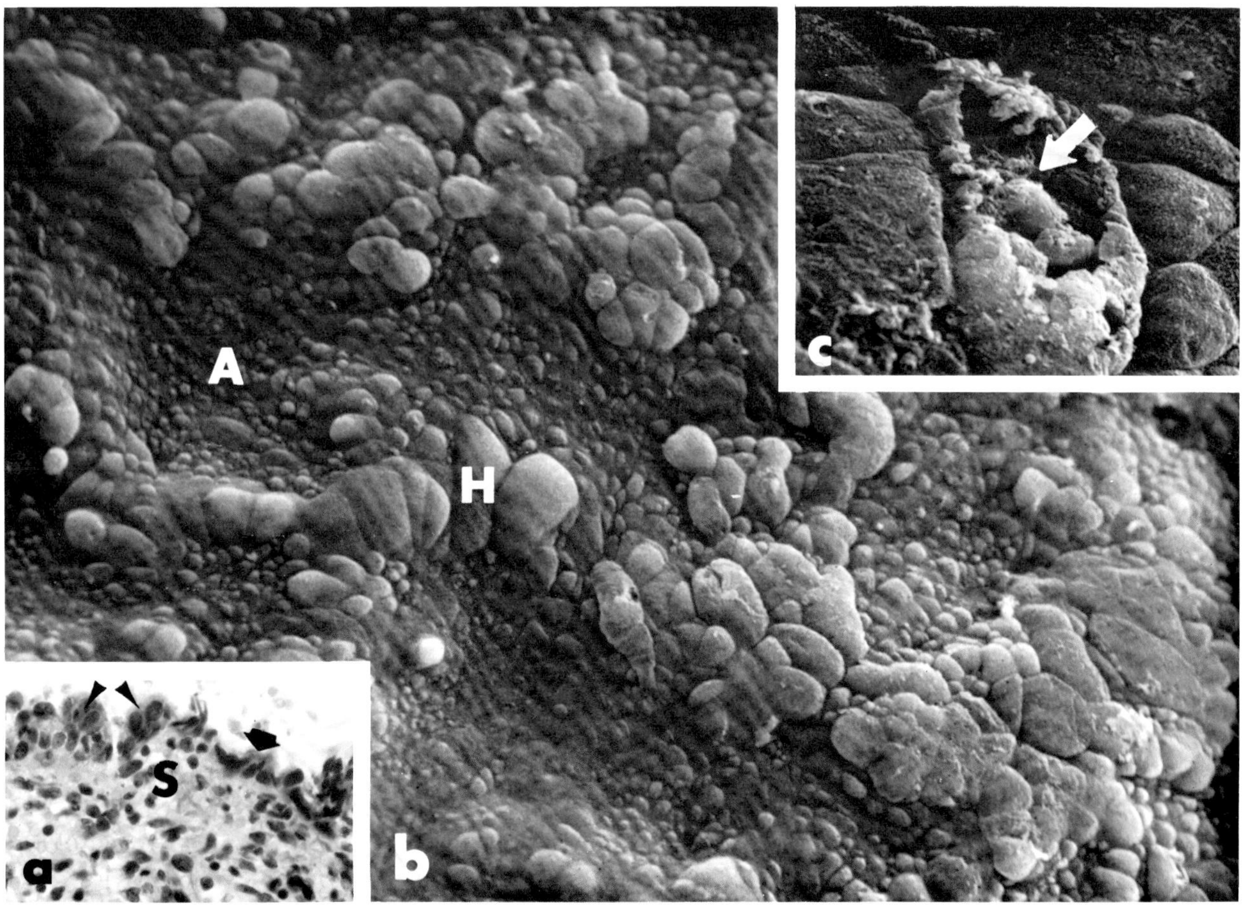

33

Endometritis

CHRONIC, NONSPECIFIC ENDOMETRITIS

Figure 129a. *Chronic, nonspecific endometritis* is a relatively common inflammatory condition which, histologically, is characterized by the presence of plasma cells (arrows). The stromal cells are enlarged, plump, and generally randomly oriented but occasionally have a whorled pattern. They are intermixed with lyphocytes and mature plasma cells. (H & E stain, × 120.)

Figure 129. *At the electron microscopic level,* mature plasma cells (P) with abundant granular endoplasmic reticulum, lymphocytes (L) with poor cytoplasmic content, and extravasated red blood cells (RBC) intermingle with clusters of predecidual cells (PD). × 5600.

REFERENCE (Figures 129–130)

1. Vasudeva, K., T. Thrasher, and R. M. Richart. Chronic endometritis: a clinical and electron microscopic study. *Am. J. Obstet. Gynecol.* **112:** 749 (1972).

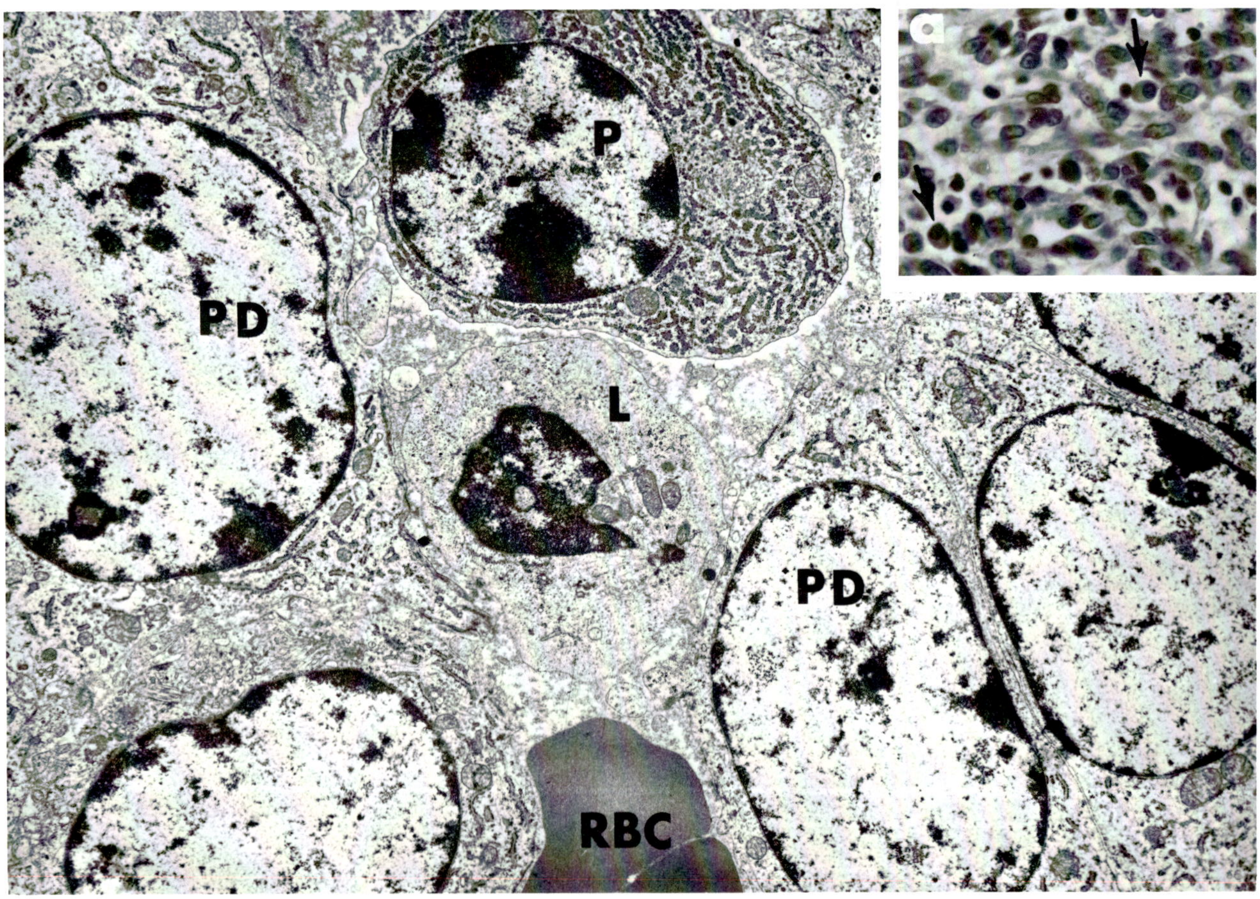

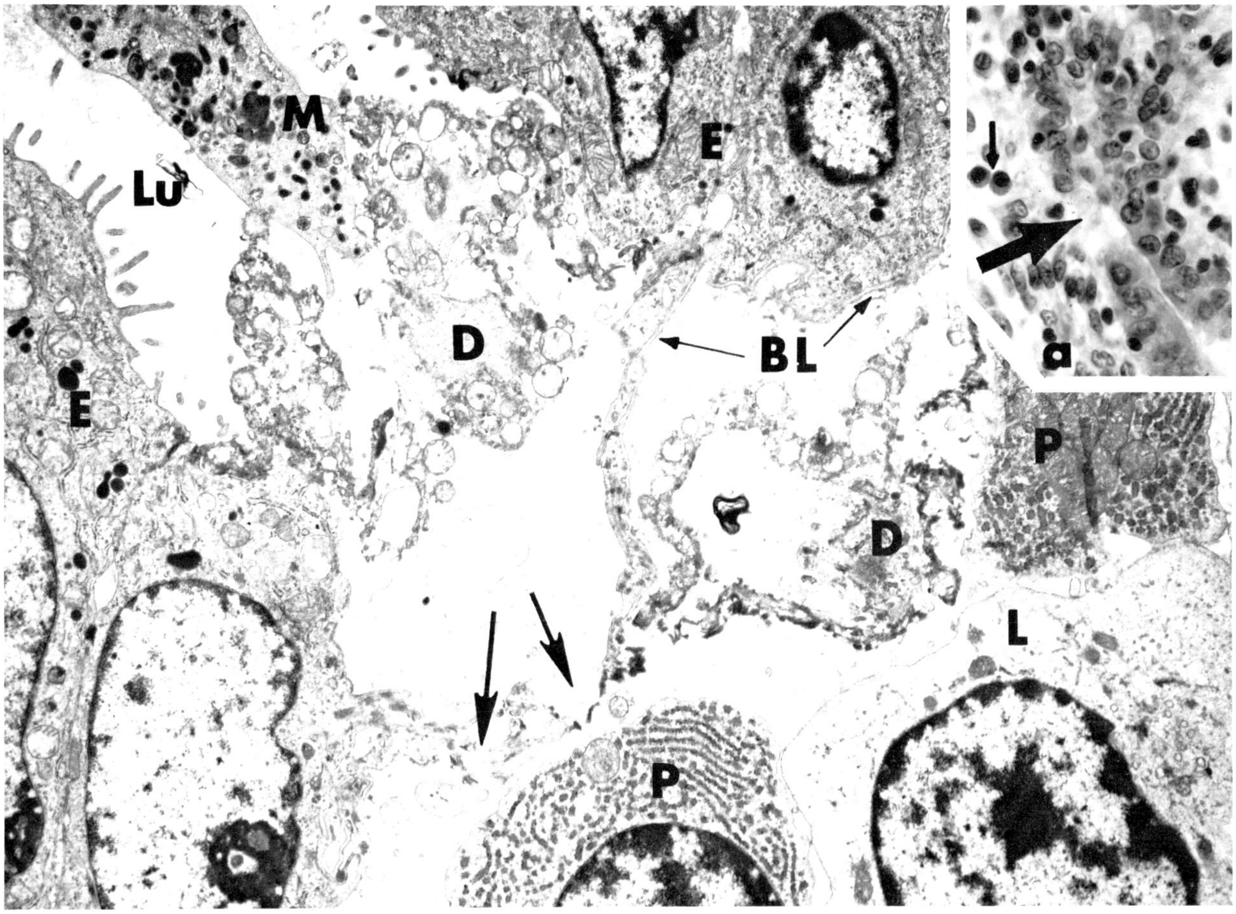

Figure 130a. *The endometrial glandular lining* in severe chronic endometritis appears inconsistent with the cycle and is often ruptured (long arrow) and permeated by polymorphonuclear cells and lymphocytes. The surrounding stroma contains numerous plasma cells (small arrow). (H & E stain, × 120.)

Figure 130. *At the ultrastructural level,* there is a considerable reduction in secretory activity and cytoplasmic glycogen, and an absence of the nucleolar channel system is noted.[1] Bacteria have not been found electron microscopically.[1] Although intraepithelial lymphocytes are numerous, plasma cells (P) are not seen within the intercellular spaces, and disruption (arrows) of the glandular basal lamina (BL) and epithelial degeneration (D) are observed only in the severe form of the disease. Epithelial glandular cells (E) adjacent to degenerating cells (D) contain numerous lysosomes. Degenerating epithelial cells and macrophages (M) are seen both in the glandular lumen (Lu) and in the stroma near the disrupted basal lamina. × 5600. L: lymphocyte in the stroma.

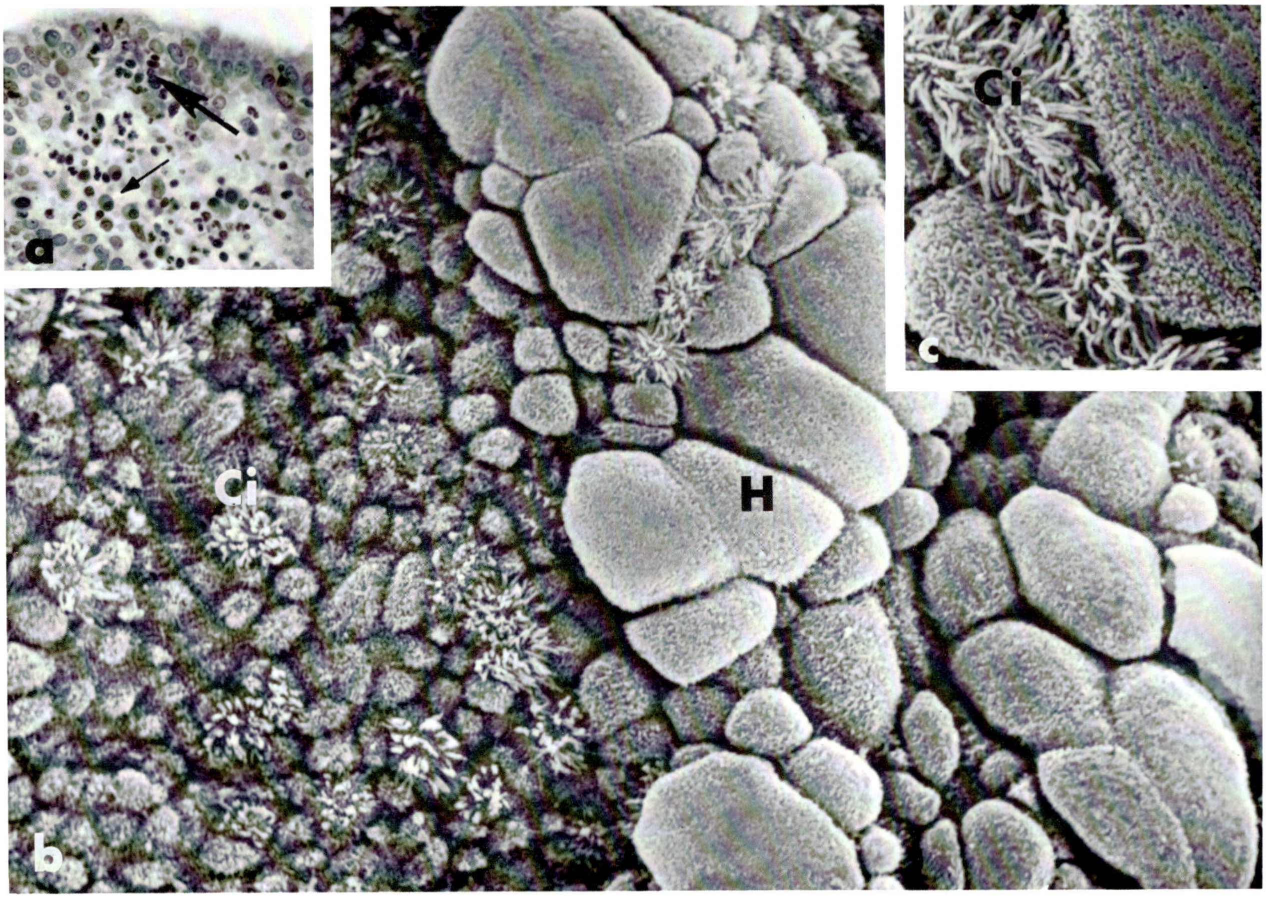

Figure 131a. *Chronic, nonspecific endometritis.* There is permeation of the surface epithelium by numerous mononuclear inflammatory cells (long arrow), and the underlying stroma contains plasma cells (short arrow) and clusters of polymorphonuclear cells. (H & E stain, × 75.)

Figure 131b. *The uterine surface epithelium* contains groups of markedly enlarged cells corresponding to hypertrophic epithelial cells (H), and the ciliated cells (Ci) have shorter and fewer ciliary shafts. × 960.

Figure 131c. *Higher magnification,* illustrating the surface plasma membrane of nonciliated, hypertrophic cells covered by abundant, but short, microvilli. Note the short and sparse cilia (Ci) on the adjacent cells. × 1920.

TUBERCULOUS ENDOMETRITIS

Tuberculous endometritis is almost always secondary to tuberculous salpingitis, and in the typical case there are stromal lymphoplasmacytic infiltrates in addition to typical granulomata with acid phosphatase-rich epithelioid and Langerhans giant cells. Tubercle bacilli and caseation necrosis are seldom observed because cyclic endometrial shedding precludes their proliferation and full development.

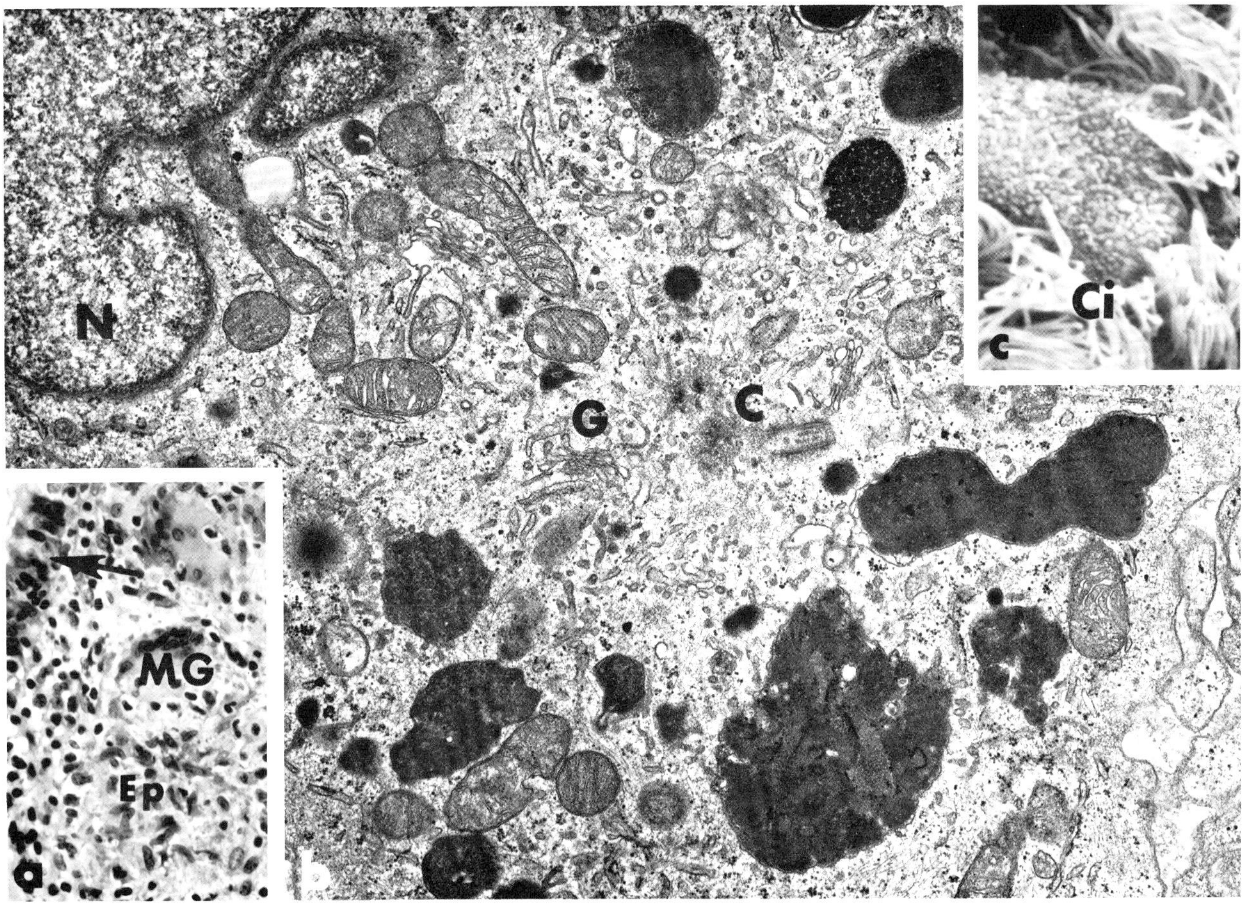

Figure 132a. *Light micrograph* of a tuberculous granuloma in the neighborhood of an endometrial gland (arrow). The lesion consists of large multinucleated giant cells (MG), clusters of epithelioid cells (Ep), and peripheral mononuclear cells. (H & E stain, × 75.)

Figure 132b. *At an ultrastructural level, the epithelioid cells* forming the granulomatous lesions appear as large interdigitating histiocytes with numerous blunt-ended, cytoplasmic extensions and intracytoplasmic lysosomes and phagosomes. The abundant organelles and dense granules contribute to their acidophilic appearance. Electron microscopic[1] and histochemical[2] studies of experimentally produced tuberculosis have suggested that destruction of the tubercle bacilli occurs in the mature macrophages (epithelioid cells), which have a high lysosomal content and are rich in β-galactosidase, microbicidins, and other digestive enzymes. The accumulated lysosomal products, stimulated by cellular immunity mediated by lymphocytes, are discharged into vacuoles containing mycobacteria. After bacillar degradation occurs, the macrophages degenerate, probably secondarily to the release of the tuberculinoid cytotoxic products. In the epithelioid cell shown in this figure tubercule bacilli are not recognized. × 16,900. G: Golgi; C: centriole, N: nucleus.

Figure 132c. *The ultrastructure of the surface* and glandular epithelium in tuberculous endometritis undergoes changes similar to those described in severe nonspecific, chronic endometritis. Cilia (Ci) as well as surface microvilli are short. × 2400.

REFERENCES (Figures 131a–132c)

1. Dumont, A. and H. Sheldon. Changes in the fine structure of macrophages in experimentally produced tuberculous granulomas in hamsters. *Lab. Invest.* **14:** 2034 (1965).
2. Shima, K., A. M. Dannenberg, M. Ando, S. Chandrasekhar, J. A. Seluzicki, and J. I. Fabrikant. Macrophage accumulation, division, maturation and digestive and microbicidal capacities in tuberculous lesions. *Am. J. Pathol.* **67:** 159 (1972).

34

Adenocarcinoma

Adenocarcinoma of the endometrium is among the most common malignant neoplasms of the female genital tract with a peak incidence at 55 to 60 years of age. Endocrine abnormalities such as postmenopausal hyperestronism[2,3] granulosa-theca cell tumors, and the Stein-Leventhal syndrome,[1] are often associated with endometrial carcinoma. Similarly, an increased conversion rate of Δ-4-androstenedione to estrone is found in postmenopausal women with carcinoma of the endometrium, as compared to normal controls.[2,3]

The concept that long-standing, unopposed estrogens are related to the development of endometrial malignancy, however, is as yet unproved, although the possibility is supported by the production of estrogen-induced uterine neoplasms in experimental animals.[4]

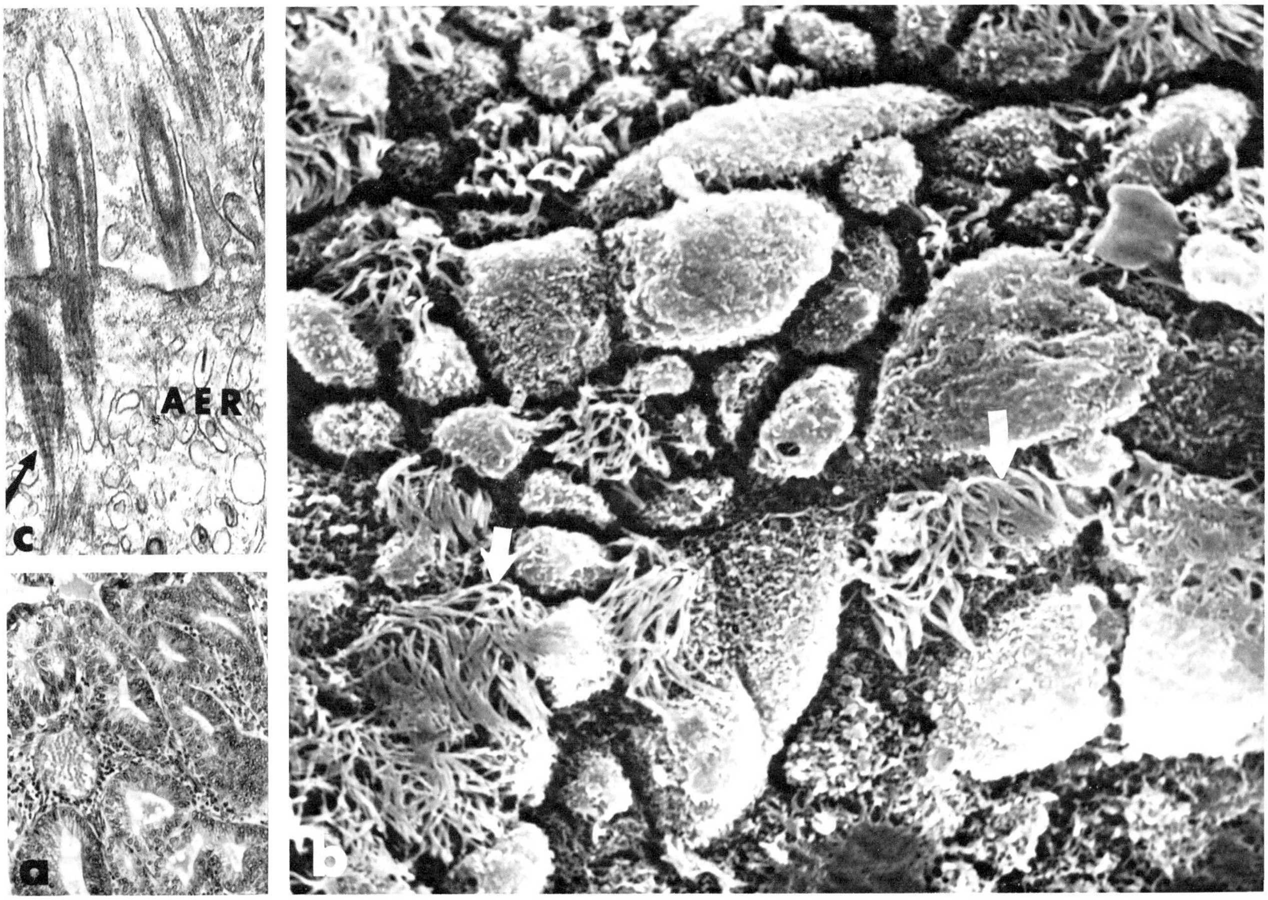

Figure 133a. *Histologically,* uterine adenocarcinoma is commonly divided into well, moderately well, and poorly differentiated types, according to the degree of glandular and cytologic differentiation. The light micrograph is of a well-differentiated adenocarcinoma. (H & E stain, × 30.)

Figure 133b. *In well-differentiated adenocarcinoma* the surface contains considerably fewer ciliated cells (arrow), as compared to hyperplastic endometria,[5] and there is cellular pleomorphism throughout. The microvilli covering the nonciliated cells are short and poorly preserved in the most superficial cells. × 1600. *From* A. Ferenczy and R. M. Richart. Scanning electron microscopy of hyperplastic and neoplastic endometria. In *Scanning Electron Microscopy/1973.* Part III: *Proceedings of the Workshop on Scanning Electron Microscopy in Pathology,* O. Johari (Ed.). IIT Research Institute, Chicago, 1973, pp. 613–620.

Figure 133c. *Ciliated cells,* morphologically similar to those seen in nonneoplastic endometria, but comparatively fewer in number,[5] are visible in the well-differentiated neoplasms.[5-7] Ciliary bodies are associated with abundant agranular endoplasmic reticulum (AER) and cross-striated ciliary rootlets (arrow). × 30,400.

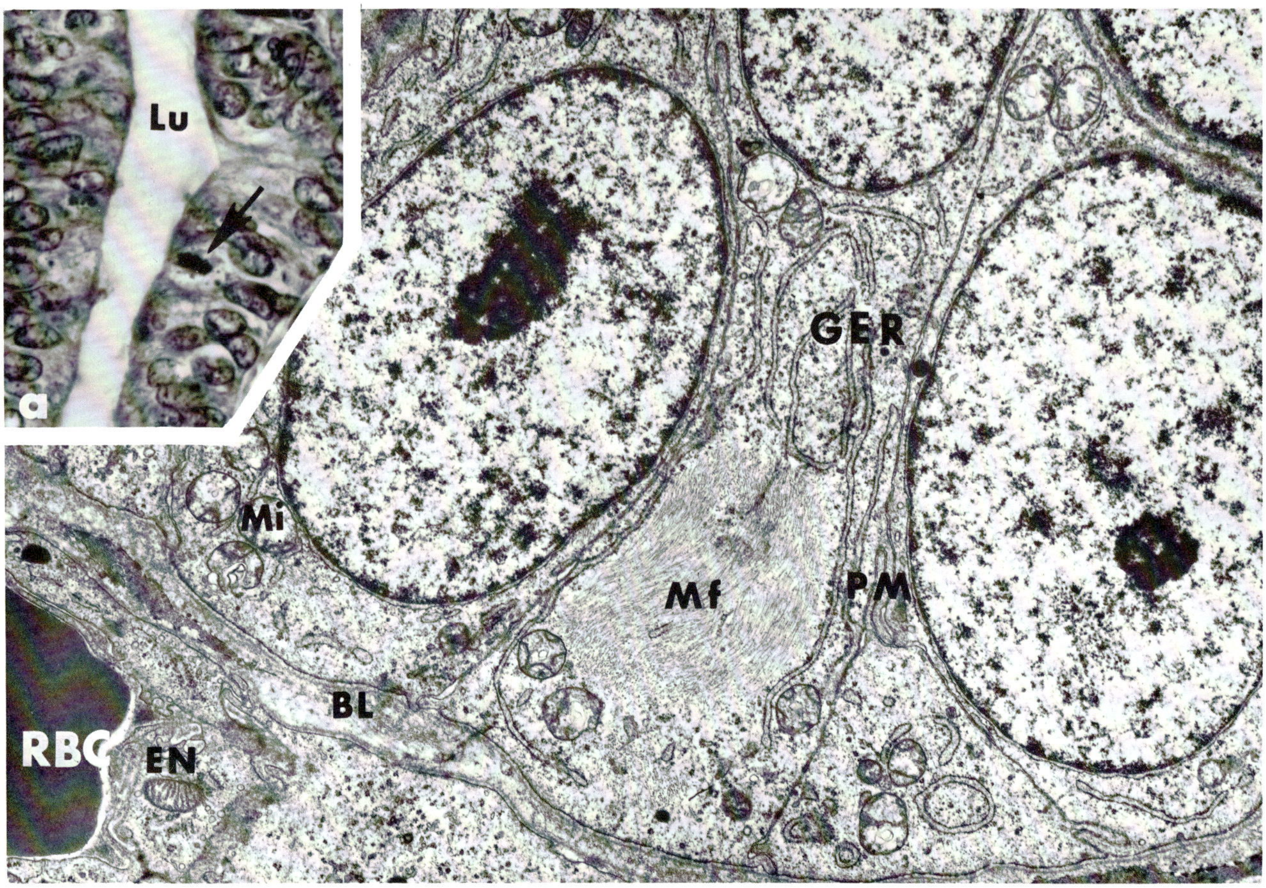

Figure 134. *At the ultrastructural level,* in the well-differentiated carcinoma cells the dominant cytoplasmic organelles are free ribosomes (polysomes) and granular endoplasmic reticulum (GER),[9-14] the latter often appearing in a complex, convoluted pattern. The Golgi are generally abundant and devoid of peripheral vesicles, [6,11,12,15,16] although occasionally there may be some secretory activity. Mitochondria (Mi) vary in size and number from cell to cell and are frequently enveloped by membranes of granular endoplasmic reticulum. Glycogen, lysosomes, and lipid droplets are sparse,[9-14] and bundles of microfilaments (Mf), [11,13,14,17] indistinguishable from those seen in normal and hyperplastic endometria, are commonly observed. The spatial relationship seen in normal endometrial cells between the microfilaments, Golgi, and glycogen is absent. The plasma membranes (PM), especially near the basal lamina, are irregular with complex infoldings[9-14] and are interconnected by a few small desmosomes. A well-developed basal lamina (BL) is always present. The intracytoplasmic glycogen, apical acid mucopolysaccharides, and alkaline phosphatase contents decrease with loss of differentiation.[1] These findings parallel a gradual loss in estrogen sensitivity, and a progressive decrease of 17-β-estradiol binding receptor content from well-differentiated (high levels) to poorly differentiated (low levels) neoplasms.[18] $\times$ 12,600. EN: capillary endothelium; RBC: red blood cells in capillary lumen.

Figure 134a. *Well-differentiated adenocarcinoma.* The nuclei are pseudostratified and the nucleoli are enlarged, usually are pleomorphic with numerous mitotic figures (arrow), and usually contain abnormal chromosome numbers and nuclear DNA values.[8] (H & E stain, $\times$ 190.) Lu: lumen.

REFERENCES (Adenocarcinoma–Figure 134)

1. Dallenbach-Hellweg, G. *Histopathology of the Endometrium.* Springer-Verlag, New York, 1971.
2. Rubin, B. L., S. B. Gusberg, J. Butterly, T. C. Han, and M. Maralit. A screening test for estrogen dependence of endometrial carcinoma. *Am. J. Obstet. Gynecol.* **114:** 660 (1972).
3. MacDonald, P. C., J. M. Grodin, and P. K. Siiteri. The utilization of plasma androstenedione for estrone production in women. In *Progress in Endocrinology: Proceedings of the Third International Congress of Endocrinology, Mexico, D.F., June 30 to July 5, 1968.* Excerpta Medica Foundation, Amsterdam, 1969, pp. 770–776.
4. Gardner, W. U., C. A. Pfeiffer, J. J. Trentin, and J. T. Wolstenholme. Hormonal factors in experimental carcinogenesis. In *The Physiopathology of Cancer,* 2nd ed., F. Homburger (Ed.). Hoeber Medical Division Harper & Row, New York, 1959.
5. Ferenczy, A. and R. M. Richart. Scanning electron microscopy of hyperplastic and neoplastic endometria. In *Scanning Electron Microscopy/1973.* Part III. *Proceedings of the Workshop on Scanning Electron Microscopy in Pathology,* O. Johari (Ed.). IIT Research Institute, Chicago, 1973, pp. 613–620.
6. Fasske, E., K. Morgenroth, H. Themann, and A. Verhagen. Electronenmikroskopische Untersuchungen menschlicher Collumcarcinome und ihres Stromas. *Arch. Gynaekol.* **197:** 511 (1960).
7. Sirtori, C. and E. Morano. *Cancer of the Uterus from Gross Appearance to Ultrastructure,* 2nd ed. Charles C Thomas, Springfield, Ill., 1963.
8. Wagner, D., R. M. Richart, and J. Y. Terner. Deoxyribonucleic acid content of presumed precursors of endometrial carcinoma. *Cancer* **20:** 2067 (1967).
9. Nilsson, O. Electron microscopy of the human endometrial carcinoma. *Cancer Res.* **22:** 492 (1962).
10. Nilsson, O., H. L. Kottmeier, and K. G. Tillinger. Some differences in the ultrastructure of normal and cancerous human uterine epithelium. *Acta. Obstet. Gynecol. Scand.* **45:** 73 (1963).
11. Hayakawa, K. Effects of dimethisterone on endometrial adenocarcinoma: Electron microscopic study. *Acta Obstet. Gynaecol. Jap.* **16:** 285 (1969).
12. Sirtori, C. Some ultrastructural aspects of human uterine physiopathology: cyclosenility, senility, antisenile and antitumoral therapies, and contraceptive drugs. In *Proceedings of International Symposium on Obstetrics and Gynaecology,* J. A. Chalmers, R. Merger, and G. B. Candiani (Eds.). Carlo Erba Foundation, Milan, 1969, pp. 129–154.
13. Gompel, C. Ultrastructure of endometrial carcinoma: review of fourteen cases. *Cancer* **28:** 745 (1971).
14. Thrasher, T. V. and R. M. Richart. An ultrastructural comparison of endometrial adenocarcinoma and normal endometrium. *Cancer* **29:** 1713 (1972).
15. Fasske, E., K. Morgenroth, H. Themann, and A. Verhagen. Elektronenmikroskopische Untersuchungen von Proliferationspase, glandularcystischer Hyperplasie und Adenocarcinom der Schleimhaut des Corpus Uteri. *Arch. Gynaekol.* **200:** 473 (1965).
16. Wessel, W. Endometriale Adenocarcinome verschiedener Differenzierungsgrade und ihr Stroma im elektronenmikroskopischen Bild. *Z. Krebforsch.* **66:** 421 (1965).
17. Hameed, K. and D. A. Morgan. Papillary adenocarcinoma of endometrium with psammoma bodies. Histology and fine structure. *Cancer* **29:** 1326 (1972).
18. Terenius, L., A. Lindell, and B. H. Persson. Binding of estradiol-17-β to human cancer tissue of the female genital tract. *Cancer Res.* **31:** 1895 (1971).

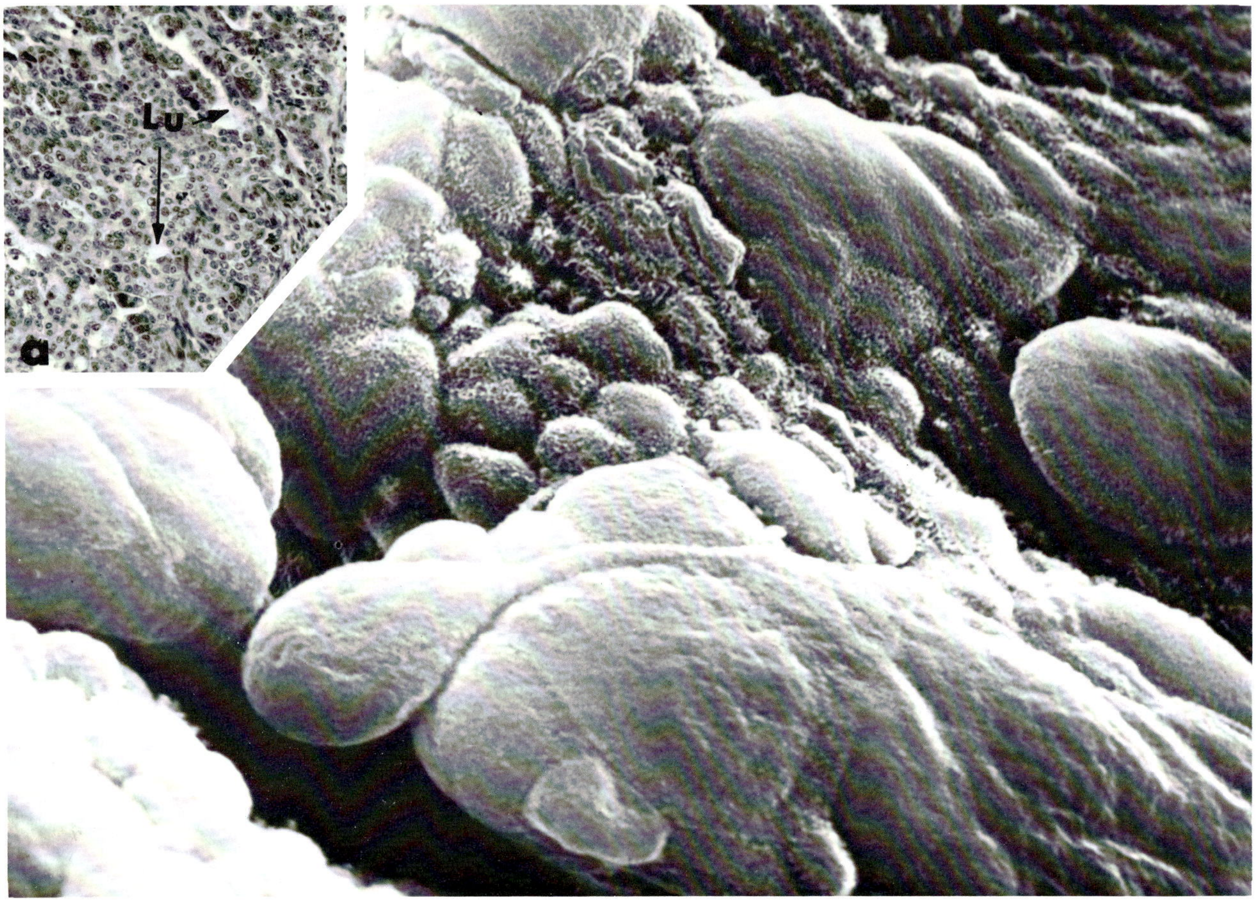

ADENOCARCINOMA ASSOCIATED WITH PROGESTIN THERAPY

The strong influence of progestational agents on endometrial cancer, observed clinically and experimentally, has also been demonstrated biochemically and morphologically. In-vitro DNA and RNA synthesis in endometrial cancer cells decreases in the presence of progestins,[7,8] and the binding of estradiol is reduced. Prolonged administration of pharmacologic doses of progestins[9] induces essentially similar morphologic alterations in well-differentiated carcinoma cells and in normal or hyperplastic endometrium (see **Cystic Glandular Hyperplasia with Progestin Effect**). Initially, a dramatic increase in the development of the endoplasmic reticulum–mitochondrial–Golgi complex and in glycogen accumulation takes place,[8,10-12] consistently with active glycoprotein synthesis. As secretory activity increases, giant autolysosomes, similar to those seen in the late luteal phase, appear,[8,9] and the neoplastic cells become low cuboidal and devoid of mitotic activity. Eventually, complete glandular atrophy and stromal decidualization may occur.

Although the precise mechanism of action of synthetic progestins on endometrial neoplasia is unclear, the presently available morphological and biochemical data suggest a direct cellular effect (not mediated by immunological mechanisms) on both the neoplastic and stromal cells, producing a "retrogressive maturation" of uterine carcinoma.[7-9,11]

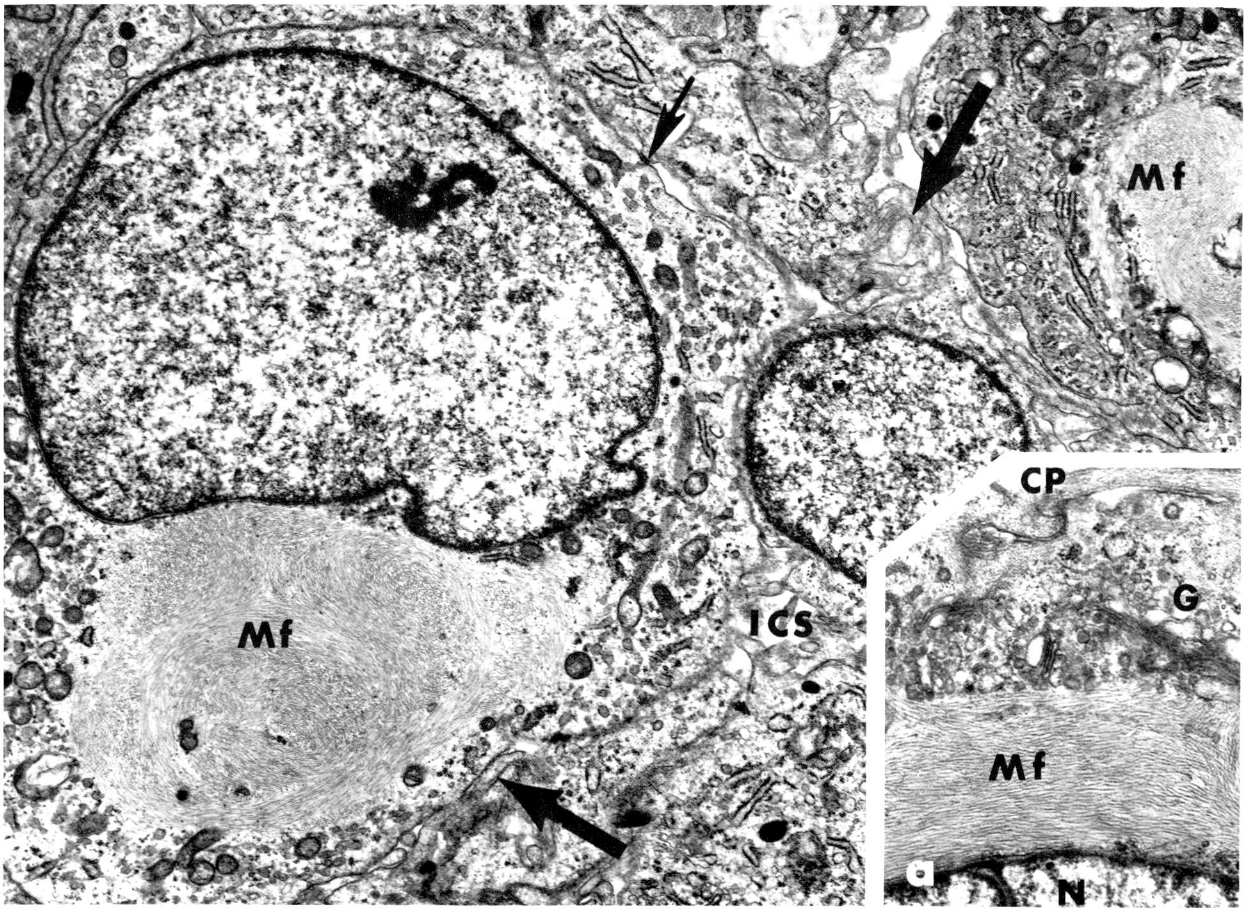

Figure 135a. *Histologic appearance* of poorly differentiated endometrial carcinoma, containing solid sheets of pleomorphic neoplastic cells and abortive gland formation (Lu). (H & E stain, × 30.)

Figure 135. *Topographically,* the surface has highly pleomorphic cells, covered by short microvillous processes, and ciliated cells are uniformly absent. × 1280. From A. Ferenczy and R. M. Richart. Scanning electron microscopy of hyperplastic and neoplastic endometria. In *Scanning Electron Microscopy/1973.* Part III. *Proceedings of the Workshop on Scanning Electron Microscopy in Pathology,* O. Johari (Ed.). IIT Research Institute, Chicago, 1973, pp. 613–620.

Figure 136. *In less mature and poorly differentiated carcinomas,* ciliated cells,[1] as well as cytoplasmic organelles, decrease in number except for the microfilamentous (Mf) structures and free and bound ribosomes, which appear even more abundant. The convolutions in the granular endoplasmic reticulum and plasma membranes are pronounced, the latter being occasionally attached by poorly developed desmosomes (short arrow). The cytoplasmic processes become extremely complex[2,3] (long arrows), and the basal lamina in many undifferentiated cells is absent.[4] Large masses of juxtanuclear microfilaments (Mf) are frequently encountered, however, even in the most undifferentiated neoplastic cells. The endometrial stroma cells between the carcinomatous glands contain well-developed ergastoplasm[4,5] and prominent Golgi with numerous peripheral vesicles. Foam cells of stromal cell derivation, similar to those observed in hyperplastic endometrial tissue, are often seen.[6] × 12,600. ICS: intercellular spaces.

Figure 136a. *Higher magnification* of perinuclear (N) microfilaments (Mf) occurring in large bundles, pushing aside the Golgi (G). × 23,060. (CP): Cytoplasmic microvillous process.

REFERENCES (The strong influence–Figure 136)

1. Ferenczy, A. and R. M. Richart. Scanning electron microscopy of hyperplastic and neoplastic endometria. In *Scanning Electron Microscopy/1973*. Part III. *Proceedings of the Workshop on Scanning Electron Microscopy in Pathology*, O. Johari (Ed.). IIT Research Institute, Chicago, 1973, p. 613.
2. Nilsson, O. Electron microscopy of the human endometrial carcinoma. *Cancer Res.* **22:** 492 (1962).
3. Nilsson, O., H. L. Kottmeier, and K. G. Tillinger. Some differences in the ultrastructure of normal and cancerous human uterine epithelium. *Acta Obstet. Gynecol. Scand.* **42:** 73 (1963).
4. Fasske, E., K. Morgenroth, H. Themann, and A. Verhagen. Elektronenmikroskopische Untersuchungen menschlicher Collumcarcinome und ihres Stromas. *Arch. Gynaekol.* **197:** 511 (1960).
5. Fasske, E., K. Morgenroth, H. Themann, and A. Verhagen. Elektronenmikroskipische Untersuchunger von Proliferationsphase, glandularcystischer Hyperplasie und Adenocarcinom der Schleimhaut des Corpus Uteri. *Arch. Gynaekol.* **200:** 473 (1965).
6. Thrasher, R. V. and R. M. Richart. An ultrastructural comparison of endometrial adenocarcinoma and normal endometrium. *Cancer* **29:** 1713 (1972).
7. Nordqvist, S. The synthesis of DNA and RNA in human carcinomatous endometrium in short term incubation in vitro and its response to oestradiol and progesterone. *J. Endocrinol.* **48:** 29 (1970).
8. Hayakawa, K., Y. Okudaira, and K. Nasu. Effect of gestagen on uterine adenocarcinoma of the endometrium in the human, with special reference to electron microscope study. *J. Jap. Obstet. Gynecol. Soc.* **20:** 1528 (1968).
9. Friedrich, E. F. Discussion of paper by D. G. Anderson. The possible mechanisms of action of progestins on endometrial adenocarcinoma. *Am. J. Obstet. Gynecol.* **113:** 208 (1972).
10. Sirtori, C. Some ultrastructural aspects of human uterine physiopathology: cyclosenility, senility, antisenile and antitumoral therapies, and contraceptive drugs. In *Proceedings of International Symposium on Obstetrics and Gynaecology*, J. A. Chalmers, R. Merger, and G. B. Candiani (Eds). Carlo Erba Foundation, Milan, 1969, pp. 129–154.
11. Anderson, D. G. The possible mechanism of action of progestins on endometrial adenocarcinoma. *Am. J. Obstet. Gynecol.* **113:** 195 (1972).
12. Kohorn, E. I. and R. Tchao. Endometrial carcinoma in organ culture. *J. Obstet. Gynaecol. Brit. Commonw.* **75:** 1262 (1968).

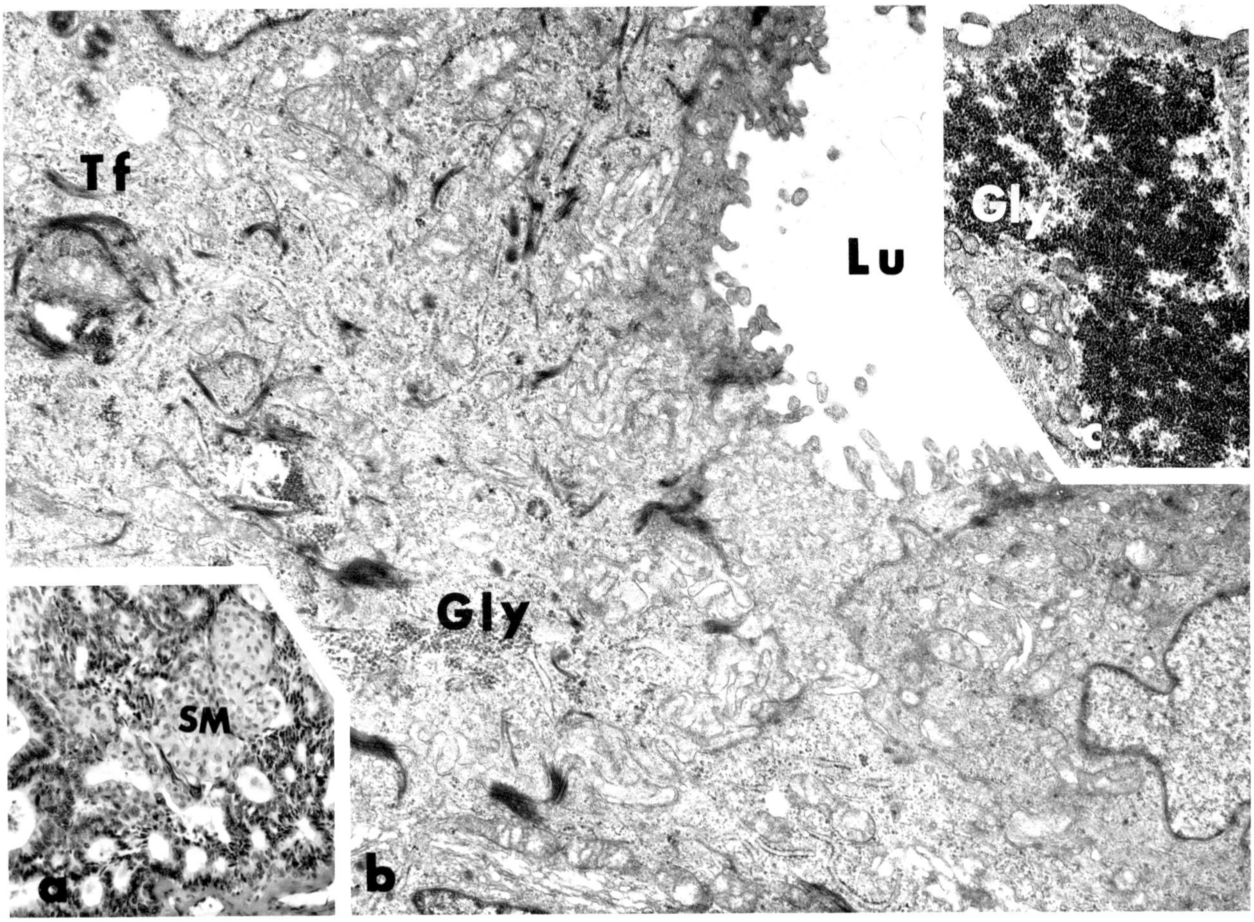

ADENOCARCINOMA WITH SQUAMOUS METAPLASIA (ADENOACANTHOMA)

Figure 137a. *Adenoacanthomas* are well-differentiated adenocarcinomas, containing foci of squamous epithelium (SM). The squamous nodules are considered to be metaplastic and are thought to arise either from indifferent reserve cells or from neoplastic columnar cells.[1] Uterine adenoacanthomas have been experimentally induced in rabbits with high doses of estrogens.[2] (H & E stain, × 30.)

Figure 137b. *Ultrastructurally,*[3] the squamous cells in the adenoacanthoma bear a close resemblance to the squamous metaplasia that occurs in the endocervical epithelium, including large aggregates of glycogen (Gly), scant bundles of tonofilaments (Tf), and small-sized desmosomes interconnecting prominent cytoplasmic processes. Intercellular spaces are enlarged, and keratohyaline granules may occur. The luminal (Lu) metaplastic squamous cells have numerous, short microvilli. × 5600.

Figure 137c. *Higher-power view* of intracytoplasmic glycogen particles (Gly) in metaplastic squamous cells. × 19,600.

REFERENCES (Figures 137a–138a)

1. Baggish, M. S. and J. D. Woodruff. The occurrence of squamous epithelium in the endometrium. *Obstet. Gynecol. Surv.* **22:** 69 (1967).
2. Meissner, W. A., S. C. Sommers, and G. Sherman. Endometrial hyperplasia, endometrial carcinoma and endometriosis produced experimentally by estrogens. *Cancer* **10:** 500 (1957).
3. Sirtori, C. and E. Morano. *Cancer of the Uterus from Gross Appearance to Ultrastructure,* 2nd ed. Charles C Thomas, Springfield, Ill., 1963.

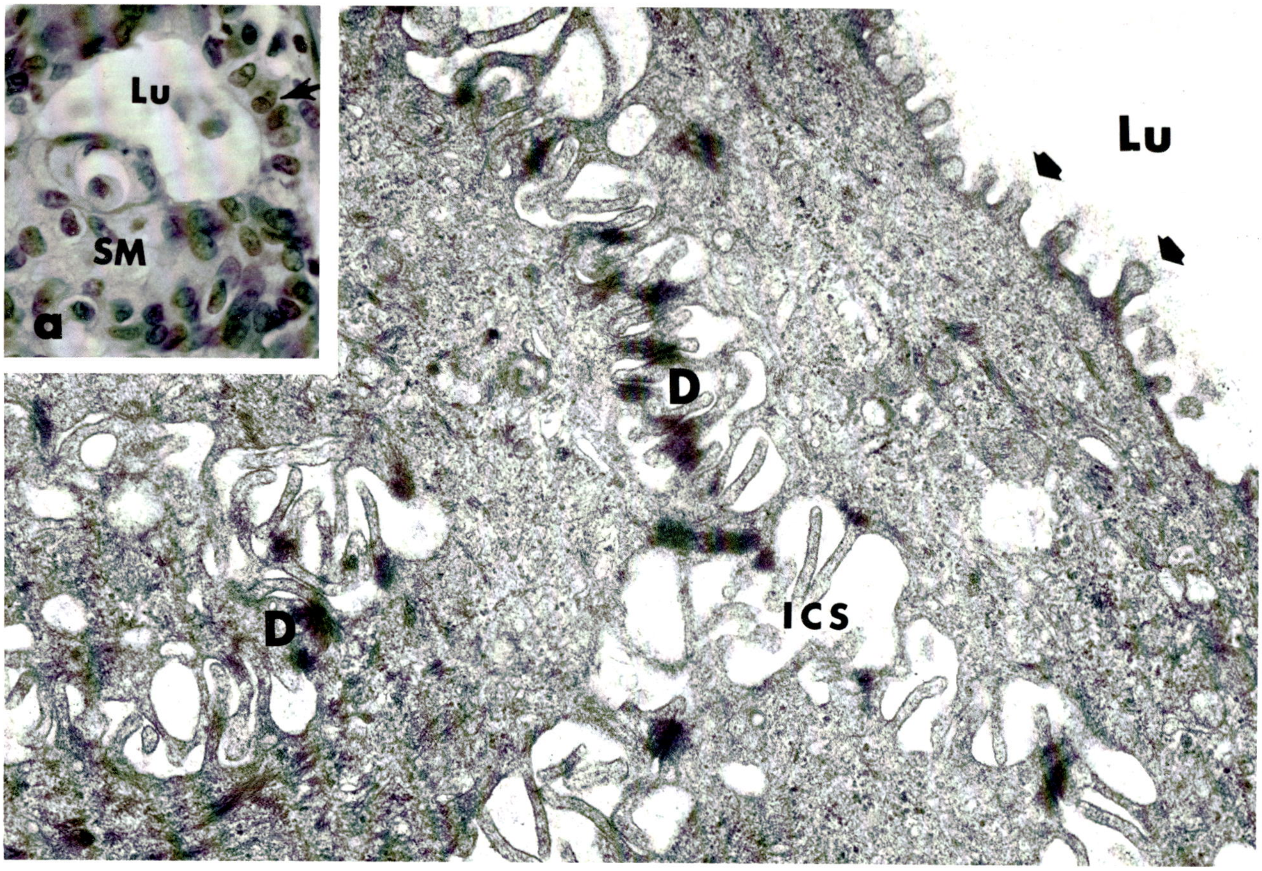

Figure 138a. *The neoplastic glandular epithelium* (arrow seems to be in direct continuity with masses of squamous cells (SM), which form one part of the glandular lumen (Lu). (H & E stain, × 120.)

Figure 138. *Ultrstructurally,* the luminal (Lu) lining cells have short microvilli (arrows) covered by filamentous material. As in normal squamous mucous membranes, the intercellular spaces (ICS) are dilated and contain numerous interdigitating microvilli, attached by poorly developed tonofilament–desmosome complexes (D). × 23,040.

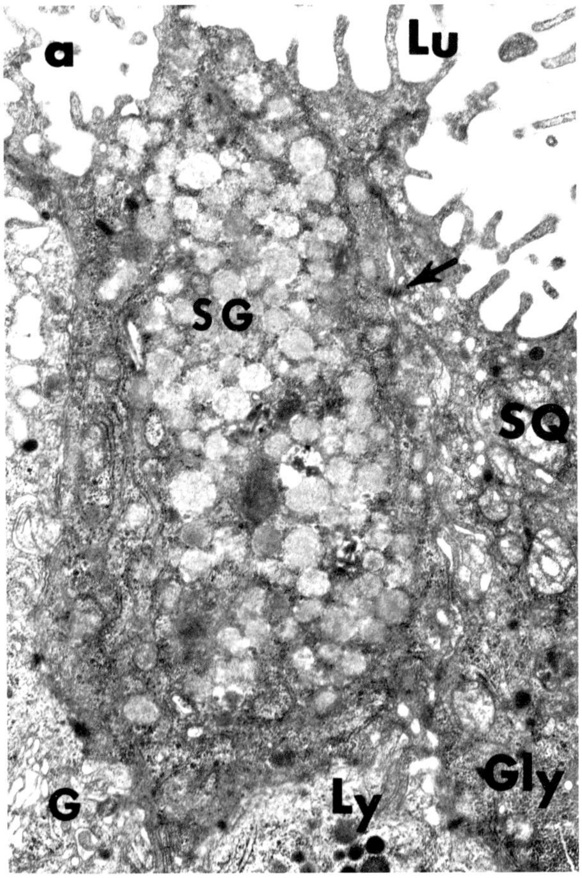

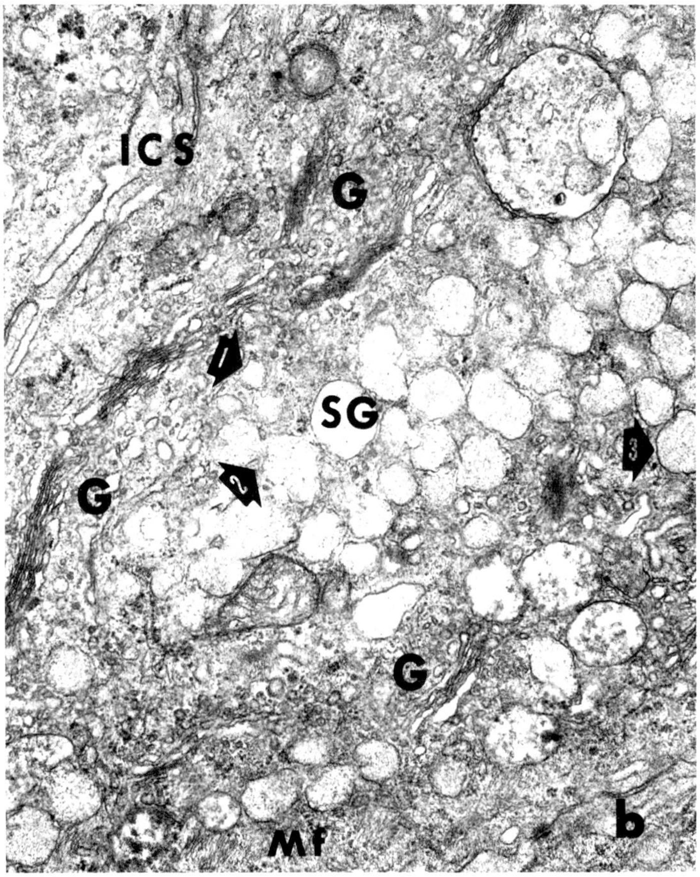

Figure 139a. *Among the squamous cells,* secretory cells with conspicuous secretory granules (SG) and Golgi (G) are occasionally seen. These occur singly or in groups, and are interconnected (arrow) with the adjacent squamous cells (SQ). Several small lumina may be formed within the metaplastic nests by both squamous and secretory cells, and cells intermediate between secretory and squamous cells that have well-equipped organelles but are devoid of secretory vacuoles, tonofilaments, and cytoplasmic processes are frequently seen. A well-defined basal lamina surrounds the squamous nests. × 12,600. Ly: lysosomes; Lu: lumen; Gly: glycogen in squamous cells.

Figure 139b. *Detail of mucogenesis with squamous metaplastic nests.* The secretory granules (SG) originate from the Golgi (G) by coalescence of small peripheral vesicles, giving rise to larger membrane-bound granules (arrow 1), which by further coalescence produce larger vesicles (arrow 2). Fully developed secretory granules (arrow 3) are enveloped by a well-defined membrane, and the secretory content appears finely granular. The peri-Golgian free and bound ribosomes and mitochondria provide the essential proteins and energy for mucopolysaccharide synthesis. × 29,200. Mf: microfilaments; ICS: intercellular space.

REFERENCE (Figures 139a–150a)

1. Ferenczy, A. and R. M. Richart. Scanning electron microscopy of hyperplastic and neoplastic endometria. In *Scanning Electron Microscopy/1973.* Part III. *Proceedings of the Workshop on Scanning Electron Microscopy in Pathology,* O. Johari (Ed.). IIT Research Institute, Chicago, 1973, pp. 613–620.

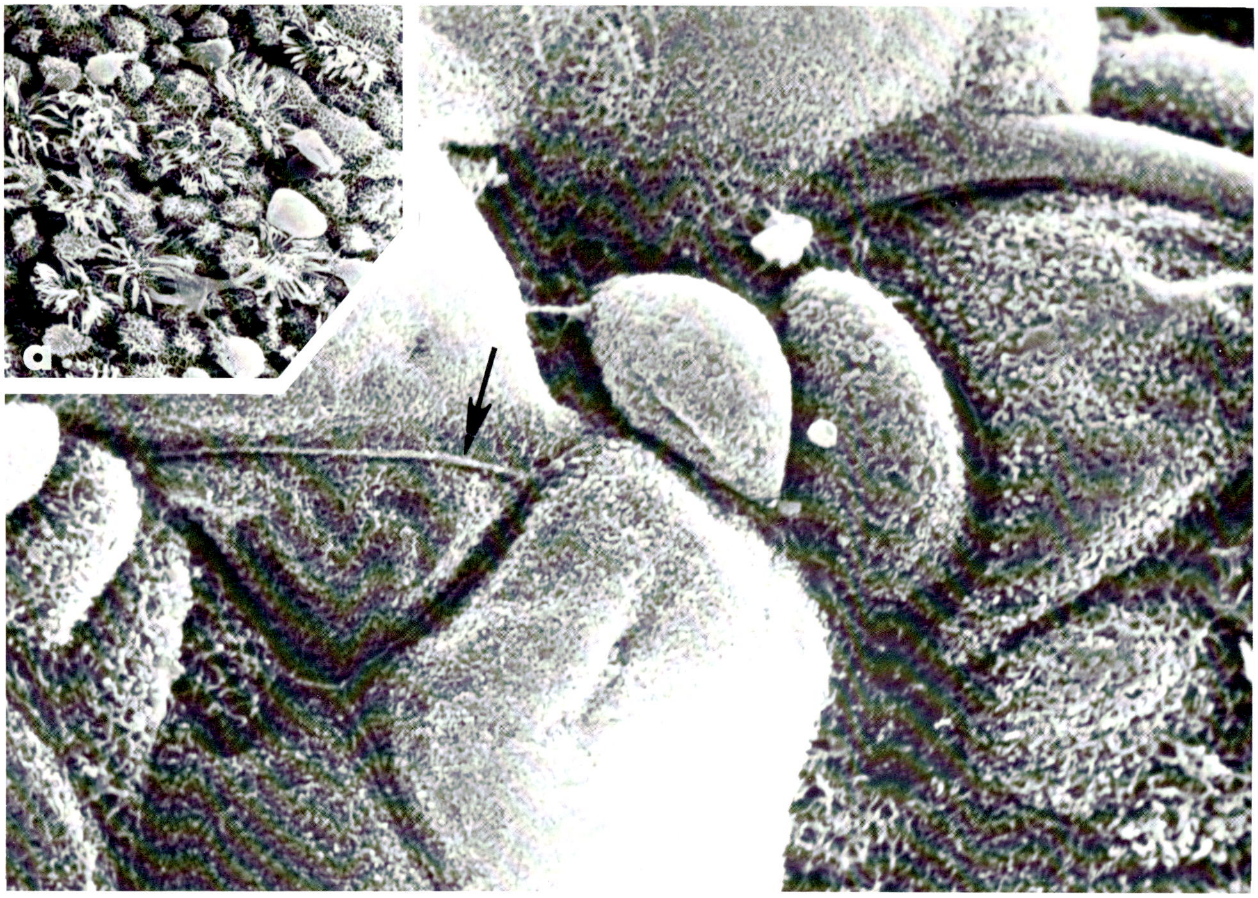

Figure 140. *Stereoscopic examination*[1] of the most superficial cells forming the metaplastic squamous epithelium reveals large polyhedral cells interconnected by prominent intercellular bridges (arrow). The surface specialization is similar in architecture to that found in the immature transformation zone and in neoplastic cervix squamous epithelia. × 1600. *From* A. Ferenczy and R. M. Richart. Scanning electron microscopy of hyperplastic and neoplastic endometria. In *Scanning Electron Microscopy/1973*. Part III. *Proceedings of the Workshop on Scanning Electron Microscopy in Pathology*, O. Jahari (Ed.). IIT Research Institute, Chicago, 1973, pp. 613–620.

Figure 140a. *The adenocarcinoma portion* of adenoacanthoma contains several ciliated cells,[1] and the nonciliated cells are covered by short microvilli. × 1000.

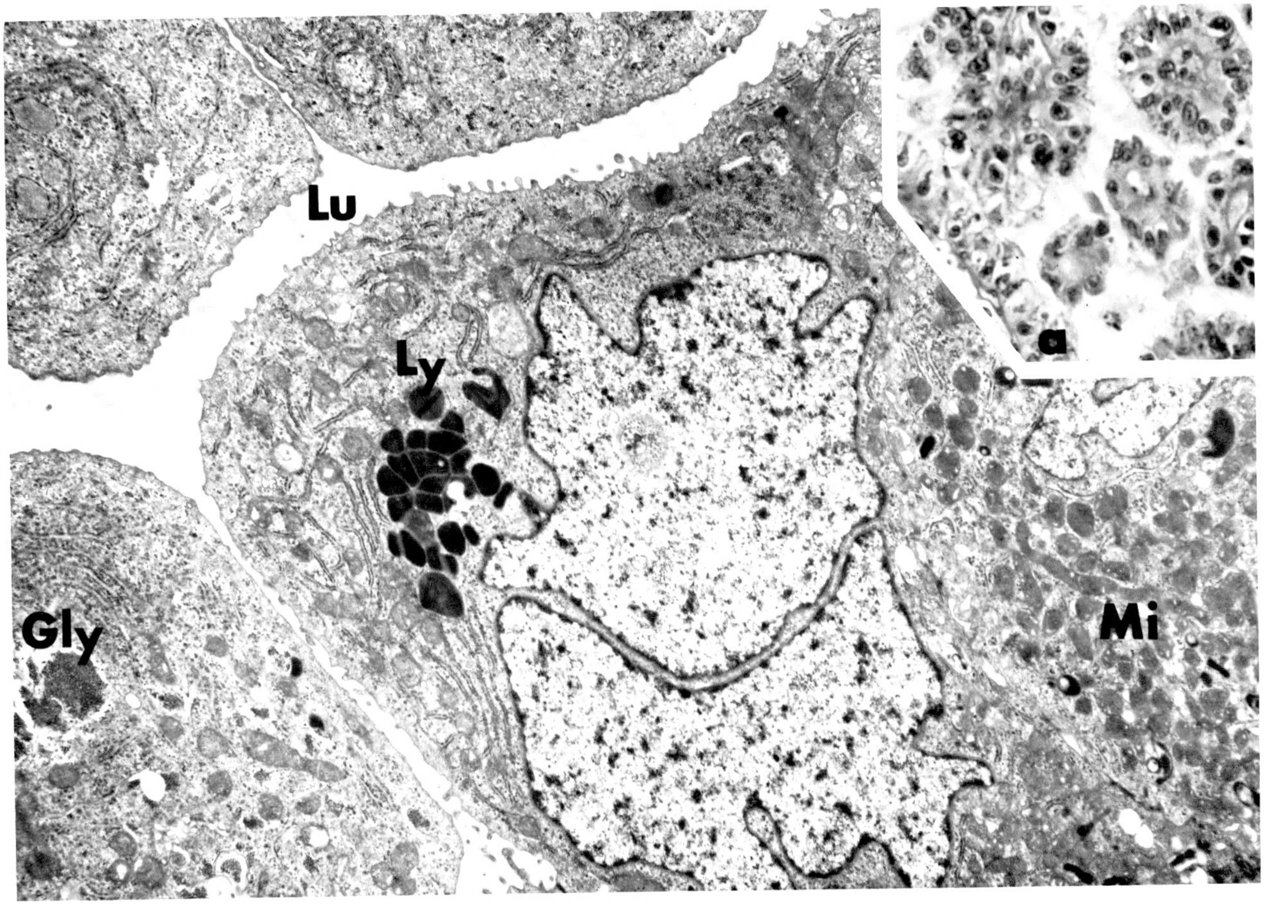

CLEAR CELL ADENOCARCINOMA
(Mesonephric Carcinoma)

Clear cell adenocarcinoma is a rare type of endometrial neoplasm, often with a papillary pattern, in which the glands, tubules, or papillae are lined by neoplastic clear cells, many of them with a "hobnail" appearance. Histochemically, as well as ultrastructurally,[1] these clear cells contain veritable pools of glycogen particles, primarily in a supranuclear location, and detached fragments of apical cytoplasm filled with glycogen are often seen in the glandular lumina. The significance and pathogenesis of the excessive glycogen synthesis and secretion in clear cell carcinoma are unknown. Similar clear cell neoplasms with conspicuous glycogen content are seen in the ovary[2] and vagina,[3] suggesting a common Müllerian, rather than mesonephric, origin.

Figure 141a. *Papillary clear cell adenocarcinoma.* The papillae are seen in transverse section covered by large, columnar clear cells. (H & E stain, × 75.)

Figure 141. *Ultrastructurally,* the glandular lining cells have prominent nuclei with markedly indented membranes and bulging cytoplasm, resulting in a narrowing of the glandular lumen (Lu). In addition to large aggregates of glycogen particles (Gly), there are prominent membranes of granular endoplasmic reticulum and Golgi, a massive, subnuclear concentration of mitochondria (Mi), and abundant free ribosomes. Occasionally, collections of tightly attached, electron-dense lysosomes (Ly) are found. × 20,600.

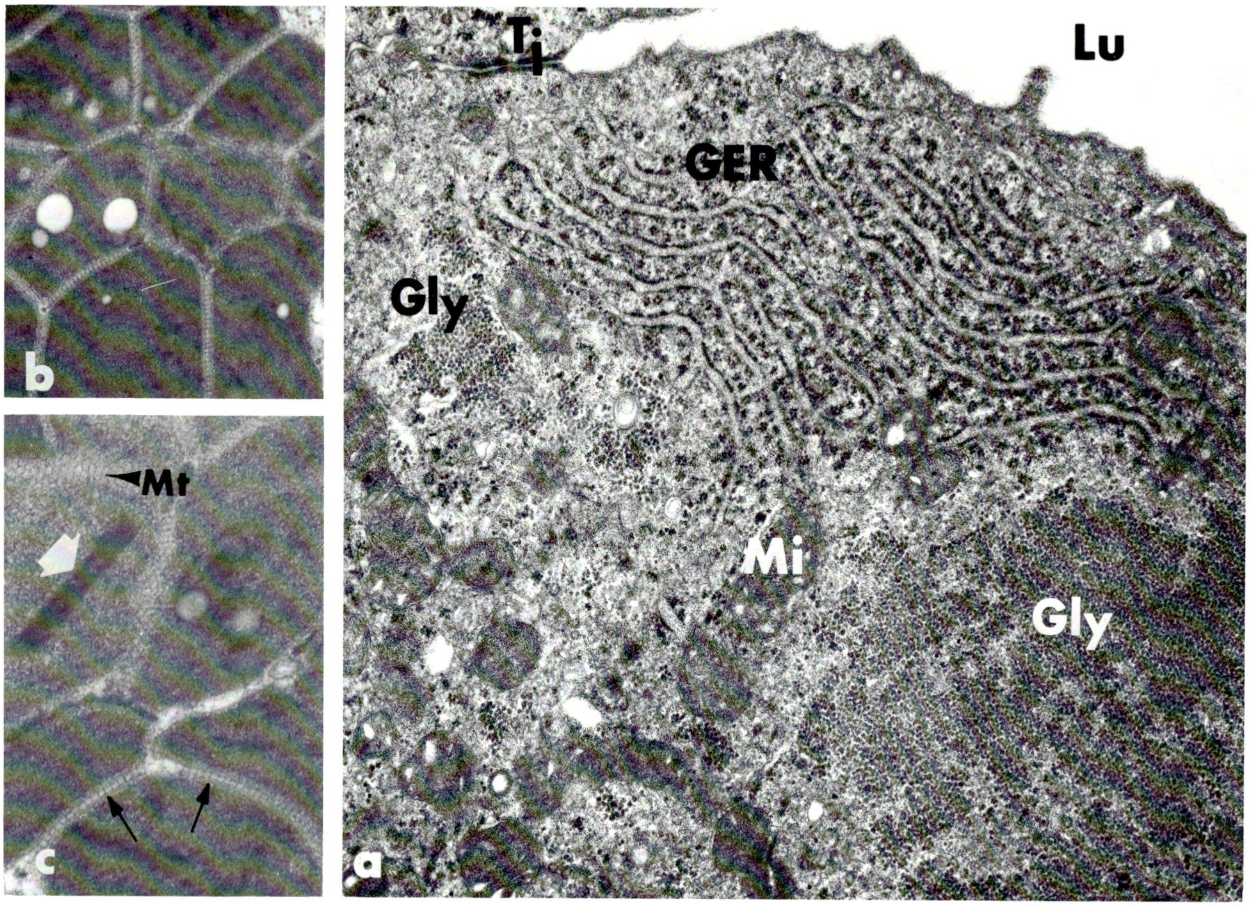

Figure 142a. *Higher magnification* of neoplastic clear cells, illustrating the close association of supranuclear glycogen particles (Gly) with parallel cisternae of granular endoplasmic reticulum (GER) and mitochondria (Mi). × 29,200. Tj: luminal tight junctional complex;; Lu: glandular lumen.

Figure 142b. *Higher magnification of Figure 141,* illustrating the polyhedral contour of electron-dense bodies, interconnected by cross-striated membrane structures. Within the bodies are lipid droplets and irregular electron-dense material. × 16,900. *From* E. Rorat, A. Ferenczy, and R. M. Richart. The ultrastructure of clear cell adenocarcinoma of endometrium. *Cancer* (in press).

Figure 142c. The cross-striated appearance (arrows) of the attachments is due to the presence of collateral membranes distributed at regular intervals, interconnecting the double-limiting membranes of adjacent dense bodies. On tangential section, these interconnections are made of tightly packed hexagonal microtubules (Mt), suggestive of crystalline material. Note the presence of needlelike structures (white arrow) within dense bodies. Similar structures have been observed in a pleural mesothelioma[4] and are regarded as related to lysosomal bodies undergoing partial crystallization. × 41,000. *From* E. Rorat, A. Ferenczy, and R. M. Richart. The ultrastructure of clear cell adenocarcinoma of endometrium. *Cancer* (in press).

REFERENCES (Clear cell adenocarcinoma–Figure 142c)

1. Rorat, E., A. Ferenczy, and R. M. Richart. The ultrastructure of clear cell adenocarcinoma of endometrium. *Cancer* (in press).
2. Okagaki, T. and R. M. Richart. Mesonephroma ovarii (hypernephroid carcinoma). Light and ultrastructural study of a case. *Cancer* **26:** 453 (1970).
3. Silverberg, S. G. and L. S. DeGiorgi. Clear cell carcinoma of the vagina. A clinical, pathologic and electron microscopic study. *Cancer* **29:** 1680 (1972).
4. Ferenczy, A., J. Fenoglio, and R. M. Richart. Observations on benign mesothelioma of the genital tract (adenomatoid tumor). A comparative ultrastructural study. *Cancer* **30:** 244 (1972).

35

Endometrial Stromal Sarcoma

Endometrial stromal sarcoma is a rare uterine neoplasm, thought to be derived from endometrial stromal cells. Two varieties are recognized: a low-grade sarcoma, referred to as *endolymphatic stromal myosis* (ELSM), and the highly malignant, true *endometrial stromal sarcoma.* The former has very few mitoses, whereas the latter characteristically has a high mitotic rate.[1] Histologically, both types have infiltrating margins and are composed of endometrial-like stromal cells resembling those seen in stromal cell hyperplasia.[1]

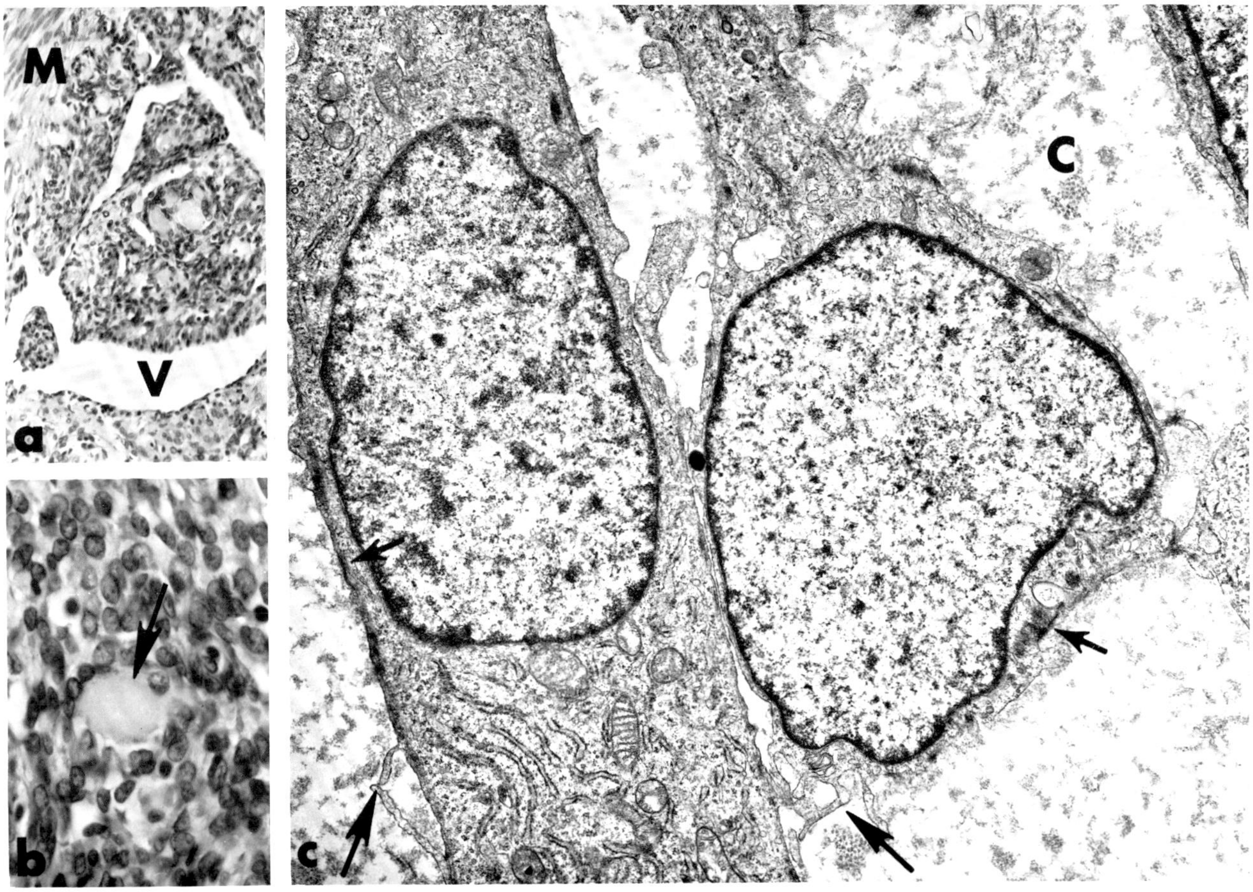

Figure 143a. *Endolymphatic stromal myosis* (low-grade endometrial stromal sarcoma). Typical of this type of neoplasm are masses of neoplastic stromal cells with hyaline nodules within and around the uterine vessels (V). (H & E stain, × 30.) M: myometrium.

Figure 143b. *Higher magnification* of a hyaline nodule (arrow) encased by plump neoplastic stromal cells. (H & E stain, × 120.)

Figure 143c. *The resemblance between the cells of endolymphatic stromal myosis and those from normal stroma* is readily appreciated at the ultrastructural level. The cells of ELSM are similar to the stromal cells of early,[2] mid-, or late proliferative endometrium, including prominent oval nuclei, and the cytoplasm contains from few to abundant organelles. In this electron micrograph, the neoplastic cells have numerous cisternae of granular endoplasmic reticulum, free ribososomes, coated vesicles, and mitochondria resembling normal endometrial stromal cells of the mid-proliferative phase of the menstrual cycle. Endolymphatic stromal myosis cells also have abundant intracytoplasmic microfibrils with peripheral condensation (short arrow) along the plasma membranes. This cytoplasmic organization in ELSM is consistent with active fibrillogenesis leading to extracellular collagen synthesis (C). The plasma membranes often exhibit complex microvillous projections (long arrows) and are uniformly devoid of a covering basal lamina. The neoplasm is highly vascular, and the cells are frequently related to small and medium-sized vessels. Myofilaments and micropinocytic vesicles are seen in periendothelial or myometrial cells but not in the neoplastic stromal cells. × 7200.

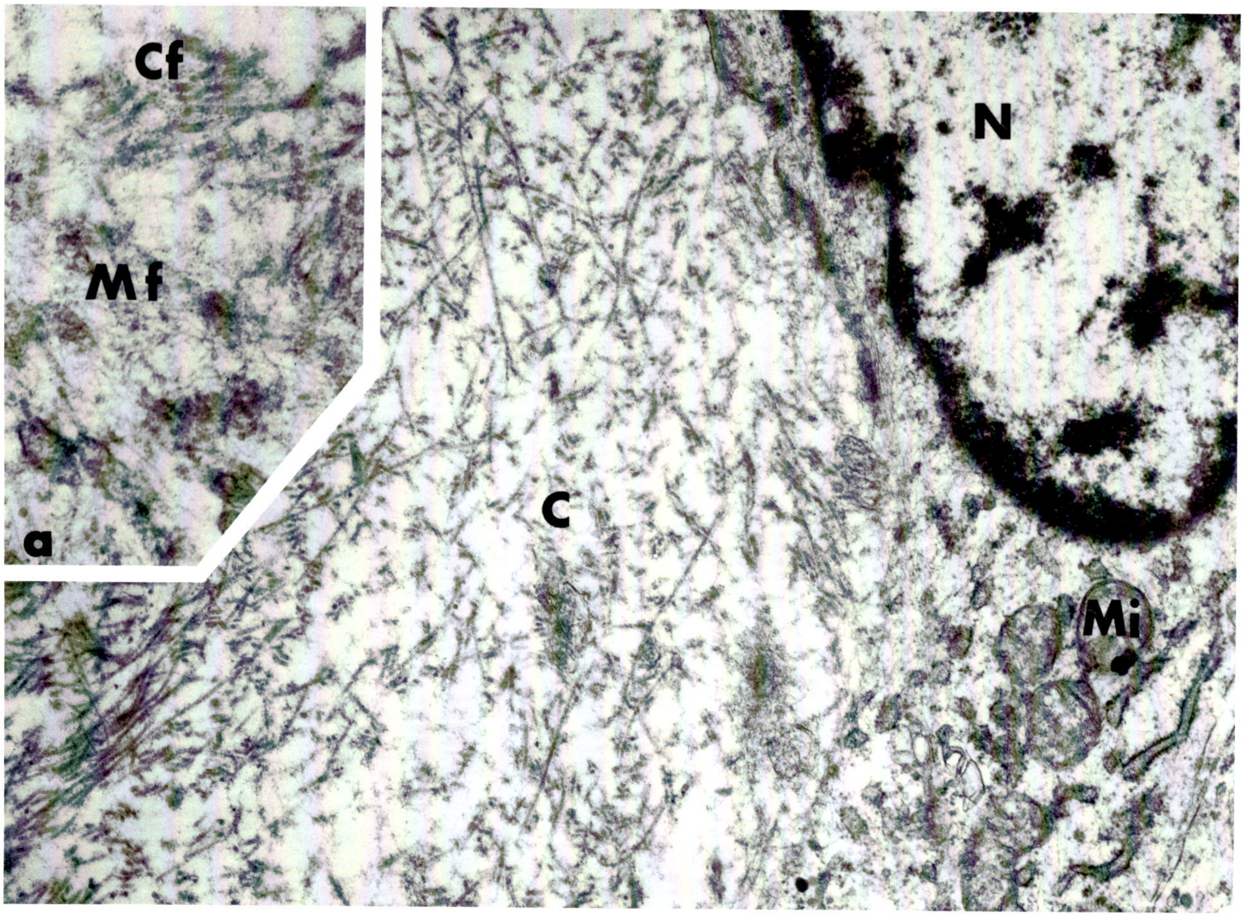

Figure 144. *Endolymphatic stromal myosis.* Electron micrograph of a hyaline nodule seen in Figure 143b. The hyaline nodules are apparently formed by neoplastic stromal cells that are rich in tropocollagen (200–300 Å thick) and precollagen (400–500Å) fibrils, associated with abundant granular endoplasmic reticulum, free ribosomes, and mitochondria (Mi). The hyaline nodules are composed predominantly of cross-striated precollagen fibers (C). × 20,600. N: nucleus of neoplastic stromal cell.

Figure 144a. *Detail view of Figure 144,* illustrating the junction between the cytoplasm (lower) and the hyaline nodule (upper). The cytoplasmic border is indistinct, and fine tropocollagen (Mf) fibrils are in close association with the extracellular cross-striated precollagen fibers (Cf). × 54,000.

REFERENCES (Endometrial Stromal Sarcoma–Figure 144a)

1. Norris, H. J. and H. B. Taylor. Mesenchymal tumors of the uterus. I. A clinical and pathological study of 53 endometrial stromal tumors. *Cancer* **19:** 755 (1966).
2. Komorowski, R. A., J. C. Garancis, and L. J. Clowry, Jr. Fine structure of endometrial stromal sarcoma. *Cancer* **26:** 1042 (1970).

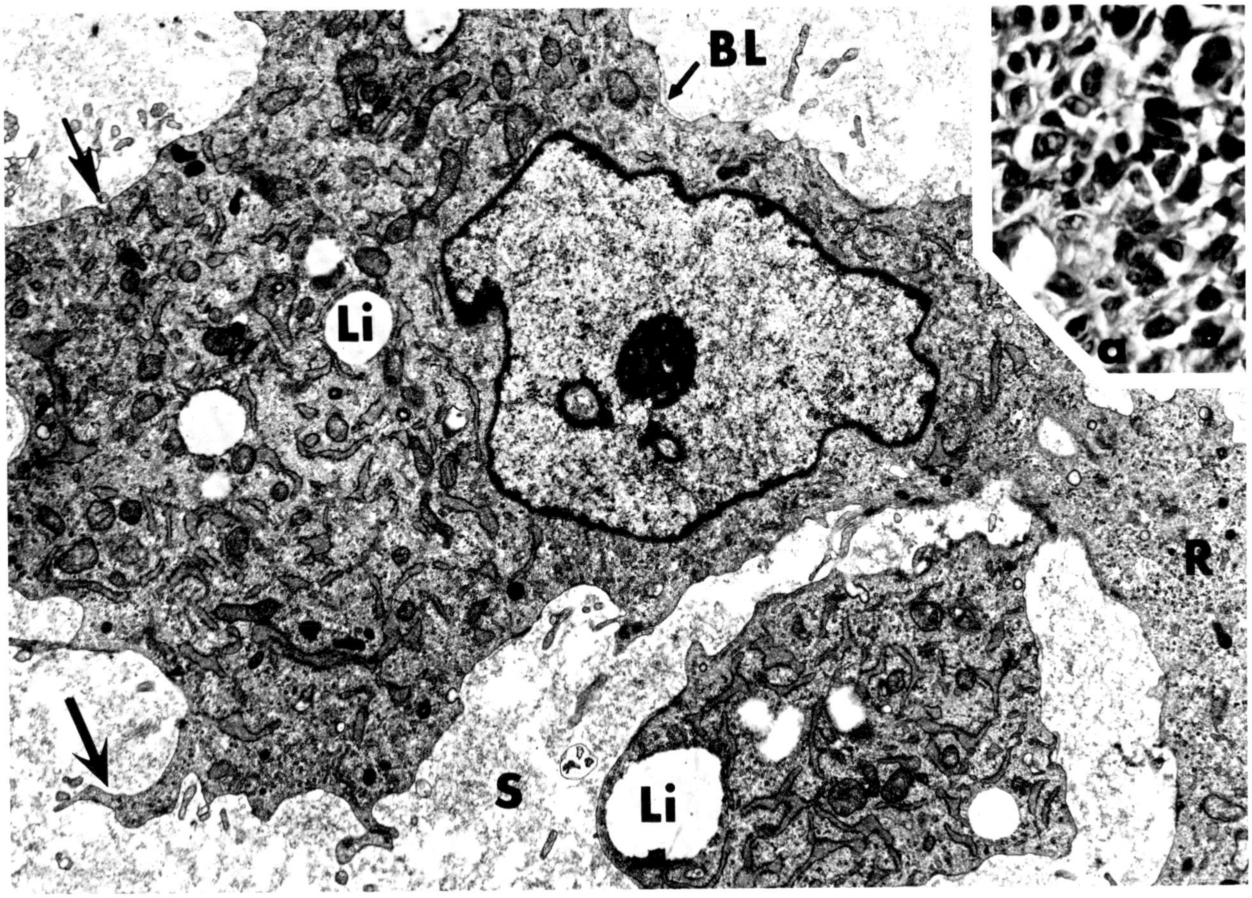

Figure 145a. *The endometrial stromal sarcoma cells* are more pleomorphic than those of endolymphatic stromal myosis and have hyperchromatic, irregular nuclei and prominent nucleoli. (H & E stain, × 120.)

Figure 145. *Ultrastructurally,* the endometrial sarcoma cells contain numerous fine cytoplasmic processes (long arrow) and abundant, slightly dilated cisternae of granular endoplasmic reticulum, filled with electron-dense amorphous material, free ribosomes (R), mitochondria, lipid droplets (Li), and microfilaments. The plasma membrane has several pinocytic invaginations (short arrow), and basal lamina (BL) formation is incomplete. In these cells, unlike those in endolymphatic stromal myosis, fibrillogenesis for intercellular (S) collagen synthesis is reduced. Note the prominent, compact nucleolus. × 10,200.

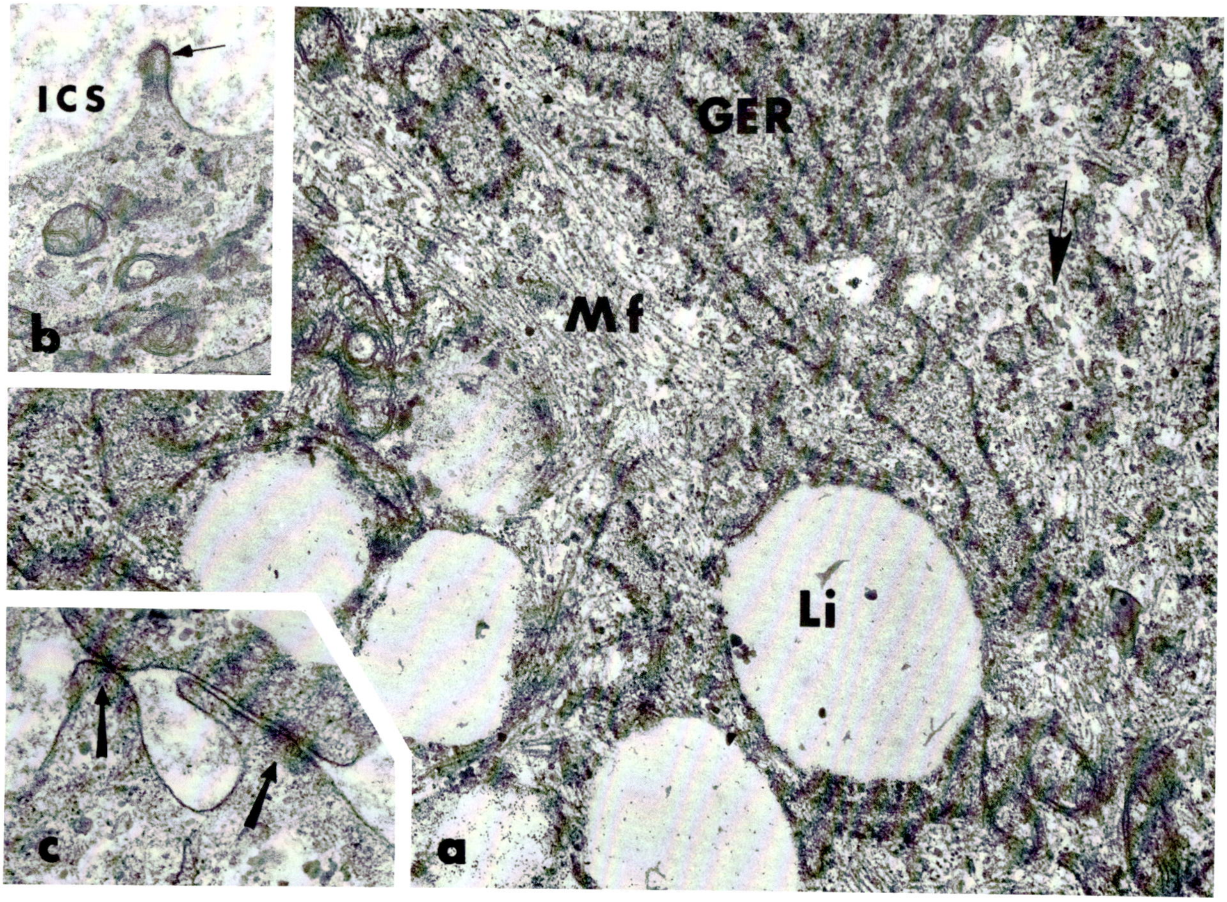

Figure 146a. *Cellular detail of endometrial stromal sarcoma.* The cytoplasm is packed with 100- to 200-Å-thick microfilaments (Mf), interspersed with granular endoplasmic cisternae (GER), lipid droplets (Li), and larger granules resembling glycogen particles (arrow). × 40,000.

Figure 146b. *Electron micrograph* illustrating a cytoplasmic microvillous process with peripheral microfilamentous condensation (arrow). ICS: intercellular space. × 18,500.

Figure 146c. *Juxtaposed* cytoplasmic processes are occasionally attached by focal microfilamentous thickenings (arrows). × 40,000.

36

Carcinosarcoma of the Uterus

Carcinosarcoma of the uterus is a malignant Müllerian neoplasm that most commonly contains adenocarcinomatous and endometrial stromal (homologous) sarcomatous elements. The fine structure of the epithelial component is similar to that of a moderately to poorly differentiated adenocarcinoma. The mesenchymal component is similar to the endometrial stromal sarcomas, in which the cells have the structural characteristics of fibrohistiocytic cells.

Figure 147a. *Histologic appearance* of uterine carcinosarcoma, in which a neoplastic endometrial gland (Gl) is surrounded by endometrial stromal sarcoma (SS) cells. (H & E stain, × 75.)

Figure 147. *Ultrastructurally,* the neoplastic glandular cells have prominent nuclei, and the cytoplasm is rich in free ribosomes (R) and membranes of granular endoplasmic reticulum (GER). The markedly convoluted plasma membranes (PM) are tightly apposed, and desmosomal attachments are infrequent. The luminal plasma membrane is covered by short and sparse microvilli (Mv). × 5600.

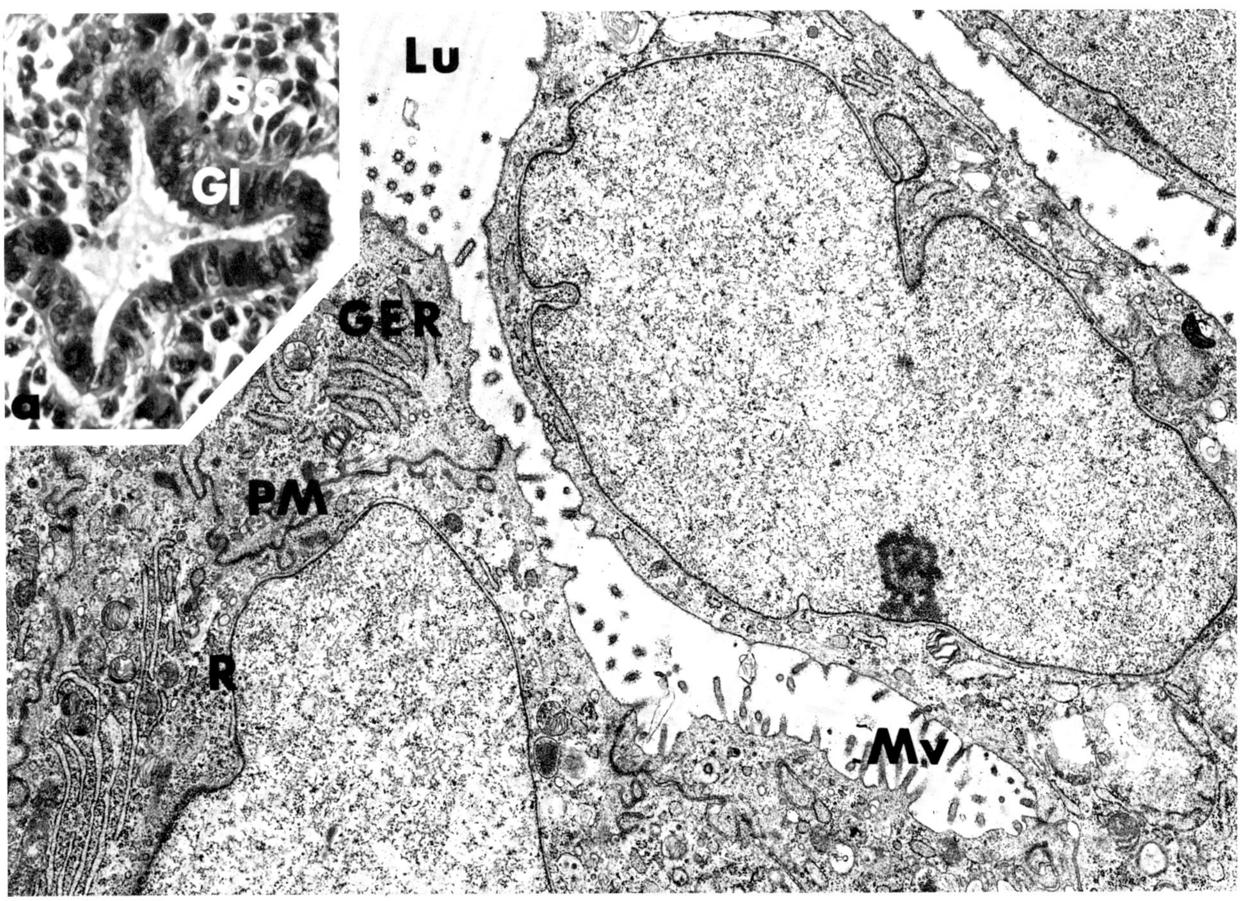

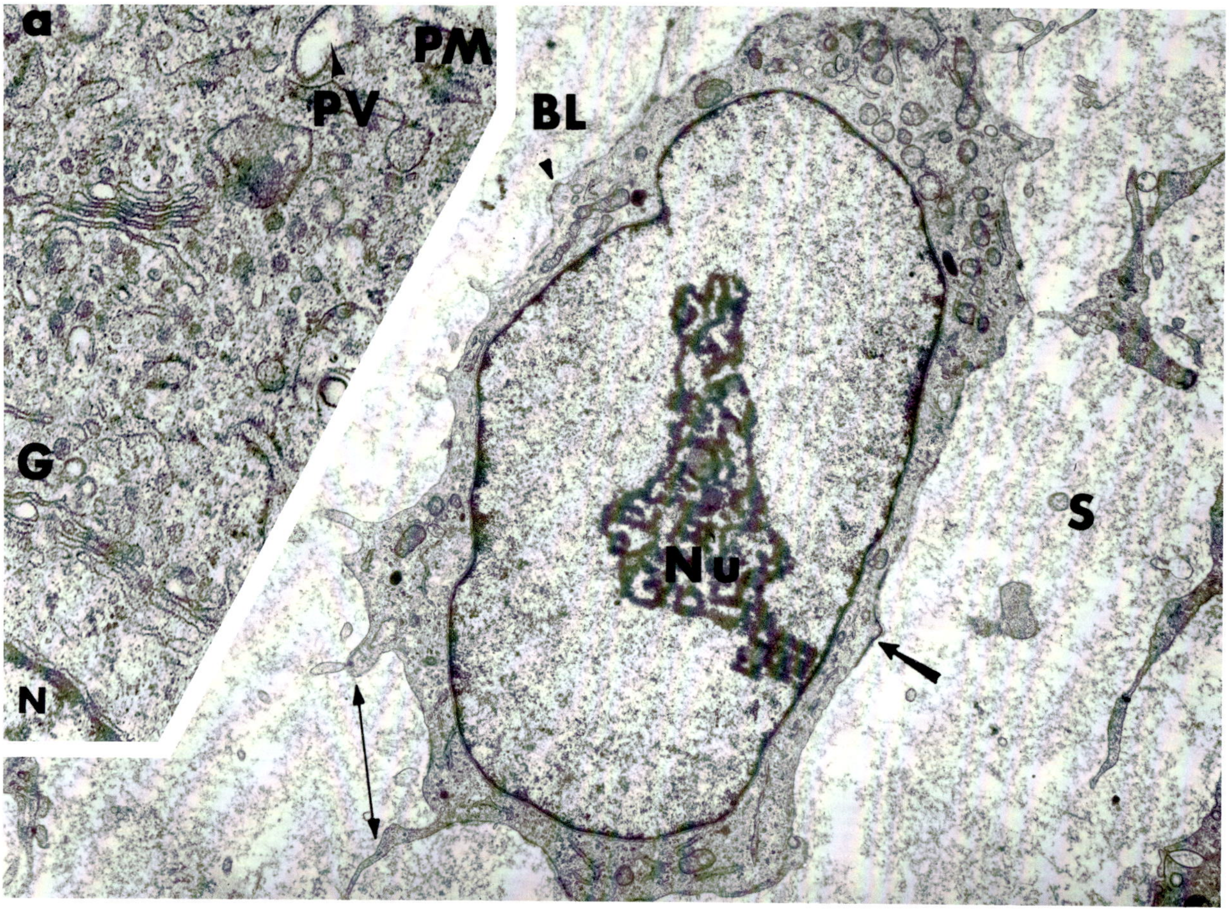

Figure 148. *Electron micrograph* of a stromal sarcoma cell representing the most common mesenchymal element of uterine carcinosarcoma. There is marked nuclear and nucleolar (Nu) enlargement, and the scant cytoplasmic substance with numerous cytoplasmic processes (double-headed arrow) contains scattered mitochondria, granular endoplasmic reticulum, and free ribosomes. Focal, peripheral microfilamentous condensations (arrow) occur along the plasma membrane, which is partially covered by a frequently interrupted basal lamina (BL). The extracellular stroma (S) is composed of amorphous ground substance. × 6000.

Figure 148a. *Occasionally, endometrial stromal sarcoma cells* have well-developed perinuclear (N) Golgi (G) with numerous peripheral vesicles, and the plasma membrane (PM) contains pinocytic invaginations (PV). × 35,000.

37
Malignant Mixed Mesodermal Tumors

Malignant mixed mesodermal tumors are distinguished from carcinosarcomas on the basis of the mesenchymal component, which contains heterologous elements, such as chondrosarcoma, rhabdomyosarcoma, and osteosarcoma. Histologically and ultrastructurally,[1,2] the adenocarcinomatous portion resembles pure endometrial adenocarcinoma, whereas the stromal portion contains immature endometrial stromal cells, chondroblasts,[1] fibroblasts, and rhabdomyoblasts[2] exhibiting varying degrees of differentiation.[1,2]

Figure 149a. *Histological appearance* of a malignant mixed mesodermal tumor composed of an admixture of neoplastic glandular epithelium (Gl) and undifferentiated, hyperchromatic, mesenchymal cells sprinkled with immature, cross-striated rhabdomyoblasts (arrow). (H & E stain, × 120.)

Figure 149. *Electron micrograph of a neoplastic rhabdomyoblast* (myofilamentous rhabdomyoblast).[2] The nuclear (N) envelope has an irregular contour with numerous pseudopodlike projections engulfing large portions of the sarcoplasm. A cluster of poorly organized, predominantly thick (175 Å in diameter) myofilaments (Mf) is seen near the nucleus. A beginning of myofilamentous organization is suggested by the presence of a few myofilamentous densities resembling primitive Z bands (Z). Numerous polyribosomes (R) and glycogen particles (Gly) are seen throughout the sarcoplasm. × 20,800. ICS: intercellular space; Mi: mitochondrion. *From* L. H. Boram, R. A. Erlandson, and S. I. Hajdu. Mesodermal mixed tumor of the uterus. A cytologic, histologic, and electron microscopic correlation. *Cancer* **30:** 1295–1306 (1972).

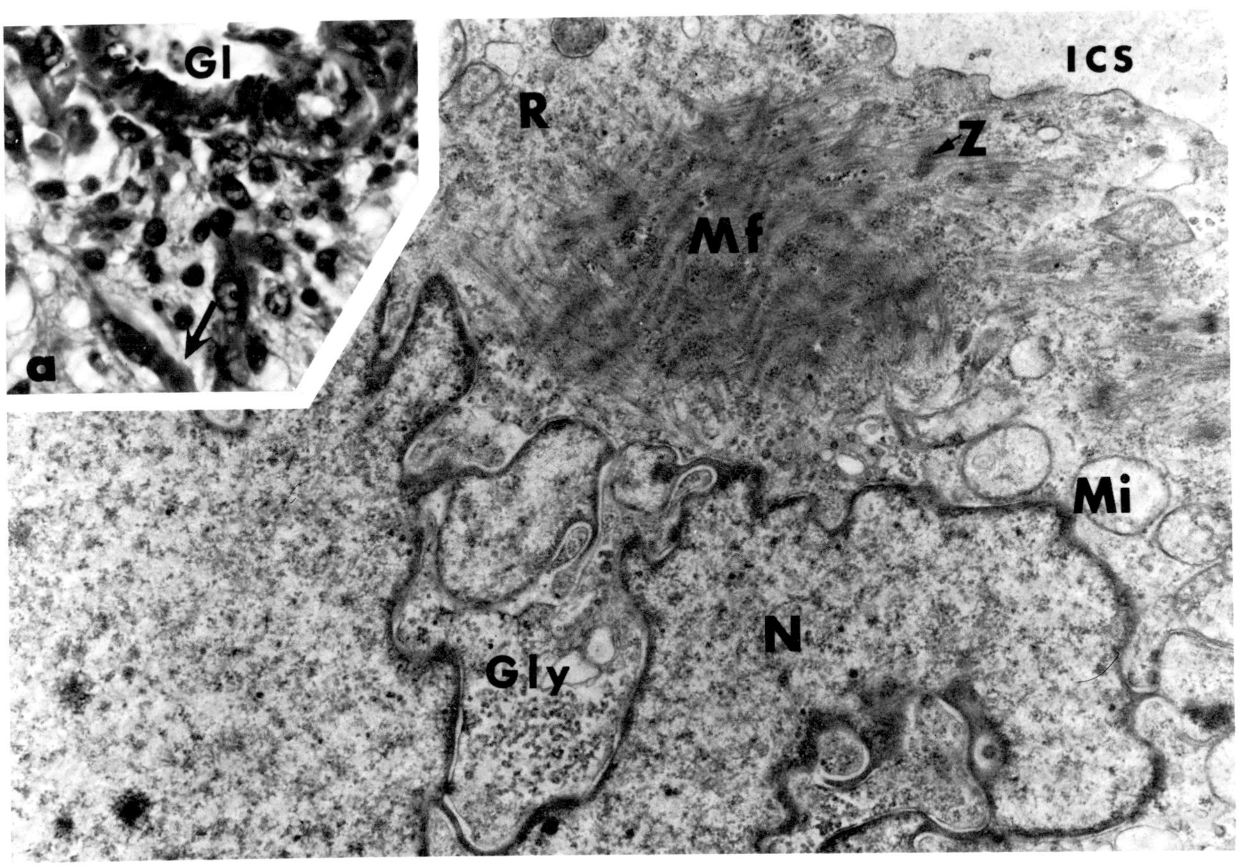

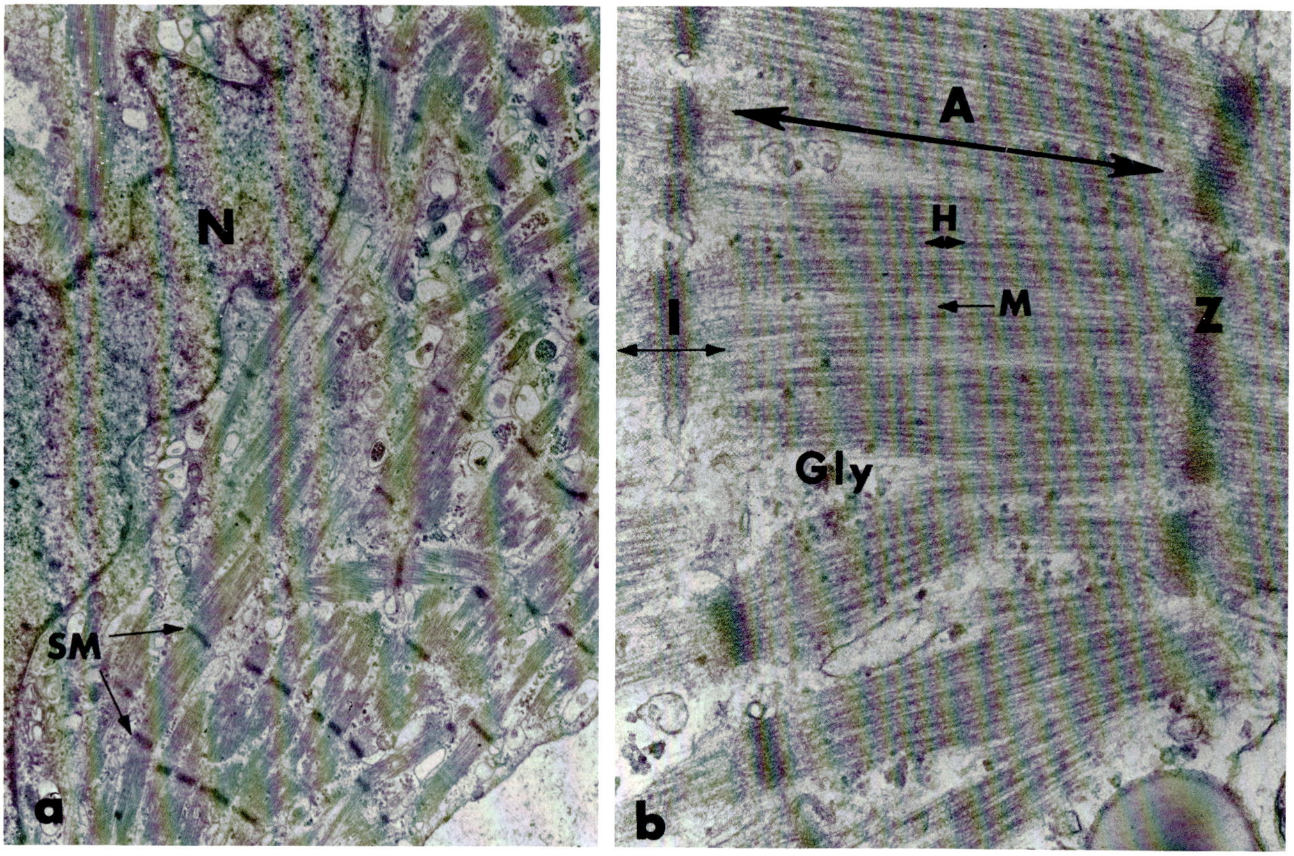

Figure 150a. *Malignant mixed mesodermal tumor.* The better-differentiated "myofibrillar rhabdomyoblast"[2] contains abundant mature, banded sarcomeres (SM), exhibiting marked alignment. This orientation is characterized by the lateral apposition of *Z* bands in register and the end-to-end alignment of sarcomeres at the approximate level of the *H* band. This alignment is responsible for the "cross striations" in straplike and tadpole-shaped rhabdomyoblasts. × 11,200. N: nucleus. *From* L. H. Boram, R. A. Erlandson, and S. I. Hajdu. Mesodermal mixed tumor of the uterus. A cytologic, histologic, and electron microscopic correlation. *Cancer* **30:** 1295–1306 (1972).

Figure 150b. *Higher magnification of a mature sarcomere* in a "myofibrillar rhabdomyoblast," composed of well-defined *I, A, H, M,* and *Z* bands. Numerous glycogen (Gly) particles are seen scattered between the myofilaments and myofibrils. × 40,000. *From* L. H. Boram, R. A. Erlandson, and S. I. Hajdu. Mesodermal mixed tumor of the uterus. A cytologic, histologic, and electron microscopic correlation. *Cancer* **30:** 1295–1306 (1972).

REFERENCES (Malignant mixed mesodermal tumors–Figure 150b)

1. Silverberg, S. G. Malignant mixed mesodermal tumor of the uterus. An ultrastructural study. *Am. J. Obstet. Gynecol.* **110:** 702 (1971).
2. Boram, L. H., R. A. Erlandson, and S. I. Hajdu. Mesodermal mixed tumor of the uterus. A cytologic, histologic, and electron microscopic correlation. *Cancer* **30:** 1295 (1972).

MYOMETRIUM

38

Normal Myometrium

The cells of the myometrium, although similar in structure to smooth muscle cells of extrauterine origin, have the unique ability to respond to ovarian hormonal stimuli. Thus the specific functions of smooth muscle cells—tension, contraction, and relaxation—are under the influence of estrogen and progesterone.

Estrogen promotes myometrial growth by stimulating RNA synthesis,[1-4] resulting in the accentuated production of contractile proteins—the actomyosin filaments. Estrogen also stimulates electrical excitability and the propagation of impulses,[5] as well as specific enzyme systems and carbohydrate metabolism, both of which are related to the generation of energy for muscular contraction. The myometrial capillaries are also subject to estrogenic influence and respond by endothelial growth and increased mucopolysaccharide synthesis.[4]

The effect of progesterone on the myometrium is not well understood. The available biochemical, electrophysiological, and morphological data suggest that progesterone has no inhibitory effect on estrogen-stimulated smooth muscle cell growth and protein synthesis. Its blocking effect on myometrial excitability during pregnancy remains an equivocal finding. From a biochemical point of view, progesterone may prevent the proteolysis of actomyosin by stabilizing the lysosomal membranes, thereby promoting uterine growth in pregnancy.[6]

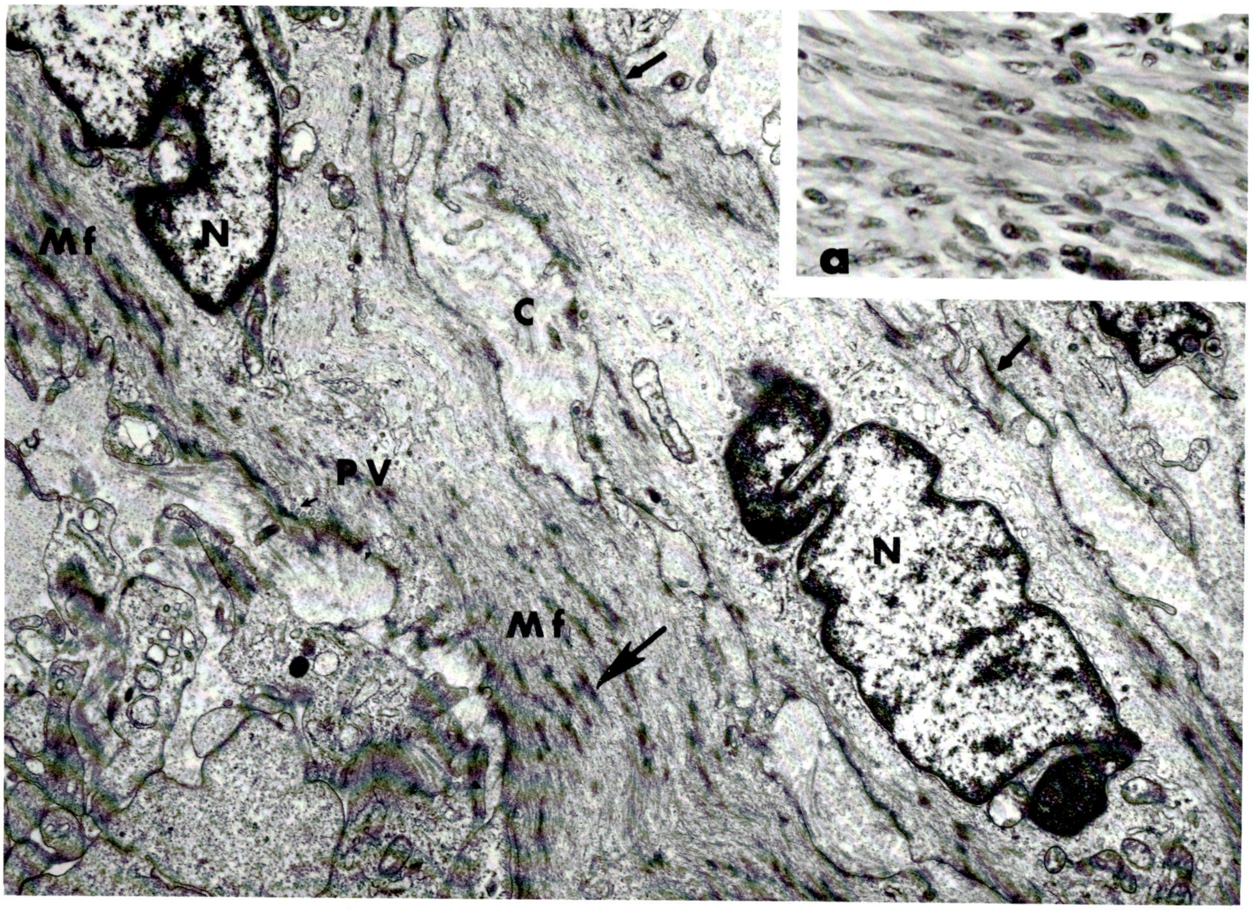

Figure 151a. *Longitudinally sectioned myometrial smooth muscle cells* during the reproductive period. The cells have blunt-ended, spindle-shaped nuclei with equally spindle-shaped cytoplasmic substance, which appears finely fibrillar. (H & E stain, × 120.)

Figure 151. *Ultrastructurally,* the normal human myometrium[7-11] consists of bundles of spindle-shaped cells with fusiform, blunt-ended nuclei (N). The myoplasm is packed with threadlike myofilaments (Mf), oriented parallel to the long axis of the cells. As is characteristic of myogenic cells, myofilaments containing numerous spindle-shaped densities (long arrow) and well-developed plasma membrane dense bodies (small arrows) are found along the plasma membranes. The latter often alternate with rows of micropinocytic vesicles (PV) approximately 60 mμ in diameter, which are apparently related to the active transport of proteins and ions, such as sodium and potassium, that are important elements in the generation of action potentials.[5] × 8000. C: extracellular collagen.

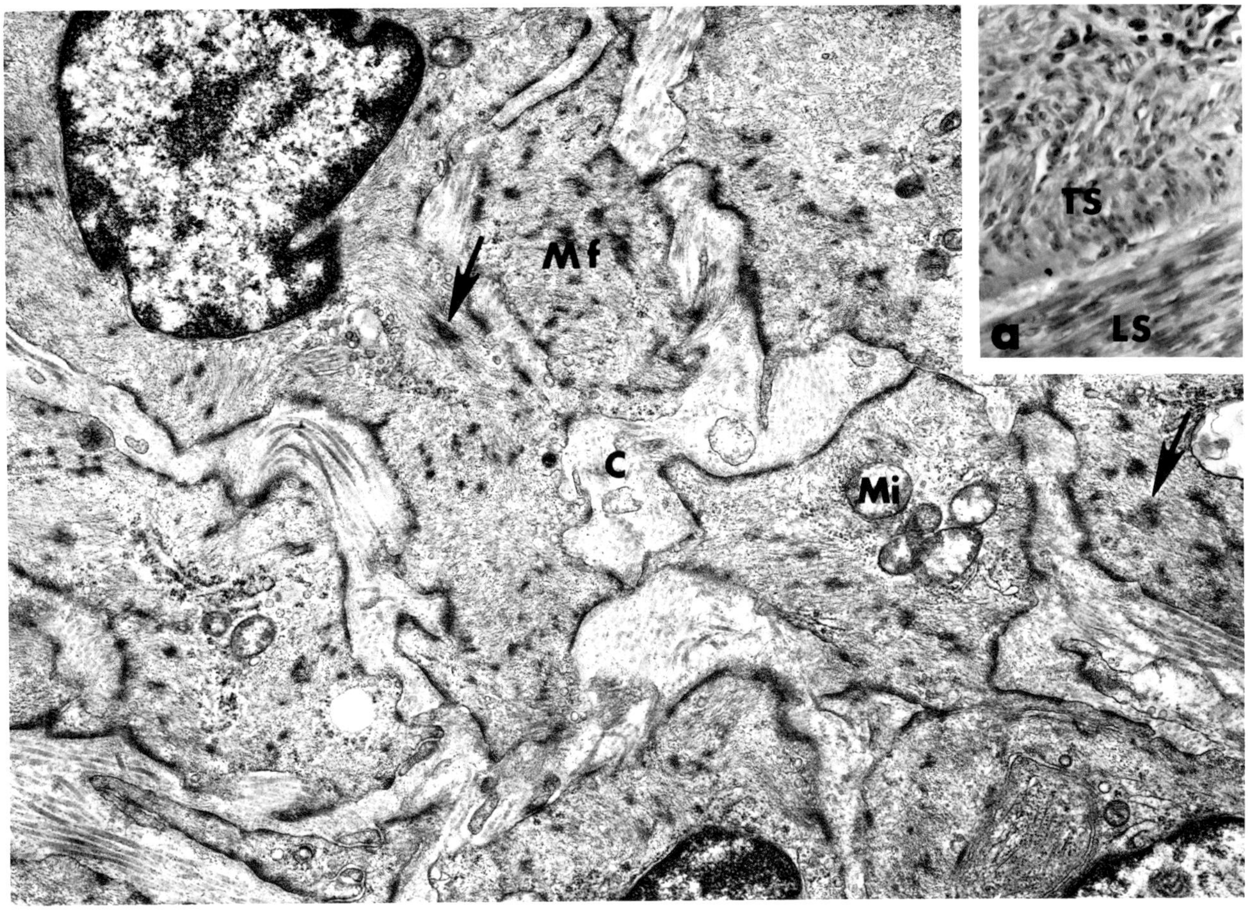

Figure 152a. *Light micrograph* of both longitudinally (LS) and tangentially (TS) sectioned myometrial smooth muscle cells. (H & E stain, × 75.)

Figure 152. *Tangentially sectioned smooth muscle cells* appear as large polygonal cells with irregular cellular outlines. Masses of threadlike myofilaments (Mf) with numerous spindle-shaped bodies (long arrow) occupy most of the myoplasm. As is characteristic of smooth muscle cells, organelles are scant and are located principally near the nuclear poles. The extracellular space is packed with collagen fibers (C). × 14,000. Mi: mitochondria.

REFERENCES (The cells of the myometrium–Figure 152a)

1. Csapo, A., T. Erdos, C. R. De Mattos E. Gramss, and C. Moscowitz. Stretch-induced uterine growth, protein synthesis and function. *Nature* **207:** 1378 (1965).
2. Laguens, R. Effect of estrogen upon the fine structure of the uterine smooth muscle cell of the rat. *J. Ultrastruct. Res.* **10:** 578 (1964).
3. Needham, D. M. and C. F. Shoenberg. The biochemistry of the myometrium. In *Cellular Biology of the Uterus,* R. M. Wynn (Ed.). Appleton-Century-Crofts, New York, 1967, pp. 291–352.
4. Friderici, H. H. R. and R. J. Decloux. The early response of immature rat myometrium to estrogenic stimulation. *J. Ultrastruct. Res.* **22:** 402 (1968).
5. Kao, C. Y. Ionic basis of electrical activity in uterine smooth muscle. In *Cellular Biology of the Uterus,* R. M. Wynn (Ed.). Appleton-Century-Crofts, New York, 1967, pp. 386–448.
6. Goodall, F. R. Progesterone retards postpartum involution of the rabbit myometrium. *Science* **152:** 356 (1966).
7. Hashimoto, M., A. Komori, M. Kosaka, Y. Mori, T. Shimoyama, and T. Akashi. Electron microscopic studies on the smooth muscle of the human uterus. *J. Jap. Obstet. Gynecol. Soc.* **7:** 115 (1960).
8. Jaeger, J. and G. Pohlmann. On the ultrastructure of human myometrium cells. *Beitr. Pathol. Anat.* **126:** 113 (1962).
9. Lo Stumbo, F. Ultrastruttura della cellula muscolare dell'utero umano in situazioni fisiologiche diverse. I. Nell-utero normale non gravido. *Riv. Ostet. Ginecol.* **20:** 436 (1965).
10. Nemetschek-Gansler, H. Ultrastructure of the myometrium. In *Cellular Biology of the Uterus,* R. M. Wynn (Ed). Appleton-Century-Crofts, New York, 1967, pp. 353–385.
11. Ferenczy, A., R. M. Richart, and T. Okagaki. A comparative ultrastructural study of leiomyosarcoma, cellular leiomyoma and leiomyoma of the uterus. *Cancer* **28:** 1004 (1971).

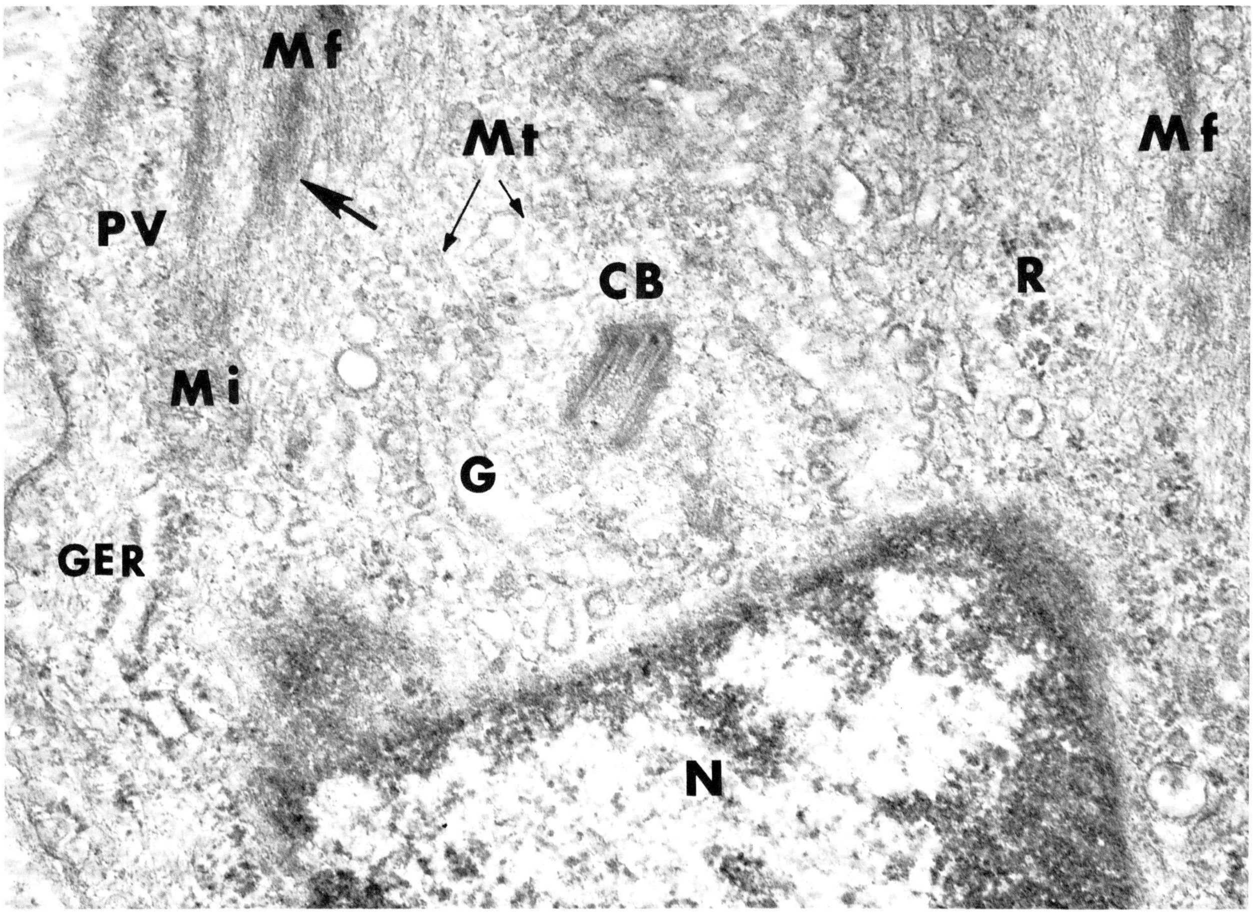

Figure 153. *The organelles in myometrial cells* are characteristically scant and occur in a cone-shaped, paranuclear location.[1-5] These organelles become prominent when stimulated by estrogen,[4] however, and have been shown by autoradiographic studies to synthesize and secrete proline, contributing to the formation of extracellular collagen and elastic fibers.[6] Human myometrial mitochondria have been reported to contain prominent calcium binding capacity (fractionation studies), indicating a possible role in the control of the uterine contraction-relaxation phenomenon.[7] A juxtanuclear (N) centriolar body (CB) is associated with a well-developed Golgi (G) with abundant peripheral vesicles, microtubules (Mt), polysomes (R), and granular endoplasmic reticulum (GER). Myofilaments (Mf) do not penetrate this region. × 61,000. PV: micropinocytic vesicles; Mi: mitochondria.

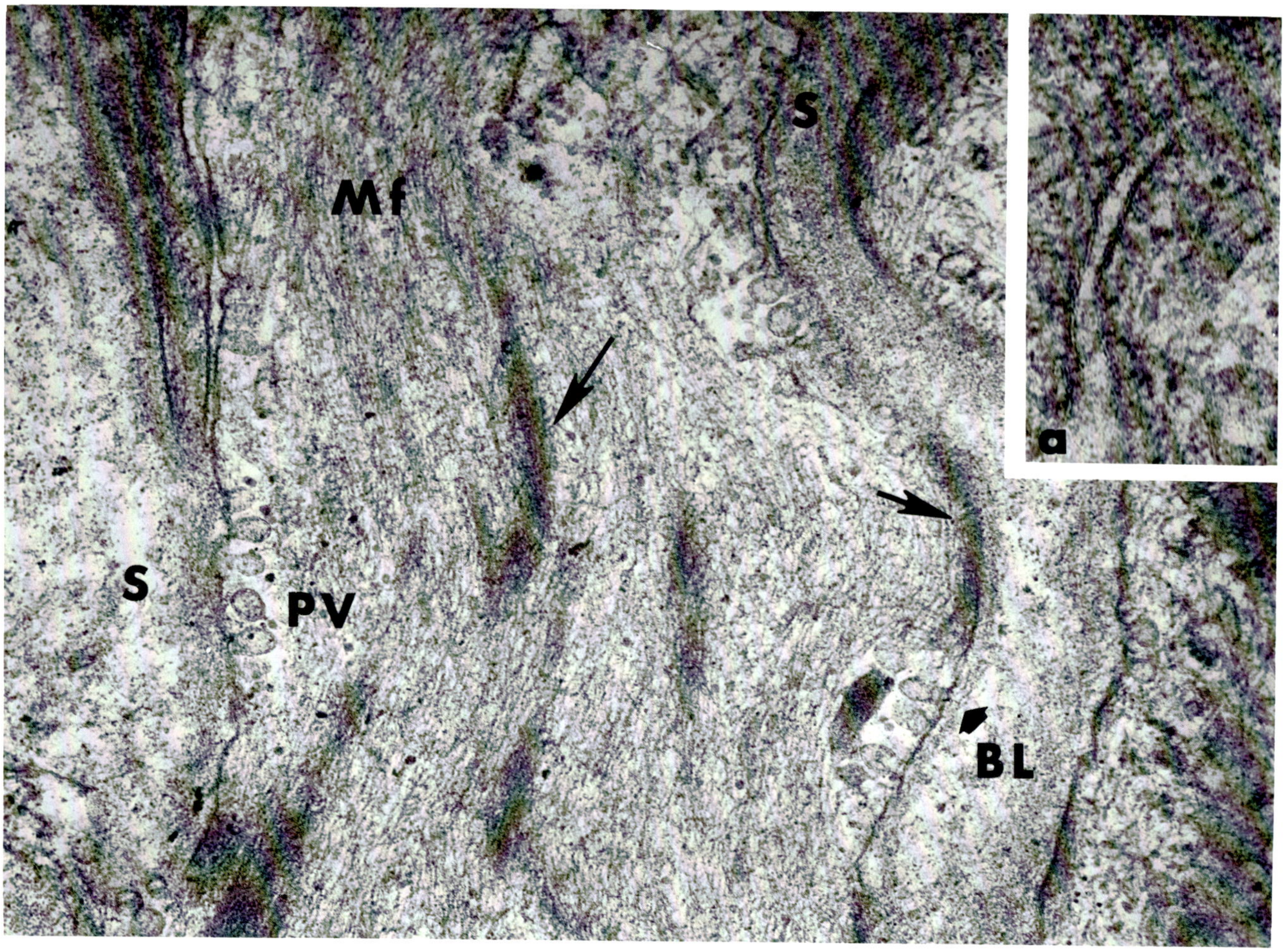

Figure 154. *The majority of the filaments* (Mf) are thin actin filaments 50 to 60 Å in diameter, which, when viewed in cross section at high magnification, are arranged in arrays in a hexagonal or square pattern.[8] The existence of thick myosin filaments in smooth muscle cells in vivo has been demonstrated convincingly by biochemical, X-ray diffraction, and electron-optical studies. These filaments appear as long ribbonlike structures 100 to 200 Å in width and are oriented parallel to arrays of actin filaments.[8-10] Interconnections occur between thin (actin) and thick (myosin) filaments in a manner similar to that which prevails in striated muscle.[10] The presence of a two-filament system with the above-mentioned spatial organization suggests that contraction in smooth muscle cells must occur via a sliding mechanism similar to that in the skeletal muscle system.[8-13] The characteristic spindle-shaped bodies (long arrow), as well as the plasma membrane densities (short arrow), are composed of actin filaments with collateral interattachments of 20-Å-thick filaments.[11] A few myosin filaments may also be identified near, and within, these spindle-shaped densities.[9] These structures serve as attachment units[11,13] of myofilaments and are considered to be analogous to the *Z*-line sarcomeres seen in striated muscle cells. The myometrial cells are embedded in an abundant connective tissue stroma, from which they are separated by a well-defined, but often interrupted, basal lamina (BL).[4,5] × 60,750. PV: micropinocytic vesicles; S: extracellular space with finely filamentous material.

Figure 154a. *Intercellular connections* are seen as closely apposed plasma membranes,[14] with or without juxtaposed plasma membrane dense bodies, and occasionally as 25- to 30-Å intermembrane gap junctions (nexuses).[15] The latter are likely to be involved in the transmission of electrical impulses between muscle cells.[16] Smooth muscle cells are innervated by the autonomic nervous system, branches of which form close contacts with the plasma membranes of the myometrial cells. The nerve fibers at these points contain membrane-bound neurovesicles (450–500 Å), the contents of which may be identified in the micropinocytotic vesicles of adjacent smooth muscle cells.[13] Direct axonal penetration into muscle cells is not seen.[14,17] × 83,250.

REFERENCES (Figures 153–154a)

1. Hashimoto, M., A. Komori, M. Kosaka, Y. Mori, T. Shimoyama, and K. Akashi. Electron microscopic studies on the smooth muscle of the human uterus. *J. Jap. Obstet. Gynecol. Soc.* **7:** 115 (1960).
2. Jaeger, J. and G. Pohlmann. On the ultrastructure of human myometrium cells. *Beitr. Pathol. Anat.* **126:** 113 (1962).
3. Lo Stumbo, F. Ultrastruttura della cellula muscolare dell'utero umano in situazioni fisiologiche diverse. I. Nell'utero normale non gravido. *Riv. Ostet. Ginecol.* **20:** 436 (1965).
4. Nemetschek-Gansler, H. Ultrastrutcure of the myometrium. In *Cellular Biology of the Uterus,* R. M. Wynn (Ed.). Appleton-Century-Crofts, New York, 1967, pp. 353–385.
5. Ferenczy, A., R. M. Richart, and T. Okagaki. A comparative ultrastructural study of leiomyosarcoma, cellular leiomyoma and leiomyoma of the uterus. *Cancer* **28:** 1004 (1971).
6. Ross, R. and S. J. Klebanoff. The smooth muscle cell. I. In vivo synthesis of connective tissue proteins. *J. Cell Biol.* **50:** 159 (1971).
7. Batra, S. The role of calcium binding by subcellular particles in the contraction and relaxation of the myometrium. *Am. J. Obstet. Gynecol.* **112:** 851 (1972).
8. Lowry, J. and J. V. Small. The organization of myosin and actin in vertebrate smooth muscle. *Nature* **227:** 46 (1970).
9. Lowy, J., F. R. Poulsen, and P. J. Vibert. Myosin filaments in vertebrate smooth muscle. *Nature* **225:** 1053 (1970).
10. Kristensen, B. I. and L. E. Nielsen. A two-filament system and interaction of heavy meromyosin (HMM) with thin filaments in smooth muscle. *Z. Zellforsch.* **122:** 350 (1971).
11. Panner, B. J. and C. R. Honig. Filament ultrastructure and organization in vertebrate smooth muscle. Contraction hypothesis based on localization of actin and myosin. *J. Cell Biol.* **35:** 303 (1967).
12. Rice, R. V., J. A. Moses, G. M. McManus, A. C. Brady, and L. M. Blasik. The organization of contractile filaments in a mammalian smooth muscle. *J. Cell Biol.* **47:** 183 (1970).
13. Needham, D. M. and C. F. Shoenberg. The biochemistry of the myometrium. In *Cellular Biology of the Uterus,* R. M. Wynn (Ed.). Appleton-Century-Crofts, New York, 1967, pp. 291–352.
14. Lane, B. P. and J. A. G. Rhodin. Cellular interrelationships and electrical activity in two types of smooth muscle. *J. Ultrastruct. Res.* **10:** 470 (1964).
15. Uehara, Y. and G. Burnstock. Demonstration of "gap junctions" between smooth muscle cells. *J. Cell Biol.* **44:** 215 (1970).
16. Kao, C. Y. Ionic basis of electrical activity in uterine smooth muscle. In *Cellular Biology of the Uterus,* R. M. Wynn (Ed.). Appleton-Century-Crofts, New York, 1967, pp. 386–448.
17. Friderici, H. H. and R. J. Decloux. The early response of immature rat myometrium to estrogenic stimulation. *J. Ultrastruct. Res.* **22:** 402 (1968).

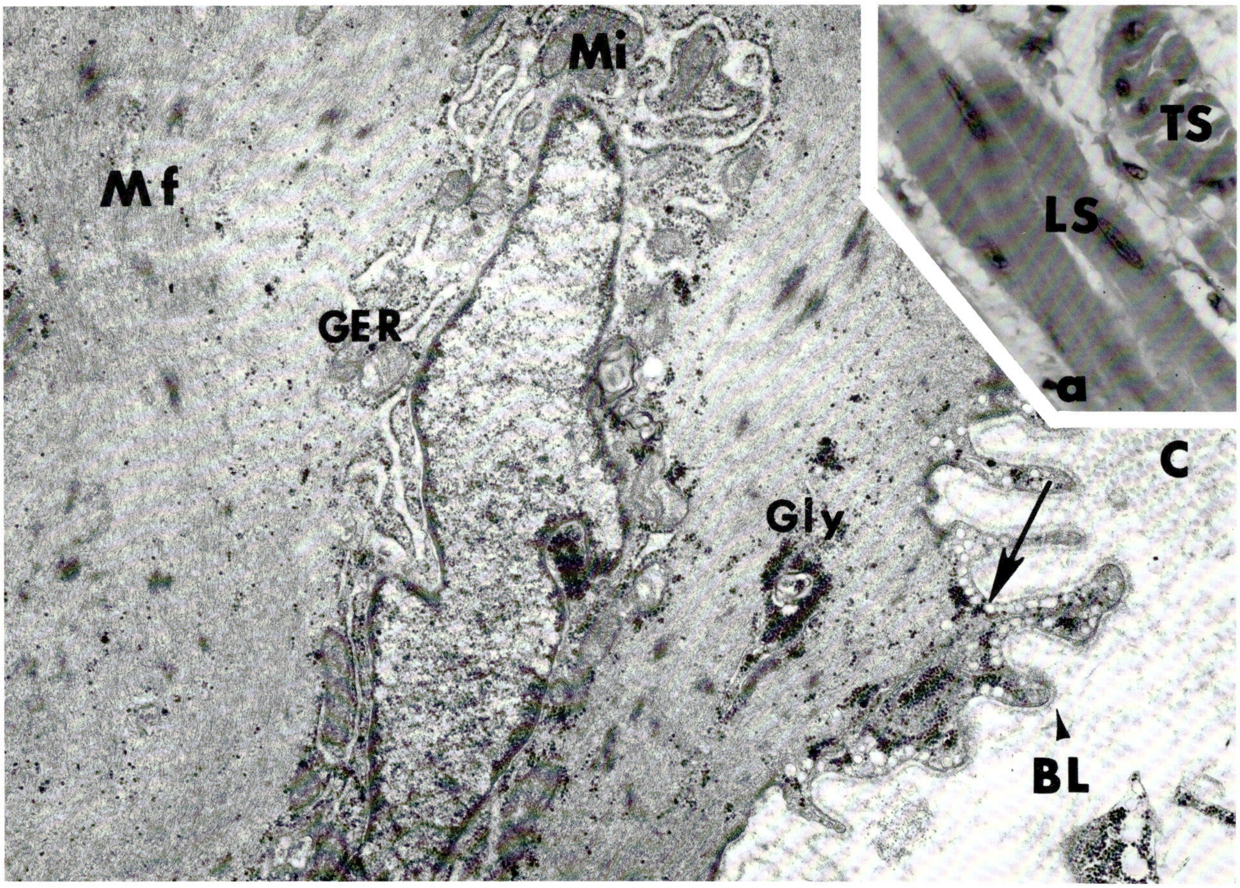

39

Myometrium of Gestation

The gravid uterus undergoes a considerable degree of myometrial hypertrophy during pregnancy.

REFERENCES (Figures 155–156a)

1. Nemetschek-Gansler, H. Ultrastructure of the myometrium. In *Cellular Biology of the Uterus,* R. M. Wynn (Ed.). Appleton-Century-Crofts, New York, 1967, pp. 353–385.
2. Mark, J. S. An electron microscope study of uterine smooth muscle. *Anat. Rec.* **125:** 473 (1956).
3. Lo Stumbo, F. Ultrastruttura della cellula muscolare dell'-utero umano in situazioni fisiologiche diverse. II. Nell'-utero gravido. *Riv. Ostet. Ginecol.* **20:** 453 (1965).
4. Dessouky, D. A. Fine structural changes of the uterine smooth muscle boundary during gestation. *Am. J. Obstet. Gynecol.* **103:** 1117 (1969).

Figure 155a. *Histology* of longitudinally (LS) and tangentially (TS) sectioned gestational myometrium (term pregnancy). The myometrial cells increase in volume, and the nuclei are enlarged. (H & E stain, × 120.)

Figure 155. *Ultrastructurally,* the number of perinuclear organelles, especially the granular endoplasmic reticulum (GER) and micropinocytic vesicles (arrow), increases,[1-4] reflecting accelerated protein synthesis. As a result, the myofilaments (Mf) also increase in number.[3,4] Characteristically, large aggregates of glycogen (Gly) accumulate and the plasma membranes become sinuous, with interdigitating cytoplasmic processes.[4] In contrast to the nonpregnant myometrium, the gestational smooth muscle cells are enveloped by a thickened and uninterrupted basal lamina (BL). The extracellular space is wider than in normal myometrium because of an increase in collagen fibers (C) and ground substance. × 16,900. Mi: mitochondria.

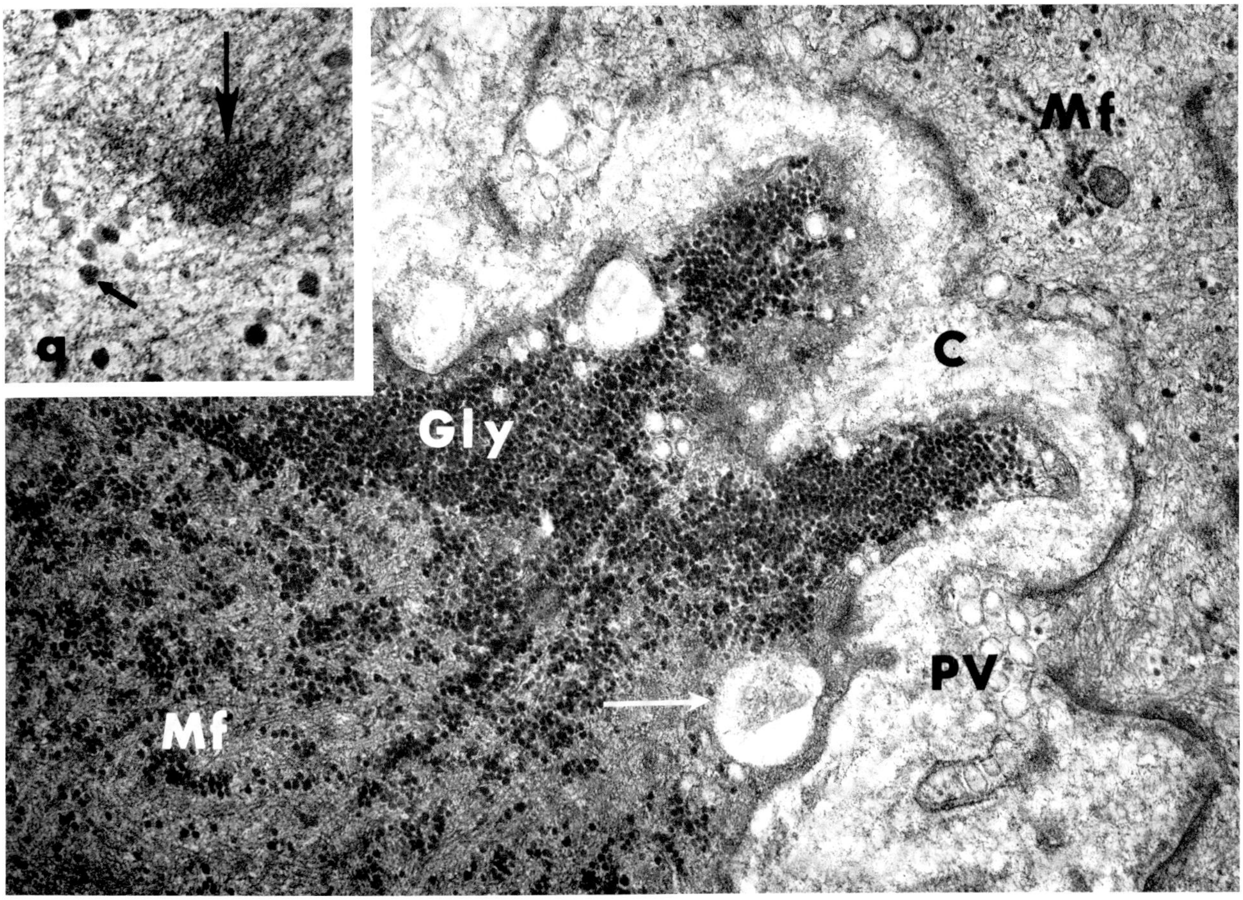

Figure 156. *Electron micrograph* of dark (left) and light (right) myometrial smooth muscle cells. Although both cell types contain abundant myofilaments (Mf), the dark cell has an electron-dense myoplasmic matrix, and the glycogen (Gly) accumulation at the periphery appears comparatively more conspicuous than in the light cell. Micropinocytic vesicles (PV) are associated with larger vesicles (arrow). The extracellular space contains collagen (C) and thinner precollagen and tropocollagen fibrils. × 48,000.

Figure 156a. *High magnification of a spindle-shaped body* (long arrow), into which thin (60 Å) actin filaments merge. Single glycogen particles (short arrow) are enmeshed between myofilaments. × 114,000.

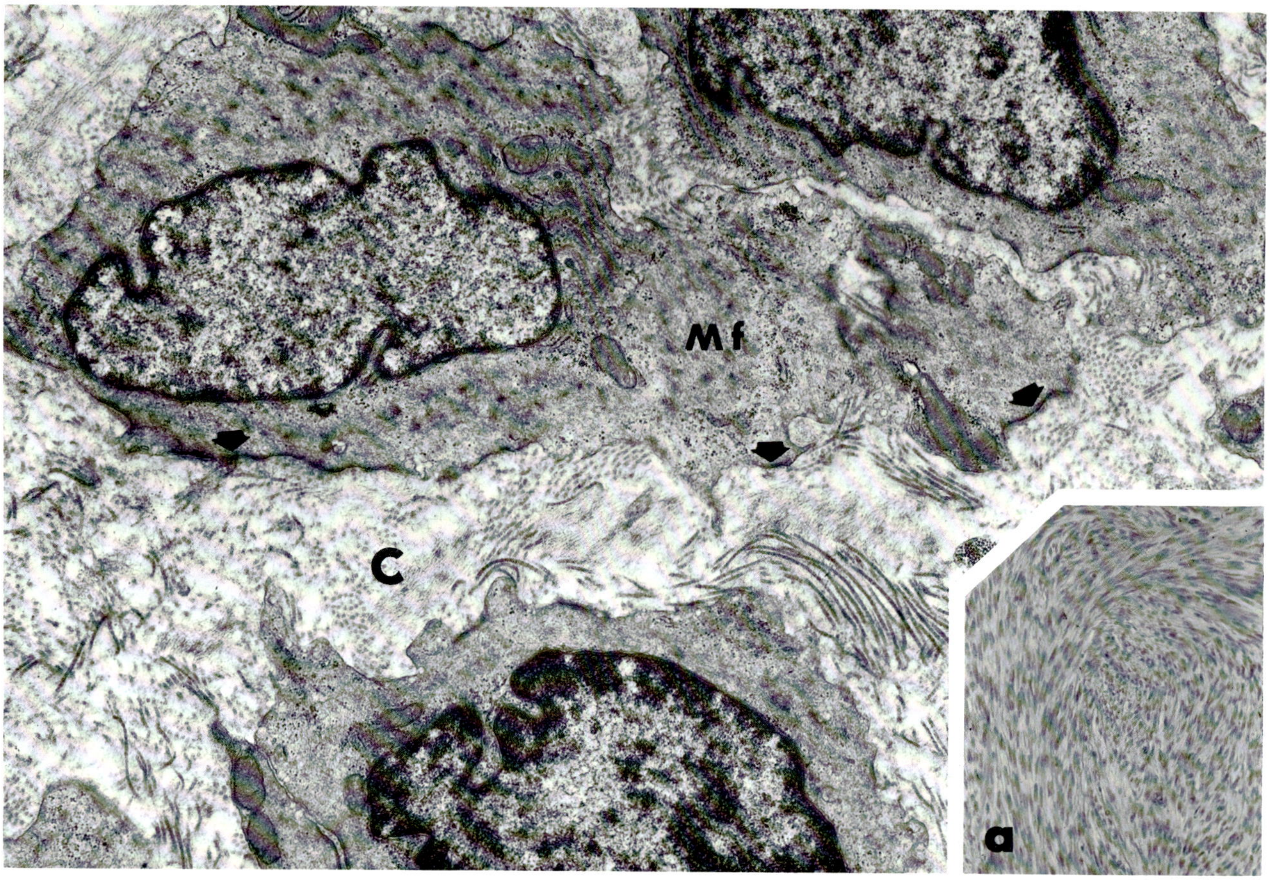

40

Leiomyoma

REFERENCES (Figures 157–158a)

1. Ferenczy, A., R. M. Richart, and T. Okagaki. A comparative ultrastructural study of leiomyosarcoma, cellular leiomyoma, and leiomyoma of the uterus. *Cancer* **28:** 1004 (1971).

Figure 157a. *The leiomyoma,* the most common uterine neoplasm, is composed of well-differentiated smooth muscle cells growing in bundles and cords and arranged in an interlacing pattern. Characteristically, the intercellular stroma contains a dense collagenous matrix. (H & E stain, × 300.)

Figure 157. *Ultrastructurally,* the neoplastic smooth muscle cells are identical in architecture and organization to normal myometrial cells.[1] The cells contain abundant myofilaments (Mf), marginal dense bodies (arrows), and micropinocytic vesicles. Characteristically, scant organelles are concentrated near the nuclear poles. The intercellular stroma (C) has bundles of collagen fibers and thinner tropocollagen fibrils. The ultrastructural similarity of leiomyoma cells to normal myometrial cells and the lack of a close relationship between neoplastic cells and perithelial cells of myometrial blood vessels suggest that the common leiomyomas are derived from uterine myometrial cells rather than from smooth muscle cells of blood vessels.[1] × 6500. *From* A. Ferenczy, R. M. Richart, and T. Okagaki. A comparative ultrastructural study of leiomyosarcoma, cellular leiomyoma, and leiomyoma of the uterus. *Cancer* **28:** 1004–1018 (1971).

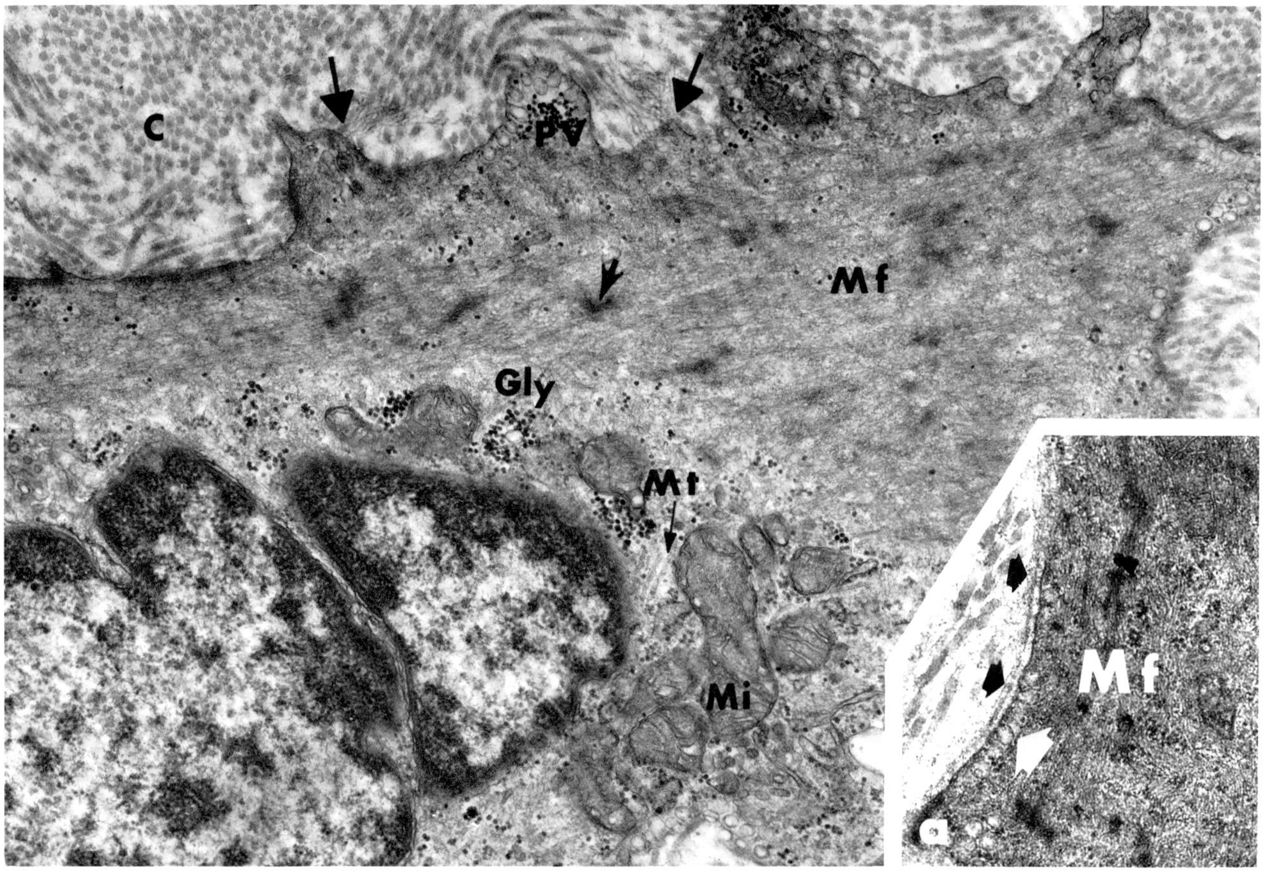

Figure 158. *Detailed view of a neoplastic smooth muscle cell* with well-developed, threadlike myofilaments and spindle-shaped dense bodies (short arrow). Perinuclear mitochondria (Mi) are associated with glycogen particles (Gly), cisternae of granular endoplasmic reticulum, and microtubules (Mt). Rows of micropinocytic vesicles (PV) with aggregates of glycogen particles and mitochondria are seen along the plasma membrane. Tufts of filaments approximately 300 Å thick resembling tropocollagen fibrils are in close relationship with the plasma membrane (large-headed arrows) and precollagen and collagen fibers (C), suggesting that smooth muscle cells are involved in collagen synthesis. × 25,000.

Figure 158a. *Leiomyoma.* The myoplasm is filled with myofilaments (Mf) containing focal densities, oriented parallel to the plasma membrane. Numerous micropinocytic vesicles (arrow) are seen, and a poorly developed basal lamina (short arrows) separates the cells from the collagenous stroma. × 44,000. *From* A. Ferenczy, R. M. Richart, and T. Okagaki. A comparative ultrastructural study of leiomyosarcoma, cellular leiomyoma, and leiomyoma of the uterus. *Cancer* **28:** 1004–1018 (1971).

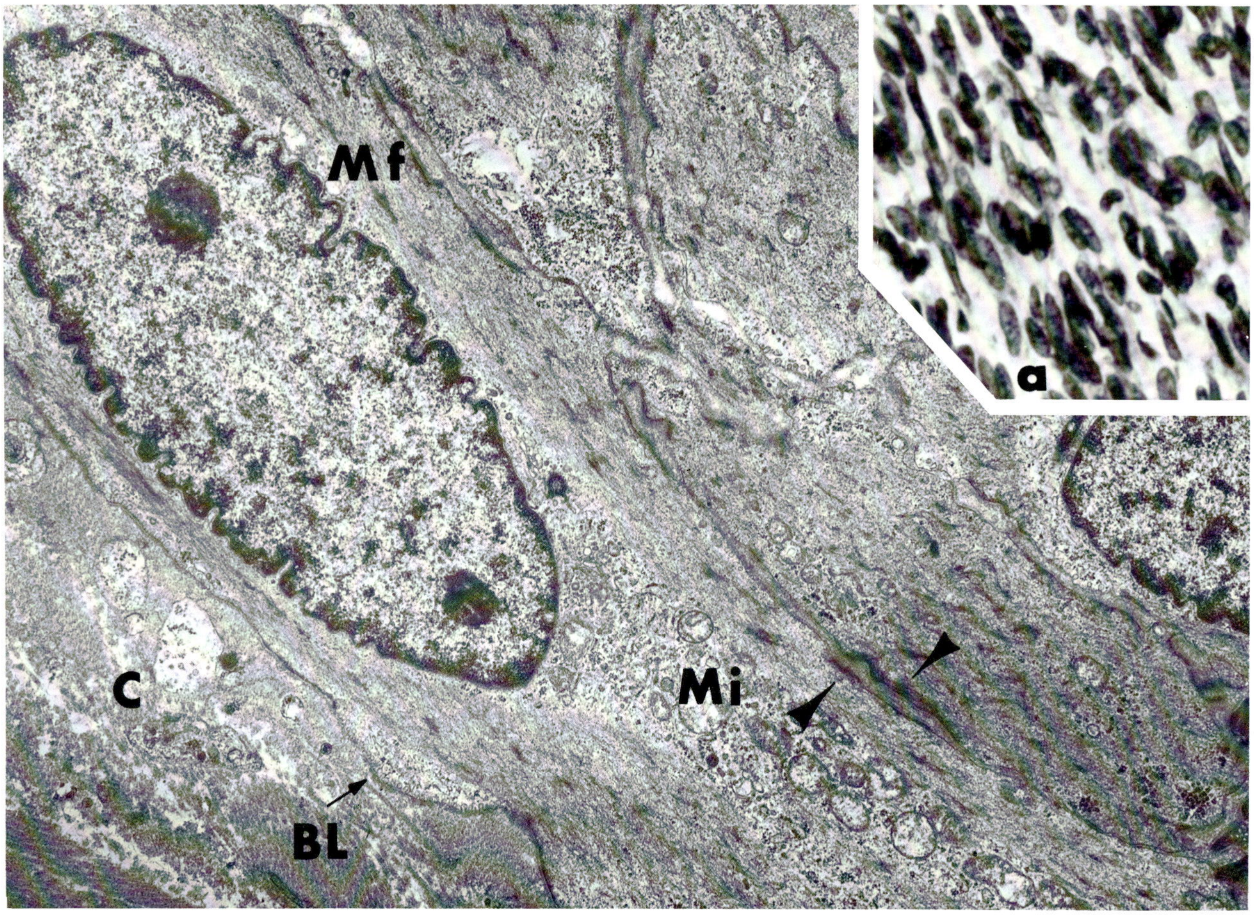

41

Cellular Leiomyoma

REFERENCE (Figures 159a–160c)

1. Ferenczy, A., R. M. Richart, and T. Okagaki. A comparative ultrastructural study of leiomyosarcoma, cellular leiomyoma, and leiomyoma of the uterus. *Cancer* **28:** 1004 (1971).

Figure 159a. *Cellular leiomyoma,* as its name implies, is a highly cellular variety of uterine leiomyoma with minimal nuclear atypia and mitotic activity. The intercellular connective tissue stroma is comparatively reduced. (H & E stain, × 240.)

Figure 159. *Electron microscopically,*[1] the cells, although essentially similar to those of the common leiomyoma and possessing abundant and diffusely distributed myofilaments (Mf), contain larger nuclei and increased, conically arranged, myoplasmic organelles such as mitochondria (Mi), polysomes, and Golgi. The myofilaments, myoplasmic and plasma membrane dense bodies (arrow heads), micropinocytic vesicles, and basal laminar (BL) are otherwise identical to those of the smooth muscle cells of leiomyoma or normal myometrium. These ultrastructural findings suggest that cellular leiomyoma represents a variety of common leiomyoma, rather than an intermediate form between leiomyoma and leiomyosarcoma.[1] × 7100. C: extracellular collagen. *From* A. Ferenczy, R. M. Richart, and T. Okagaki. A comparative ultrastructural study of leiomyosarcoma, cellular leiomyoma, and leiomyoma of the uterus. *Cancer* **28:** 1004–1018 (1971).

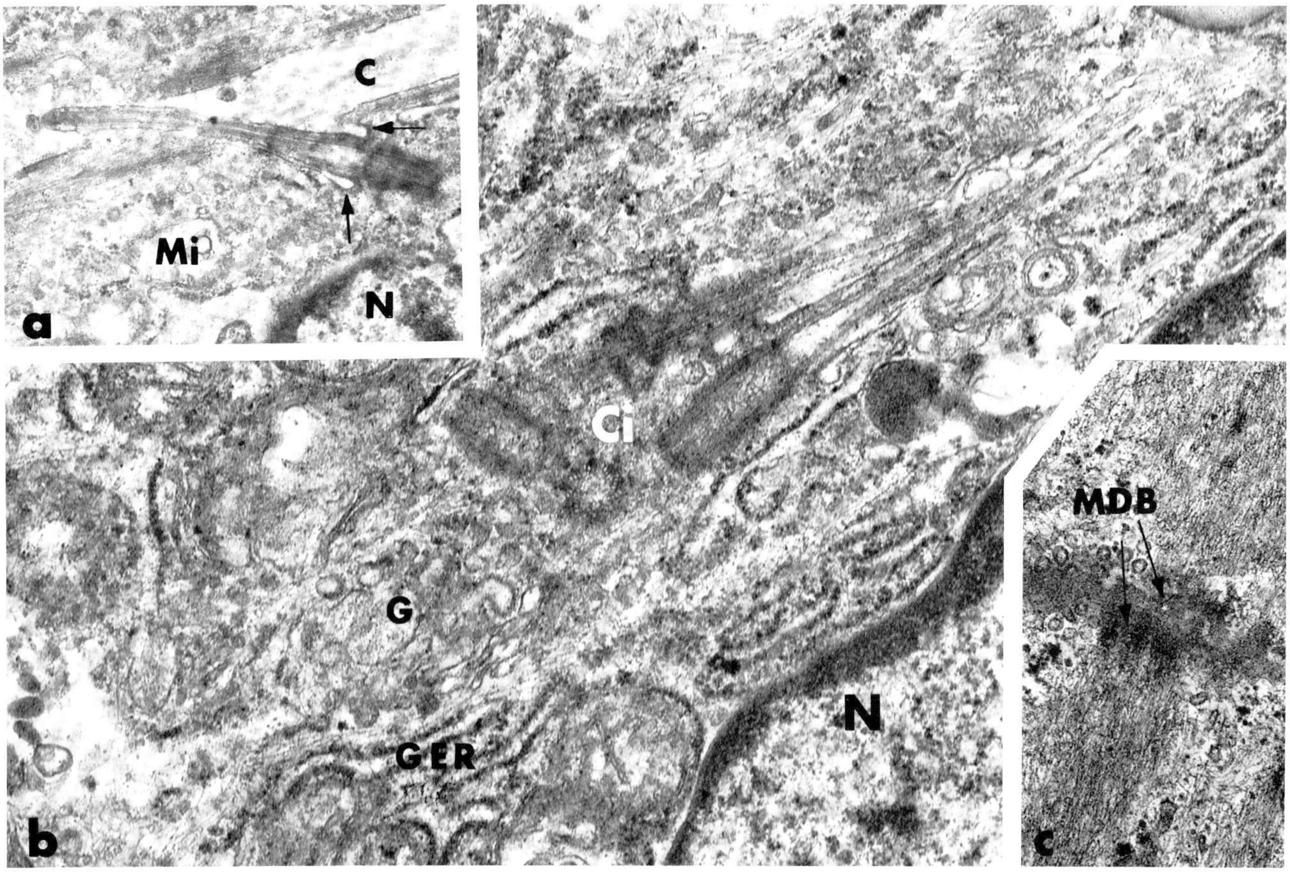

Figure 160a. *Single cilia* are more frequently seen in cellular than in ordinary leiomyoma.[1] A well-developed, supranuclear (N), single cilium with ciliary vesicles (arrow) is emerging into the extracellular space (C). × 25,000. Mi: mitochondria. *From* A. Ferenczy, R. M. Richart, and T. Okagaki. A comparative ultrastructural study of leiomyosarcoma, cellular leiomyoma, and leiomyoma of the uterus. *Cancer* **28:** 1004–1018 (1971).

Figure 160b. *Cellular leiomyoma.* Occasionally, two intracytoplasmic cilia with a centriolar apparatus (Ci) and a Golgi complex (G) are encountered. Note the well-developed, slightly dilated cisternae of granular endoplasmic reticulum (GER). × 32,000. *From* A. Ferenczy, R. M. Richart, and T. Okagaki. A comparative ultrastructural study of leiomyosarcoma, cellular leiomyoma, and leiomyoma of the uterus. *Cancer* **28:** 1004–1018 (1971).

Figure 160c. *Cellular leiomyoma.* Bundles of myofilaments appear to converge into juxtaposed marginal dense bodies (MDB), in consistency with the concept that such bodies may serve as attachment sites for myofilaments. × 28,000. *From* A. Ferenczy, R. M. Richart, and T. Okagaki. A comparative ultrastructural study of leiomyosarcoma, cellular leiomyoma, and leiomyoma of the uterus. *Cancer* **28:** 1004–1018 (1971).

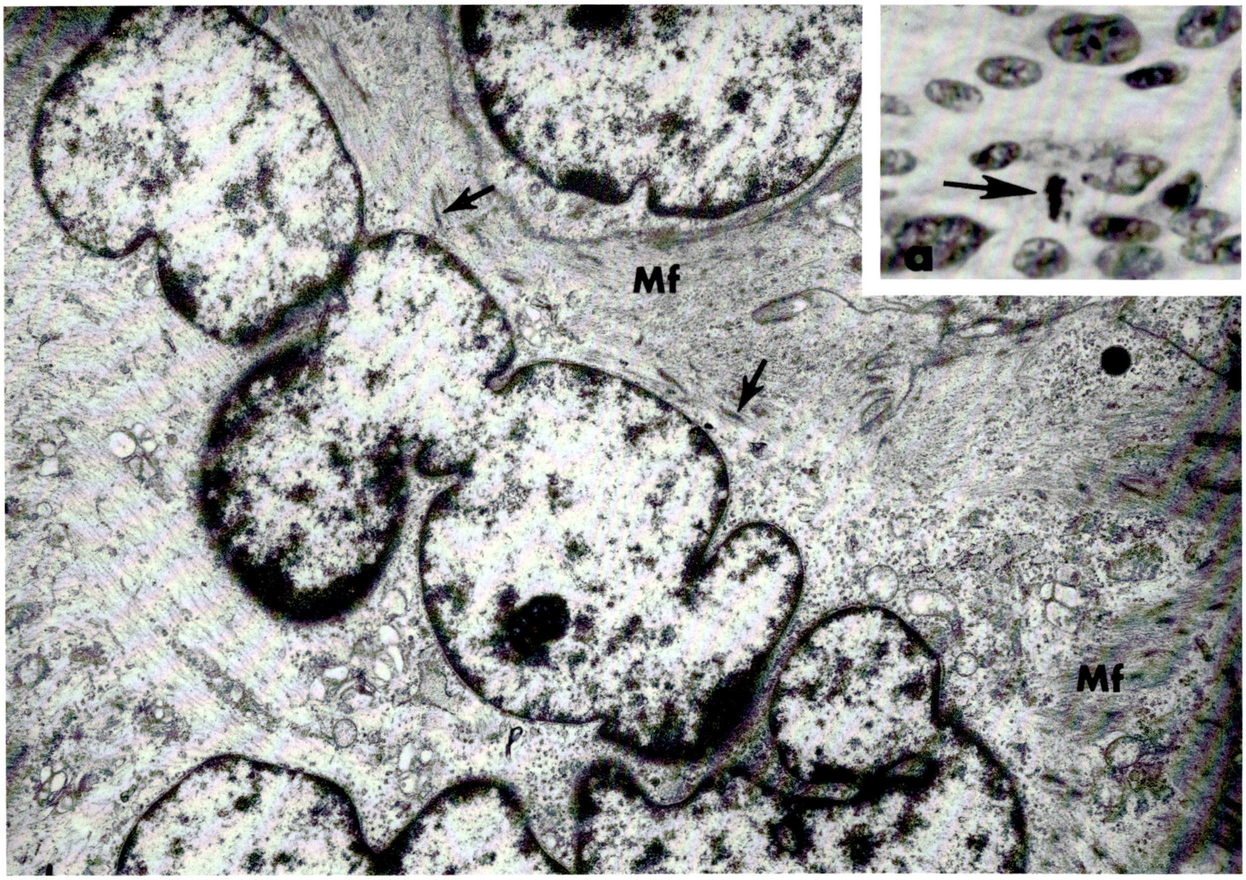

42

Leiomyosarcoma

Leiomyosarcoma, the most common uterine sarcoma, generally grows in a diffuse and infiltrating fashion and is highly malignant.

REFERENCE (Figures 161–162c)

1. Ferenczy, A., R. M. Richart, and T. Okagaki. A comparative ultrastructural study of leiomyosarcoma, cellular leiomyoma, and leiomyoma of the uterus. *Cancer* **28:** 1004 (1971).

Figure 161a. *Histologically,* there are generally striking nuclear pleomorphism and significantly mitotic activity (arrow). (H & E stain, × 400.)

Figure 161. *Leiomyosarcoma.* In addition to nuclear abnormalities, there is ultrastructural evidence of disturbed cellular organization and an abnormal formation of myofilaments (Mf),[1] which usually appear as short bundles with spindle-shaped densities (arrow) and are often arranged in a haphazard manner. Many cells are completely devoid of myofilaments. Despite the reduction in myofilaments, other organelles, including mitochondria, polysomes, and granular endoplasmic reticulum, are prominent in many cells. In others, however (the so-called light cells), the cytoplasmic matrix is poor in cytoplasmic organelles. Glycogen is inconspicuous in leiomyosarcoma cells but is seen in both cellular and ordinary leiomyoma. Micropinocytic activity, together with basal lamina formation, is comparatively reduced in the leiomyosarcomas, and the complicated cytoplasmic processes often seen in other malignant uterine mesenchymal neoplasms do not occur. The stroma between sarcoma cells is strikingly reduced, and the adjacent plasma membranes are often in close apposition for considerable distances.[1] × 6600.

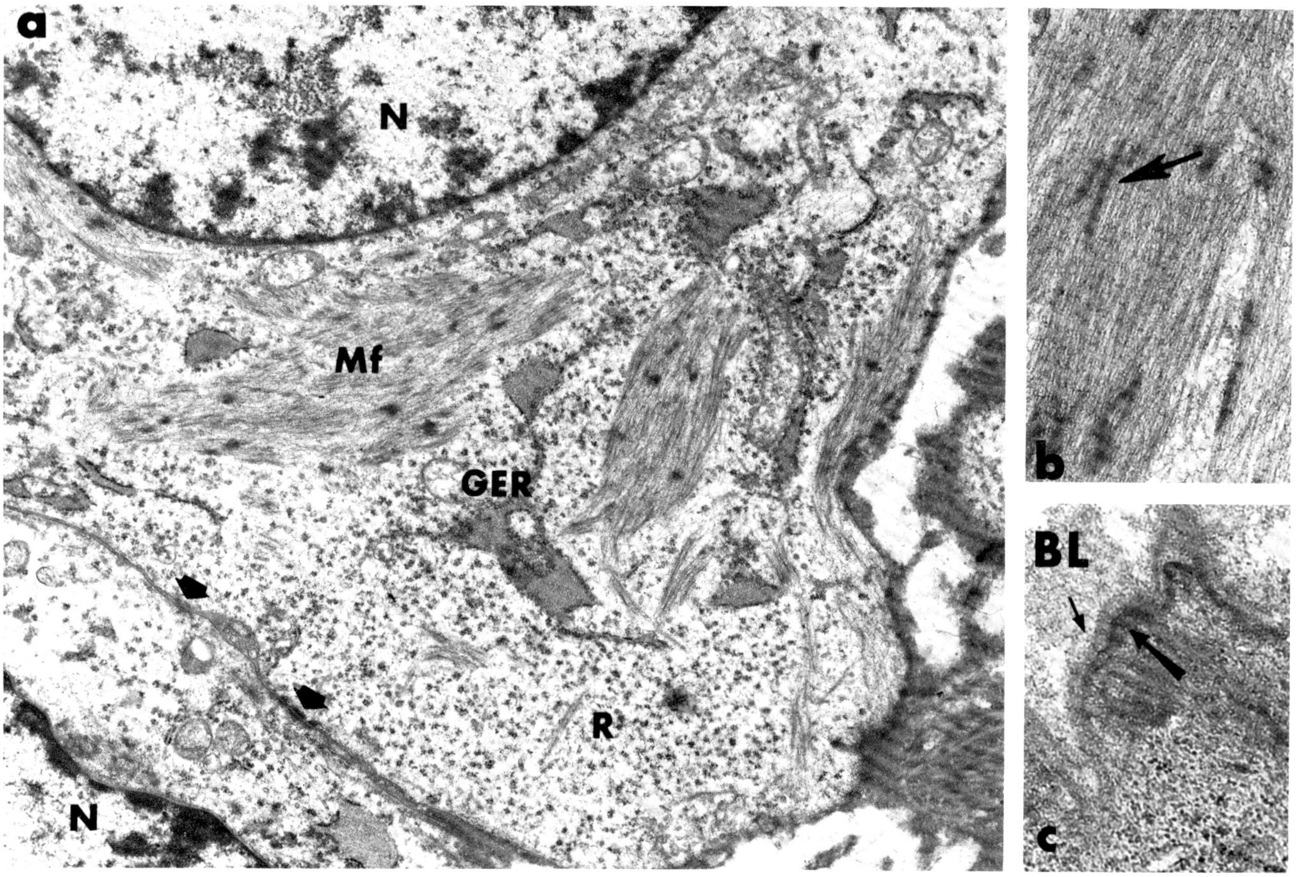

Figure 162a. *Leiomyosarcoma.* Cellular detail of a "light cell." The clear cytoplasmic background is obscured by numerous polysomes (R). Dilated cisternae of granular endoplasmic reticulum with electron-dense amorphous content (GER) and haphazardly oriented short bundles of myofilaments (Mf) with focal periodicity are the characteristic features of this cell type. Note the presence of occasional juxtaposed, poorly formed, marginal dense bodies (arrows) simulating desmosomal attachments. × 22,000. N: nucleus. *From* A. Ferenczy, R. M. Richart, and T. Okagaki. A comparative ultrastructural study of leiomyosarcoma, cellular leiomyoma, and leiomyoma of the uterus. *Cancer* **28:** 1004–1018 (1971).

Figure 162b. *Higher magnification* of myofilaments with spindle-shaped dense bodies (arrow). × 30,000. *From* A. Ferenczy, R. M. Richart, and T. Okagaki. A comparative ultrastructural study of a leiomyosarcoma, cellular leiomyoma, and leiomyoma of the uterus. *Cancer* **28:** 1004–1018 (1971).

Figure 162c. *Leiomyosarcoma.* Bundles of myofilaments appear to terminate on a plasma membrane dense body (large arrow), which is covered by a well-defined basal lamina (BL). × 25,000. *From* A. Ferenczy, R. M. Richart, and T. Okagaki. A comparative ultrastructural study of leiomyosarcoma, cellular leiomyoma, and leiomyoma of the uterus. *Cancer* **28:** 1004–1918 (1971).

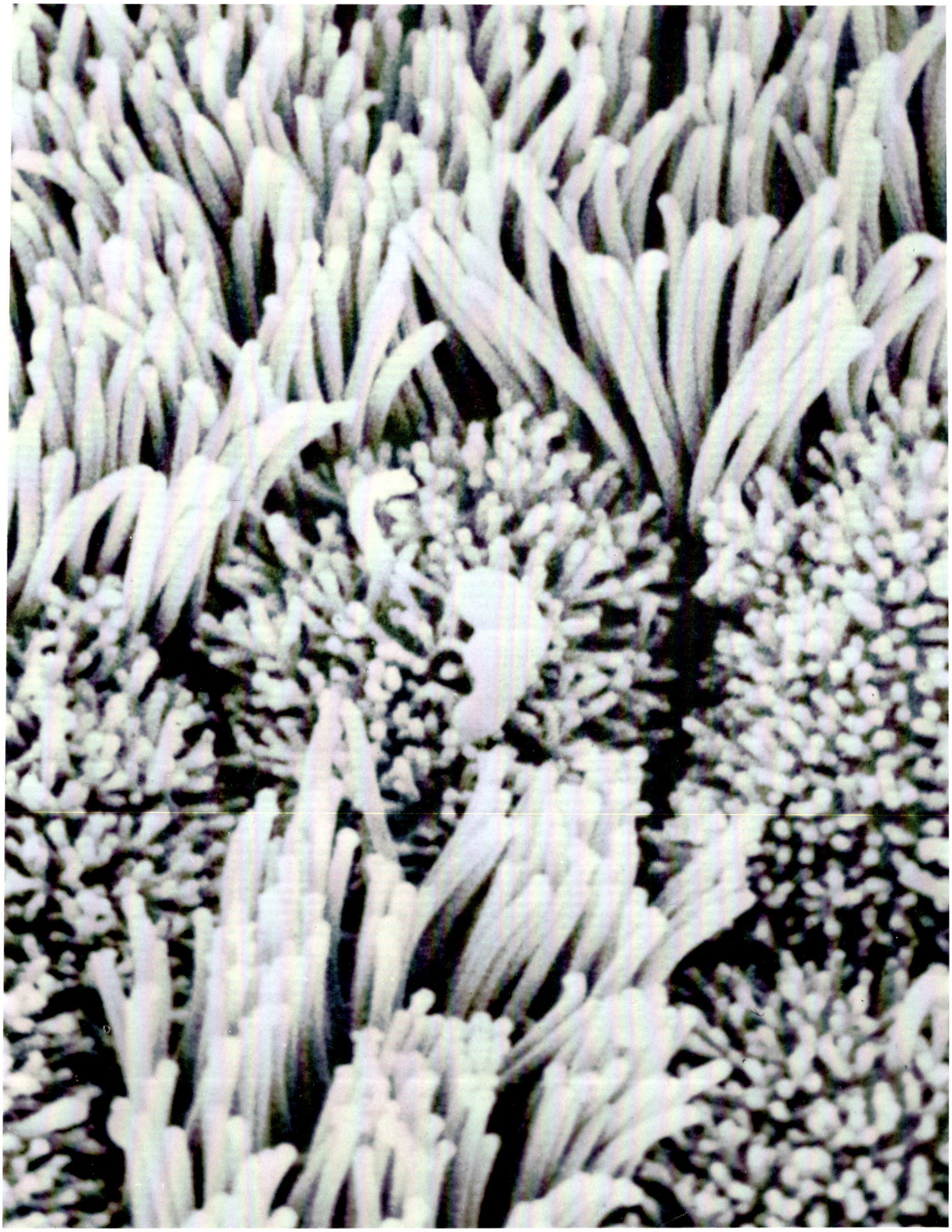

The Fallopian tube during the early proliferative phase of the menstrual cycle. Numerous ciliated cells alternate with dome-shaped microvillous secretory cells. × 12,500.

FALLOPIAN TUBE (OVIDUCT)

43

Normal Menstrual Cycle

The paired uterine tubes extend from the fundus of the uterus to both ovaries. Their primary function is to conduct the fertilized ovum to its endometrial bed for nidation.

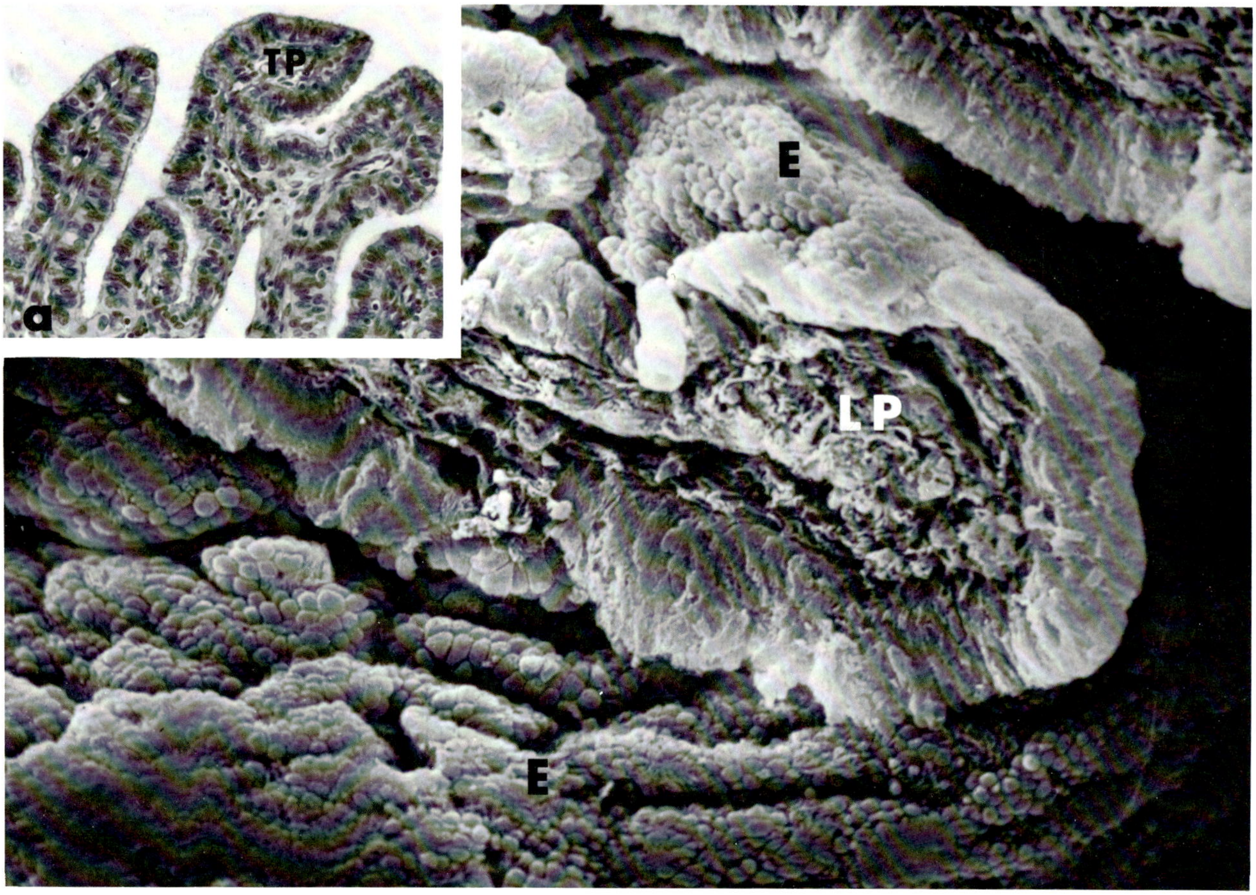

Figure 163a. *Fallopian tube (ampulla).* The oviductal mucosa is composed of numerous branching mucosal plicae (TP), or folds, projecting into the tubal lumen. The plicae are covered by a single-layered columnar epithelium supported by a loose fibrovascular lamina propria. (H & E stain, × 48.)

Figure 163. *Fallopian tube (ampulla).* Scanning electron microscopy of a cross-sectioned, blunt-ended, tubal plica, the covering epithelium (E) of which has a cobblestone appearance. The lamina propria (LP) contains interlacing collagen fibers. × 288.

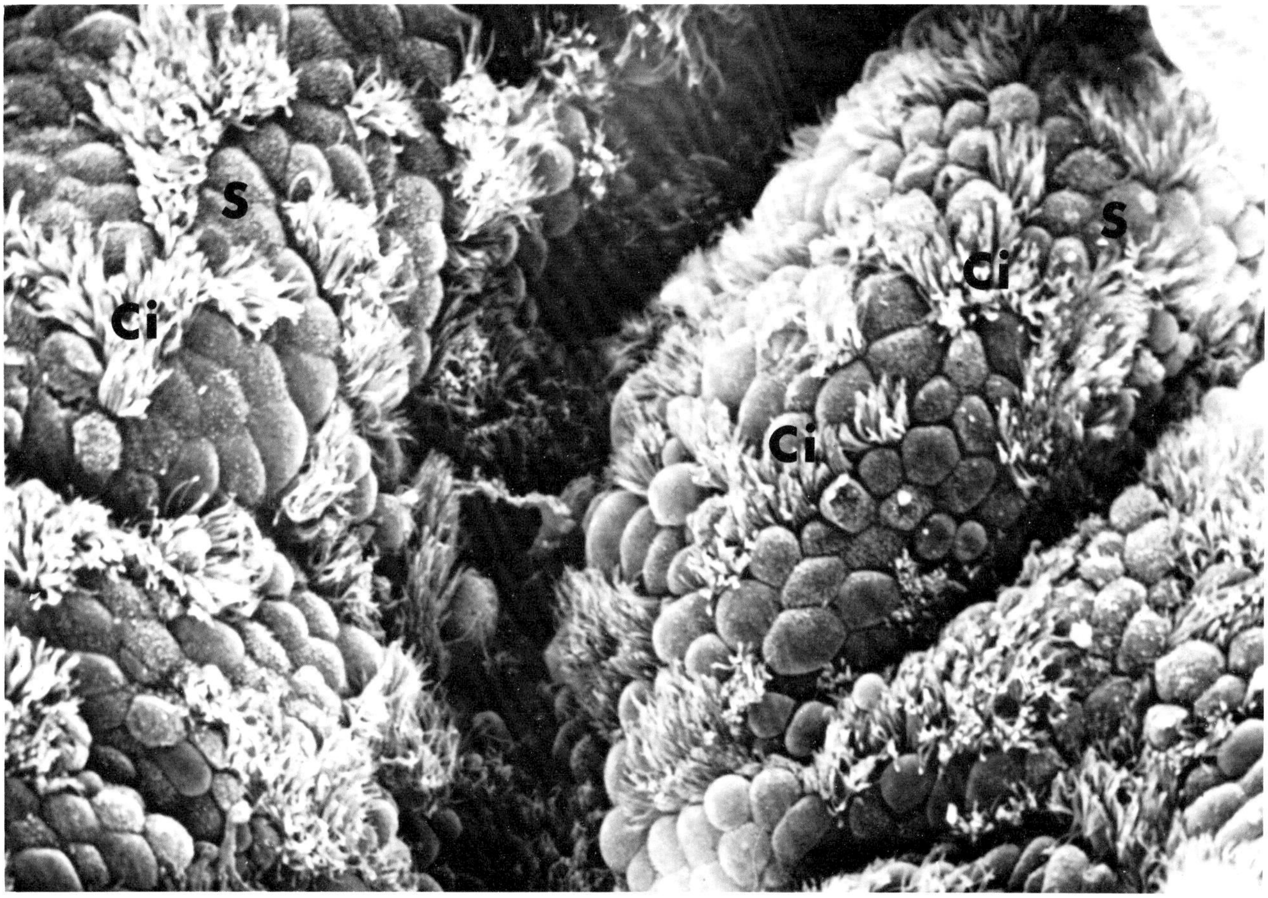

Figure 164. *Fallopian tube (ampulla).* Higher-magnification scanning electron micrograph, illustrating the summit of two adjacent tubal plicae. The covering epithelium contains numerous clusters of ciliated cells (Ci) alternating with nonciliated, dome-shaped secretory cells (S). Although ciliated and nonciliated cells occur in approximately equal numbers and proportions along different segments of the human oviduct,[1] ciliated cells are more prominent on the plical plateaus than in the crypts.[1,2] × 2000.

REFERENCES (Figures 163–164)

1. Ferenczy, A., R. M. Richart, F. J. Agate, Jr., M. L. Purkerson, and E. W. Dempsey. Scanning electron microscopy of the human Fallopian tube. *Science* **175:** 783 (1972).
2. Patek, E., L. Nilsson, and E. Johannisson. Scanning electron microscopic study of the human Fallopian tube. Report I. The proliferative and secretory stages. *Fertil. Steril.* **23:** 459 (1972).

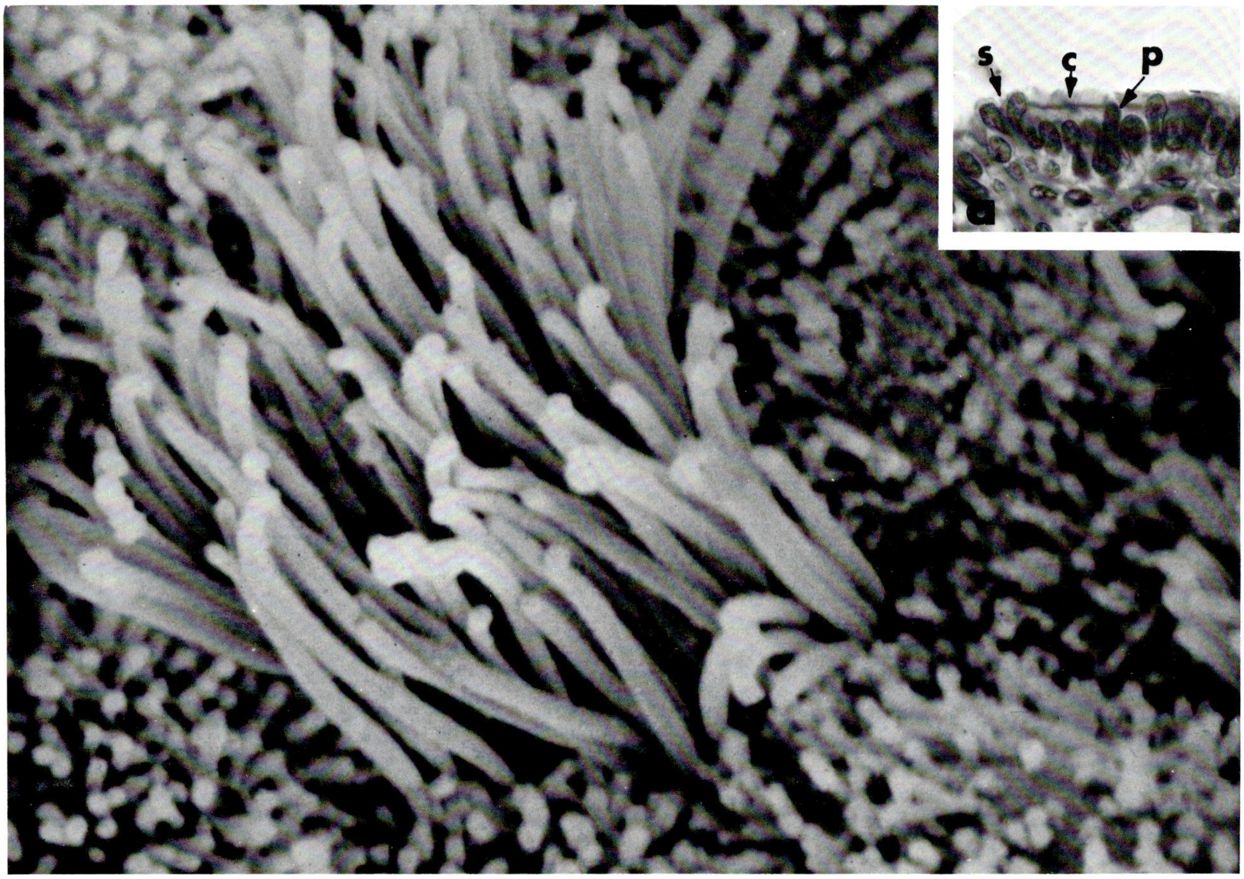

Figure 165a. *Fallopian tube (fimbria).* During the reproductive years the human oviductal mucosa contains ciliated (C), secretory (S), and peg (P) cells (*Stiftchenzellen*), as well as reserve or indifferent cells.[1] The ciliated and secretory units are the principal cell types and occur in an approximately equal ratio. The peg cells represent degenerating or exhausted secretory cells. The reserve cells, which have a high ^{3}H-thymidine uptake,[1] are located near or on the basal lamina and are believed to be the precursors of both the secretory and the ciliated cells. The existence of tubal reserve cells remains highly controversial, however, and many investigators regard these cells as emperiopoietic lymphocytes or degranulating mast cells of stromal origin.[2] (H & E stain, × 75.)

Figure 165. *Scanning electron microscopy of a small cluster of ciliated cells.* There are well-developed ciliary shafts with folded bulbous apices. Each cilium measures 3 to 4μ in length, and there are approximately 50 cilia per cell. The surrounding secretory cells are covered by numerous slender microvilli. × 13,600.

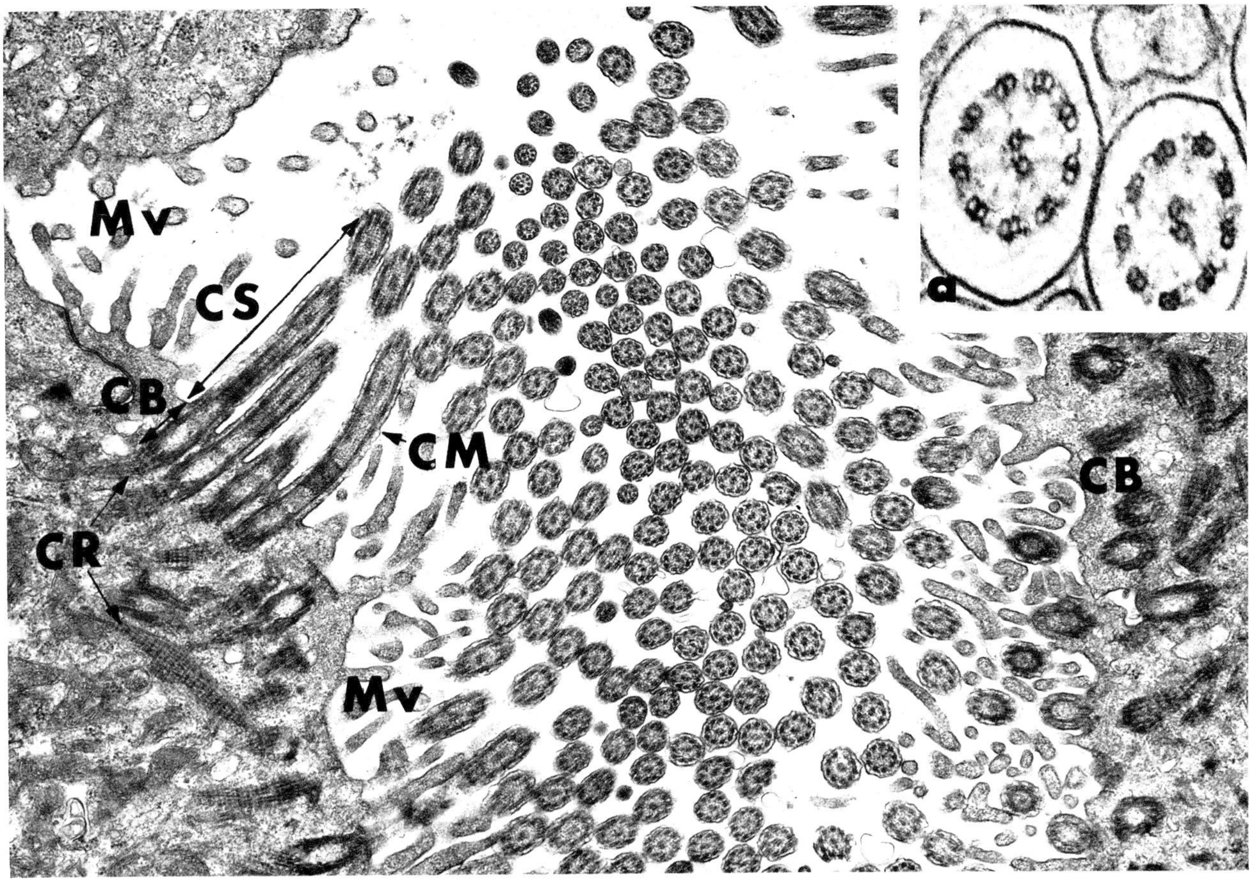

Figure 166. *Fallopian tube (isthmus).* Tangential section of the apical portion of ciliated cells containing numerous cilia and surface microvillous (Mv) processes. The cilial basal bodies (CB) are cylindrical structures, composed of nine sets of three tubules embedded in an amorphous matrix. The nine sets are equally pitched to the left at a 10 to 15° angle to the longitudinal axis.[3] The basal bodies often have identifiable accessory structures associated with them. These include the basal foot, or satellite, process, a pyramidal fibrous structure projecting at right angles from the mid-region of the basal body, and cross-striated rootlets (CR), structures attached to the base of basal bodies, which extend for a short distance into the cytoplasm. The ciliary shaft (CS), or cilium, originates from the apex of basal bodies and is composed of nine sets of peripheral double tubules surrounding a central pair of tubules. Each ciliary shaft is enveloped by the ciliary membrane (CM), which is in continuity with the surface plasma membrane. × 20,600.

Figure 166a. *Transverse section of ciliary shafts,* containing nine double peripheral tubules and two double central tubules. × 120,000. *From* L. Overbeck. Die Feinstruktur des Tubenepithels im mensuellen Zyklus. *Z. Geburtsh. Gynaekol.* **171:** 241–260 (1969).

REFERENCES (Figures 165–166a)

1. Woodruff, J. D. and C. J. Pauerstein. The epithelium. In *The Fallopian Tube: Structure, Function, Pathology and Management.* Williams & Wilkins, Baltimore, 1969, pp. 22–46.
2. Rasweiler, J. J. The basal or indifferent cell and the ciliary vacuole in the oviductal epithelium of the long-tongued bat, *Glossophaga soricina. J. Reprod. Fertil.* **30:** 191 (1972).
3. Anderson, R. G. W. The three-dimensional structure of the basal body from the rhesus monkey oviduct. *J. Cell Biol.* **54:** 246 (1972).

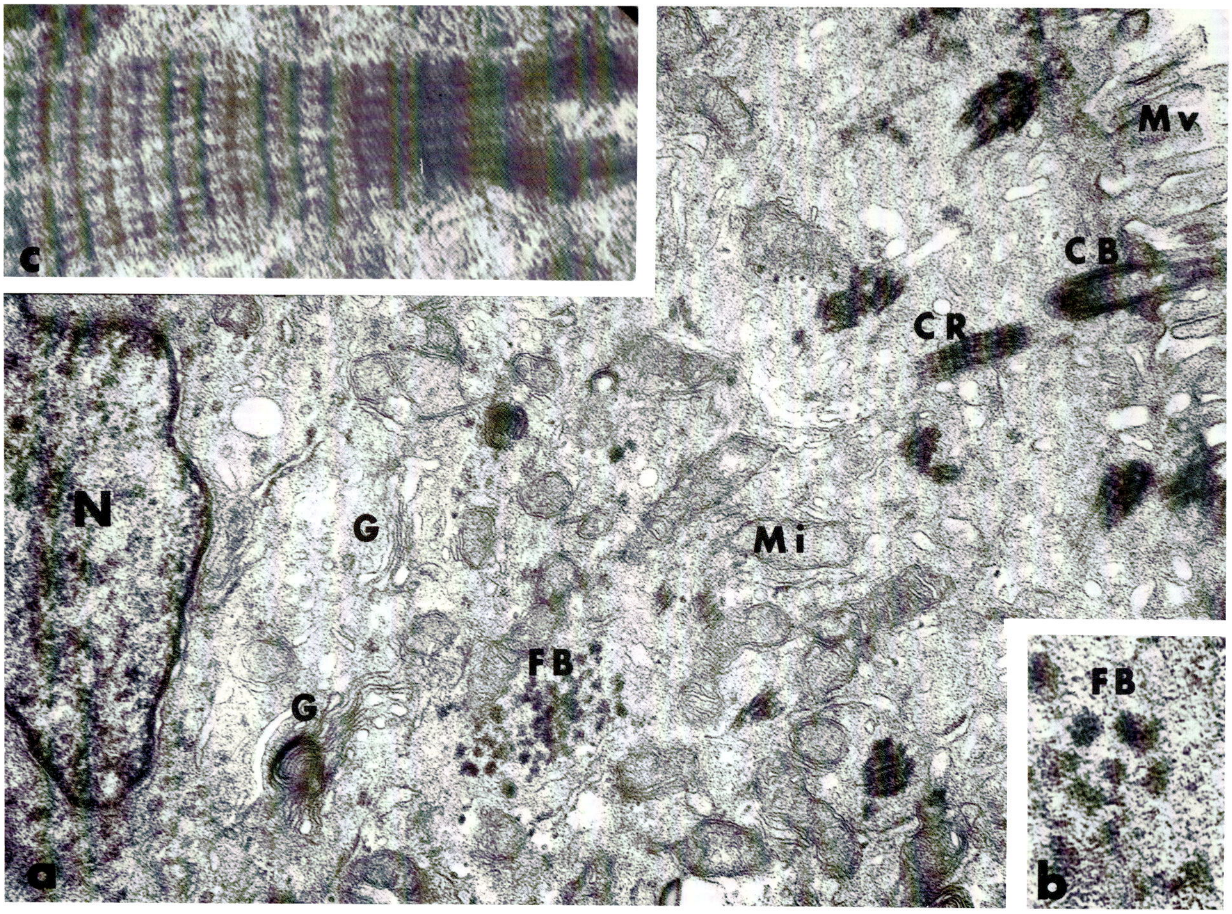

Figure 167a. *The cilial basal bodies* (CB) are most commonly formed by acentriolar body formation but may be formed by centriolar body formation. In the former case procentrioles are generated from a "spherical aggregate of fibers" (FB) often found near the Golgi (G), and in the latter, from the "diplosomal centrioles."[1] The cilium has a similar end structure irrespective of the mechanism of ciliogenesis. Although the exact significance of ciliary motion remains to be clarified, it is probably directed toward the mobilization and distribution of secretory material, rather than toward gamete transport, which is thought to be mediated by muscular contractions of the oviduct. × 36,000. N: nucleus; Mi: mitochondria; CR: ciliary rootlet; Mv: microvilli associated with pinocytic vesicles.

Figure 167b. *Higher magnification* of the spherical bodies (FB), illustrating their fibrous nature. × 75,000.

Figure 167c. *Detail of a cross-striated ciliary rootlet.* The rootlet (left) is continuous with the base of the basal body (right) and is composed of longitudinally arranged fibers alternating with clear, amorphous spaces. At regular intervals, electron-dense bands or plates approximately 500 Å in diameter are disposed perpendicularly to the longitudinal fibers. The precise function of ciliary rootlets is not clear. × 87,500.

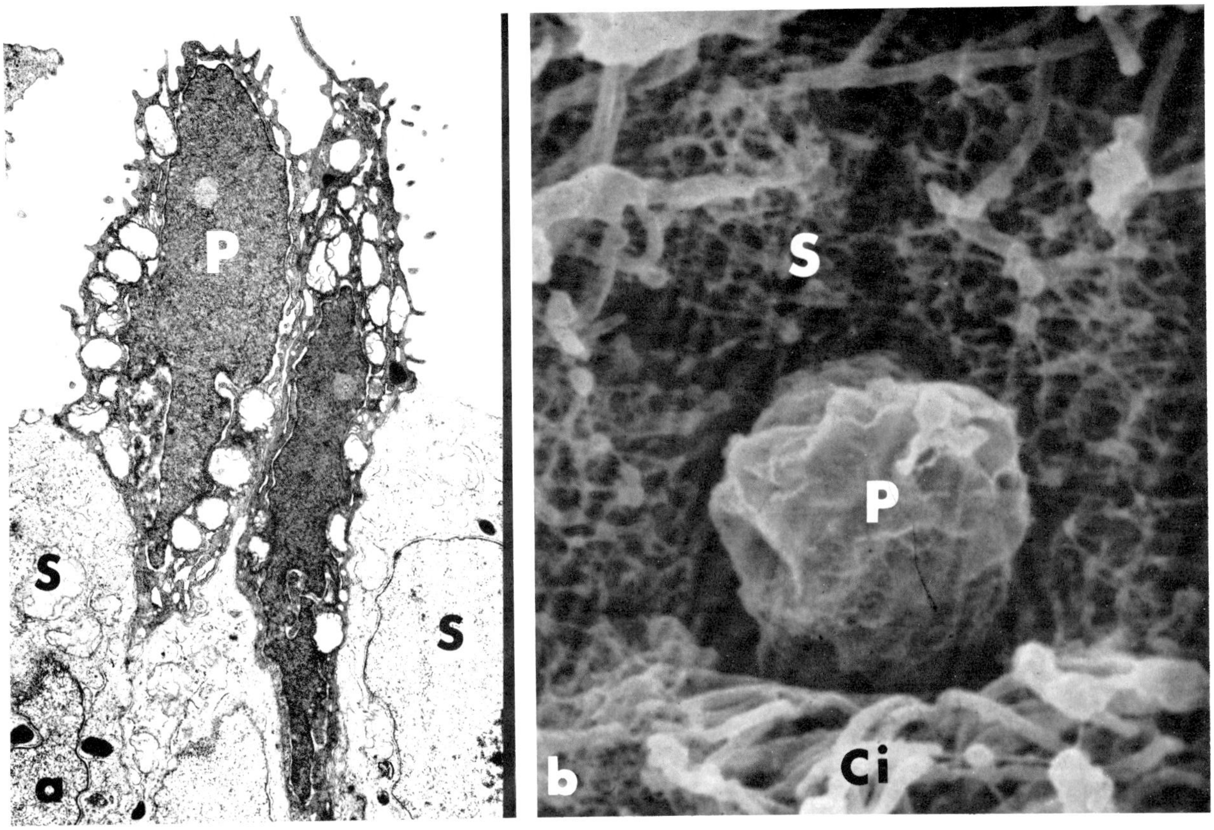

Figure 168a. *Eletcron microscopic appearance of degenerated secretory or peg (P) cells.* The cells are protruding and have shrunken nuclei with condensation of nuclear chromatin, and the narrow, electron-dense cytoplasmic substance contains markedly swollen mitochondria with ruptured cristae. The adjacent secretory cells (S) have abundant and well-preserved organelles and scattered electron-dense lysosomes. × 5800.

Figure 168b. *Topographic appearance of a degenerated peg cell (P).* The protruding cell membrane is wrinkled and devoid of surface microvillous processes. By virtue of cellular shrinkage the intercellular space around the peg cell is enlarged. By contrast, the adjacent secretory cells (S) have dome-shaped surface plasma membranes covered by abundant microvilli. A ciliated cell (Ci) is seen in the lower center. × 8000.

REFERENCE (Figures 167a–168b)

1. Anderson, R. G. W. and R. M. Brenner. The formation of basal bodies (centrioles) in the rhesus monkey oviduct. *J. Cell Biol.* **50:** 10 (1971).

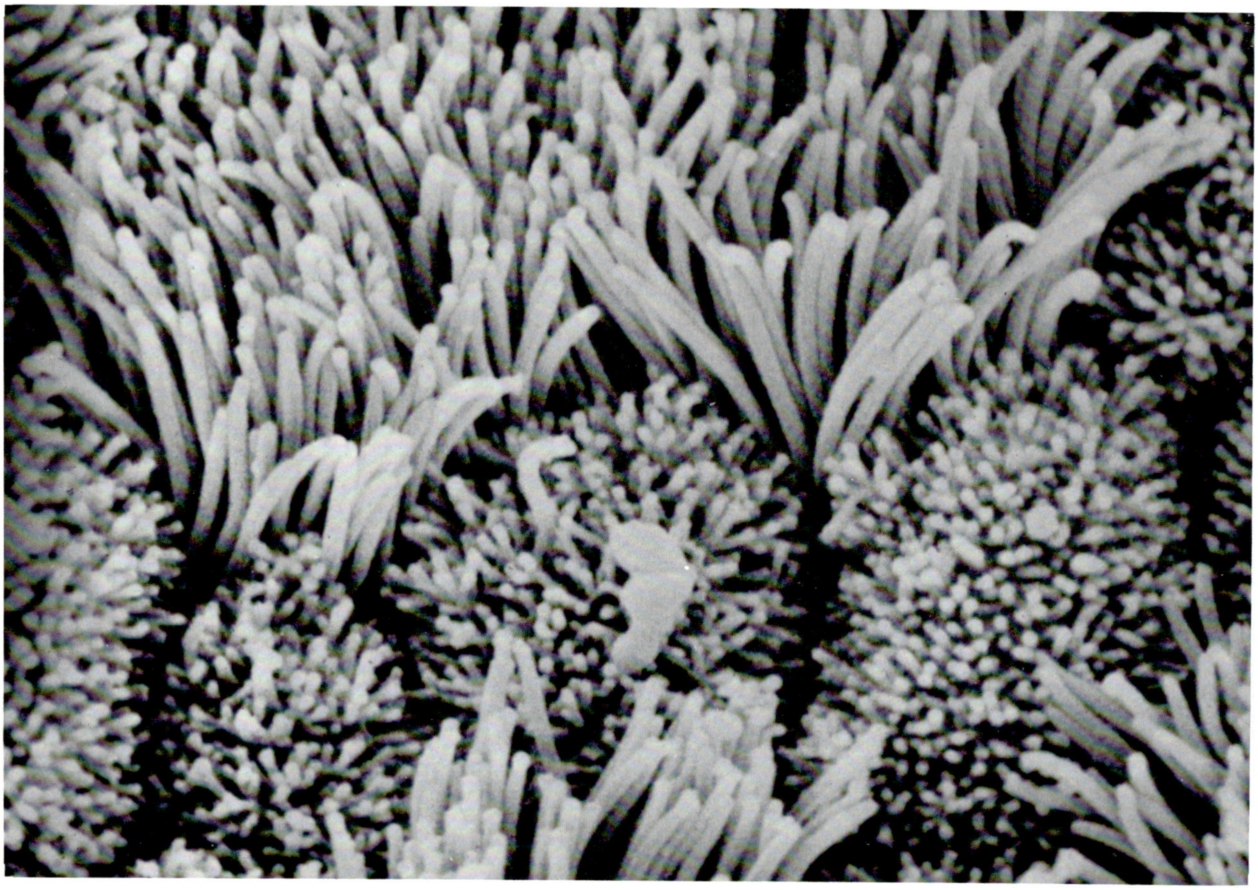

Figure 169. *Fallopian tube (isthmus). Early proliferative phase (4–7th days) of the menstrual cycle.* Ciliated and non-ciliated cells occur in approximately equal ratio. Tufts of cilia having a slightly wavy appearance project well above the adjacent secretory cells and result in an irregular surface pattern. In the early phase of the menstrual cycle, surface secretory activity appears inconspicuous. Note the well-developed microvillous covering of the secretory cells. × 9600.

Although tubal ciliogenesis has been described in the 70-mm embryo[1] and fetus,[2] no significant cyclical or geographical morphologic variations in ciliated cells are seen during the menstrual cycle.[3-5] In contrast to the human case, the ciliated cells in the oviducts of subprimates and rodents are unevenly distributed, and there is a gradual proportional increase from the isthmus (30%) to the ampulla (50%). The fimbria is abundantly ciliated (85%).[6-8]

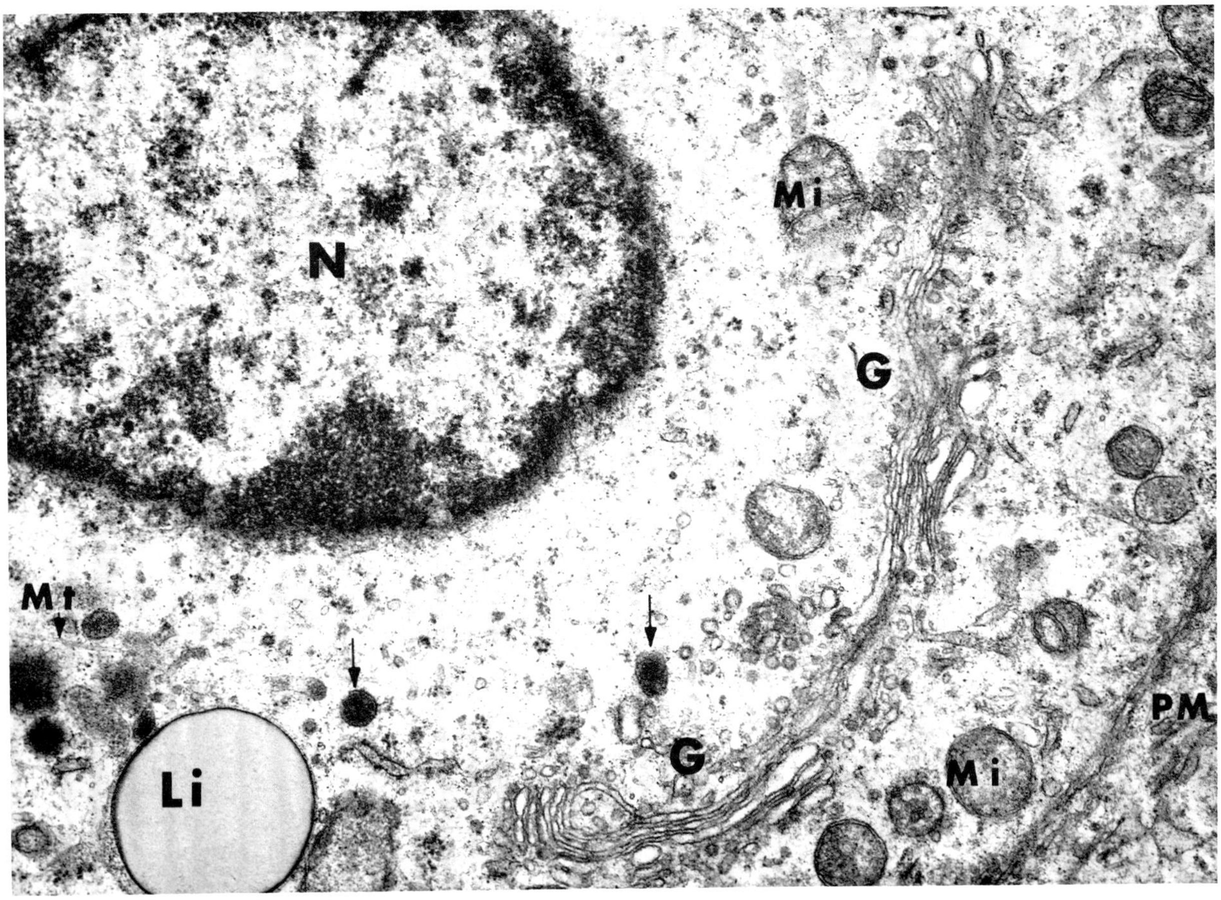

Figure 170. *Fallopian tube (isthmus). Early proliferative phase of the menstrual cycle.* Although secretory activity is not evident at the scanning electron microscopic level, with the transmission electron microscope several nonciliated cells are found to contain well-developed, perinuclear (N) Golgi (G) with prominent layers of saccules and peripheral coated vesicles, indicating that glyocoprotein synthesis begins in the early menstrual period. The associated polyribosomes and mitochondria (Mi) are the necessary organelles for protein synthesis, and the membrane-bound, dense granules (arrows) probably represent secretory end products. × 20,600. Li: lipid droplet; Mt: microtubule; PM: plasma membrane.

REFERENCES (Although tubal ciliogenesis—Figure 170)

1. Overbeck, L. On the ultrastructure of tubal epithelium. *Arch. Gynaekol.* **204:** 58 (1967).
2. Patek, E., L. Nilsson, and E. Johanisson. Scanning electron microscopic study of the human Fallopian tube. Report II. Fetal life, reproductive life and postmenopause. *Fertil. Steril.* **23:** 719 (1972).
3. Hashimoto, M., T. Shimoyama, M. Kosaka, A. Komori, T. Hirasawa, Y. Yokoyama, N. Kawase, and T. Nakamura. Electron microscopic studies on epithelial cells of the human Fallopian tube (11). *J. Jap. Obstet. Gynec. Soc.* **11:** 92 (1964).
4. Clyman, M. J. Electron microscopy of the human Fallopian tube. *Fertil. Steril.* **17:** 281 (1966).
5. Ferenczy, A., R. M. Richart, F. J. Agate, Jr., M. L. Purkerson, and E. W. Dempsey. Scanning electron microscopy of the human Fallopian tube. *Science* **175:** 783 (1972).
6. Kanagawa, H., E. S. E. Hafez, W. C. Pitchford, C. A. Paechler, and M. I. Barhart. Surface patterns in the reproductive tracts of the rabbit observed by scanning electron microscopy. *Anat. Rec.* **174:** 205 (1972).
7. Hafez, E. S. E. Scanning electron microscopy of rabbit and monkey female reproductive tract epithelium. *J. Reprod. Fertil.* **30:** 293 (1972).
8. Hafez, E. S. E. Scanning electron microscopy of female reproductive tract. *J. Reprod. Med.* **9:** 119 (1972).

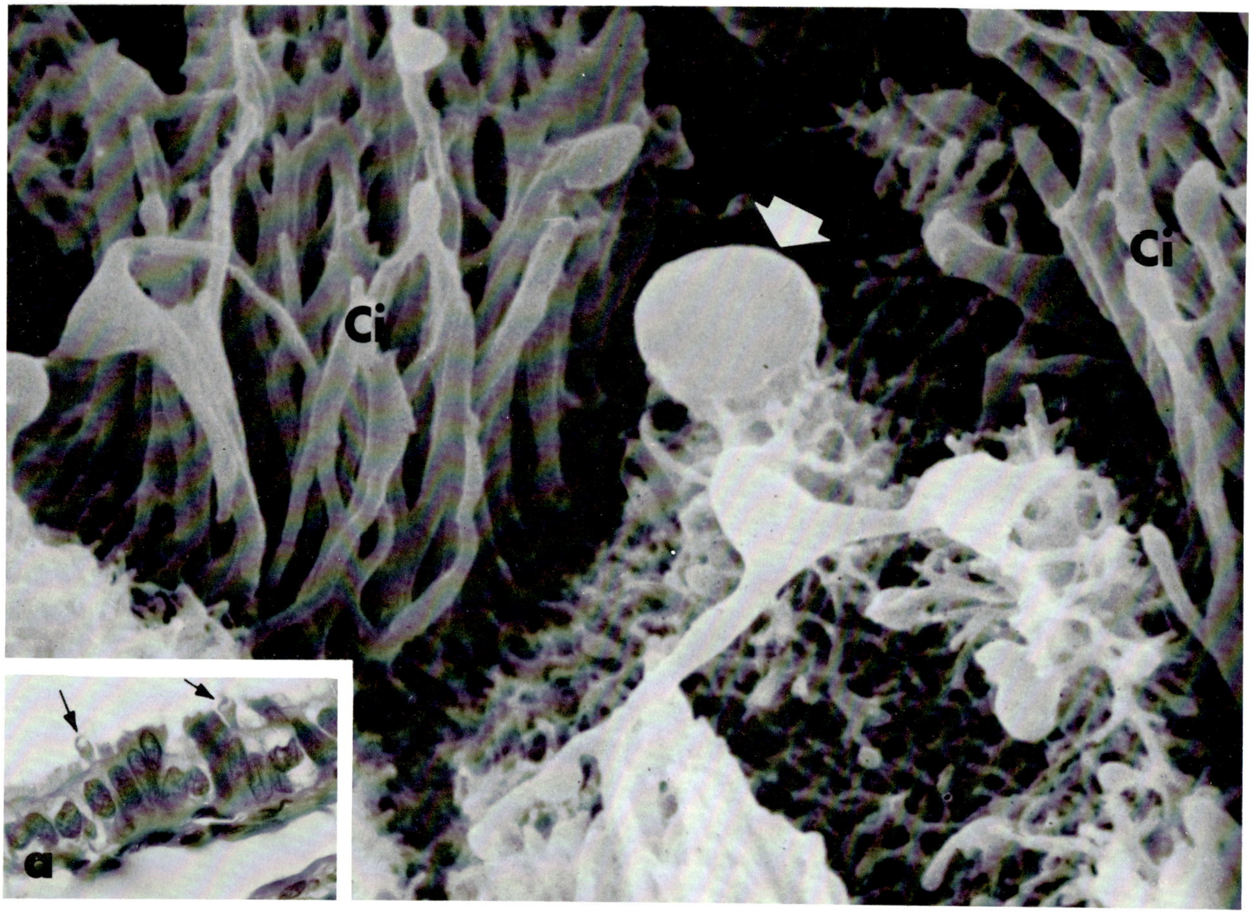

The Fallopian tube is of Müllerian origin and its epithelium is subject to cyclical variations, although its response is considerably less dramatic than that of the endometrial glandular epithelium. The cyclical morphological changes are seen principally in the secretory cells, in which the peak of secretory activity, with an increase in the Golgi, endoplasmic reticulum, and apical secretory vacuoles, occurs at about the time of ovulation,[1-9] suggesting that tubal secretion is under the influence of the ovarian steroid hormones. Tubal secretion is of the apocrine type, and secretory activity is evenly distributed in all segments of the human oviduct.[6] The secretory material, both in the cells and in the tubal lumen, is composed of alcian blue–periodic acid–Schiff-positive, diatase- and hyaluronidase-resistant acid mucopolysaccharides, electrolytes, and various enzymes,[8,10] providing an optimal environment for spermatozoa and ova.

Figure 171a. *Fallopian tube (fimbria). Late proliferative–early secretory phase (14–16th days) of the menstrual cycle.* Several secretory cells contain prominent apocrine cytoplasmic protrusions (arrows), whereas others with bulging, spindle-shaped nuclei have emptied most of their apical cytoplasmic substance, exhibiting secretory exhaustion. A dilated lymphatic vessel is seen beneath the lining epithelium. (H & E stain. × 150.)

Figure 171. *Fallopian tube (fimbria). Late proliferative–early secretory phase (14–16th days) of the menstrual cycle.* Scanning electron microscopy of a microvillous secretory cell in which apocrine secretory activity occurs by prominent apical, bulbous cytoplasmic protrusions (arrow). The neighboring cilia (Ci) are partly agglutinated by the secretory fluid. × 8000. *From* A. Ferenczy and R. M. Richart. Scanning electron microscopy of the human female genital tract. *N. Y. State J. Med.* (in press).

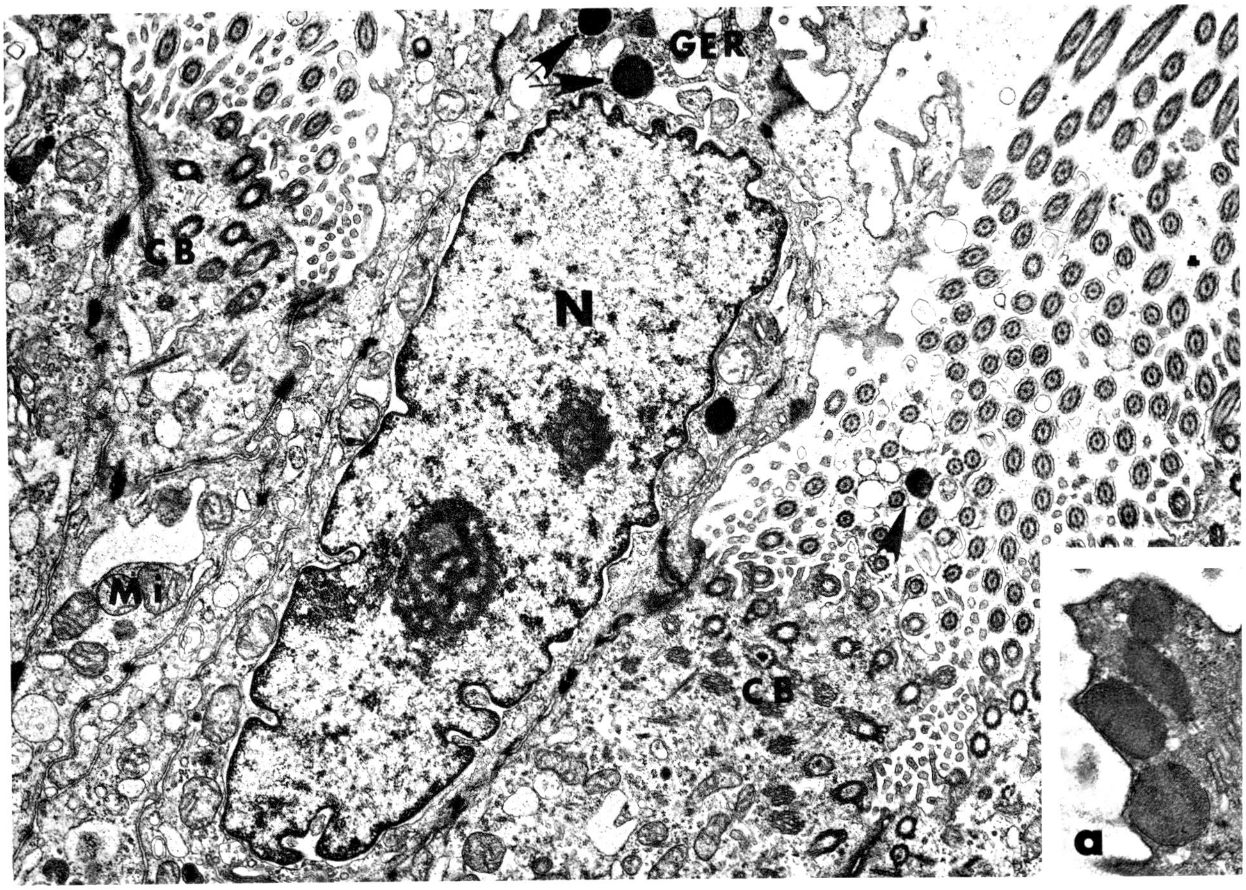

Figure 172. *Fallopian tube (fimbria). Late proliferative–early secretory phase (14–16th days) of the menstrual cycle.* At the transmission electron microscopic level, secretory cells engaged in apocrine secretion have protruding nuclei (N), as well as cytoplasmic apices, and are rich in dilated cisternae of granular endoplasmic reticulum (GER), free ribosomes, and membrane-bound, dense secretory granules (arrows). After the release of portions of cytoplam and its contents, clusters of organelles and secretory granules (arrow head) are found in the lumen, which will be incorporated into the tubal secretions. Both secretory and ciliated cells contain an increased quantity of dilated granular endoplasmic reticulum, mitochondria (Mi), polyribosomes, and Golgi, corresponding to maximum secretory activity. × 12,600. CB: cilial basal bodies.

Figure 172a. *Higher magnification* of membrane-bound secretory granules, located beneath the surface plasma membrane with finely granular, electron-dense content. × 23,060.

REFERENCES (The Fallopian tube–Figure 172a)

1. Fredricsson, B. and L. Bjorkman. Studies on the ultrastructure of the human oviduct epithelium in different functional states. *Z. Zellforsch.* ***58:*** 387 (1962).
2. Hashimoto, M., T. Shimoyama, M. Kosaka, A. Komori, T. Hirasawa, Y. Yokoyama, N. Kawase, and T. Nakamura. Electron microscopic studies on epithelial cells of the human Fallopian tube (II). *J. Jap. Obstet. Gynecol. Soc.* **11:** 92 (1964).
3. Clyman, M. J. Electron microscopy of the human Fallopian tube. *Fertil. Steril.* **17:** 281 (1966).
4. Overbeck, L. Ultrastructure of Fallopian tube epithelium during the menstrual cycle. *Z. Geburtsh. Gynaekol.* **171:** 241 (1969).
5. Overbeck, L. Ultrastructure of the Fallopian tube epithelium in the female menstrual cycle. *Arch. Gynaekol.* **207:** 165 (1969).
6. Ferenczy, A., R. M. Richart, F. J. Agate, Jr., M. L. Purkerson, and E. W. Dempsey. Scanning electron microscopy of the human Fallopian tube. *Science* **175:** 783 (1972).

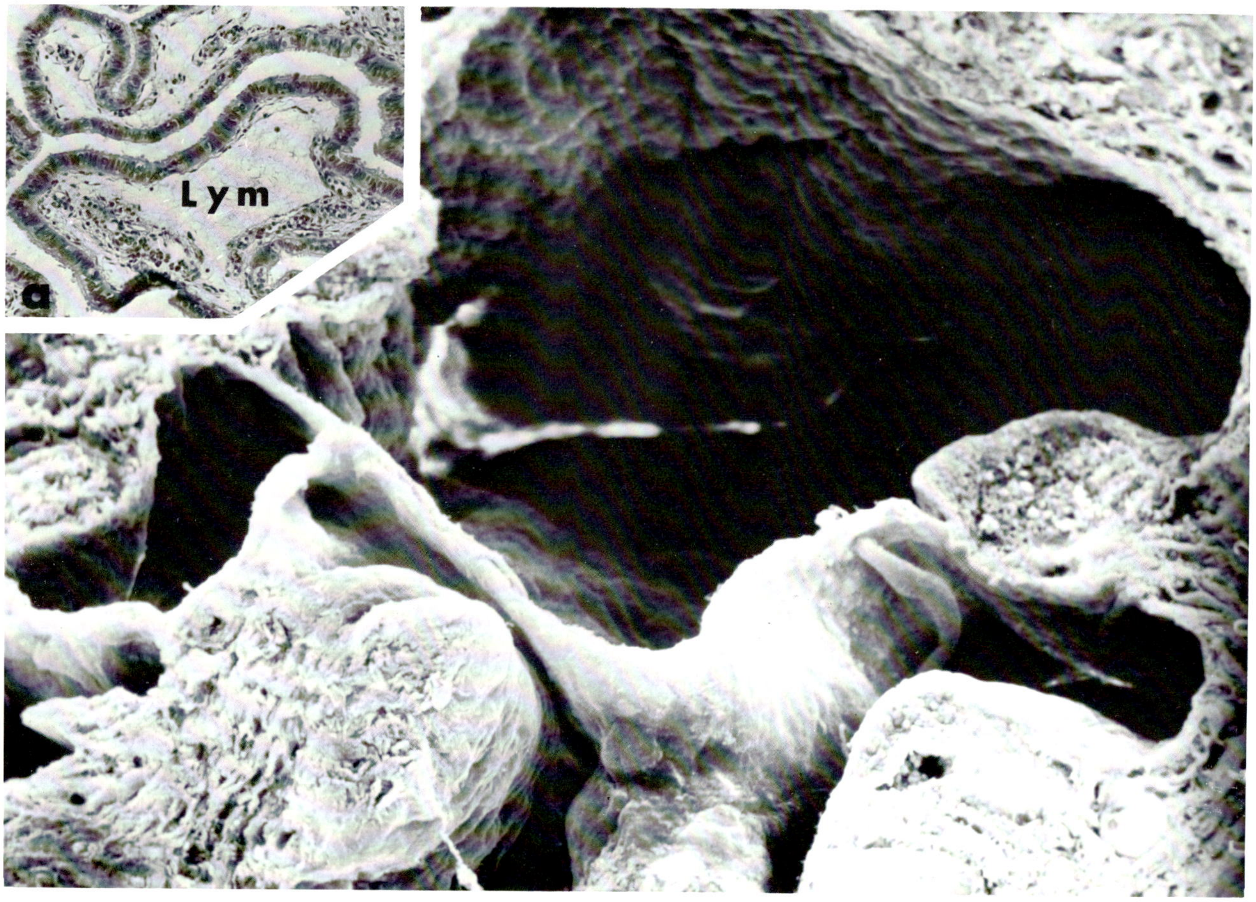

7. Patek, E., L. Nilsson, and E. Johanisson. Scanning electron microscopic study of the human Fallopian tube. Report I. The proliferative and secretory stages. *Fertil. Steril.* **23:** 459 (1972).
8. Lippes, J., R. G. Enders, D. A. Pragan, and W. R. Bartholomew. The collection and analysis of human Fallopian tubal fluid. *Contraception* **5:** 85 (1972).
9. Ludwig, H., H. Wolf, and H. Metzger. Scanning electron microscopy of the luminal surface in the human Fallopian tube. *Arch. Gynaekol.* **212:** 380 (1972).
10. Fredricsson, B. Histochemistry of the oviduct. In *The Mammalian Oviduct: Comparative Biology and Methodology,* E. C. E. Hafez and R. J. Blandau (Eds.). University of Chicago Press, Chicago, 1969, pp. 311–322.

Figure 173a. *Fallopian tube (fimbrial). During the ovulatory period* the lymphatic vessels (Lym) in the lamina propria of the fimbria become greatly distended by the rapid accumulation of lymph. The dilatation of the lymphatic vasculature in the fimbriated end is thought to contribute to the fimbrial "erection" in grasping the ovary as follicles rupture at the time of ovulation. (H & E stain, × 30.)

Figure 173. *Fallopian tube (fimbria).* Scanning electron microscopy of greatly dilated, labyrinthine lymphatic channels at the time of ovulation. × 200.

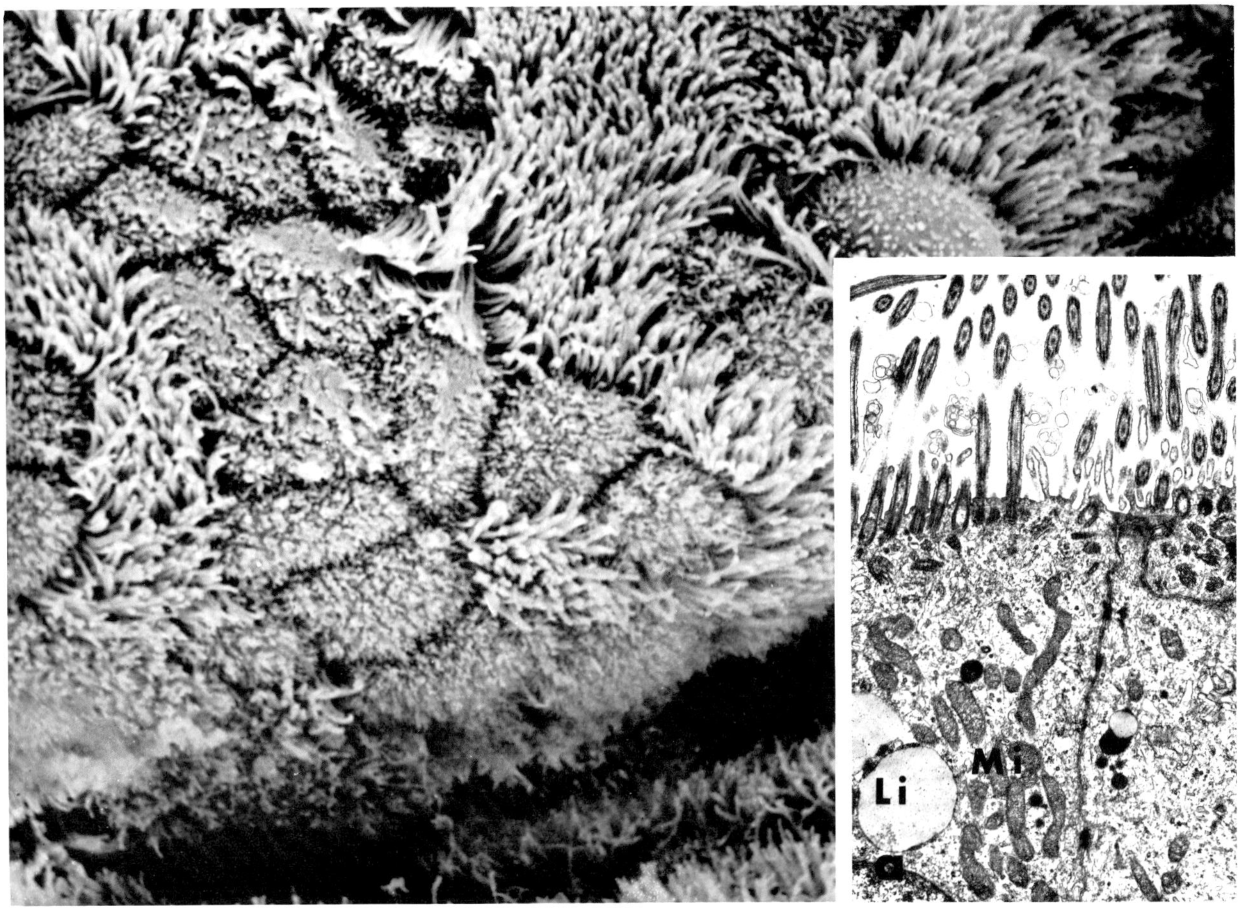

Figure 174. *Fallopian tube (ampulla). Mid-menstrual period (2nd–3rd days).* Unlike the endometrium, in the tubal epithelium no significant morphologic changes are observed, as indicated by the essentially similar ciliated–nonciliated cell ratio and distribution during the menstrual cycle. Note the presence of abundant and well-developed ciliary shafts arranged in large clusters in the summit of a tubal fold, interspersed with dome-shaped microvillous secretory cells. × 2720.

Figure 174a. *Fallopian tube (fimbria). Mid-menstrual period (2nd–3rd days).* Ciliated cells contain abundant mitochondria (Mi), associated with polyribosomes, membrane-bound dense bodies, and lipid droplets (Li). There is no evidence of cellular involution, and the tightly apposed lateral plasma membranes are reinforced by well-developed desmosomal belts. × 6400.

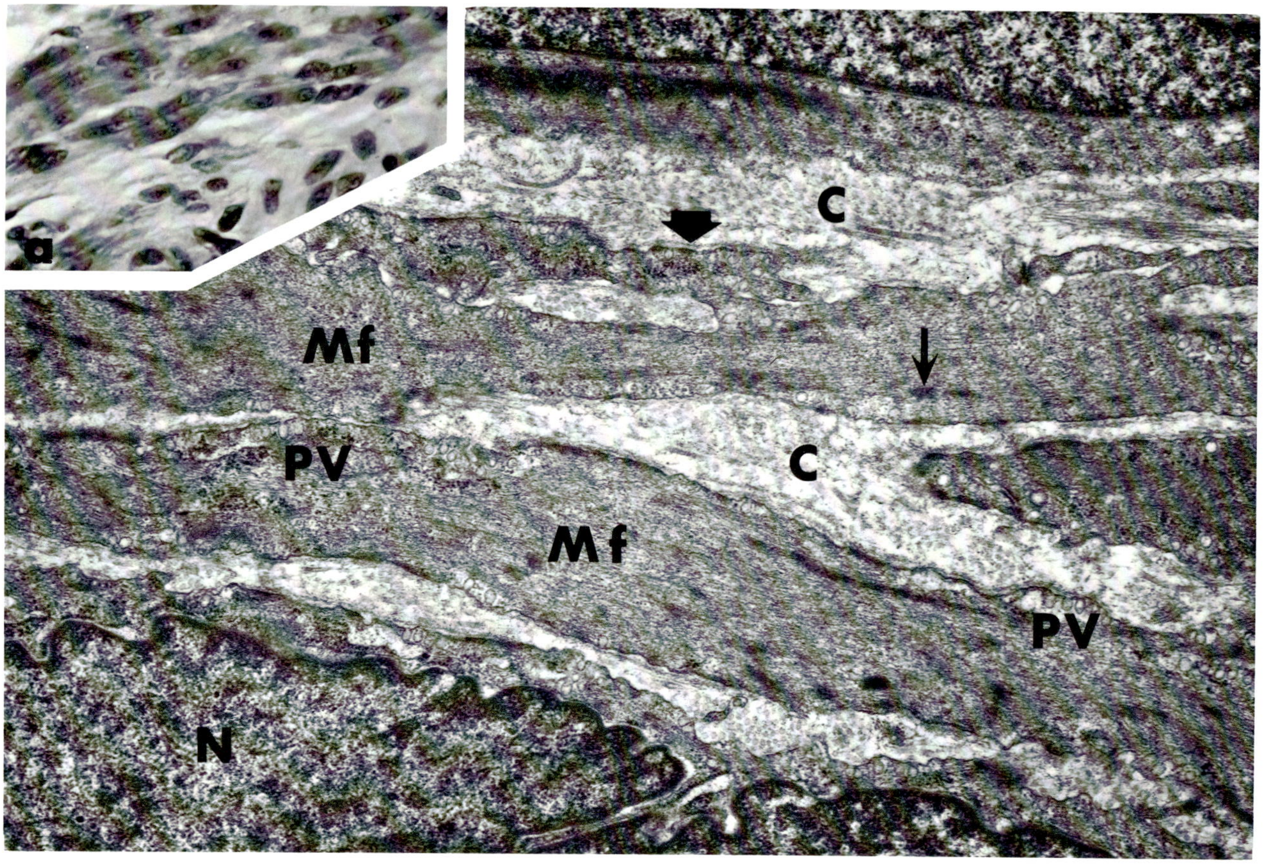

44
Myosalpinx

The tubal musculature[1] is composed of an inner longitudinal, a middle circular, and an outer longitudinal layer at the intramural and isthmic portions of the oviduct. The inner longitudinal layer becomes indistinct in the ampulla and fimbria and is continued as haphazardly arranged muscle bundles within the lamina propria of the tubal plicae. The tubal muscular wall contains two functional, rather than anatomical sphincters at both the uterotubal junction and the abdominal ostium, which, together with muscular contractions, are related to the mobilization and transport of sperm and ova.

Figure 175a. *Fallopian tube, myosalpinx (ampulla).* Histologically, the muscle coat (myosalpinx) of the oviducts is composed of spindle-shaped, smooth muscle cells arranged in bundles with cigar-shaped, blunt-ended nuclei and fusiform, finely fibrillar myoplasm. The narrow intercellular space contains collagen. (H & E stain, × 120.)

Figure 175. *Fallopian tube, myosalpinx (ampulla).* Ultrastructurally, as is typical of smooth muscle cells, the myoplasm is packed with threadlike myofilaments (Mf) with numerous spindle-shaped densities (long arrow). Organelles are sparse. The plasma membrane contains rows of micropinocytic vesicles (PV), which alternate with plasma membrane dense bodies. A well-developed, but often interrupted, basal lamina (short arrow) separates the smooth muscle cells from the stroma. The latter is rich in collagen (C) and tropocollagen fibrils (upper right corner). The close interrelationship between tropocollagen fibrils and plasma membranes suggests that smooth muscle cells are responsible at least in part for collagen synthesis. × 20,600. N: nucleus.

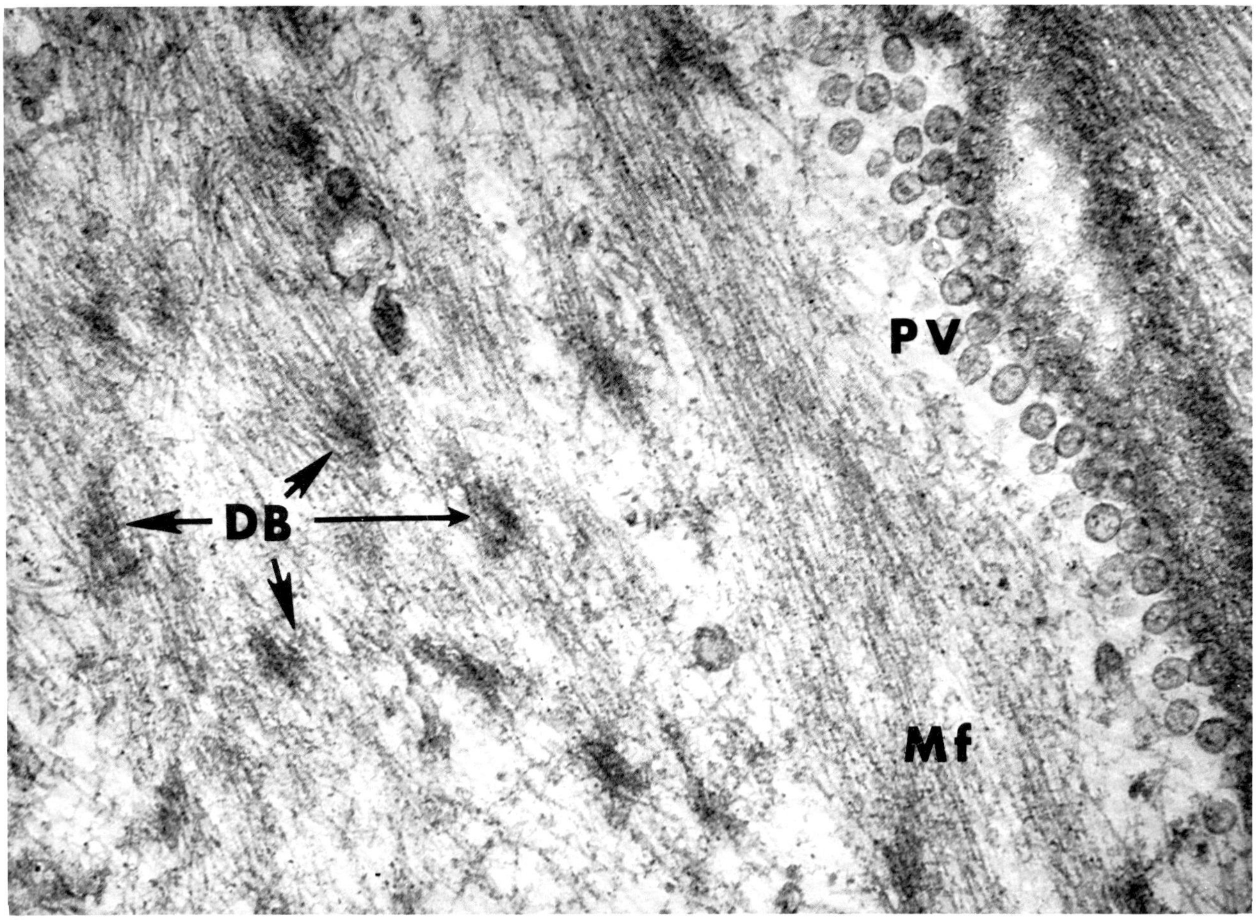

Figure 176. *Fallopian tube, myosalpinx (ampulla).* Cellular detail of tangentially sectioned, tubal, smooth muscle cells, in which myofilaments (Mf) approximately 60 to 80 Å thick run parallel to the plasma membrane. Spindle-shaped dense bodies (DB) represent focal condensation of thin actin filaments reinforced by 20-Å-thick collateral filaments, and are regarded with the plasma membrane dense bodies as attachment sites for myofilaments (see **Normal Myometrium**). Numerous pinocytic vesicles (PV) (60 mμ in diameter) are aligned along the plasma membrane. × 60,000.

REFERENCE (The tubal musculature–Figure 176)

1. Woodruff, J. D. and C. J. Pauerstein. Anatomy. In *The Fallopian Tube: Strutcure, Function, Pathology and Management.* Williams & Wilkins, Baltimore, 1969, pp. 22–45.

45

Fallopian Tube in Pregnancy

Distinct changes in cellular morphology and function are not seen during the first two-thirds of gestation,[1] but in the third trimester[2] the epithelium becomes lower. Ciliated cells decrease in number and become shorter in the postpartum period, when estrogen levels are comparatively low. Estrogen-dependent secretory activity is also depressed.

Figure 177a. *Fallopian tube (ampulla). Between the 10th and 12th weeks of gestation* the lining epithelium has morphologic characteristics essentially similar to those found in nongestational tubal epithelium, including active apocrine (arrows) secretion. (H & E stain, × 190.)

Figure 177. *Fallopian tube (ampulla). First trimester of pregnancy (10–12th weeks).* Clusters of nonciliated, microvillous, secretory cells are covered by numerous granules and droplets (arrows) of varying size, presumably secretory in nature. Similar secretory material is seen on the tips of the neighboring cilia. × 4800.

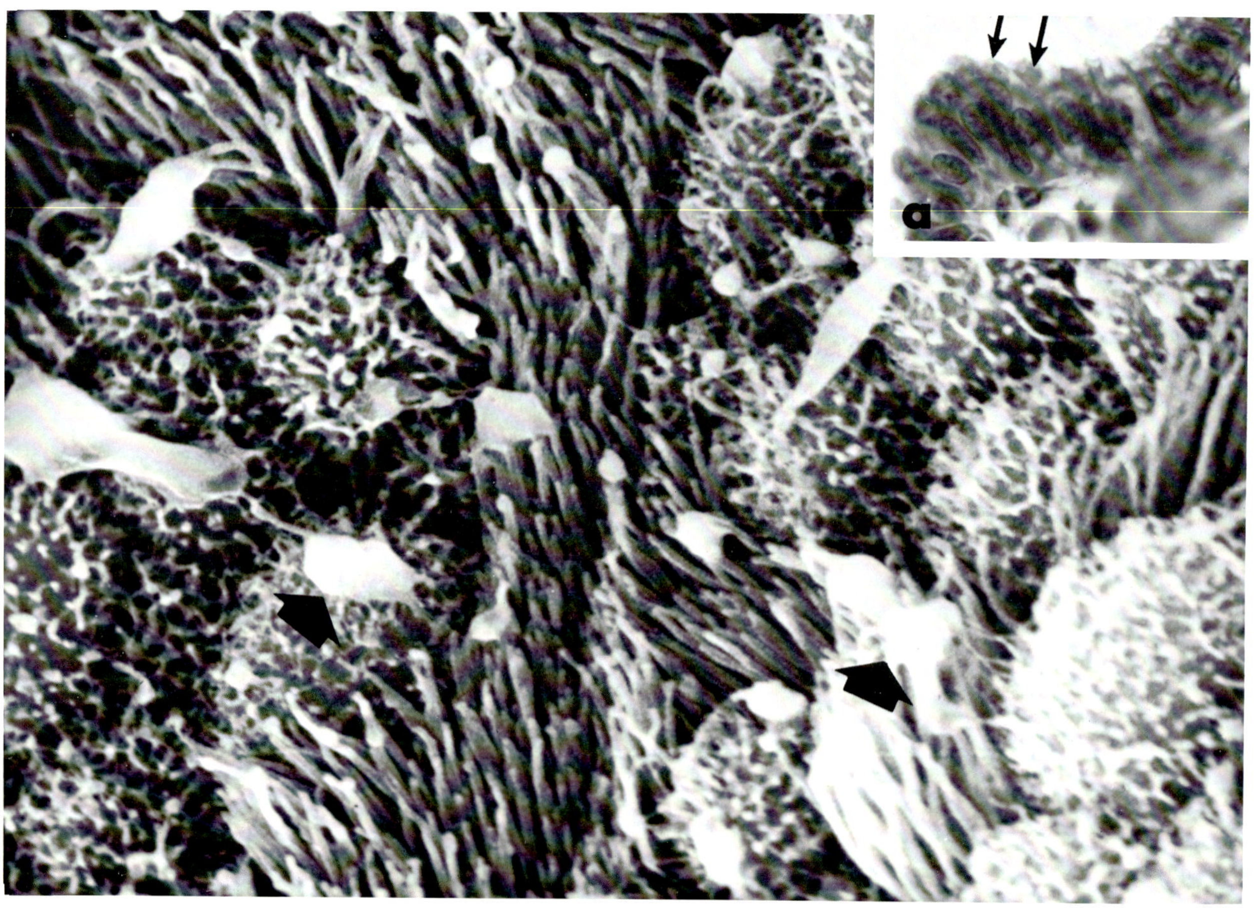

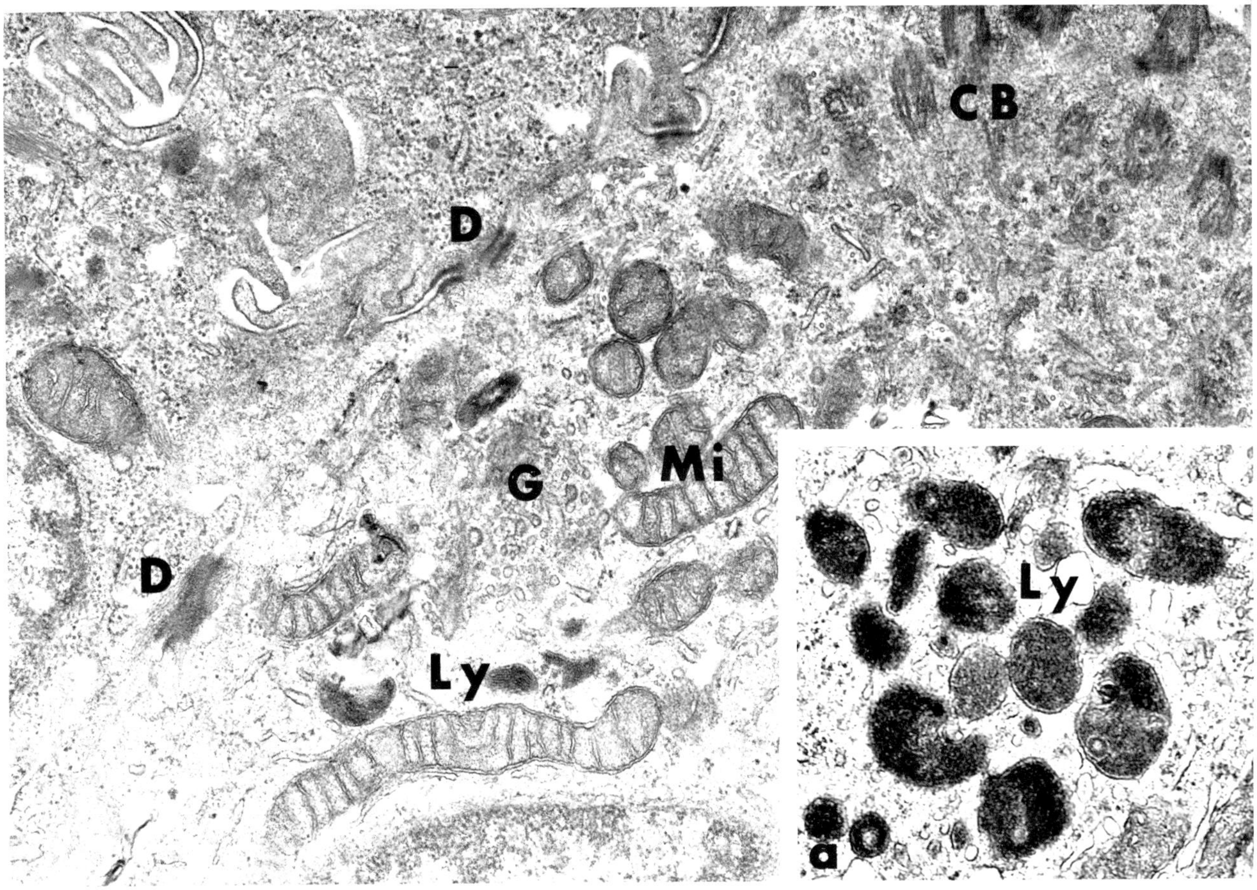

Figure 178. *Fallopian tube (isthmus). First trimester of pregnancy (10–12 weeks).* Electron micrograph of a ciliated cell with numerous cilial basal bodies (CB) and well-developed supranuclear Golgi (G) and mitochondria (Mi). Several dense lysosomes (Ly) with lamellated matrix are seen in the immediate vicinity of the Golgi. As is characteristic of ciliated cells, the apical portion is rich in cytoplasmic microtubules, tubular granular and agranular endoplasmic reticulum, polyribosomes, and multivesicular bodies. The adjacent secretory cell (left) has abundant free ribosomes and interdigitating microvillous cytoplasmic processes. × 6400. D: desmosomes.

Figure 178a. *Fallopian tube (isthmus). First trimester of pregnancy (10–12 weeks).* Cellular detail of a secretory cell containing clusters of membrane-bound lysosomes (Ly) with electron-dense amorphous and lamellated matrix and occasionally spherical inclusions: residual bodies (lower right). Most of these dense bodies are believed to contain secretory products generated from the Golgi zone. × 41,000.

REFERENCES (Distinct changes in cellular morphology–Figure 178a)

1. Fredricsson, B. and L. Bjorkman. Studies on the ultrastructure of the human oviduct epithelium in different functional states. *Z. Zellforsch.* **58:** 387 (1962).
2. Horbelt, D. V. Ultrastructural changes in Fallopian tube epithelium at term gestation and during postpartum period. *Texas J. Med.* **66:** 76 (1970).

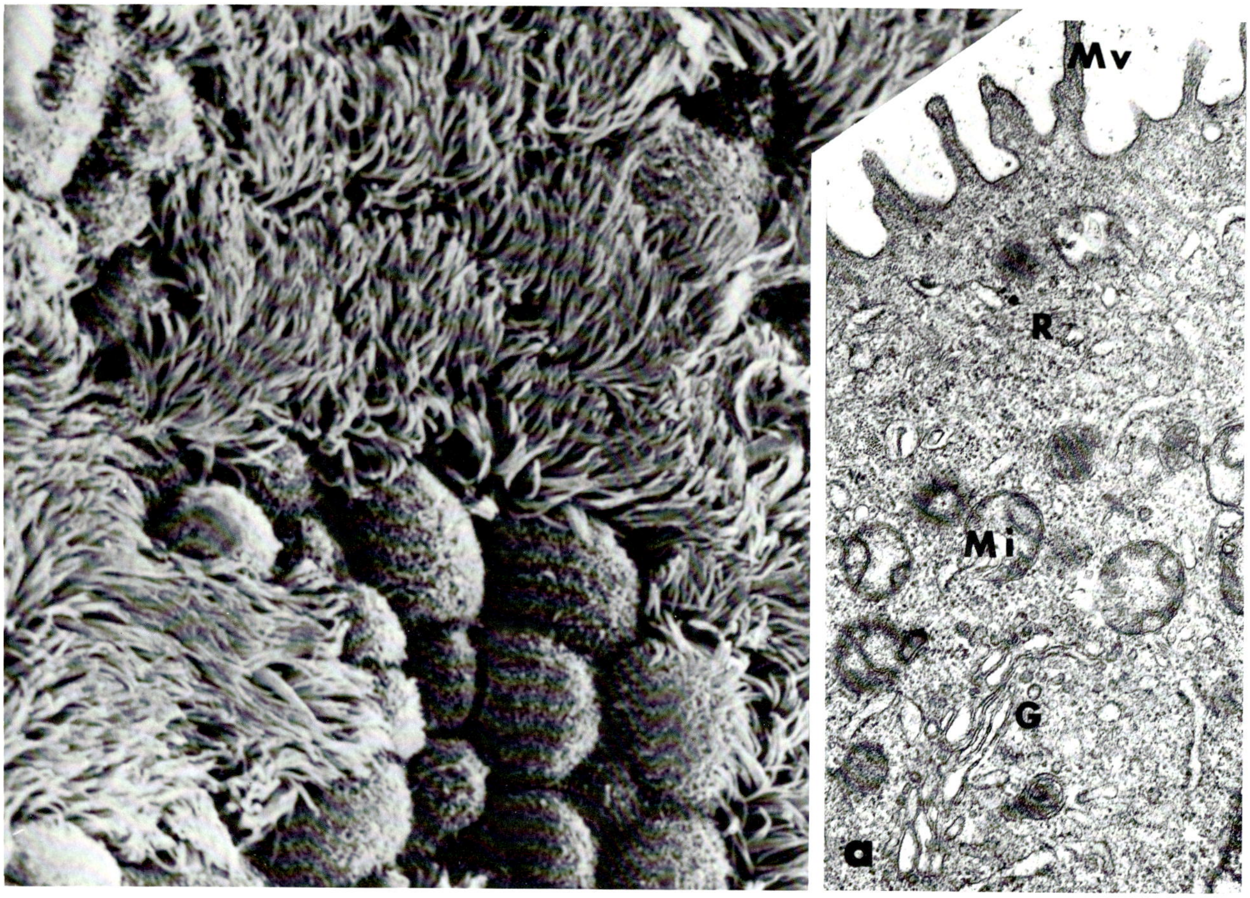

Figure 179. *Fallopian tube (ampulla)—full-term pregnancy.* Although the lining epithelium is reduced from tall columnar to cuboidal during the third trimester of gestation, ciliated cells remain numerous with well-developed ciliary shafts, and the adjacent secretory cells have prominent dome-shaped surface plasma membranes. The latter are uniformly devoid of secretory activity. × 1840.

Figure 179a. *Fallopian tube (ampulla)—full-term pregnancy.* Electron micrograph of a nonciliated microvillous (Mv) cell, in which the Golgi (G) are associated with peripheral vesicles, mitochondria (Mi), bound and free ribosomes (R), and occasional membrane-bound bodies. Despite this relatively well-developed cytoplasmic organization, apocrine secretion and accumulation of secretory granules are not observed. × 29,200.

REFERENCES (Figures 179–180c)

1. Hashimoto, M., T. Shimoyama, M. Kosaka, A. Komori, T. Hirasawa, Y. Yokoyama, N. Kawase, and T. Nakamura. Electron microscopic studies on epithelial cells of the human Fallopian tube (II). *J. Jap. Obstet. Gynecol. Soc.* **11:** 92 (1964).
2. Patek, E., L. Nilsson, and E. Johanisson. Scanning electron microscopic study of the human Fallopian tube. Report II. Fetal life, reproductive life and postmenopause. *Fertil. Steril.* **23:** 719 (1972).
3. Ferenczy, A., R. M. Richart, F. J. Agate, Jr., M. L. Purkerson, and E. W. Dempsey. Scanning electron microscopy of the human Fallopian tube. *Science* **175:** 783 (1972).
4. Anderson, R. G. W. and R. M. Brenner. The formation of basal bodies (centrioles) in the rhesus monkey oviduct. *J. Cell Biol.* **50:** 10 (1971).

46

Fallopian Tube in Menopause

Although the oviductal epithelium remains unaffected for a long period of time atfer the cessation of menstruation,[1,2] in the later postmenopausal period progressive deciliation occurs.[1-3] That this effect is principally hormonal rather than age related is supported by the marked loss of cilia in reproductive-aged oophorectomized monkeys.[4] The administration of exogenous estrogen stimulates cilioneogenesis in such animals, whereas exogenous progesterone inhibits it.[4] The disappearance of ciliated cells is accompanied by the gradual decrease and eventual arrest of the production of secretions in the secretory cells, which are also apparently under hormonal control.

Figure 180a. *Fallopian tube (fimbria).* In advanced menopause, epithelial atrophy is manifested by the presence of low columnar to low cuboidal epithelium, exhibiting a marked decrease in the cytoplasmic volume. Ciliated cells are absent. (H & E stain, × 120.)

Figure 180b. *Fallopian tube (fimbria).* With the scanning electron microscope the surface of atrophic tubal epithelium has a monotonous cobblestone appearance due to the presence of flat-surfaced cells covered by short and sparse microvilli. Apocrine secretory activity is uniformly absent. × 1600.

Figure 180c. *Fallopian tube (ampulla)—advanced menopause.* Scanning electron micrograph of a poorly developed ciliated cell (Ci) with few and short ciliary shafts. The surrounding cells have short and sparse microvillous (Mv) processes. × 8000.

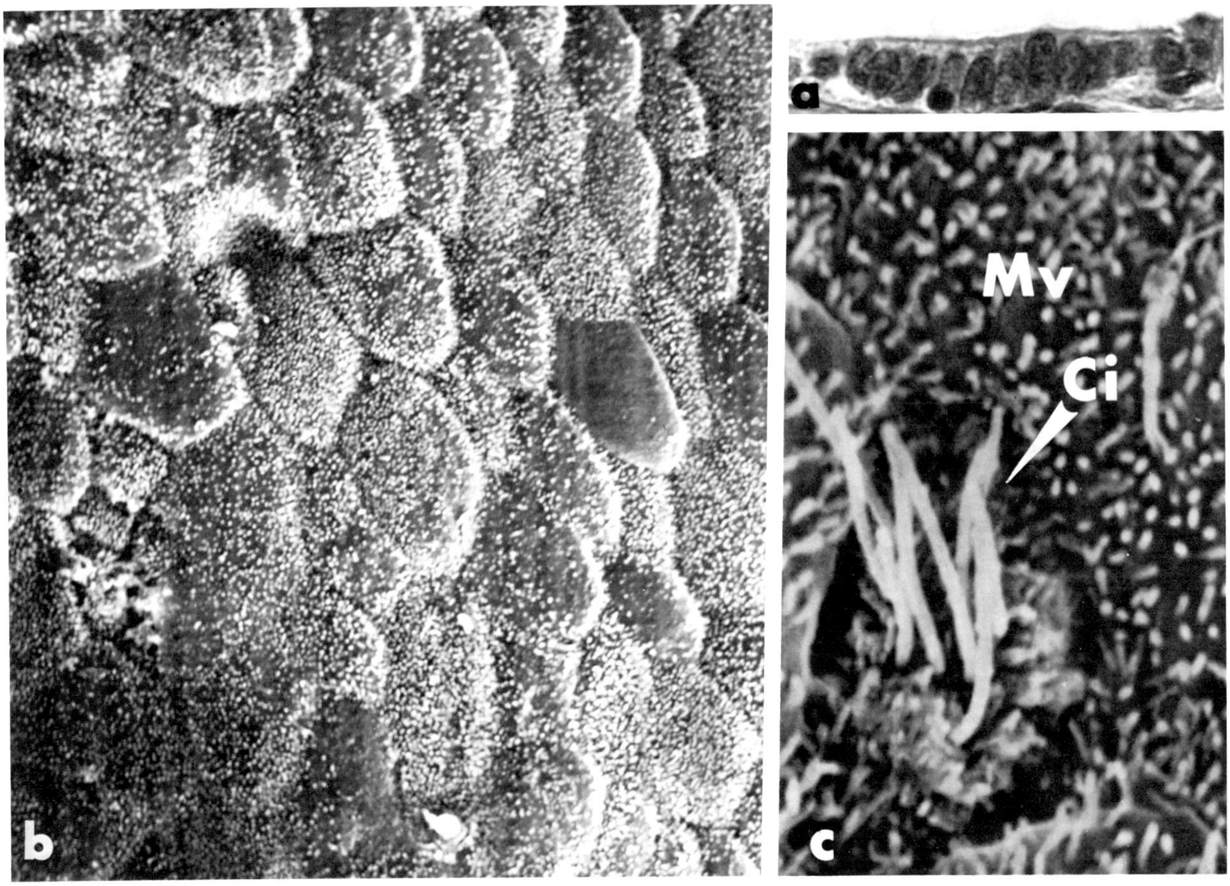

47

Fallopian Tube in Abnormal Hormonal States

HYPERESTROGENISM

Although the effect of prolonged or elevated levels of estrogens on the endometrium is well recognized (proliferative or hyperplastic endometrium), the tubal epithelium does not seem to be similarly affected.[1,2]

Figure 181. *Fallopian tube (ampulla).* At the ultrastructural level, secretory cells possess well-developed Golgi (G) and mitochondria (Mi) but electron-dense secretory granules are uniformly absent. Note the convoluted configuration of tightly apposed plasma membranes (PM), which are attached by numerous desmosomes and tight junctional complexes near the lumen. × 4400. Mv: luminal microvilli; N: nucleus: Li: lipid droplets.

Figure 181a. *Fallopian tube (fimbria).* Surface specializations, such as ciliary shafts (Ci) and microvillous processes (Mv), in hyperestrogenic conditions are unchanged from the normal. × 8000.

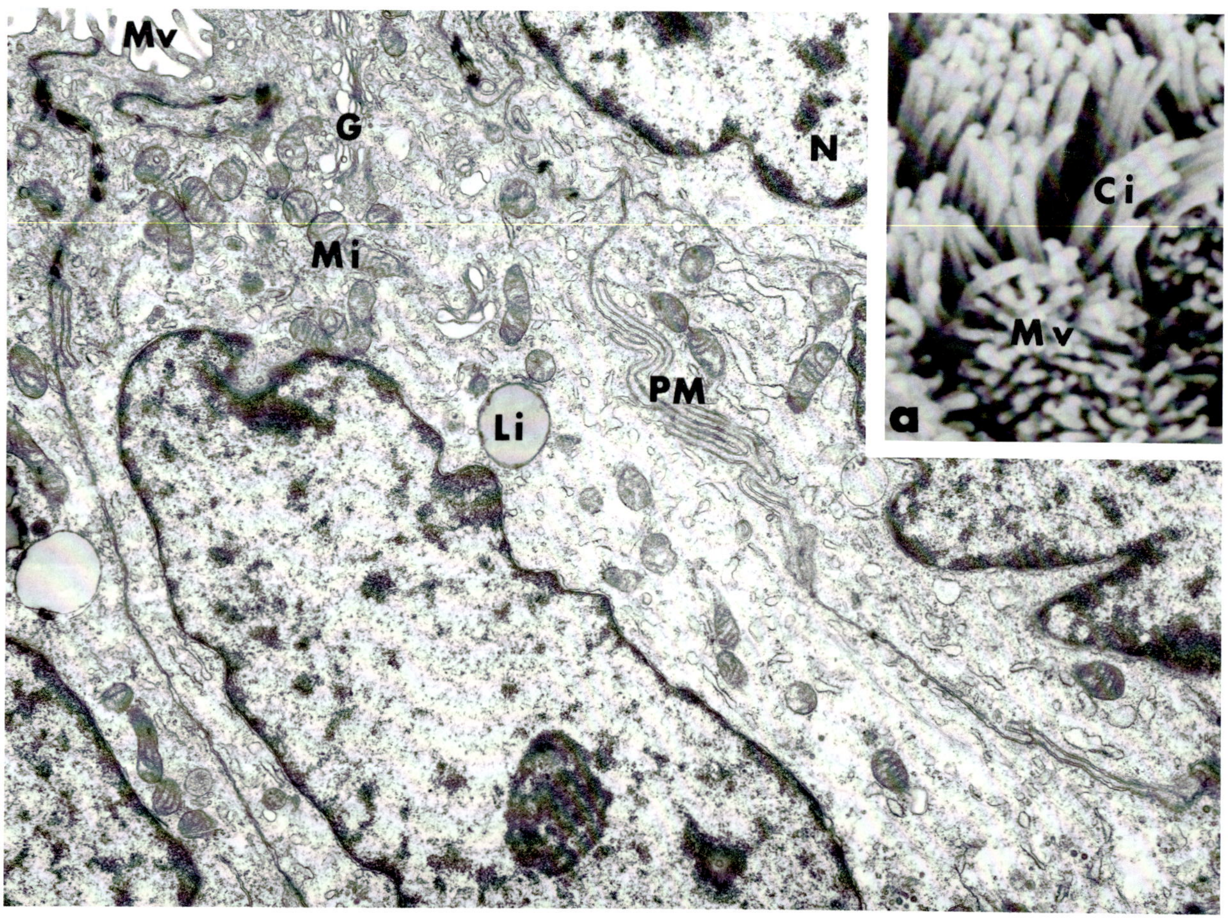

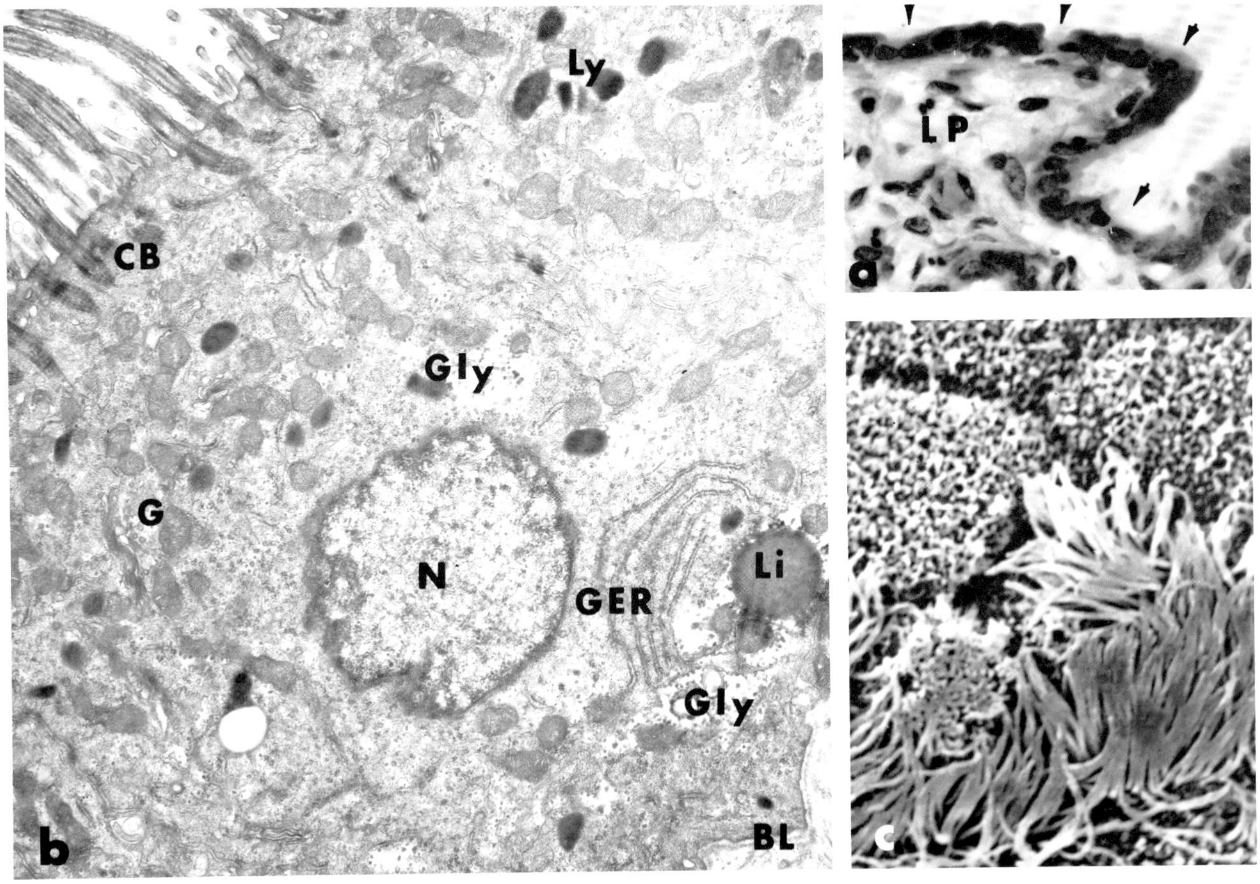

PROGESTERONE EFFECT

In patients using combination or sequential oral contraceptives or pure progestogen therapy the tubal mucosa remains essentially within the normal limits in regard to fine structural morphology and organization, as well as secretory activity and the formation of ciliary apparatuses.[2] The long-standing use of progestogens, however, results in a considerable decrease in the height of the tubal epithelium, a diminution in secretory activity, and a reduction in the number of cilia.[1] The overall pattern resembles that of the full-term pregnant or postpartum "resting" oviductal epithelium.

REFERENCES (Although the effect–Figure 182c)

1. Fredricsson, B. and N. Bjorkman. Morphologic alterations in the human oviduct epithelium induced by contraceptive steroids. *Fertil. Steril.* **24:** 19 (1973).
2. Patek, E., L. Nilsson, E. Johannisson, M. Hellema, and J. Bout. Scanning electron microscopic study of the human fallopian tube. Report III. The effect of midpregnancy and of various steroids. *Fertil. Steril.* **24:** 31 (1973).

Figure 182a. *Fallopian tube (ampulla).* Histologically, the tubal lining epithelium associated with long-standing use of progestogens (Depo-Provera® or medroxyprogesterone acetate) appears to be low cuboidal with few ciliated cells arrows). (H & E stain, × 120.)

Figure 182b. *Fallopian tube (fimbria).* At the ultrastructural level, the only significant, detectable cellular alterations that accompany the exogenous progestogenic state are accumulations of aggregates of glycogen particles (Gly), cytoplasmic free ribosomes, and parallel membranes of granular endoplasmic reticulum (GER) in both secretory and ciliated cells.[1] These changes are especially pronounced in cases in which high doses of progestogens are administered during a relatively short period of time. × 6000. CB: cilial basal bodies; Ly: lysosomes; G: Golgi; BL: basal lamina; N: nucleus of ciliated cell; Li: lipid droplets.

Figure 182c. *Fallopian tube (ampulla).* Scanning electron microscopic appearance of ciliated and nonciliated cells. The latter are covered by abundant short microvilli. × 7000.

48

Fallopian Tube in Inflammatory Conditions

Salpingitis may be acute, subacute, or chronic and may be primarily interstitial or primarily mucosal. The interstitial type is more commonly found postpartum or postabortal and is associated with streptococci, pneumococci, or other common pathogens. Mucosal salpingitis may be found at any time and is most commonly due to *Neisseria gonorrhea.*

ACUTE SALPINGITIS

Figure 183a. *Fallopian tube (ampulla)—acute salpingitis.* In the early phases of acute salpingitis there are an abundance of polymorphonuclear cells (P) in the lamina propria and a predominantly lymphocytic (L) permeation of the tubal epithelium and muscularis. Ciliated cells (Ci) remain intact. (H & E stain, × 120.)

Figure 183. *Fallopian tube (ampulla)—acute salpingitis.* The epithelium that is not degenerating has a normal ultrastructural appearance, including the distribution, number, and height of secretory and ciliated cells. × 3200.

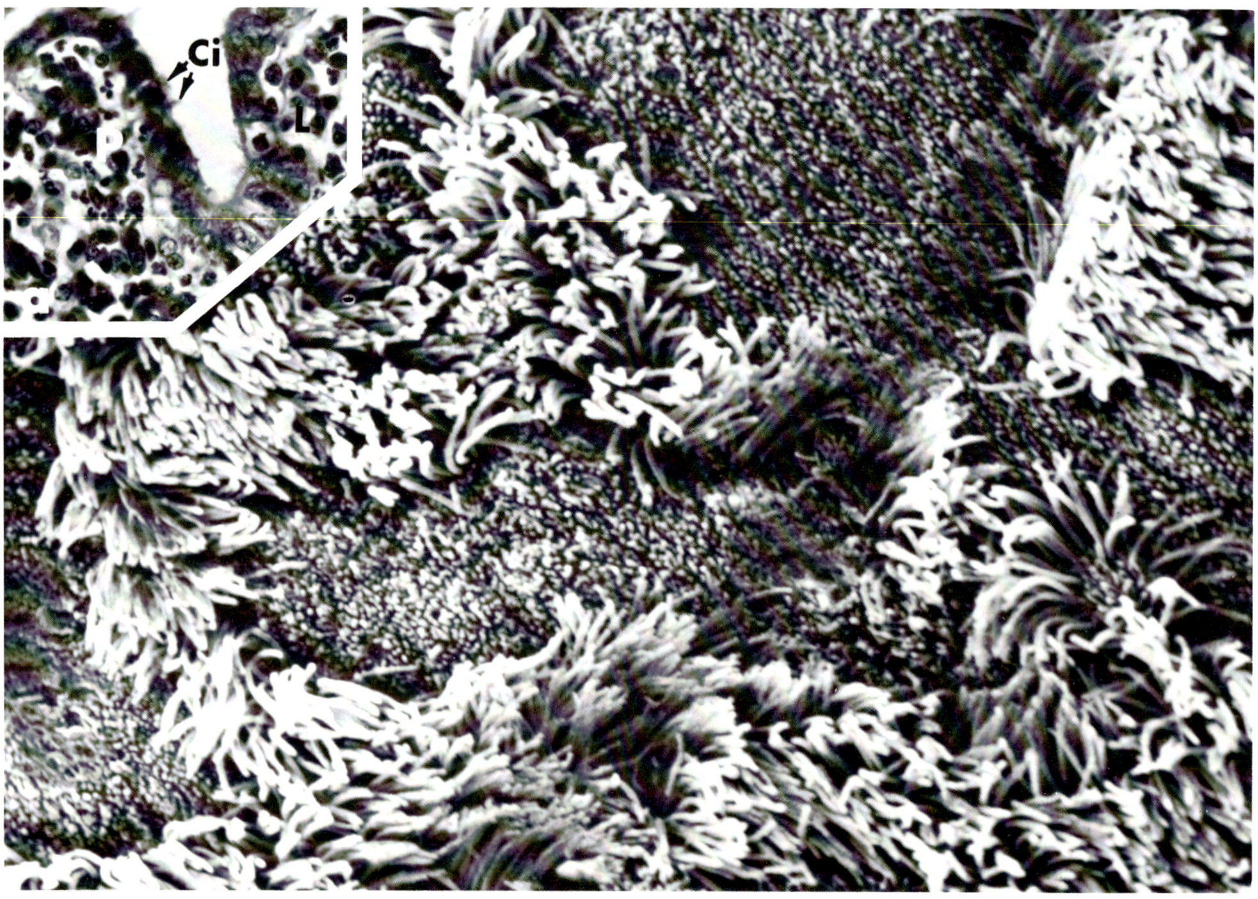

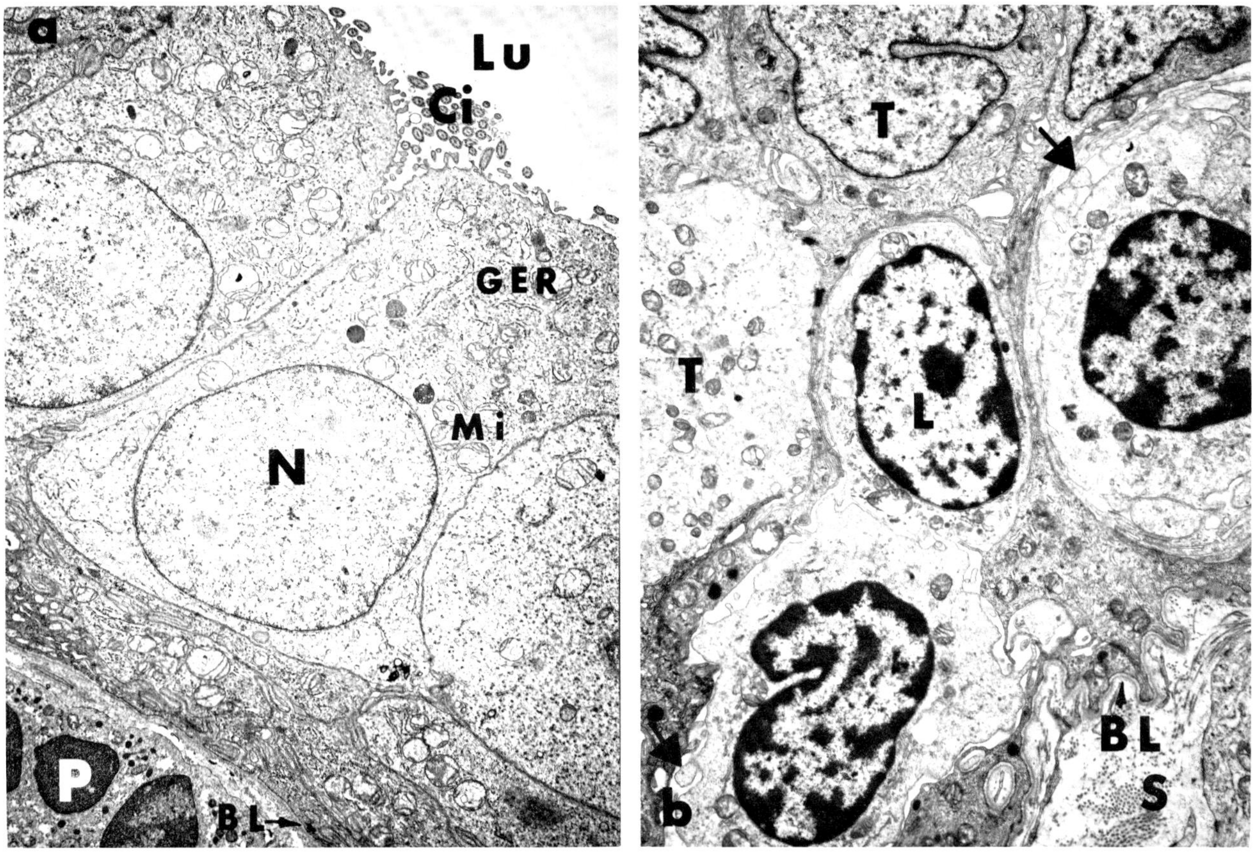

Figure 184a. *Fallopian tube (isthmus)—acute salpingitis.* Initially collections of polymorphonuclear cells (P) accumulate beneath the epithelial basal lamina (BL). The lining cells have abundant organelles throughout the cytoplasmic substance. Mitochondria (Mi) appear enlarged with disrupted cristate, but there is no evidence of intracellular degeneration. × 3360. N: nucleus; GER: granular endoplasmic reticulum; Ci: tangentially sectioned ciliary shafts; Lu: tubal lumen.

Figure 184b. *Fallopian tube (fimbria)—subacute salpingitis.* Ultrastructurally, there are phagocytic leukocytes which contain large intracytoplasmic phagosomes or phagocytic vacuoles. The morphological features of the transepithelial passage of leukocytes (L) are similar to those of vascular leukodiapedesis except for a reversed migratory direction. Clusters of mature lymphocytes (L) with prominent pseudopods (arrows) occupy the intercellular space. The adjacent tubal epithelial cells (T) are compressed or degenerated (lower left corner). The epithelial basal lamina (BL) appears intact. Although the significance of inflammation-associated intraepithelial lymphocytes is still obscure, the available data suggest an immunologic defense mechanism, probably related to delayed sensitivity to foreign proteins, rather than to the formation of circulating antibodies.[1] In the later phases of salpingitis there is progressive dilatation of the mitochondria and endoplasmic reticulum, as well of the intercellular spaces, and the epithelium undergoes segmental degeneration involving fields of one to four lining cells. The degeneration is especially pronounced in the areas of intraepithelial and subepithelial leukocytic infiltration. × 3000. S: collagenous stroma.

REFERENCE (Figures 183a–184b)

1. Dustin, P. L'inflammation et les phénomènes de défense. I. Réaction inflammatoire élémentaire. In *Leçons d'Anatomie Pathologique Générale,* P. Dustin (Ed.). Presses Académiques Européennes, Brussels, Belgium, 1966, pp. 293–341.

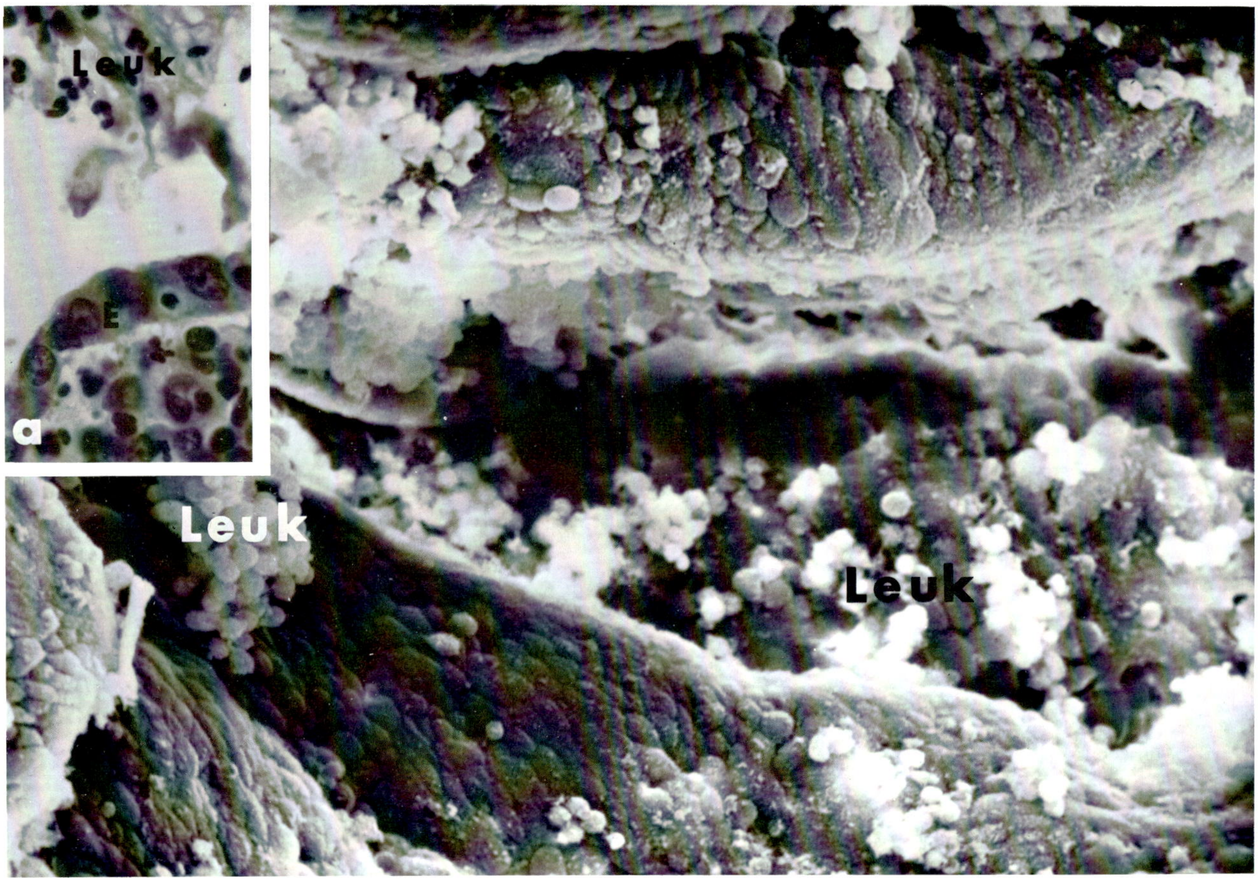

CHRONIC SALPINGITIS

When the acute phase of salpingitis has subsided, interplical and fimbrioovarian adhesions may occur, resulting in *pyosalpinx, follicular salpingitis,* and *hydrosalpinx.*

REFERENCE (Figures 185a–186b)

1. Ferenczy, A. and R. M. Richart. Scanning electron microscopy of the human female genital tract. *N.Y. State J. Med.* (in press).

Figure 185a. *Fallopian tube (ampulla).* In *pyosalpinx* the tubal lumen, as well as the lamina propria of enlarged tubal plicae, is filled with a collection of acute and chronic inflammatory exudate (Leuk). The lining epithelium (E) is low to columnar or cuboidal and often contains focal degeneration with dissolution of the basal lamina. (H & E stain, × 190.)

Figure 185. *Fallopian tube (ampulla). Pyosalpinx.* Topographically, large fields are devoid of ciliated cells, and there is a massive leukocytic exudate (Leuk) in the lumen. The focal ciliary loss appears to be directly related to the presence and extent of the inflammatory exudate,[1] suggesting that acute inflammation may lead to direct destruction of ciliary shafts or may cause profound alterations in the response of ciliated cells to hormonal stimuli, which result in the indirect inhibition of active ciliary regeneration.[1] This decrease in ciliated cells and the segmental epithelial degeneration may be the mechanisms through which the interplical adhesions are produced and may be of critical importance in the production of the late sequella of acute salpingitis (follicular salpingitis).[1] × 320.

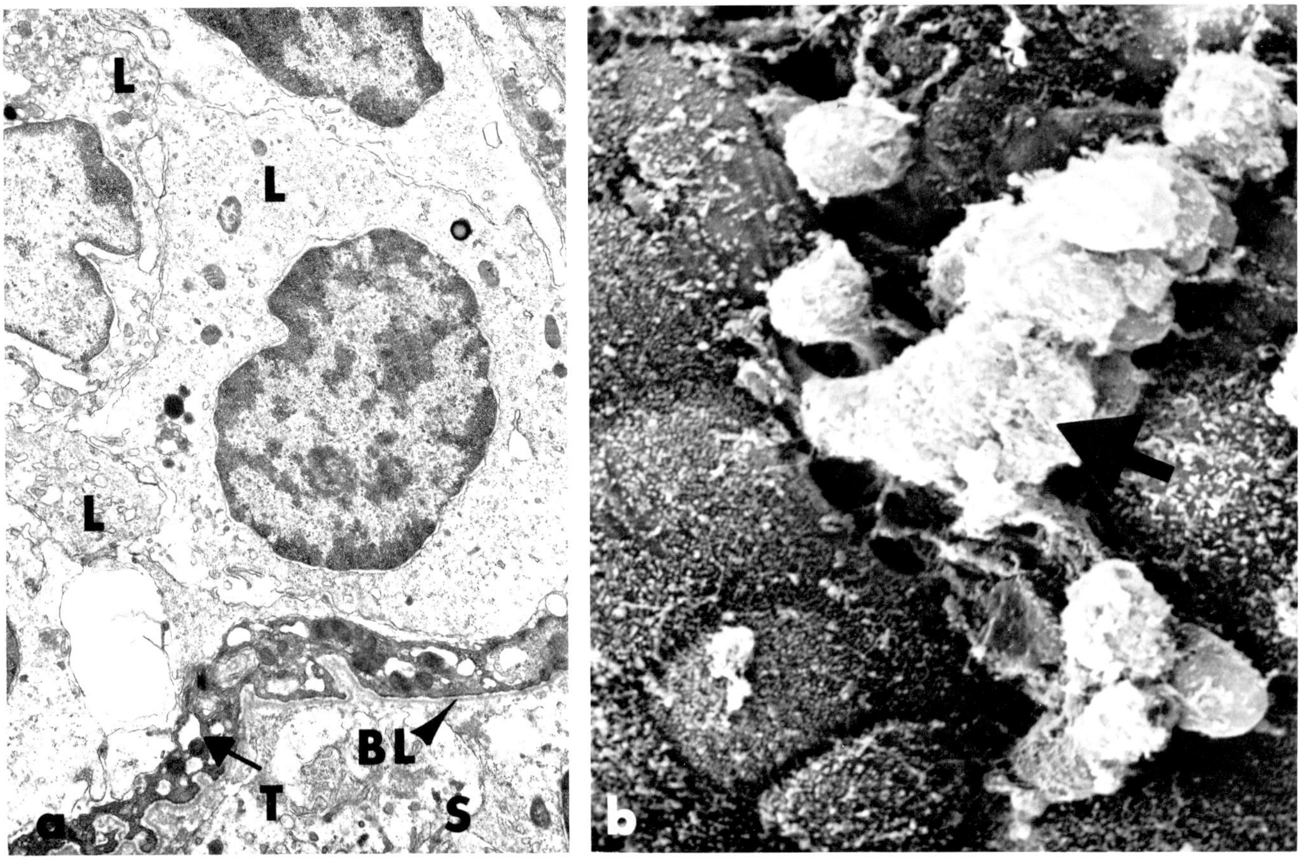

Figure 186a. *Fallopian tube (ampulla). Pyosalpinx.* Ultrastructurally, there is a massive lymphocytic (L) permeation of the lining epithelium. Epithelial degenerative (T) changes are more conspicuous than in the acute phase, and there is a segmental collapse of the lining epithelium. Focal disruption of the basal lamina in degenerated regions is often encountered. The lymphatic vessels in the lamina propria are dilated, and inflammatory cells, extravasated red blood cells, and fibroblasts are seen in the loose, edematous, connective tissue stroma. Although numerous plasma cells may be found intermingled with other types of inflammatory cells in the lamina propria, plasma cells have not been identified within the tubal epithelium. × 5600. BL: epithelial basal lamina; S: stroma of lamina propria.

Figure 186b. *Fallopian tube (ampulla). Pyosalpinx.* The tubal lining cells adjacent to clusters of adherent leukocytes (arrow) appear intact, but, characteristically, the surface microvilli are short and cilia are absent. × 1600. *From* A. Ferenczy and R. M. Richart. Scanning electron microscopy of the human female genital tract. *N. Y. State J. Med.* (in press).

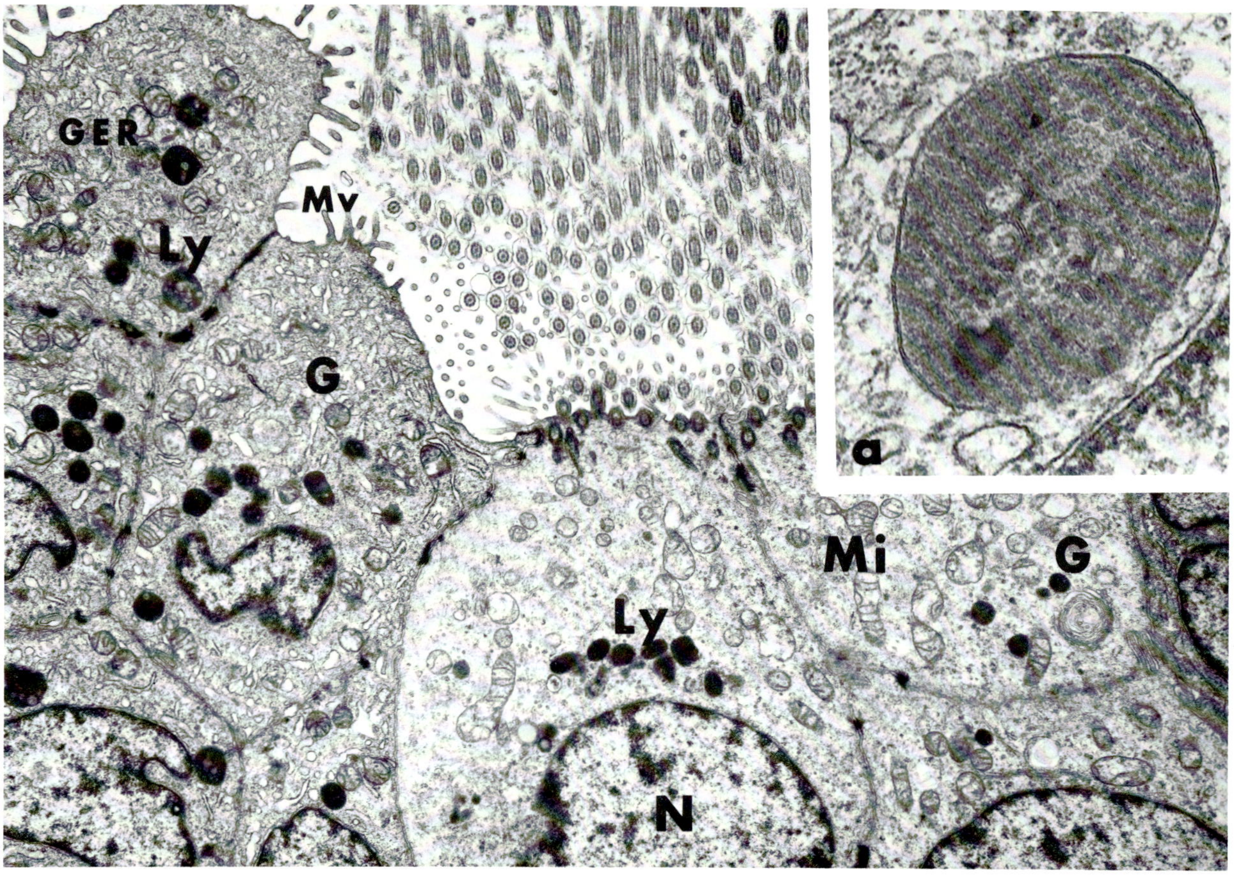

Figure 187. *Fallopian tube (fimbria). Pyosalpinx.* In the epithelial regions adjacent to degenerating cells there is a comparative increase in cytoplasmic free ribosomes, granular endoplasmic reticulum (GER), and Golgi (G), suggesting an accentuated metabolic activity, probably related to the inflammation and regeneration. Numerous intraepithelial lysosomes (Ly), cytolysosomes, and lipid droplets are seen in both the ciliated and nonciliated secretory cells. × 6800. Mi: mitochondria; Mv: luminal microvilli; N: nucleus.

Figure 187a. *High magnification* of an autophagic cytolysosome containing angular arrays of polyhedral membranes representing partially digested cytoplasmic material. × 74,200.

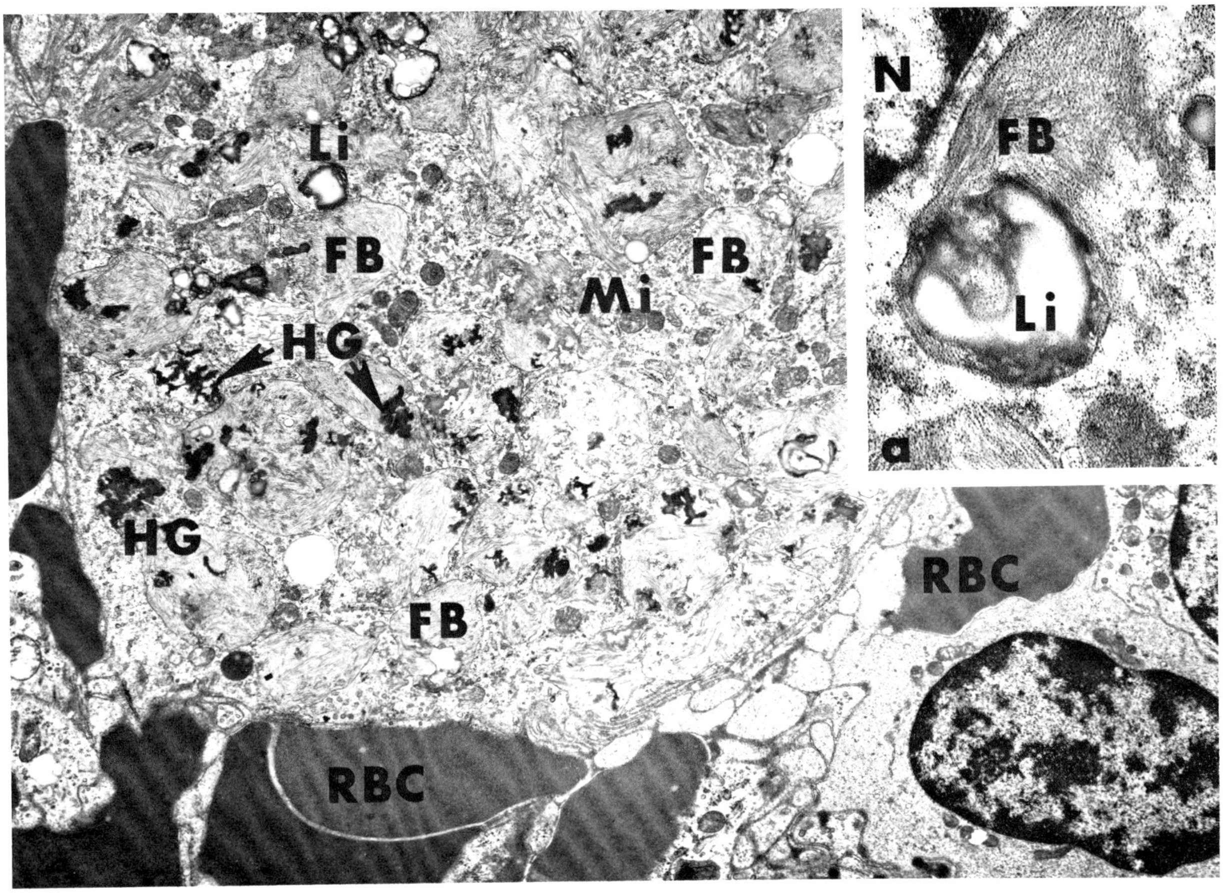

Figure 188. *Fallopian tube (ampulla). Pyosalpinx.* Electron micrograph of a siderophage in response to red blood cell extravasation into the lamina propria of inflamed tubal plicae. A siderophage is a macrophage in which the cytoplasm is packed with membrane-bound fibrillar bodies (FB) of varying size and engulfed electron-dense hemosiderin granules (HG). Note that numerous extravasted red blood cells (RBC) are in tight apposition with the convoluted plasma membrane of the siderophage. × 5600. Mi: mitochondria; Li: lipid droplet.

Figure 188a. *Detail of a perinuclear (N) fibrillar body (FB) with a lipid (Li) inclusion.* × 35,000.

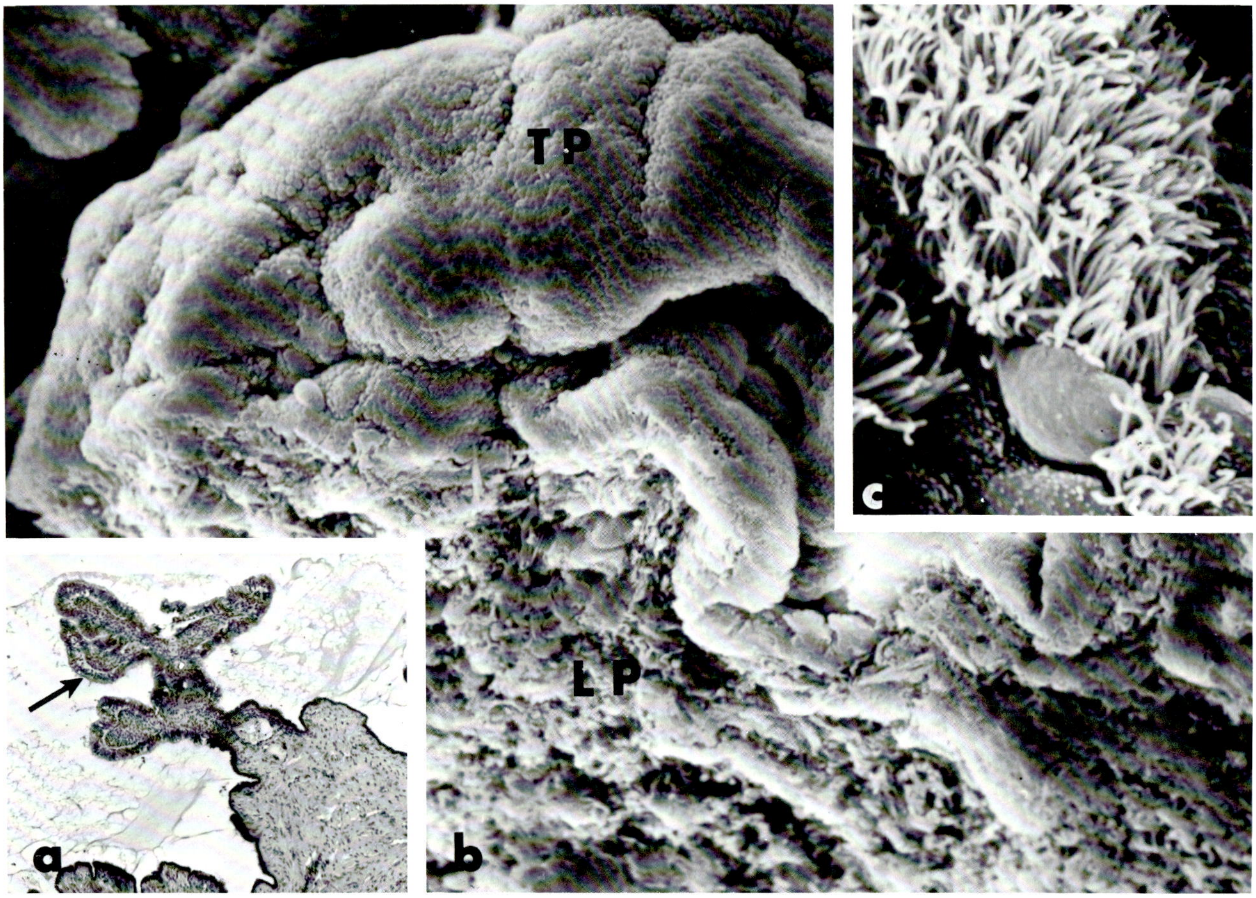

Figure 189a. *Fallopian tube (ampulla).* In *hydrosalpinx* (simplex), there is a striking decrease and atrophy of the tubal plicae, on which the covering epithelium, including the cilia, is characteristically well preserved (arrow). The epithelium directly lining the thin fibromuscular wall is generally compressed and has a low cuboidal to flattened mesothelial configuration. (H & E stain, × 30.)

Figure 189b. *Fallopian tube (ampulla). Hydrosalpinx.* Scanning electron micrograph of a club-shaped tubal fold (TP), covered by a well-preserved cellular population and supported by a fibrovascular lamina propria (LP). × 160.

Figure 189c. *Cellular detail of Figure 189b,* illustrating the normal cell surface characteristics, including the preservation of the ciliated–nonciliated cell ratio. Note the well-developed and tightly packed ciliary shafts. × 2400.

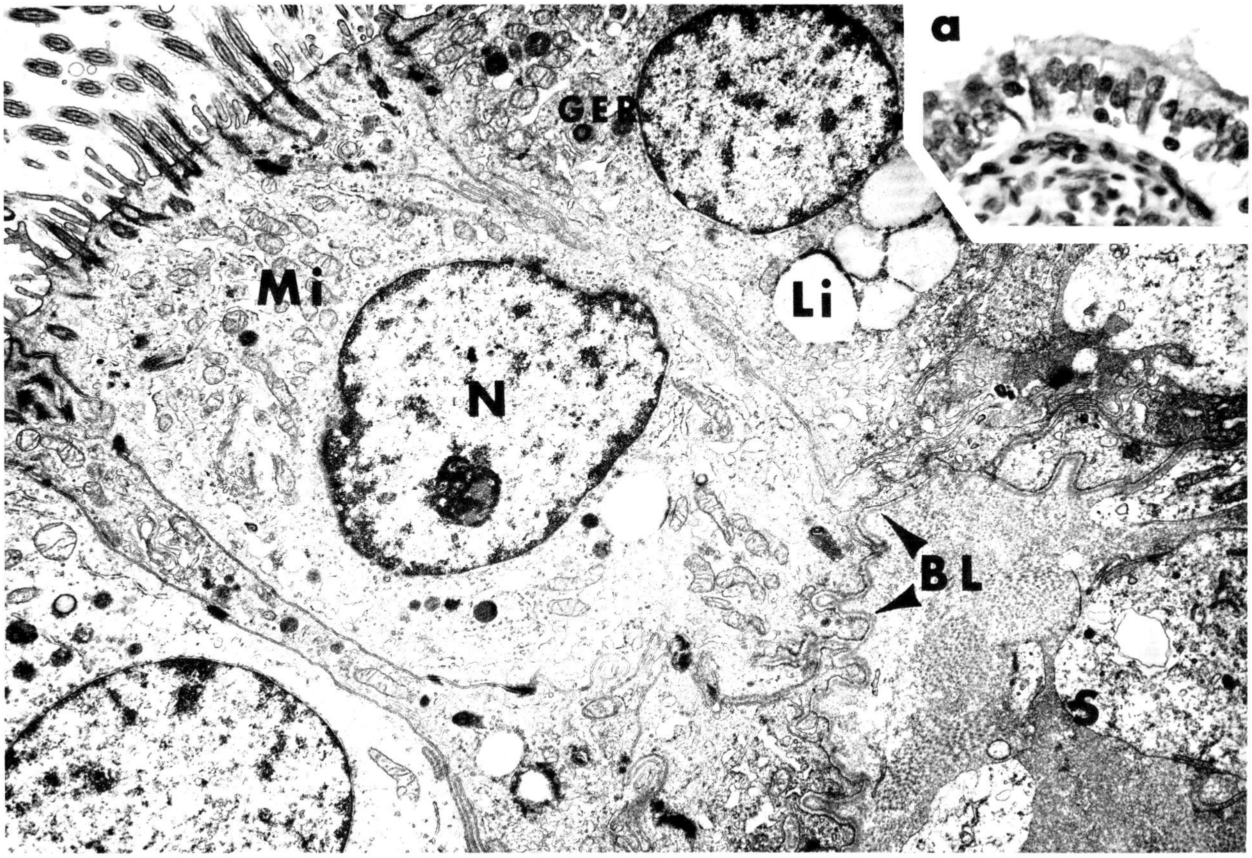

Figure 190a. *Fallopian tube (ampulla). Hydrosalpinx.* High-power micrograph of Figure 189a, in which the protruding tubal fold is covered by an intact tall columnar epithelium with abundant ciliated cells. (H & E stain, × 78.)

Figure 190. *Fallopian tube (ampulla). Hydrosalpinx.* Ultrastructurally, the epithelium lining the mucosal plicae has subcellular characteristics similar to those of normal tubal epithelium, including abundant mitochondria (Mi), granular endoplasmic reticulum (GER), and free ribosomes. Lipid droplets (Li) and electron-dense lysosomes tend to accumulate in the microvillous secretory cells. × 5600. N: nucleus; BL: epithelial basal lamina; S: collagenous stroma of lamina propria.

49

Adenocarcinoma

Primary adenocarcinoma of the human oviduct is one of the least common neoplasms of the female genital tract, accounting for less than 1% of all gynecologic malignancies. These lesions range in histologic appearance from neoplasms that are well differentiated and papillary to those that have a poorly differentiated or undifferentiated solid or trabecular pattern, closely resembling that of ovarian serous cystadenocarcinoma. This resemblance between tubal and ovarian serous neoplasms is apparent by both scanning and transmission electron microscopy, and it is possible to identify ciliated and nonciliated tubal-type cells, as well as a small population of endocervical- and endometrial-like cells. The last two cell types, however, cannot be identified in poorly differentiated carcinomas.

Characteristically, in both tubal and ovarian serous adenocarcinomas, there are large numbers of ciliated cells in well-differentiated lesions, fewer in less differentiated ones, and a complete disappearance in undifferentiated neoplasms. This progressive decrease in ciliated cells is consistent with the observation that ciliogenesis is a highly complex cellular function that may be retained in benign and well-differentiated neoplasms, but is eventually lost in undifferentiated neoplastic cells.

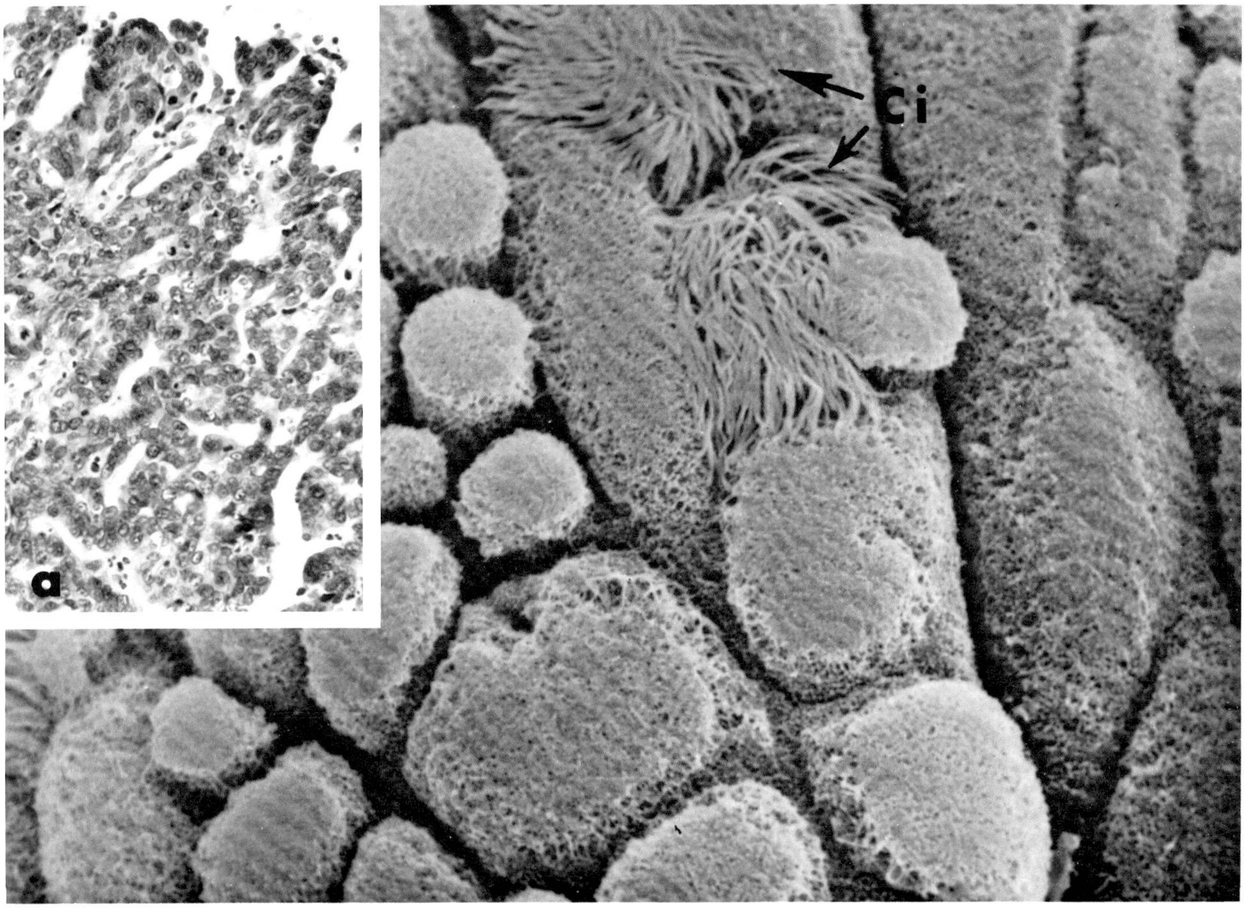

Figure 191a. *Fallopian tube. Moderately well-differentiated papillary adenocarcinoma,* composed of delicate papillary fronds lined by several layers of pleomorphic neoplastic cells with prominent nucleoli, and mitotic figures. The formation of abortive glandular structures is seen in the mid-lower portion of the photomicrograph. (H & E stain, × 30.)

Figure 191. *Fallopian tube. Moderately well-differentiated papillary adenocarcinoma.* With the scanning electron microscope occasional ciliated cells (Ci) with well-developed ciliary shafts are seen, interspersed with pleomorphic, nonciliated, neoplastic cells. The latter are covered by a thick layer of secretory material. × 3000.

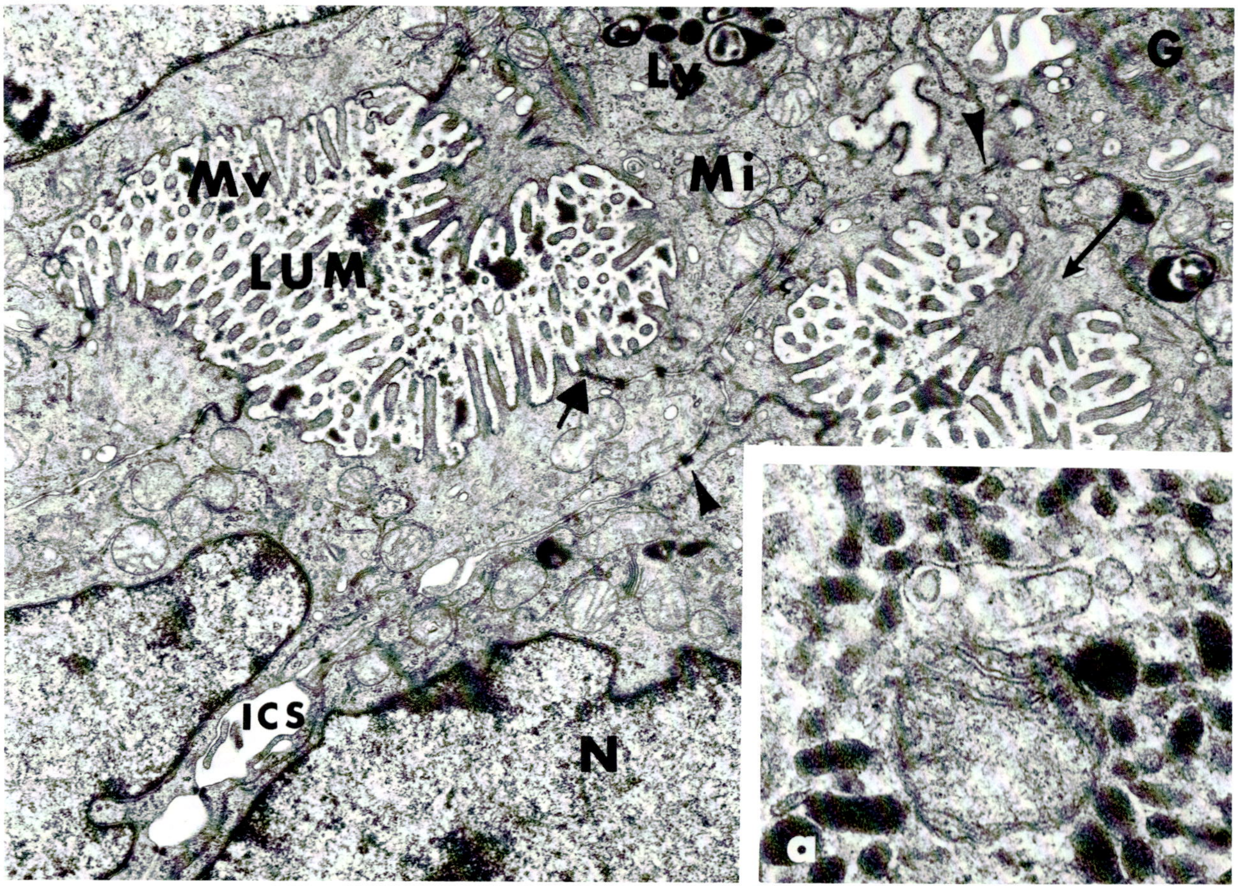

Figure 192. *Fallopian tube. In poorly differentiated adenocarcinoma,* the lumina (LUM) are small with numerous microvillous (Mv) projections and contain granular, electron-dense, secretory material. Most of the microvilli are supported by microfilaments, which extend deep into the subjacent cytoplasmic substance (long arrow). The neoplastic cells are rich in mitochondria (Mi), bound and free ribosomes, Golgi (G), pinocytic vesicles, and membrane-bound dense bodies (Ly), many of them cytolysosomes. The lateral plasma membranes are reinforced by poorly developed desmosomes (arrow head) and, near the lumina, by tight junctional complexes (short arrow). × 12,600. ICS: dilated intercellular space; N: nucleus.

Figure 192a. *Fallopian tube. Poorly differentiated adenocarcinoma.* Another typical finding in tubal and ovarian serous carcinomas is the presence of large aggregates of membrane-bound dense bodies, which are especially numerous in the basal portion of the cytoplasm. These granules are present in even the least differentiated neoplasms and are also commonly found in normal tubal epithelium. × 54,000.

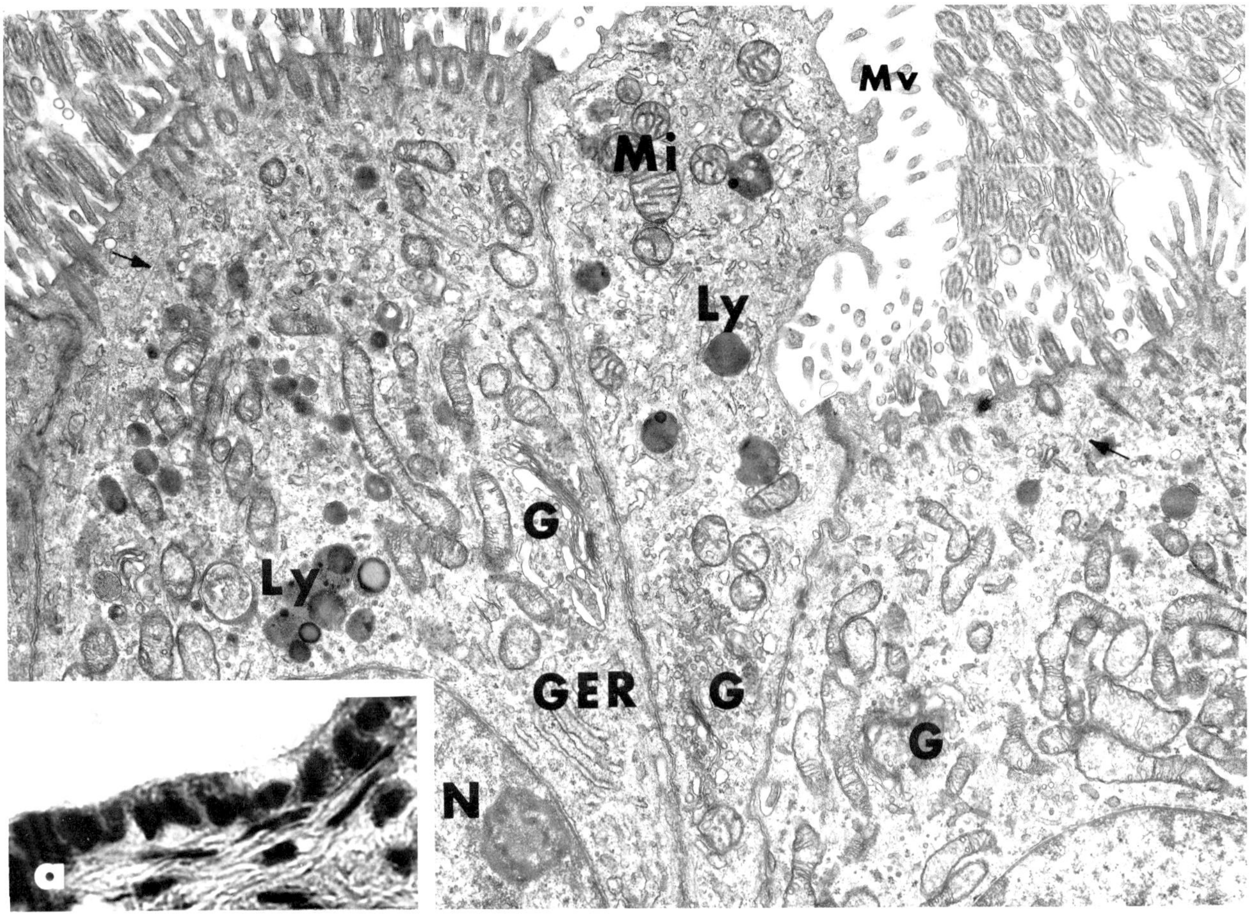

Figure 193a. *Histologic appearance* of the hydatid lining epithelium during the proliferative phase of the menstrual cycle. It is composed of rows of ciliated cells alternating with nonciliated cells of approximately equal height. (H & E stain, × 205). *From* B. R. Bransilver, A. Ferenczy, and R. M. Richart. Female genital tract remnants. An ultrastructural comparison of hydatid of Morgagni and mesonephric ducts and tubules. *Arch. Pathol.* **96:** 255–261 (1973). Copyright, 1973, American Medical Association.

Figure 193. *Hydatid of Morgagni (proliferative phase of the menstrual cycle).* A nonciliated cell (center) covered by microvilli (Mv) is flanked by two ciliated cells. Both cell types contain numerous supranuclear (N) mitochondria (Mi), Golgi (G), and electron-dense lysosomes (Ly), many of them associated with lipid droplets. The secretory cell, in addition, has more granular endoplasmic reticulum (GER) and peripheral Golgi vesicles. Scattered microtubules (arrows) and microfilaments are seen in the ciliated and nonciliated cells. × 11,000. *From* B. R. Bransilver, A. Ferenczy, and R. M. Richart. Female genital tract remnants. An ultrastructural comparison of hydatid of Morgagni and mesonephric ducts and tubules. *Arch. Pathol.* **96:** 255–261 (1973). Copyright, 1973, American Medical Association.

50

Hydatids of Morgagni

Hydatids of Morgagni are pedunculated cysts which are attached to the fimbriated ends of the Fallopian tube. The cysts are probably of Müllerian, rather than mesonephric,[1] origin, based on the histologic and ultrastructural resemblance of the hydatids to the tubal epithelium and the observation that similar morphologic changes take place during the menstrual cycle and in the postmenopausal period[2] in both the hydatid and oviductal mucosa.

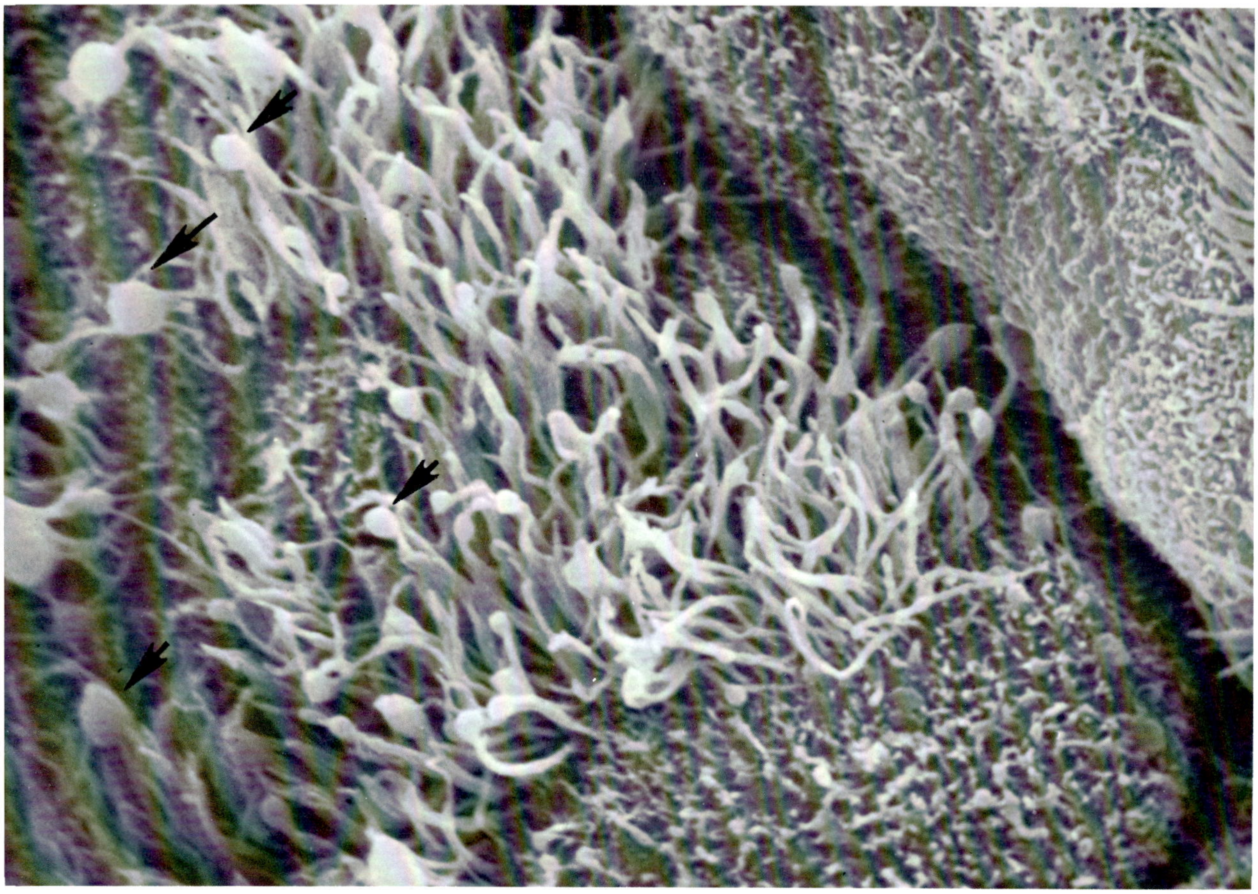

Figure 194. *Hydatid of Morgagni (17th day of the menstrual cycle).* Scanning electron micrograph of groups of ciliated cells surrounded by microvillous secretory cells. The latter have several small cytoplasmic outpouchings (long arrow) representing apocrine secretory activity, and the tips of many cilia contain agglutinated secretory material (short arrows). × 4000. *From* B. R. Bransilver, A. Ferenczy, and R. M. Richart. Female genital tract remnants. An ultrastructural comparison of hydatid of Morgagni and mesonephric ducts and tubules. *Arch. Pathol.* **96:** 255–261 (1973). Copyright, 1973, American Medical Association.

REFERENCES (Hydatids of Morgagni—Figure 194)

1. Changus, G. W., J. E. Towne, C. J. Smith, and T. N. Yonan. Fine structure of the so-called mesonephric carcinoma (abstract). *Lab. Invest.* **20:** 579 (1969).
2. Bransilver, B. R., A. Ferenczy, and R. M. Richart. Female genital tract remnants. An ultrastructural comparison of hydatid of Morgagni and mesonephric ducts and tubules. *Arch. Pathol.* **96:** 255 (1973).

51

Paratubal Mesonephric Ducts and Tubules

Paratubal mesonephric ducts and tubules are vestigial remnants of the mesonephric duct and are commonly found in the tuboovarian region. Both the ducts and tubules are lined by a single-layered cuboidal to columnar epithelium that is separated from the surrounding muscle coat by a well-defined basal lamina. The major histologic and ultrastructural difference between the two adnexal structures is the presence of ciliated cells in the mesonephric tubules and their absence in the ducts. Although intracytoplasmic glycogen particles and organelles are well developed, secretory activity is comparatively less pronounced than in the tubal epithelium, and it is not subject to cyclical variations.[1]

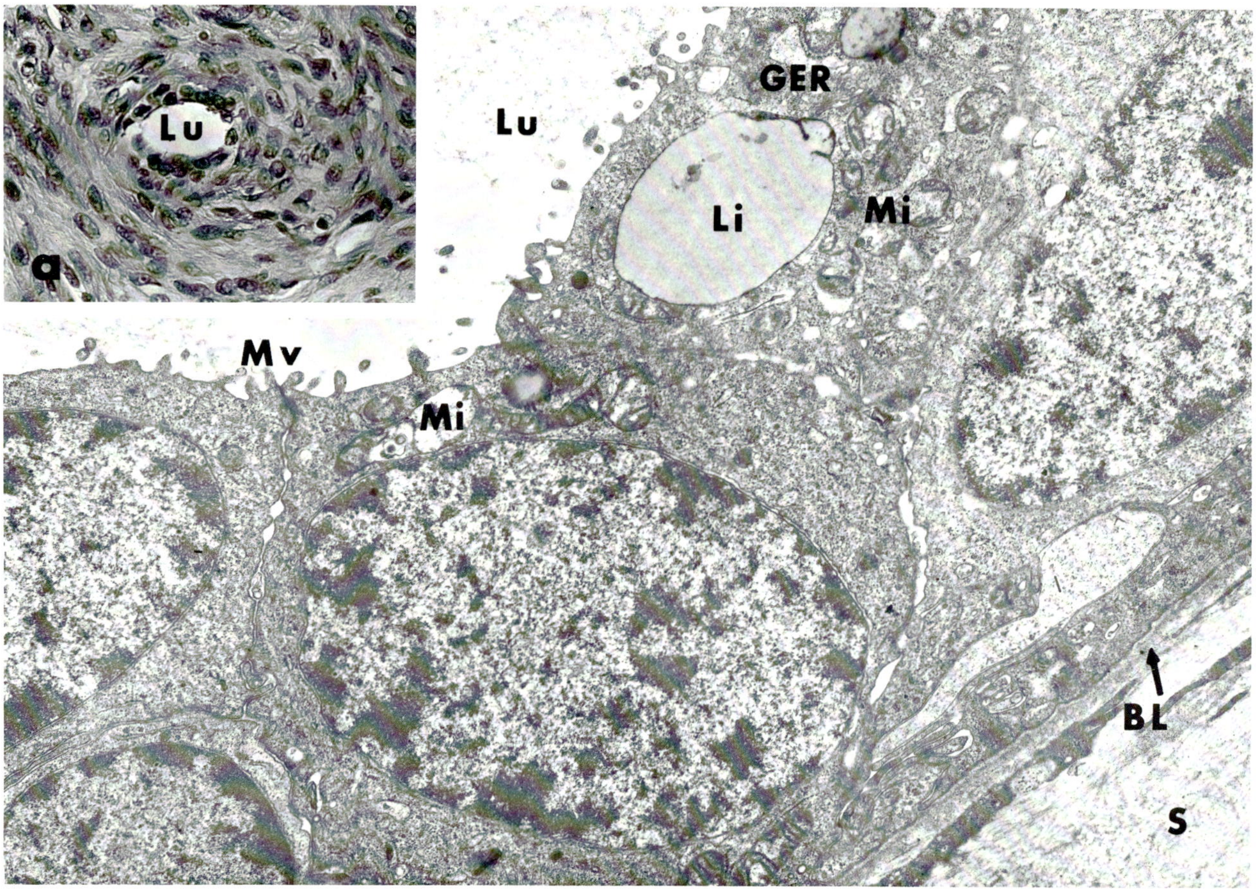

Figure 195a. *Mesonephric duct.* Histologically, the mesonephric duct is lined by a single row of nonciliated cuboidal cells. Characteristically, well-developed smooth muscle coats encircle the duct. (H & E stain, × 86.) Lu: ductal lumen. *From* B. R. Bransilver, A. Ferenczy and R. M. Richart. Female genital tract remnants. An ultrastructural comparison of hydatid of Morgagni and mesonephric ducts and tubules. *Arch. Pathol.* **96:** 255–261 (1973). Copyright, 1973, American Medical Association.

Figure 195. *Mesonephric duct.* The nuclei occupy a large portion of the cytoplasmic substance, which is poor in organelles. Lipid (Li) droplets are prominent. The luminal microvilli (Mv) are sparse and short, and desmosomes are infrequent. Note the convoluted configuration of adjacent plasma membranes near the basal lamina (BL). × 4600. Lu: ductal lumen: Mi: mitochondria; GER: granular endoplasmic reticulum; S: collagenous stroma. *From* B. R. Bransilver, A. Ferenczy, and R. M. Richart. Female genital tract remnants. An ultrastructural comparison of hydatid of Morgagni and mesonephric ducts and tubules. *Arch. Pathol.* **96:** 255–261 (1973). Copyright, 1973, American Medical Association.

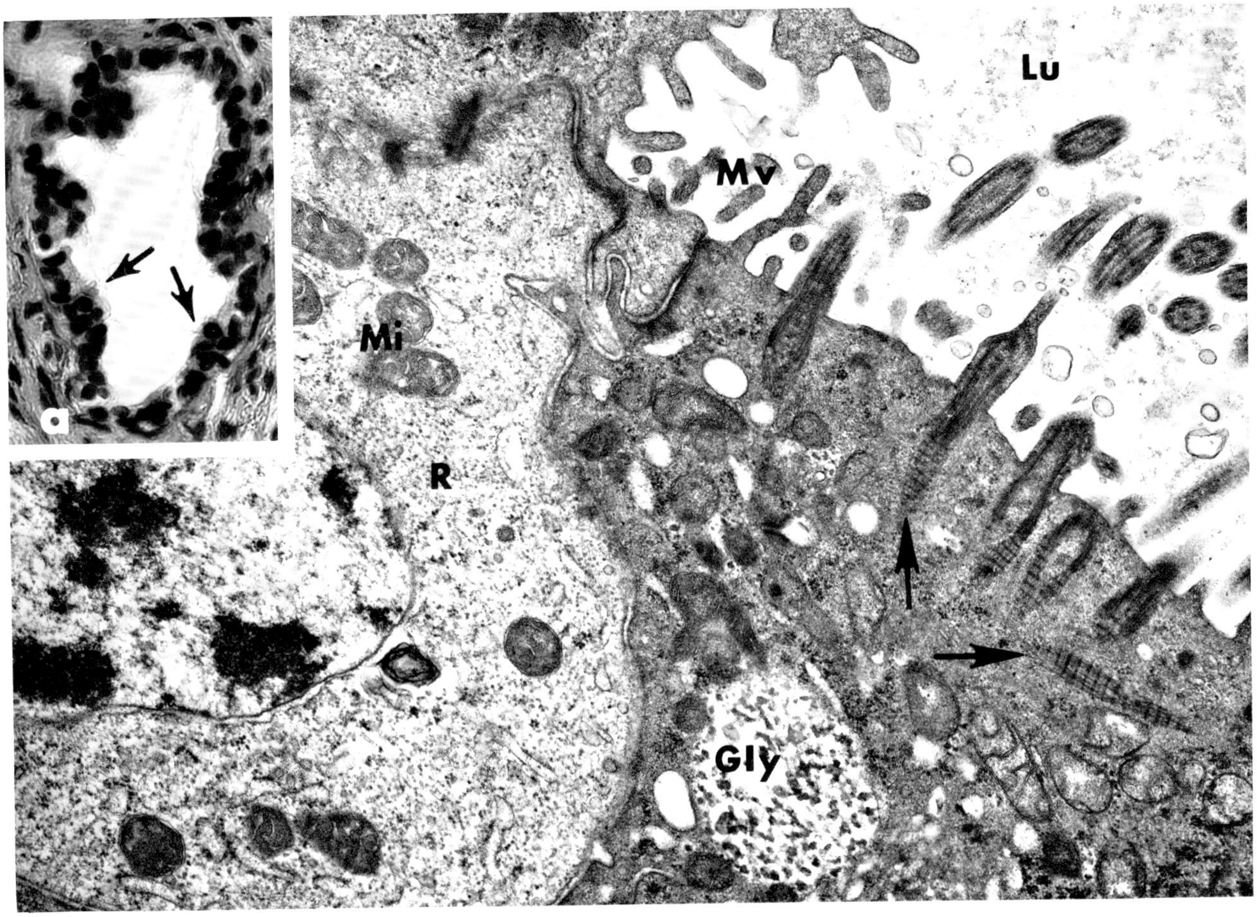

Figure 196a. *Mesonephric tubule.* The lining epithelium of the tubule is often pseudostratified with focal intraluminal projections, and ciliated cells (arrows) are numerous. (H & E stain, × 105.) *From* B. R. Bransilver, A. Ferenczy, and R. M. Richart. Female genital tract remnants. An ultrastructural comparison of hydatid of Morgagni and mesonephric ducts and tubules. *Arch. Pathol.* **96:** 255–261 (1973). Copyright, 1973, American Medical Association.

Figure 196. *Mesonephric tubule.* A dark-staining ciliated cell with abundant mitochondria and clusters of glycogen particles (Gly) is adjacent to a nonciliated cell with a light cytoplasmic matrix in which free ribosomes (R) are abundant. The cross-striated ciliary rootlets (arrows) are visible. × 12,000. Lu: tubular lumen; Mv: microvilli; Mi: mitochondria. *From* B. R. Bransilver, A. Ferenczy, and R. M. Richart. Female genital tract remnants. An ultrastructural comparison of hydatid of Morgagni and mesonephric ducts and tubules. *Arch. Pathol.* **96:** 255–261 (1973). Copyright, 1973, American Medical Association.

REFERENCE (Paratubal mesonephic ducts–Figure 196)

1. Bransilver, B. R., A. Ferenczy, and R. M. Richart. Female genital tract remnants. An ultrastructural comparison of hydatid of Morgagni and mesonephric ducts and tubules. *Arch. Pathol.* **96:** 255 (1973).

52

Walthard Cell Nests

Walthard cell nests are commonly seen on the serosal surfaces of the Fallopian tube, mesosalpinx, and mesovarium. They occur both as small, solid protuberances and as cysts, generally measuring less than 3 mm in diameter. Histologically and ultrastructurally, both the solid and cystic Walthard cell nests are composed of stratified, transitional-type epithelium, closely resembling that of the urinary tract mucosa.[1] The characteristic findings include wide intercellular spaces with numerous microvillous projections, which are occasionally attached by small desmosomes; an increasing number of organelles and autophagic lysosomes (telolysosomes) with increasing proximity to the central or luminal portion; pinocytic vesicles and surface microvilli within the luminal lining cells of cystic Walthard cell nests; and frequent central cellular degeneration in the solid variety. The last phenomenon is presumably responsible for the origin of the cystic Walthard cell nests. In addition there are deep nuclear indentations ("coffee-bean nuclear pattern") and a well-developed basal lamina. Although some cell contain bundles of tonofilaments, keratinization and prominent desmosomal belts of the type seen in epidermal cells do not occur.

The morphological similarity of the Walthard cell nests to the transitional epithelium of the urinary tract[1] and its direct continuity with genital and extragenital serosal coverings favor an origin from transitional cell metaplasia of the celomic epithelium, rather than a derivation from mesonephric or urothelial remnants. This postulate is further supported by the dissimilarity of the Walthard cell nests to the adnexal mesonephric ducts and tubules,[2] and their resemblance to the celomic epithelium.

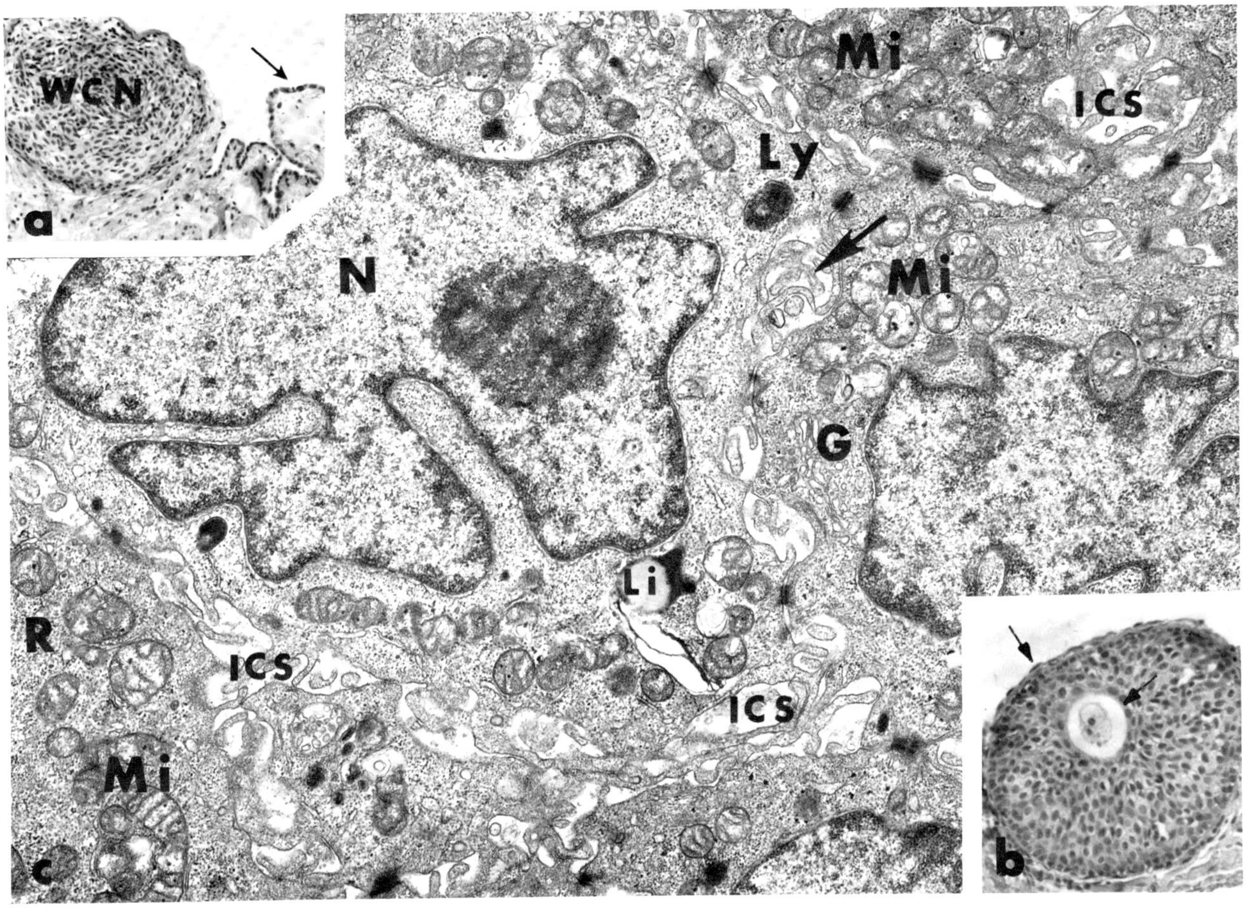

Figure 197a. *Histologically,* Walthard cell nests (WCN) form solid protuberances of stratified transitional epithelium and are most commonly found just beneath the mesothelial serosal (arrow) lining of the oviducts. (H & E stain, × 30.)

Figure 197b. *Histologic appearance of another solid Walthard cell nest.* Note the central lumen formation containing degenerated desquamated cells and the close relationship between the serosal lining (arrow) and the Walthard cell nest epithelium. (H & E stain, × 48.)

Figure 197c. *Basal portion of solid Walthard cell nest.* The nuclei (N) have deeply infolding membranes and large nucleoli. The cytoplasmic matrix contains groups of mitochondria (Mi), abundant free ribosomes (R), and microfilaments. Scattered multivesicular and dense bodies (Ly) and lipid droplets (Li) are seen. The Golgi (G) are inconspicuous. Interdigitating microvilli project into enlarged intercellular spaces (arrow), and randomly distributed small desmosomes (ICS) reinforce cellular integrity. × 16,900. *From* B. R. Bransilver, A. Ferenczy, and R. M. Richart. Brenner tumors and Walthard cell nests. A comparative ultrastructural study (in preparation).

REFERENCES (Walthard cell nests–Figure 197c)

1. Bransilver, B. R. A. Ferenczy, and R. M. Richart. Brenner tumors and Walthard cell nests. A comparative ultrastructural study (in preparation).
2. Bransilver, B. R., A. Ferenczy, and R. M. Richart. Female genital tract remnants. An ultrastructural comparison of hydatid of Morgagni and mesonephric ducts and tubules. *Arch. Pathol.* **96:** 255 (1973).

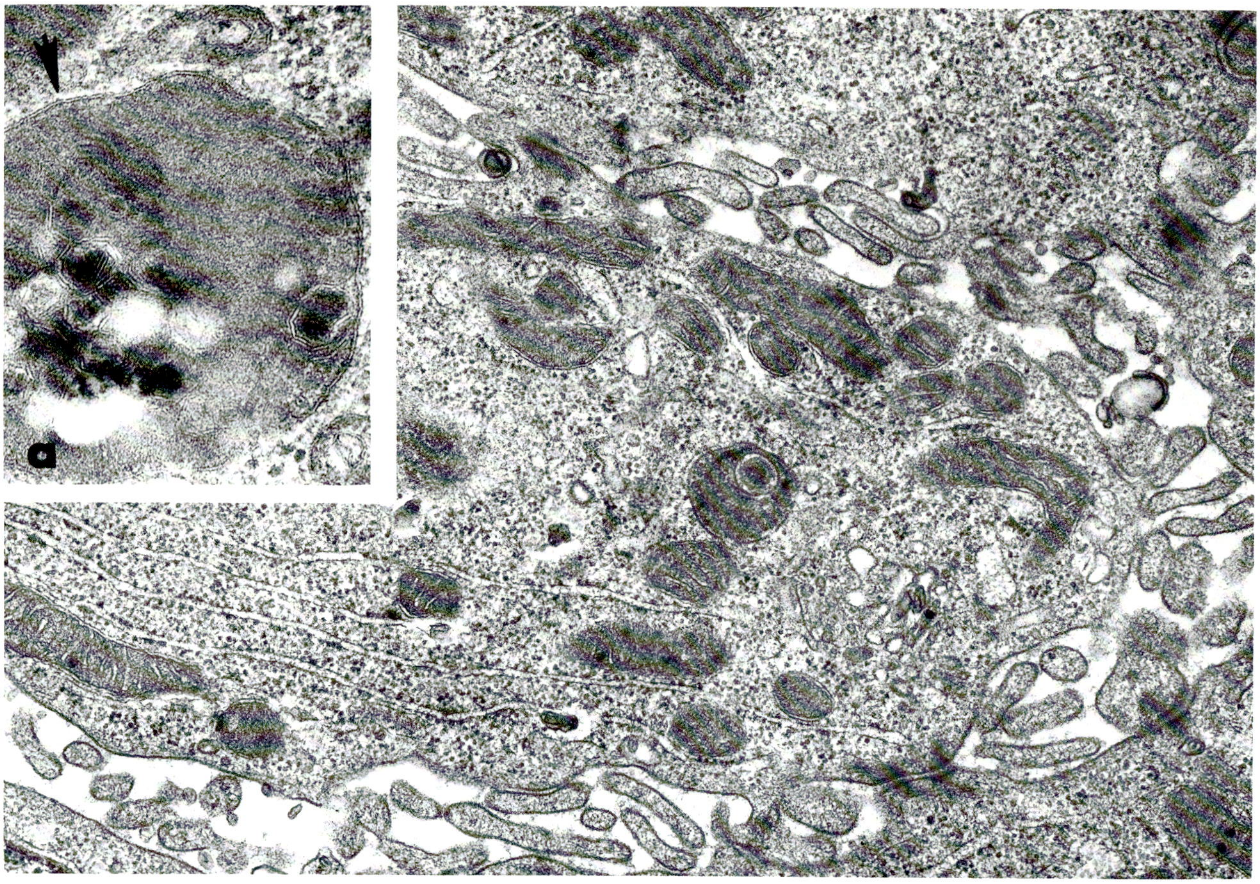

Figure 198. *Mid-portion of solid Walthard cell nest.* There is an increase in free ribosomes, and parallel membranes of granular endoplasmic reticulum are in close relationship with groups of mitochondria and Golgi. The intercellular space has numerous interdigitating microvilli. × 37,000.

Figure 198a. *High magnification of membrane-bound* (arrow) *giant autophagic cytolysosome* containing an admixture of polyhedral lamellated bodies and finely granular electron-dense material. × 50,000.

Figure 199a. *Cystic Walthard cell nest.* Histologic appearance of cystic Walthard cell nests, lined by flattened stratified transitional-like epithelium and separated from the stroma by a well-defined basal lamina (BL). (H & E stain, × 85.) Lu: lumen.

Figure 199b. *Survey electron micrograph of fully formed cystic Walthard cell nest.* The luminal plasma membrane contains stubby microvilli (Mv) associated with pinocytic infoldings (arrow head) and vesicles (arrows), and the cytoplasm has scattered groups of mitochondria (Mi), Golgi (G), and bundles of microfilaments (Mf). Free ribosomes (R) are abundant throughout. The nuclear membranes have deep infoldings, and the focally dilated and tortuous intercellular spaces (ICS) contain numerous microvilli. A well-defined basal lamina (BL) is visible. × 7975. Lu: cyst lumen; N: nucleus. *From* B. R. Bransilver, A. Ferenczy, and R. M. Richart. Brenner tumors and Walthard cell nests. A comparative ultrastructural study (in preparation).

Figure 199c. *Cellular detail of the Walthard epithelium lining a cyst.* The short microvillous projections are surrounded by stellate, fibrillar material, and the subjacent pinocytic vesicles contain similar filamentous material. Small lysosomes and larger membrane-bound dense bodies with granular and lamellated material are found near the surface plasma membrane, and the cytoplasm is rich in free ribosomes and microfilaments. × 35,000. *From* B. R. Bransilver, A. Ferenczy, and R. M. Richart. Brenner tumors and Walthard cell nests. A comparative ultrastructural study (in preparation).

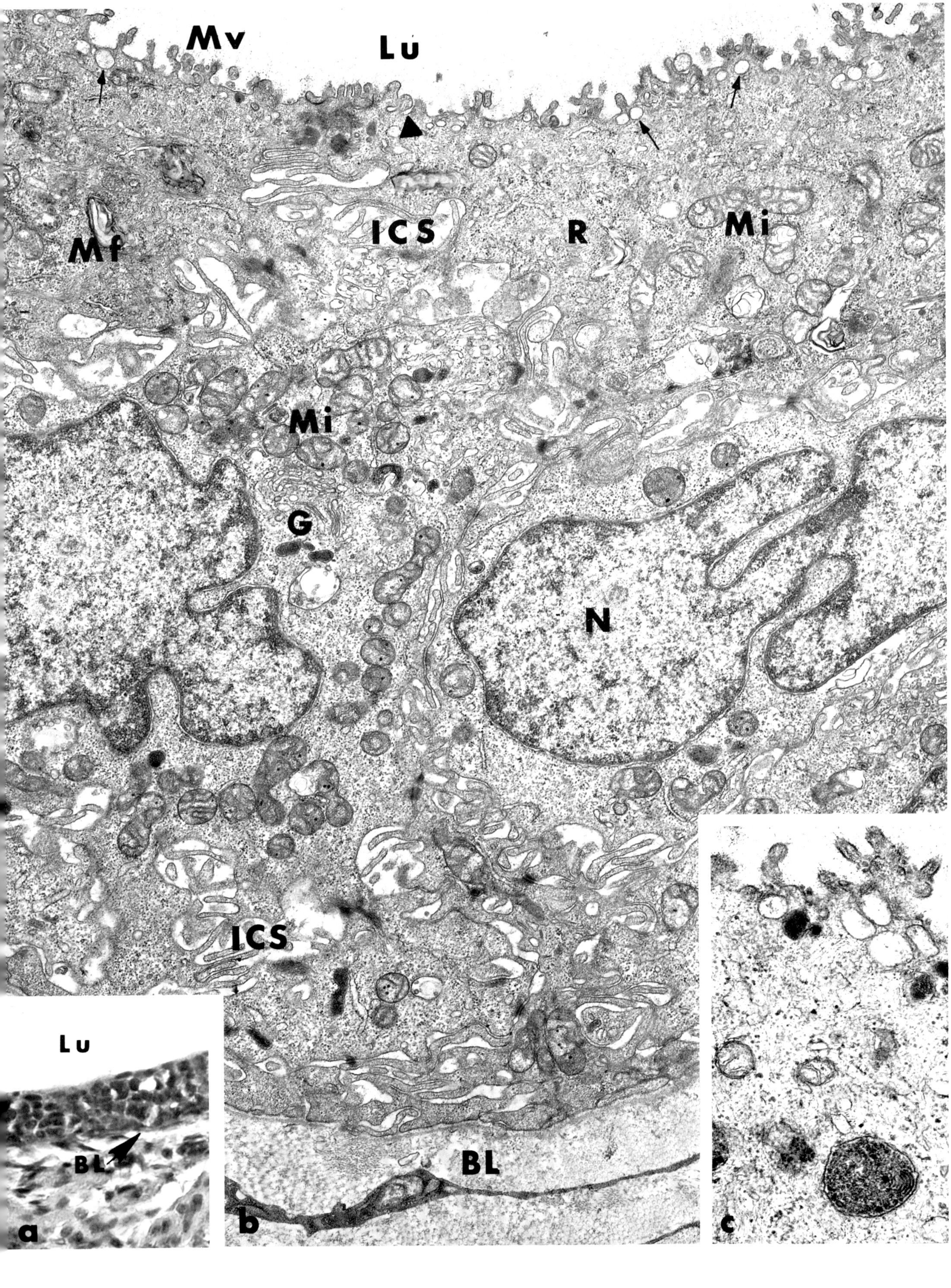
Mv
Lu
ICS
R
Mi
Mf
Mi
G
N
ICS
BL
b
Lu
BL
a
c

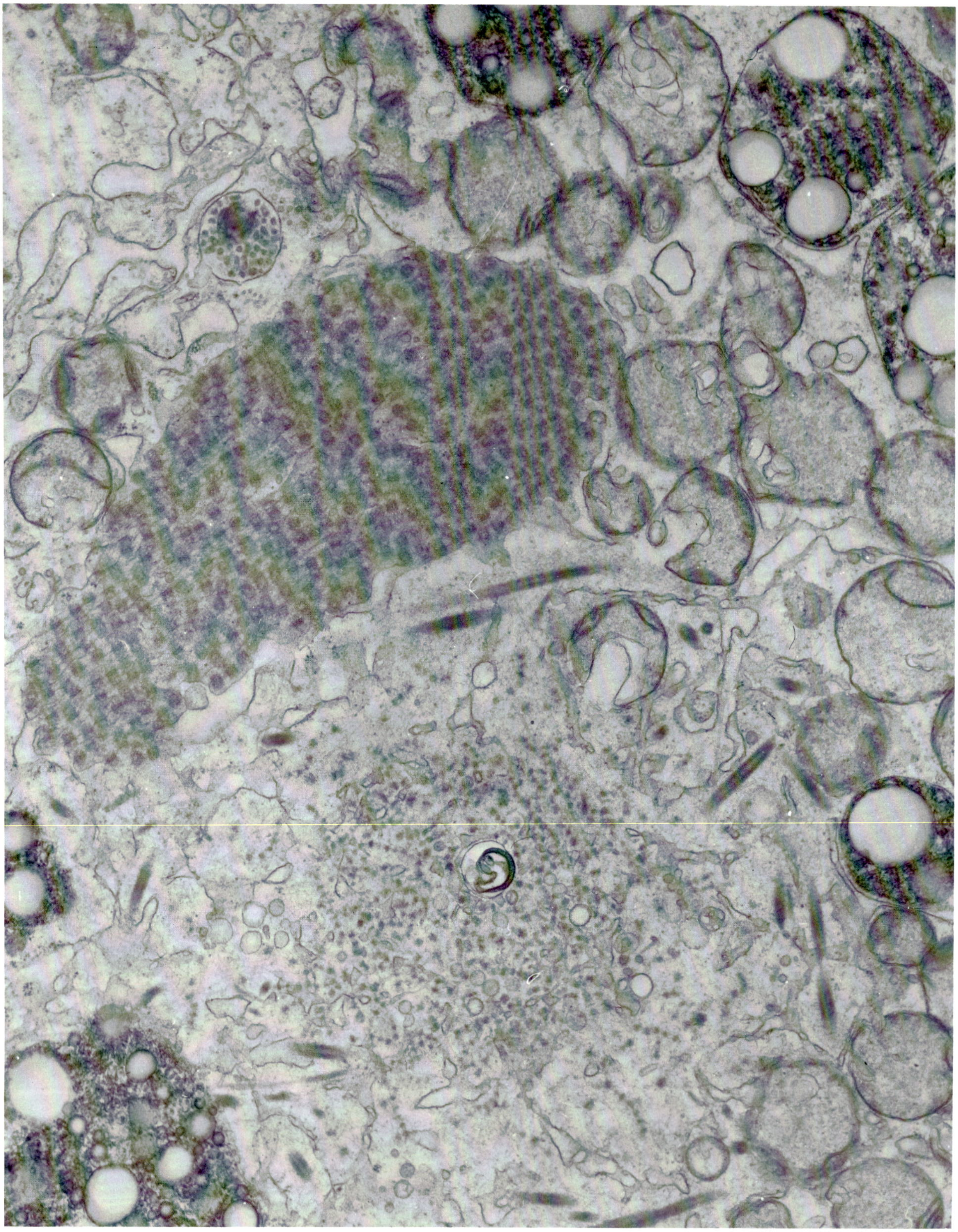

Electron micrograph illustrating the cytocentrum of Balbiani's vitelline body of a primary human oocyte. The cytocentrum is composed of central dense granules, some arranged periodically on fine fibers, and small vesicles with a peripheral zone of endoplasmic reticulum and dense fibers. Surrounding the cytocentrum are mitochondria and residual bodies. A stock of annulate lamellae is cut tangentially. × 20,000. *From* A. T. Hertig. The primary human oocyte: some observations on the fine structure of the Balbiani's vitelline body and the origin of the annulate lamellae. *Amer. J. Anat.* **122:** 107–138 (1968).

OVARY

53
Oogenesis

The primitive germ cells migrate from the endoderm of the yolk sac to the gonadal primordia of the paired urogenital ridges and undergo a series of changes during the first half of gestation (7–20 weeks),[1-3] including multiplication, meiosis, degeneration, and the formation of primordial follicles. *The primitive germ cells* are distributed singly within the genital parenchymal cells between the 7th and 9th intrauterine weeks and have abundant cytoplasmic organelles for protein synthesis and transport.[3] The complex cytoplasmic processes that are present during migration are preserved during the early phase of gonadal development,[3,4] but in the following few (10–12th) weeks *the oogonia* become organized as aggregates of large, pale cells connected by intercellular bridges and containing numerous mitotic figures.[3,5] By the 20th week, most of the germ cells enter meiosis, as indicated by the trabecular arrangement of granular chromosomes[2,5] associated with synaptinemal (axial) complexes,[3,4] and, characteristically, mitochondria are arranged in a perinuclear location.[1-3]

These cells are referred to as *oocytes*. Between the 16th and 20th weeks a large number of germ cells degenerate and are phagocytized by the neighboring granulosal cells,[3] whereas others enter meiotic prophase, assume a pachytene pattern, and become surrounded by flattened granulosa cells to form the primordial follicles.[3] Oocytes in fetal primordial follicles reach the diplotene ("resting stage") of prophase by the time of birth and remain meiotically quiescent (10–30 years) until follicle maturation preparatory to ovulation.

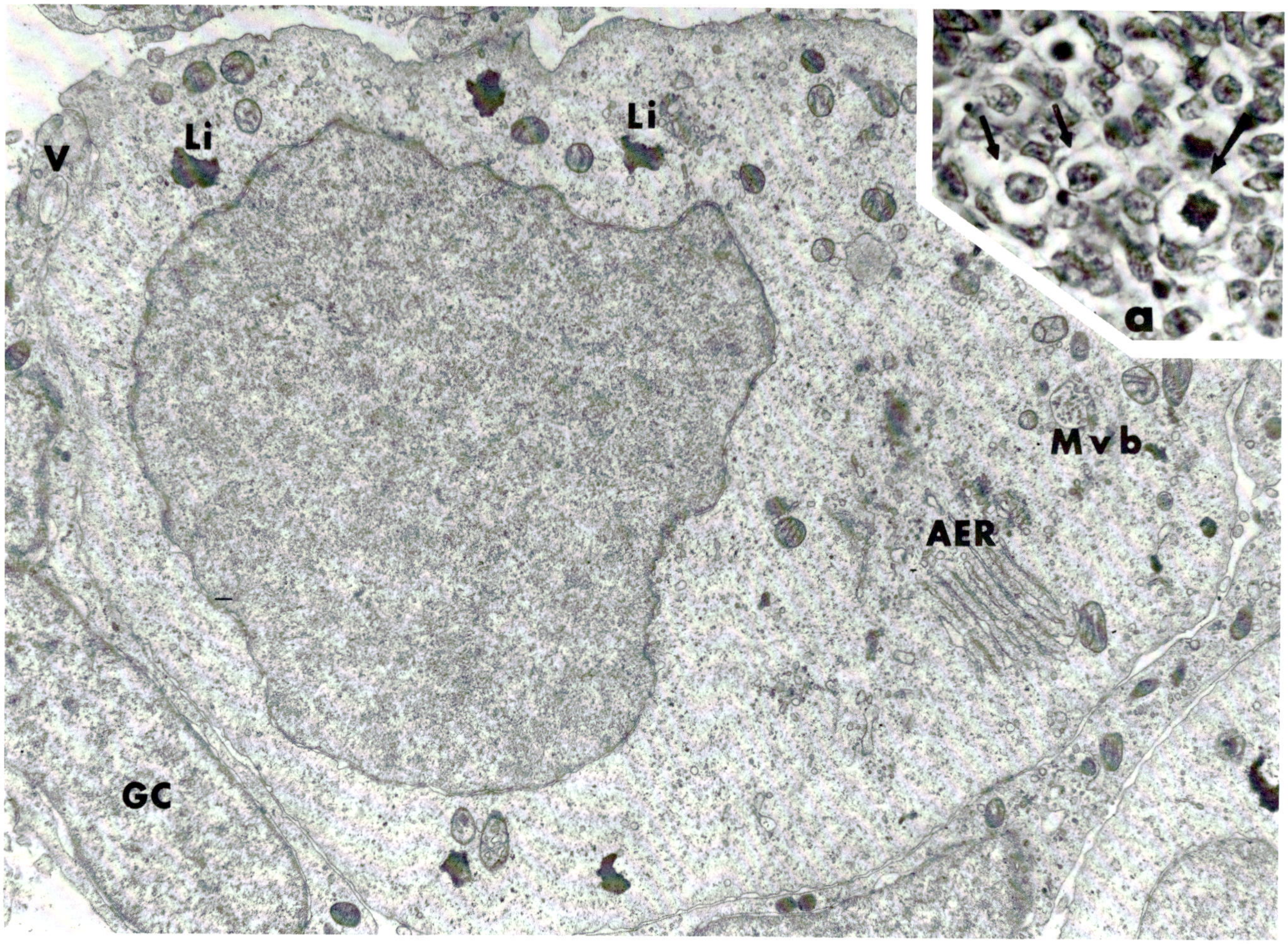

Figure 200a. *Fetal ovary (10th week of gestation).* Fetal germ cells (arrows) are recognized by their abundant pale cytoplasm and prominent nuclei. A germ cell is in mitosis (long arrow). Several germ cells contain a crown of flattened granulosa cells. (H & E stain, × 120.)

Figure 200. *Primitive germ cell, human fetal ovary (9 weeks gestation).* Cell is large and oval, with prominent villuslike extensions (V) at one pole. The nucleus, eccentrically located, is filled with dense, homogeneous chromatin granules. The cytoplasm contains loosely scattered ribosomes, spherical mitochondria, lipid droplets (Li), multivesicular bodies (Mvb), and elements of agranular endoplasmic reticulum (AER). × 8500. GC: Primitive granulosa cells. *From* B. Gondos, P. Bhiraleus, and C. J. Hobel. Ultrastructural observations on germ cells in human fetal ovaries. *Am. J. Obstet. Gynecol.* **110:** 644–652 (1971).

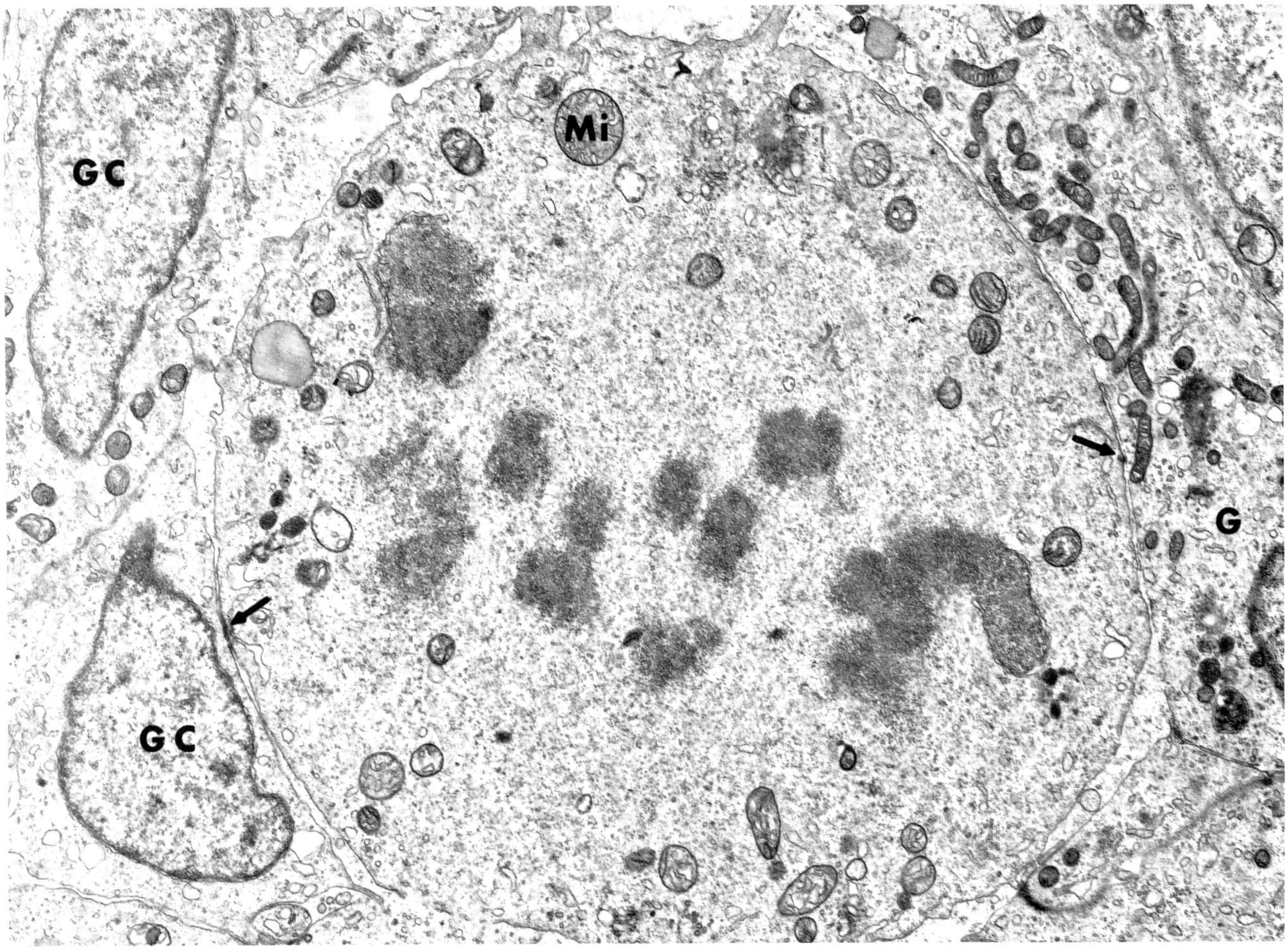

Figure 201. *Oogonium in mitosis, human fetal ovary (13 weeks gestation).* The dividing cell is completely surrounded by developing granulosa cells (GC) with tight junctions present at several points (arrows). Note contrasting appearance of spherical germ cell mitochondria (Mi) and elongated mitochondria of adjacent granulosa cells. × 9000. G: Golgi. *From* B. Gondos, P. Bhiraleus, and C. J. Hobel. Ultrastructural observations on germ cells in human fetal ovaries. *Am. J. Obstet. Gynecol.* **110:** 644–652 (1971).

REFERENCES (The primitive germ cells–Figure 201)

1. Stegner, H. E. and H. H. Wartenberg. Elektronenmikroskopische Untersuchungen an Eizellen des Menschen in verschiedenen Stadien des Oogenese. *Arch. Gynaekol.* **199:** 515 (1963).
2. Baker, T. G. and L. L. Franchi. The fine structure of oogonia and oocytes in human ovaries. *J. Cell Sci.* **2:** 213 (1967).
3. Gondos, B., P. Bhiraleus, and C. J. Hobel. Ultrastructural observations on germ cells in human fetal ovaries. *Am. J. Obstet. Gynecol.* **110:** 644 (1971).
4. Blandau, R. J. Observations on living oogonia and oocytes from human embryonic and fetal ovaries. *Am. J. Obstet. Gynecol.* **104:** 310 (1969).
5. Baker, T. G. and L. L. Francni. The structure of the chromosomes in human primordial oocytes. *Chromosoma* **22:** 358 (1967).

54

Folliculogenesis

Figure 202. *Oocyte in meiotic prophase, human fetal ovary (15 weeks gestation).* The nuclear chromatin is clumped, and several synaptinemal complexes (arrows) are visible. Note the close association between the mitochondria and the nuclear envelope. × 9000. GC: primitive granulosa cells. *From* B. Gondos, P. Bhiraleus, and C. J. Hobel. Ultrastructural observations on germ cells in human fetal ovaries. *Am. J. Obstet. Gynecol.* **110:** 644–652 (1971).

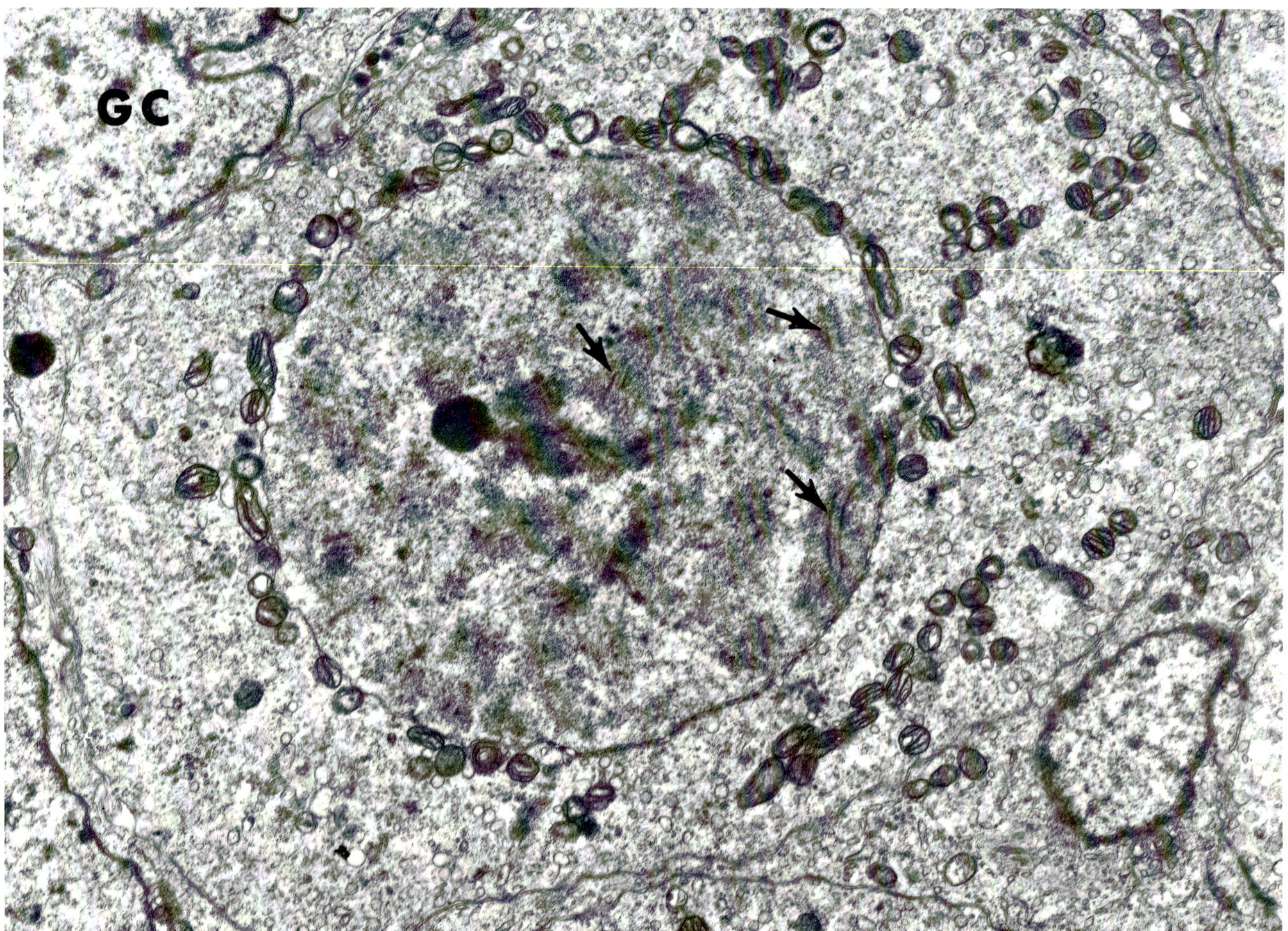

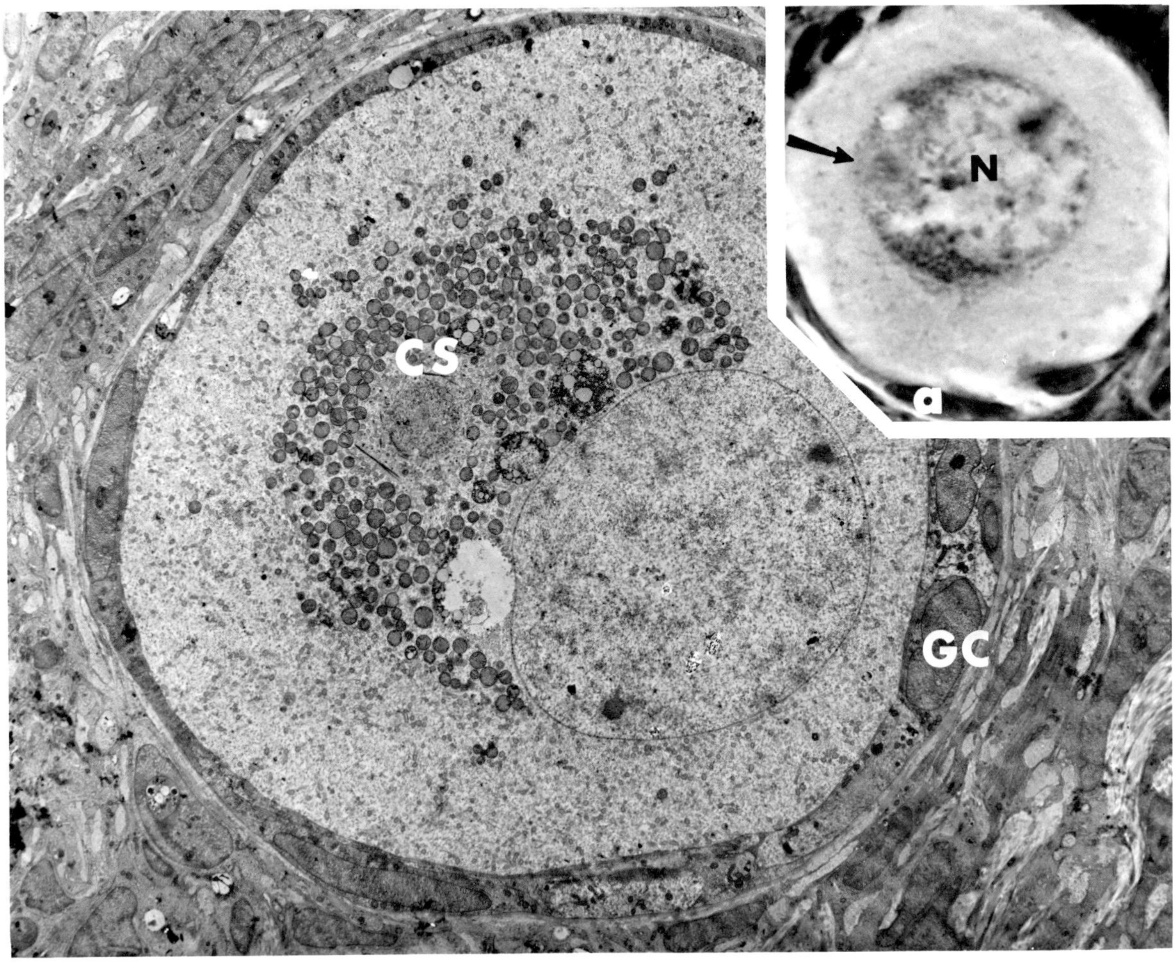

Figure 203a. *The primary oocyte of the adult human primordial follicle* (unilaminar follicle) often has a crescent-shaped perinuclear zone, referred to as the archplasm (idiosome) or Balbiani's vitelline body (arrow), closely applied to the spherical nucleus (N). The cytocentrum (centrosome) is the dark spot surrounded by a halo, which in turn is flanked by masses of mitochondria. (H & E stain, × 1200.) *From* A. T. Hertig. The primary human oocyte: some observations on the fine structure of Balbiani's vitelline body and the origin of the annulate lamellae. *Am. J. Anat.* **122:** 107–138 (1968).

Figure 203. *Primordial human oocyte.* Balbiani's vitelline body at the ultrastructural level[1-4] contains a juxtanuclear condensation of mitochondria, Golgi, endoplasmic reticulum, lysosomes, annulate lamellae, and a cytocentrum (CS), reflecting the "nuclear polarization"[4] of primary oocyte metabolic activity. The granulosa cells (GC) are of variable thickness and density. × 2400. *From* A. T. Hertig. The primary human oocyte: some observations on the fine structure of Balbiani's vitelline body and the origin of the annulate lamellae. *Am. J. Anat.* **122:** 107–138 (1968).

REFERENCES (Figures 202–203)

1. Baca, M. and L. Zamboni The fine structure of human follicular oocytes. *J. Ultrastruct. Res.* **19:** 354 (1967).
2. Hertig, A. T. and E. C. Adams. Studies on the human oocyte and its follicle. I. Ultrastructural and cytochemical observations on the primordial follicle stage. *J. Cell Biol.* **34:** 647 (1967).
3. Hertig, A. T. The primary human oocyte: some observations on the fine structure of Balbiani's vitelline body and the origin of the annulate lamellae. *Am. J. Anat.* **122:** 107 (1968).
4. Zamboni, L. *Fine Morphology of Mammalian Fertilization,* Harper & Row, New York, 1971.

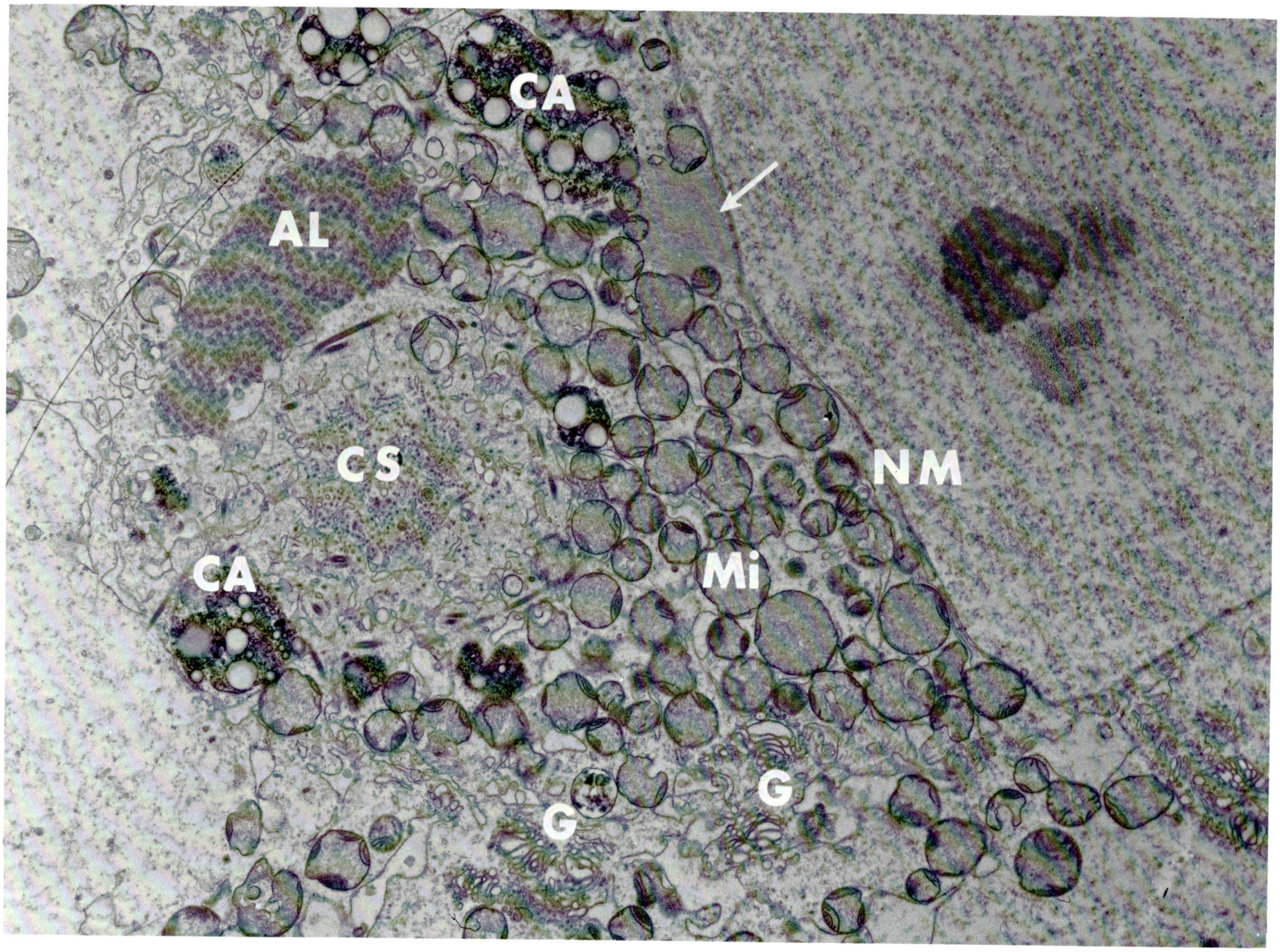

Figure 204. *Human primary oocyte from an early primary follicle. Detailed view of Balbiani's vitelline body.* A cluster of closely packed spiral fibrils (arrow) is attached to the nuclear envelope (NM). The cytocentrum (CS) is composed of dense granules, some arranged periodically on fine fibers, and small vesicles, with a peripheral zone of endoplasmic reticulum and dense fibers. Surrounding the cytocentrum are masses of mitochondria (Mi) and compound aggregates (CA). A stack of annulate lamellae (AL) is seen tangentially. Note the prominent endoplasmic reticulum and dense fibers. Surrounding the cytocentrum are masses of mitochondria (Mi) and compound aggregates (CA). A stack of annulate lamellae (AL) is seen tangentially. Note the prominent endoplasmic reticulum in close association with multiple Golgi complexes (G) at the periphery of Balbiani's vitelline body. × 7900. *From* A. T. Hertig. The primary human oocyte: some observations on the fine structure of Balbiani's vitelline body and the origin of the annulate lamellae. *Am. J. Anat.* **122:** 107–138 (1968).

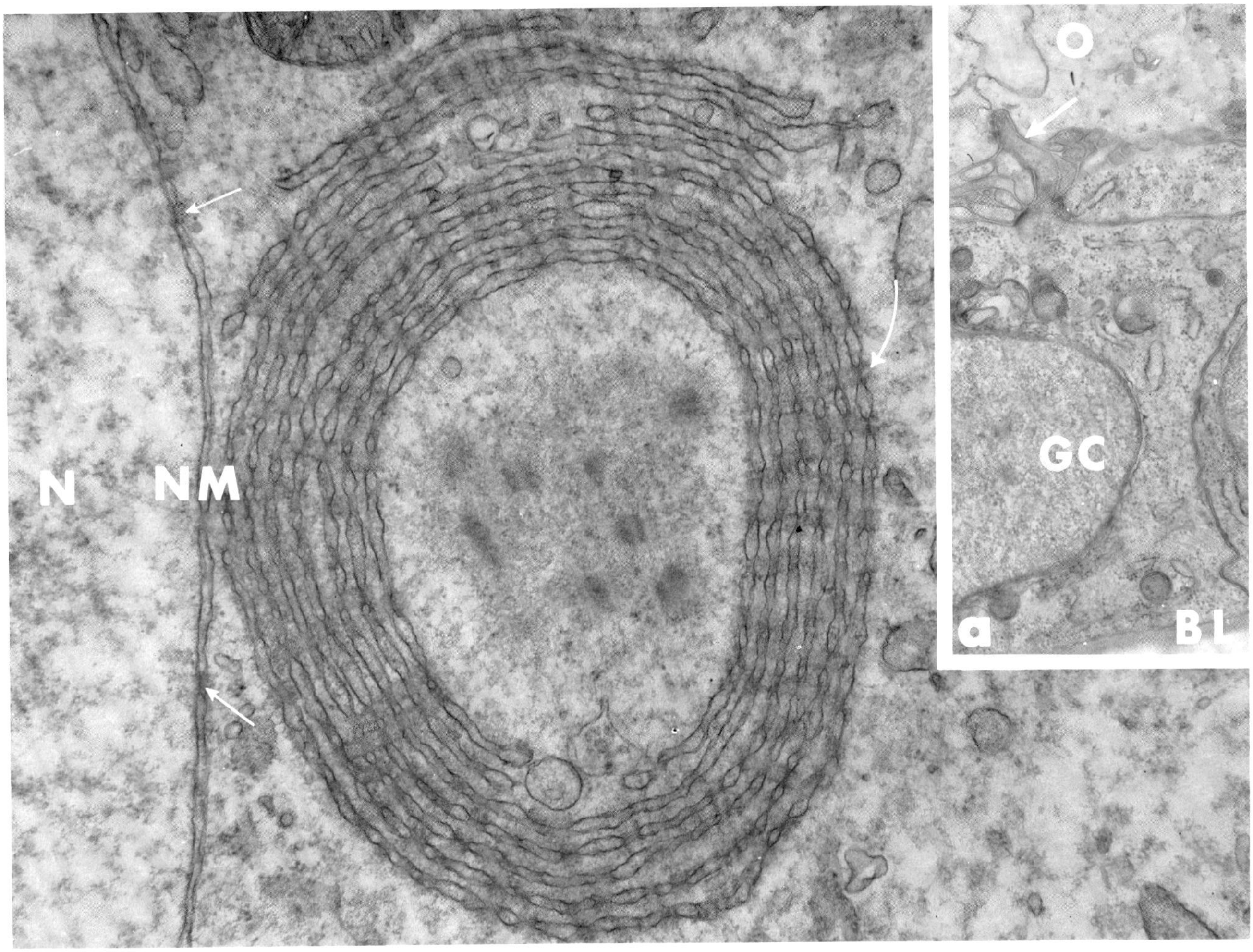

Figure 205a. *The granulosa (GC), or follicular, cells of the primordial follicles* are spindle-shaped, low cuboidal follicles. They have cytoplasmic simplicity, an absence of mitotic activity, and several microvillous projections (arrow), which are attached to the oocyte (O) through tight apposition.[1,6] × 20,000. BL: basal lamina. *From* A. T. Hertig. The primary human oocyte: some observations on the fine structure of Balbiani's vitelline body and the origin of the annulate lamellae. *Am. J. Anat.* **122:** 107–138 (1968).

Figure 205. *A coiled stack of annulate lamellae from a primordial follicle.* Annulate lamellae, located either free in the cytoplasm or attached[1-3] to the nuclear membrane (NM), are constantly present in the primary oocytes[1,4-6] and appear as collections of smooth, paired, parallel membranes 30 to 50 μ wide with areas of tight apposition (long arrow) at regular intervals resembling nuclear pore complexes (short arrows). These peculiar structures are generally considered to be formed by blebbing from the outer lamellae of the nuclear membranes[2,3] and have been demonstrated to interdigitate[1] with the intracytoplasmic endoplasmic reticulum (upper center). Although the functional significance of the annulate lamellae is unknown, their special ultrastructural organization and their presence in rapidly growing and differentiating cells, such as germinal, embryonal, and neoplastic cells,[6] suggest that they may have a role in the nucleocytoplasmic exchange of substances necessary for special and increased metabolic activity or transfer of genetic information.[1] The numerous masses of amorphous material possibly represent concentrations of core material lying within the ooplasm enclosed by the coiled annulate lamellae. × 31,250. N: nucleus. *From* A. T. Hertig. The primary human oocyte: some observations on the fine structure of Balbiani's vitelline body and the origin of the annulate lamellae. *Am. J. Anat.* **122:** 107–138 (1968).

REFERENCES (Figures 204–205a)

1. Hertig, A. T. The primary human oocyte: some observations on the fine structure of Balbiani's vitelline body and the origin of the annulate lamellae. *Am. J. Anat.* **122:** 107 (1968).
2. Kessel, R. G. Intranuclear and cytoplasmic annulate lamellae in tunicate oocytes. *J. Cell Biol.* **24:** 471 (1965).
3. Kessel. R. G. Annulate lamellae. *J. Ultrastruct. Res.* **25** (Suppl. 10) (1968).
4. Baca, M. and L. Zamboni. The fine structure of human follicular oocytes. *J. Ultrastruct. Res.* **19:** 354 (1967).
5. Hertig, A. T. and E. C. Adams. Studies on the human oocyte and its follicle. I. Ultrastructural and cytochemical observations on the primordial follicle stage. *J. Cell Biol.* **34:** 647 (1967).
6. Zamboni, L. *Fine Morphology of Mammalian Fertilization.* Harper & Row, New York, 1971.

Under the influence of follicle-stimulating hormone, follicular growth[1] is stimulated; the granulosal cells divide by mitosis, and a multilayered cell population is gradually produced. As a result of the accumulation of liquor folliculi secreted by the granulosa cells, the distended intercellular spaces coalesce, resulting in the formation of the follicular antrum[2] of the young Graafian follicle. Under the combined stimulatory effect of estrogen and luteinizing hormone,[1] follicular fluid containing glycogen and acid mucopolysaccharides continues to be secreted and accumulates in the antrum, contributing to the enlargement of the preovulatory follicle. The oocyte, encased in a thick filamentous envelope (25 μ), the zona pellucida, which is rich in acid mucopolysaccharides and glycogen; assumes an eccentric location and is surrounded by a hillock of granulosa cells called the cumulus oophorus. The bordering layer of cuboidal granulosa cells (corona radiata) develops slender cytoplasmic extensions traversing the zona pellucida and establishes close contacts (by means of tight intercellular junctions) with the surface plasma membrane of the oocyte.[2-4] During follicular development, small cystic spaces referred to as Call-Exner bodies[5] are found within masses of granulosa cells. These spaces are delimited from the surrounding granulosa cells by a basal lamina, and the lumina contain filamentous, periodic acid–Schiff-positive material probably representing sequestrated follicular fluid and precursors of the zona pellucida, both of which are eventually released into the follicular cavity.[2]

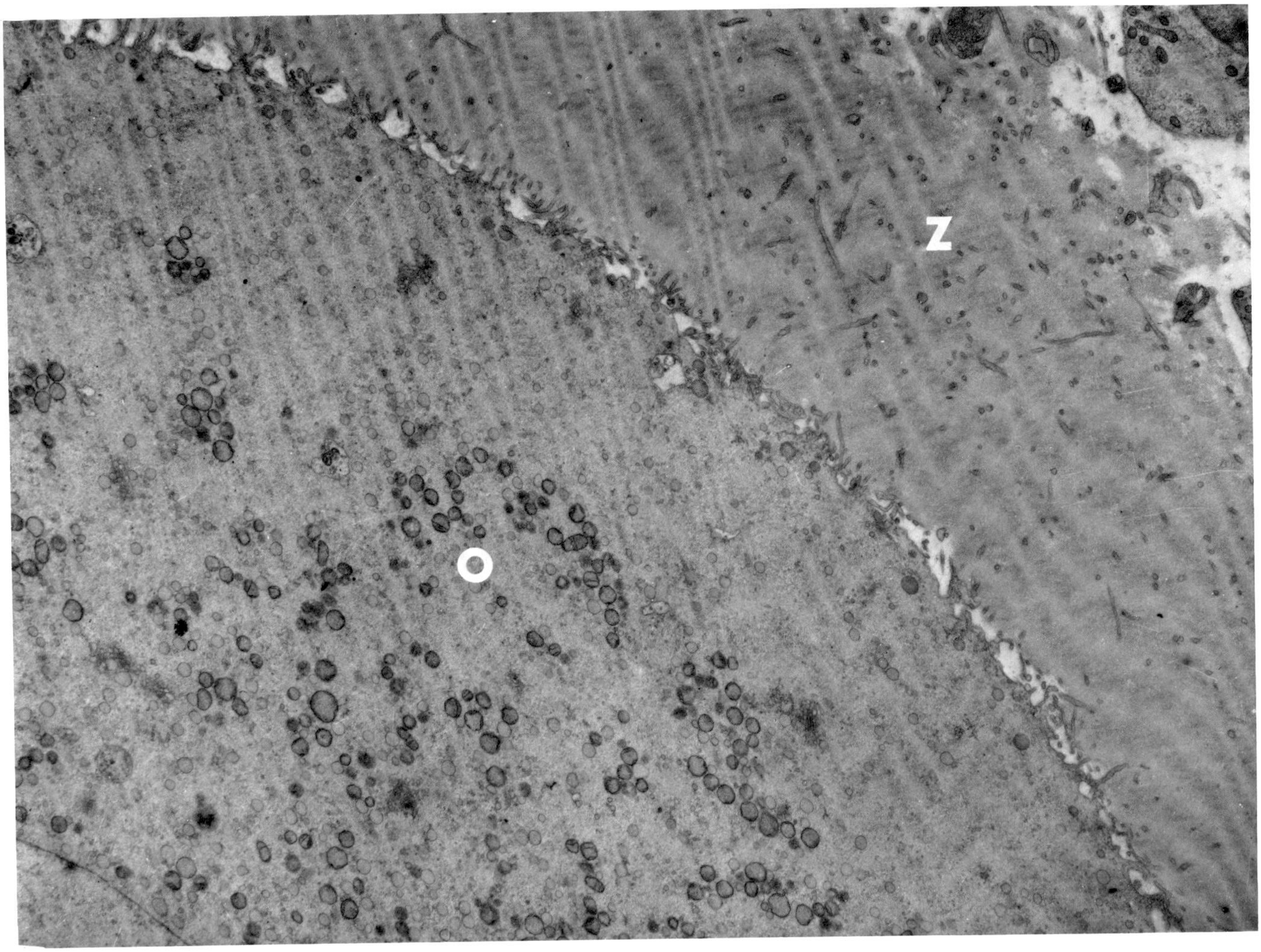

Figure 206. *Zona pellucida of human follicular oocyte.* At the end of its formation, the zona pellucida (Z) is seen as a 20- to 25-μ-thick membrane enveloping the oocyte surface. In specimens prepared for electron microscopy, the zona consists of a finely filamentous material of medium electron density. The irregular structures pervading this layer are the cytoplasmic projections of the cells of the cumulus oophorus, which traverse the zona to reach the surface of the oocyte (O), where they anchor by means of tight intercellular junctions. $\times$ 7500. *From* M. Baca and L. Zamboni. The fine structure of human follicular oocytes. *J. Ultrastruct. Res.* **18:** 354–391 (1967).

Coincidentally with the formation of the zona pellucida, the oocyte increases approximately threefold in its volume and its surface microvilli become prominent as they establish a close relationship with the villous extensions of the cumulus cells, suggesting a metabolic interrelationship.[2]

The maturing oocyte cytoplasm has numerically increased and better developed organelles (mitochondria, endoplasmic reticulum, and Golgi complexes) than do quiescent oocytes, reflecting increased protein synthesis.[2,3,6] Late in follicular growth the oocyte, surrounded by cumulus cells, detaches from the follicular wall and floats in the antral fluid. The oocyte destined to be ovulated enters telophase of the first meiotic division. Chromosomal reduction occurs by the formation of the first polar body, which contains one-half of the

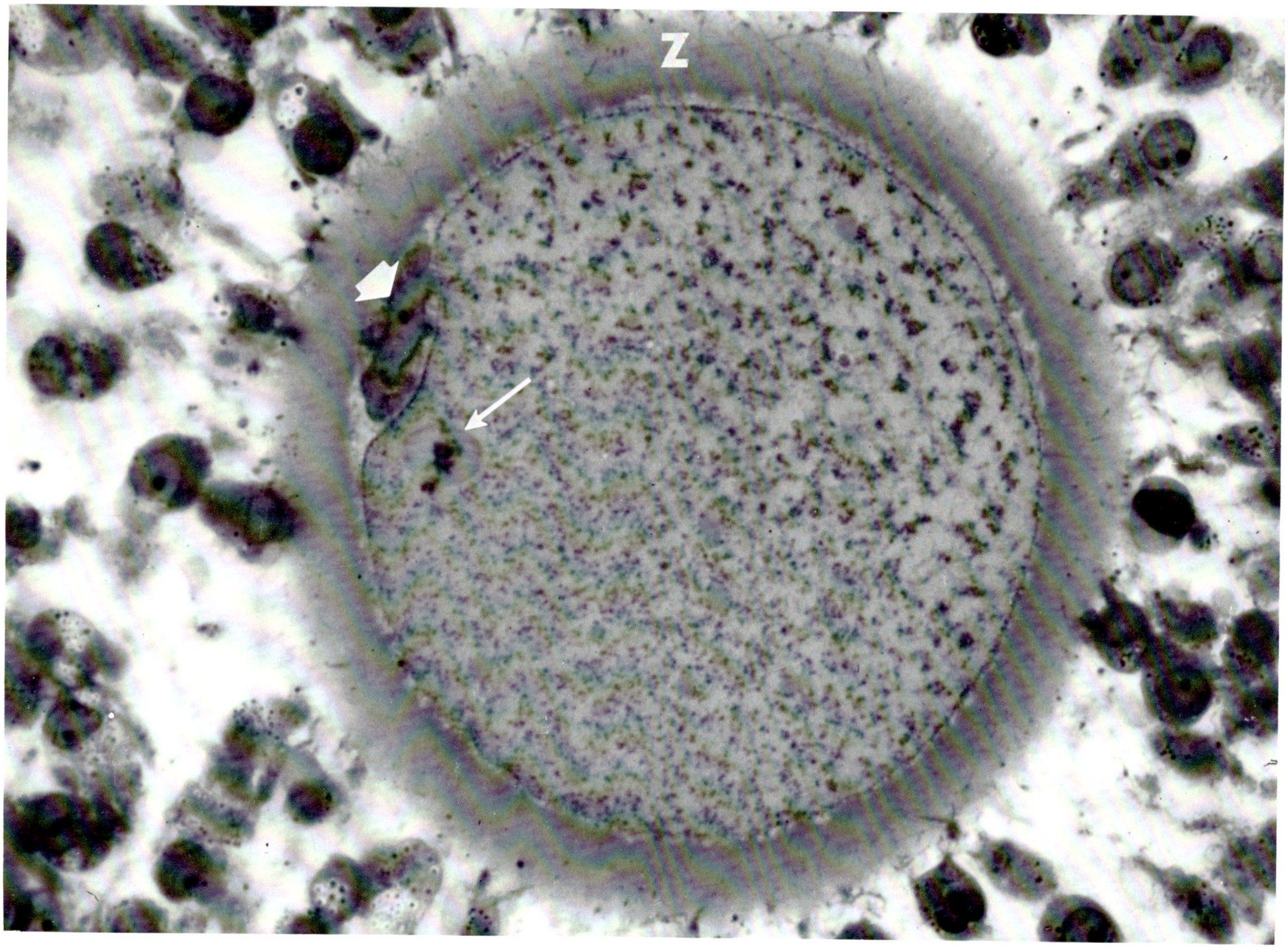

oocyte chromosomes and mucopolysaccharide-rich "cortical granules."[2,3] In the Fallopian tube the cumulus cells degenerate, leading to a gradual denudation of the oocyte, which contains the chromosomes arrested in metaphase on the equator of the meiotic spindle.

Figure 207. *Light micrograph of a human follicular oocyte.* The first polar body (short arrow) has been liberated and lies in the perivitelline space, which separates the oocyte from the zona pellucida (Z). The oocyte chromosomes are aligned on the equator of the meiotic spindle (long arrow). They will remain in this position until penetration of the fertilizing spermatozoon, when the second meiotic division will resume. The cells of the cumulus oophorus are more dispersed than in the previous stages. Some of them are undergoing regression, as shown by the presence of numerous fat droplets in the cytoplasm and pyknosis of nuclei. These features represent the onset of the denudation of the oocyte, a process that will be completed in the oviduct. × 1500. *From* M. Baca and L. Zamboni. The fine structure of human follicular oocytes. *J. Ultrastruct. Res.* **19:** 354–381 (1967).

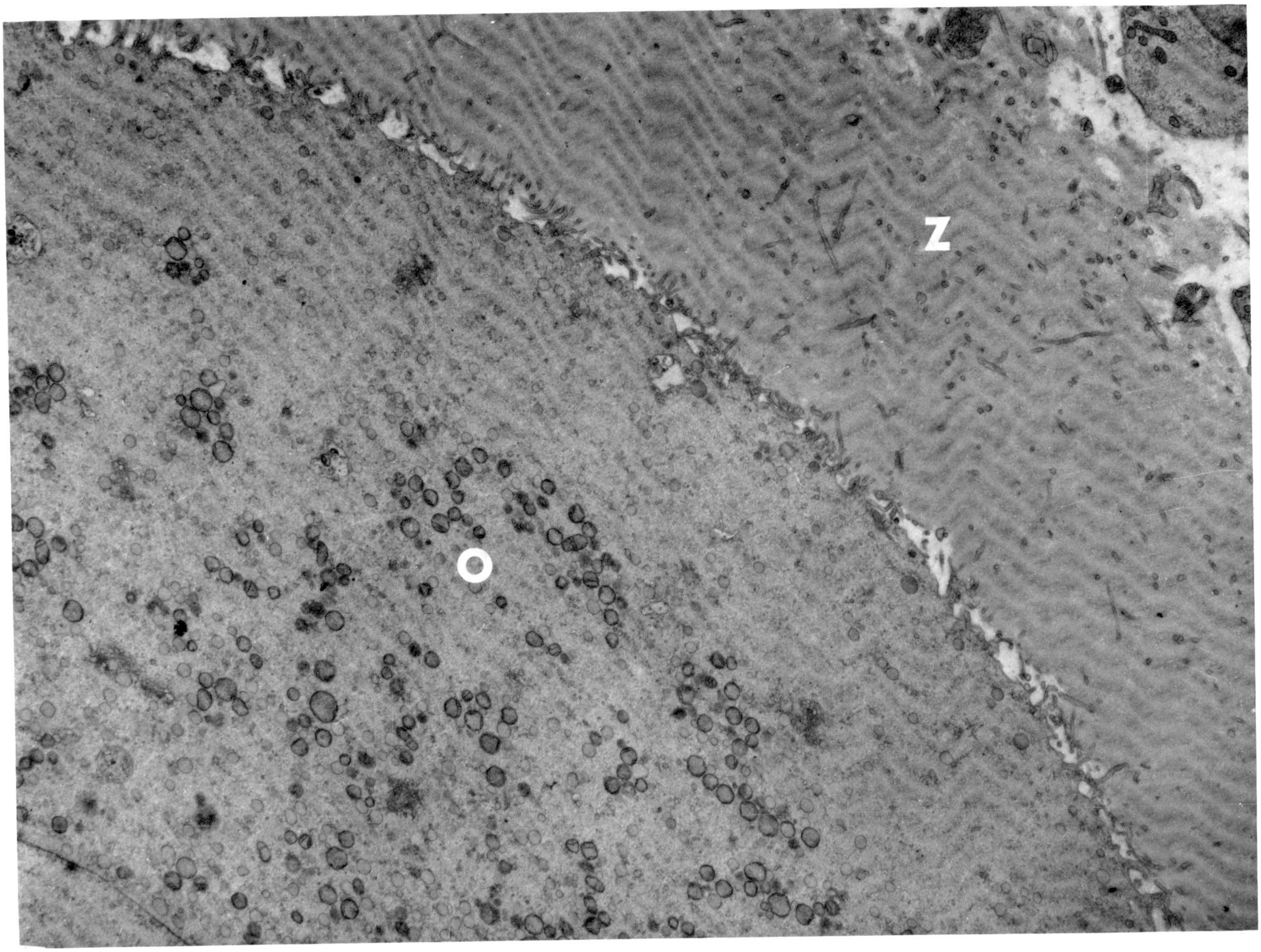

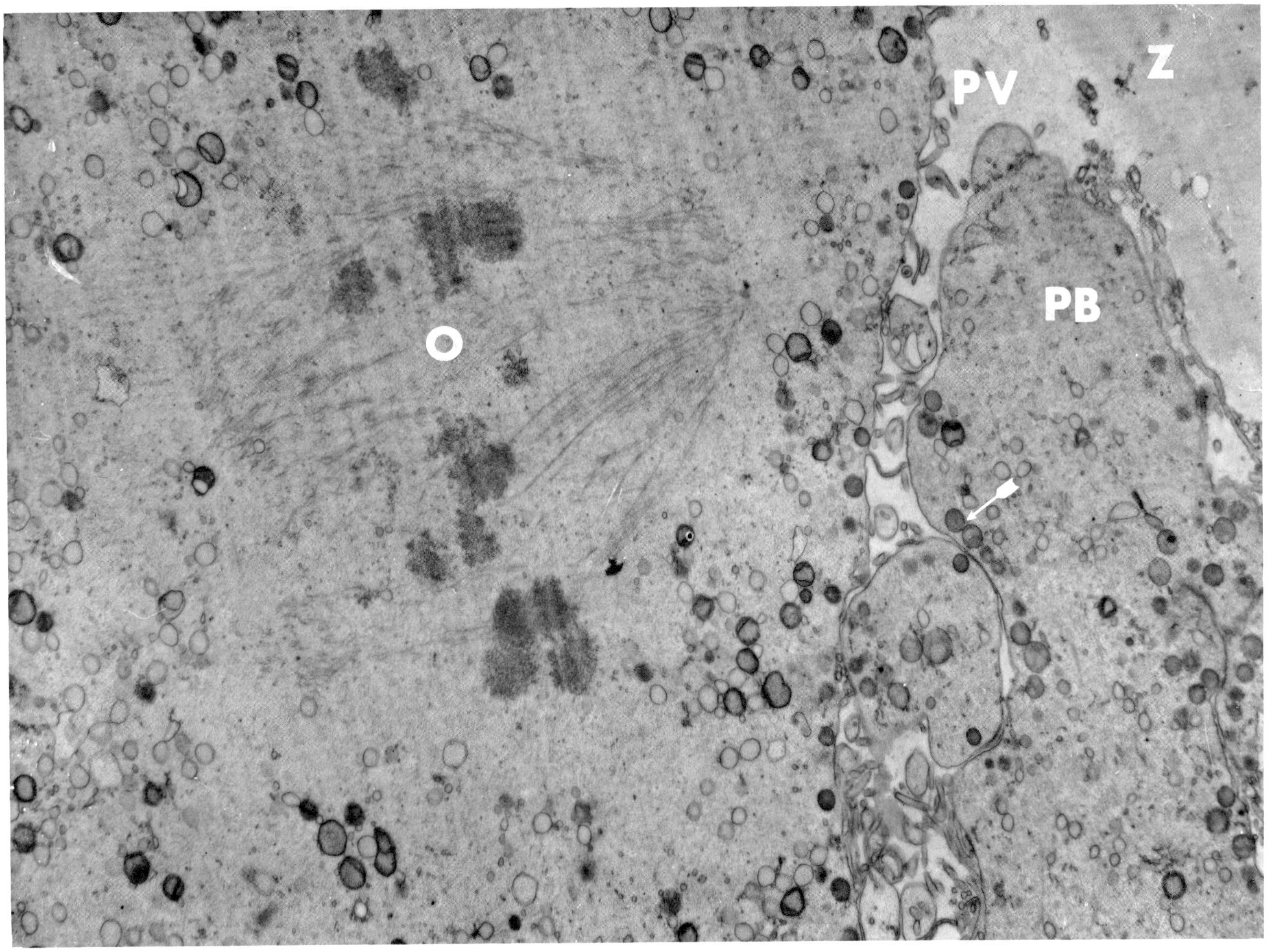

REFERENCES (Under the influence of FSH–Figure 207)

1. Bogumil, R. J., M. Ferin, J. Rootenberg, L. Speroff, and R. L. Vande Wiele. Mathematical studies of the human menstrual cycle. I. Formulation of a mathematical model. *J. Clin. Endocrinol Metab.* **35:** 126 (1972).
2. Zamboni, L. *Fine Morphology of Mammalian Fertitlization.* Harper & Row, New York, 1971.
3. Baca, M. and L. Zamboni. The fine structure of human follicular oocytes. *J. Ultrastruct. Res.* **19:** 354 (1967).
4. Wartenberg, H. and H. E. Stegner. Uber die elektronenmikroskopische Feinstruktur des menschlichen Ovarialeies. *Z. Zellforsch.* **52:** 450 (1960).
5. Motta, P. and E. Nesci. The "Call and Exner bodies" of mammalian ovaries with reference to the problem of rosette formation. *Arch. Anat. Microsc. Morphol. Exp.* **58:** 283 (1969).
6. Zamboni, L., D. R. Mishell, Jr. J. H. Bell, and M. Baca. Fine structure of the human ovum in the pronuclear stage. *J. Cell Biol.* **30:** 579 (1966).

Figure 208. *Electron micrograph illustrating a portion of the oocyte* shown in Figure 207. The first polar body (PB) and the zona pellucida (Z) are separated from the oocyte (O) by a distended perivitelline space (PV). The oocyte chromosomes appear as clumps of dense chromatin and lie on the equator of the metaphase spindle. Note the absence of centrioles at the spindle poles. A few cortical granules (arrow) are contained in the polar body. The presence of cortical granules is a criterion that can be utilized to differentiate the first polar body from the second, where cortical granules are usually absent[1] since they are liberated in the perivitelline space as soon as the sperm establishes contact with the egg, that is, before formation of the second polar body. × 16,000. *From* L. Zamboni (Ed.). *Fine Morphology of Mammalian Fertilization.* Harper & Row, New York, 1971, pp. 110–111.

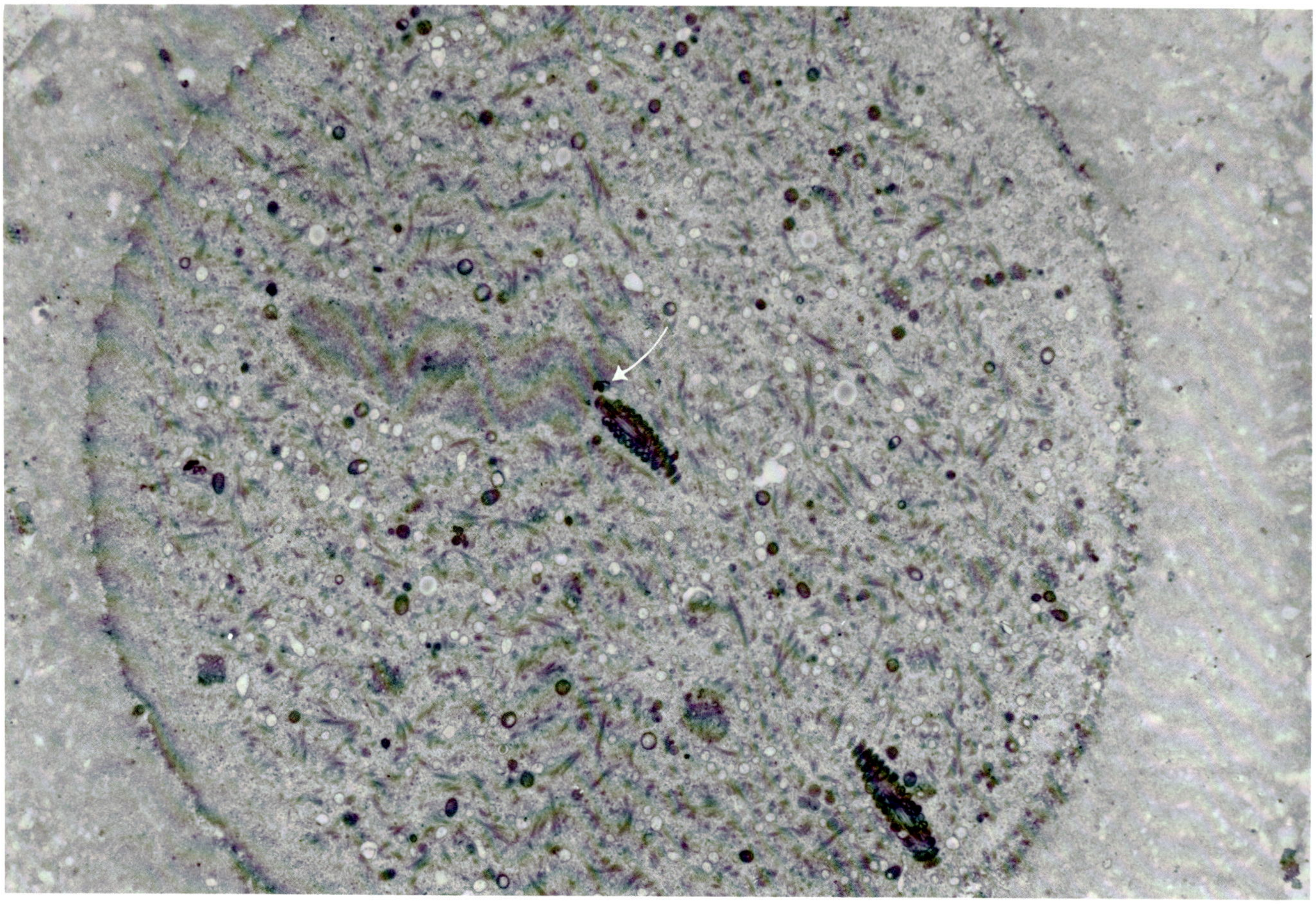

Figure 209. *Micrograph illustrating an early stage of activation of a mouse egg.* The ovum has been sectioned close to one pole and through an area containing the sperm head and middle piece. The male chromatin is dispersed but has retained its original, elongated shape. It is still associated with the middle piece through the interposition of the basal plate and proximal centriole (arrow). This micrograph was prepared from a mouse perfused 7 hours and 50 minutes after copulation and at an unknown interval after spontaneous ovulation. × 7000. *From* L. Zamboni (Ed.). *Fine Morphology of Mammalian Fertilization.* Harper & Row, New York, 1971, pp. 164–165.

REFERENCE (Figures 208–209)

1. Zamboni, L., D. R. Mishell, Jr., J. H. Bell, and M. Baca. Fine structure of the human ovum in the pronuclear stage. *J. Cell Biol.* **30:** 579 (1966).

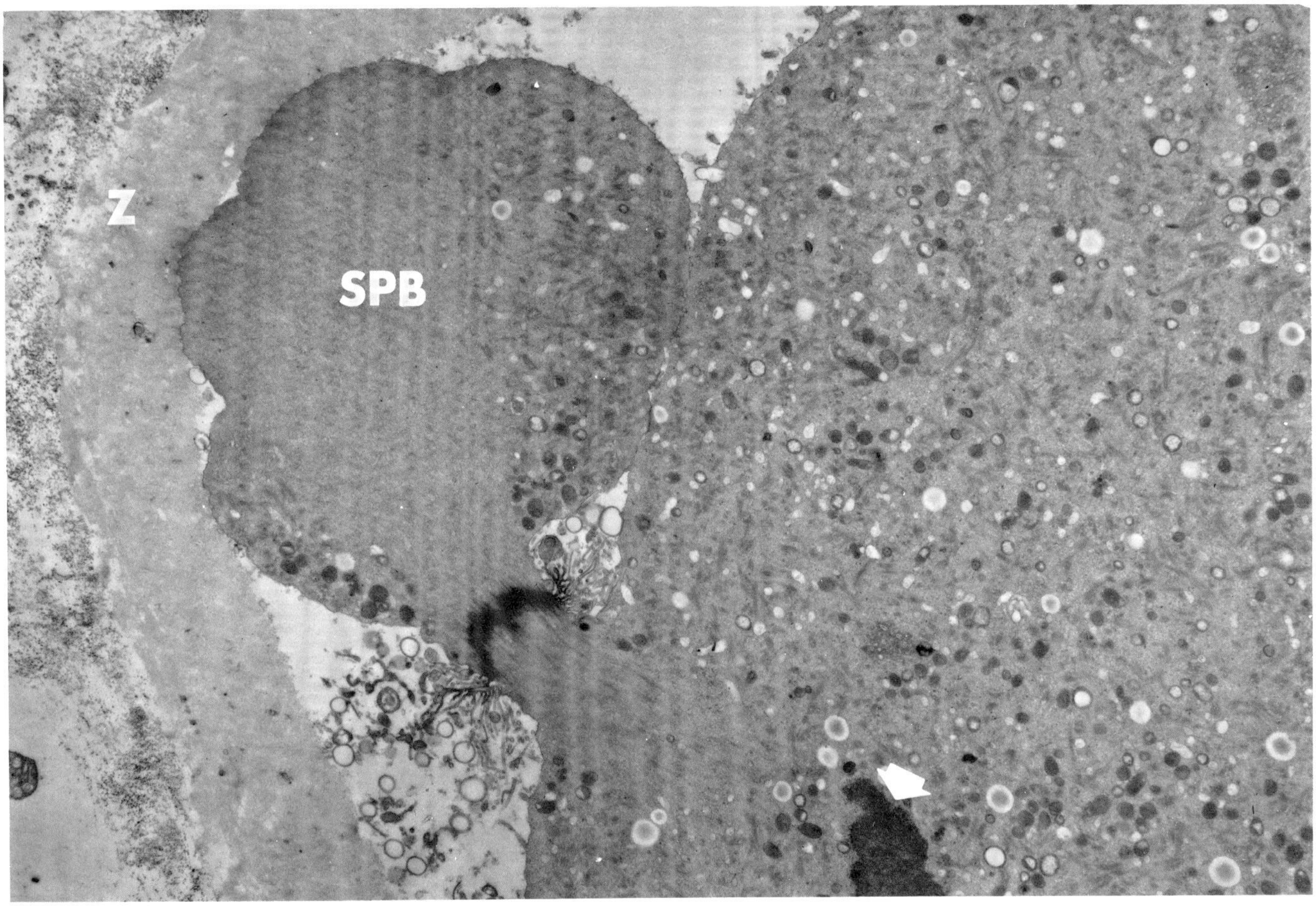

Figure 210. *Electron micrograph,* illustrating the liberation of the second polar body (SPB) into the perivitelline space (mouse ampulla). The polar body remains connected to the egg for a relatively long period of time, usually until the advanced pronuclear stage is reached.[4] The connection is seen in the form of an elongated cytoplasmic bridge containing the coated microtubules of the equatorial region of the spindle. As the polar body is being liberated, the maternal chromosomes remaining in the egg (arrow) begin to undergo the changes leading to their transformation into a female pronucleus. This micrograph was prepared from a mouse perfused 6 hours and 35 minutes after copulation and 4 hours and 15 minutes after induced ovulation. × 6000. Z: zona pellucida. *From* L. Zamboni (Ed.). *Fine Morphology of Mammalian Fertilization.* Harper & Row, New York, 1971, pp. 178–179.

55

Fertilization

After sperm penetration, the activated ovum (egg) enters the second meiotic division,[1,2] which occurs by the longitudinal division of each preactivated chromosome, half of which will be incorporated into the *second polar body.*[2] After the release of the latter, characteristically devoid of cortical nodules,[2] the egg enters the "pronucleus stage,"[2,3] resulting in the development of fertilization male and female pronuclei associated with prominent Golgi apparatuses.[1,2] In the subsequent metaphase of the first cleavage division, the diploid chromosomal content is reestablished and is followed by the formation of the first two blastomeres (or two-cell embryo).[2]

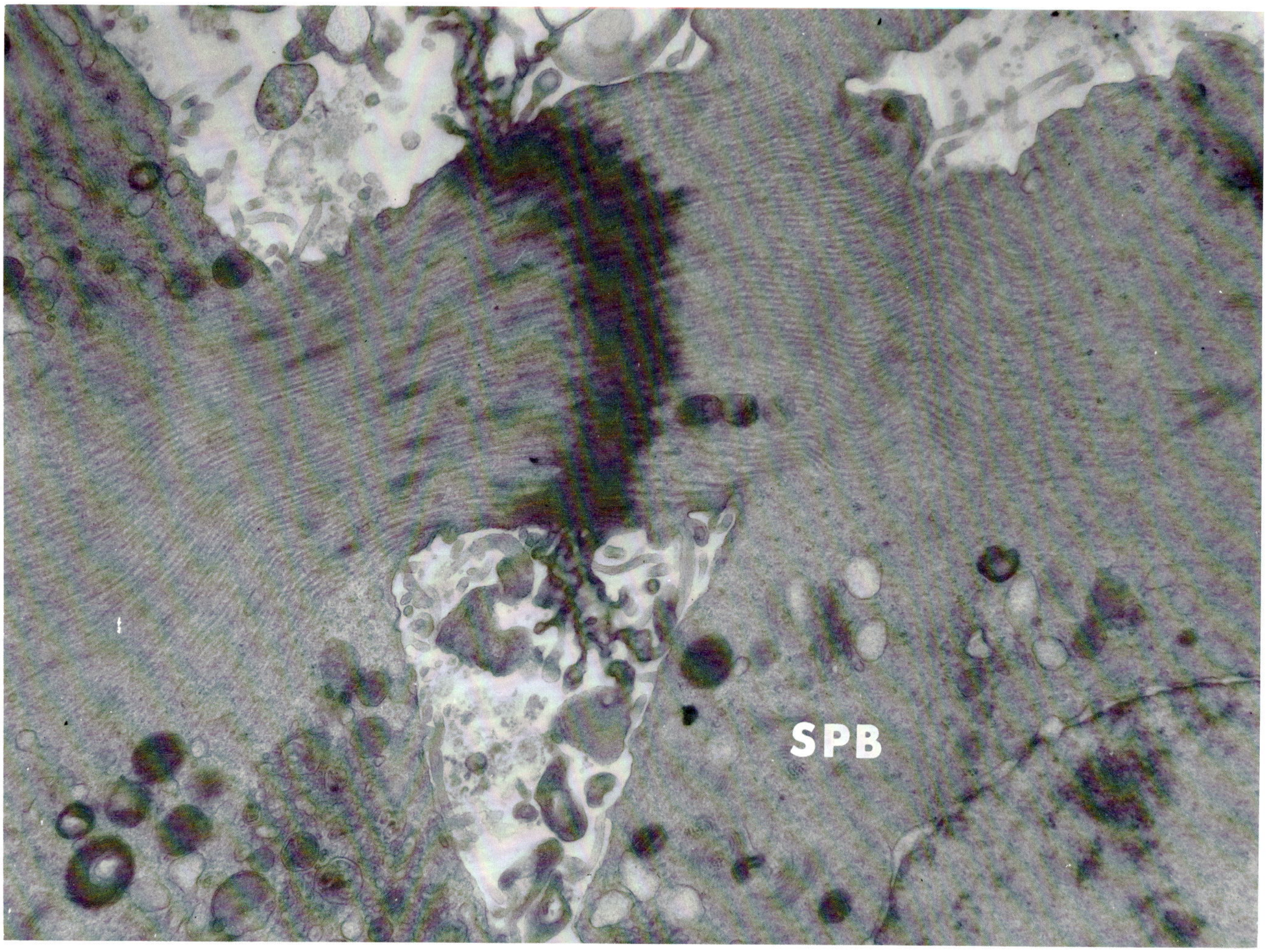

Figure 211. *The cytoplasm of the bridge connecting the egg to the second polar body* (SPB) is occupied almost exclusively by the microtubules of the meiotic spindle, coated in their equatorial segment and forming the structure referred to as the "mid-body." The compact arrangement of the microtubules in the central region of the bridges results from their inward sliding over one another at the time of the second polar body formation. At the stage illustrated in this micrograph, the sliding capacity of these microtubules has become saturated, and further contraction is prevented. This explains the persistence of the cytoplasmic bridge until late stages of activation.[4] A portion of the spheroidal nucleus of the polar body is visible in the lower right corner of the figure. This micrograph was prepared from a mouse perfused 6 hours and 35 minutes after copulation and 4 hours and 15 minutes after induced ovulation. × 26,500. *From* L. Zamboni (Ed.). *Fine Morphology of Mammalian Fertilization.* Harper & Row, New York, 1971, pp. 180–181.

REFERENCES (After sperm penetration–Figure 211)

1. Baca, M. and L. Zamboni. The fine structure of human follicular oocytes. *J. Ultrastruct. Res.* **19:** 354 (1967).
2. Zamboni, L. *Fine Morphology of Mammalian Fertilization.* Harper & Row, New York, 1971.
3. Zamboni, L., D. R. Mishell, Jr., J. H. Bell, and M. Baca. Fine structure of the human ovum in the pronuclear stage. *J. Cell Biol.* **30:** 579 (1966).
4. Stefanini, M., C. Oura, and L. Zamboni. Meiotic cleavage of the mammalian ovum. *J. Cell Biol.* **43:** 138a (1969).

56

Corpus Luteum

The corpus luteum is the principal site of progesterone synthesis with a peak of secretion between the 19th and 23rd days of the menstrual cycle. Its function is to prepare the endometrium for the reception of a prospective blastocyst. After the luteinizing hormone peak and the release of the ovulatory ovum,[1] the cells of both the granulosa and theca interna layers undergo a series of biomorphologic modifications called luteinization, through which the ovulated follicle is transformed into a corpus luteum. In addition to progesterone production, the corpus luteum is the site of estrogen biosynthesis, as indicated by the presence of aromatizing enzymes[2] in the microsomal fraction of lutein cells, principally of thecal origin, and by the in-vitro synthesis of estrone and 17-β-estradiol[3] by this fraction.

In the first few days (proliferative stage) after ovulation the granulosa cells enlarge, with a gradual increase in their organellar content, especially of agranular endoplasmic reticulum.[4] The theca interna cells have greater mitotic activity and vascularity, and their cytoplasmic organelles also increase in number and complexity.

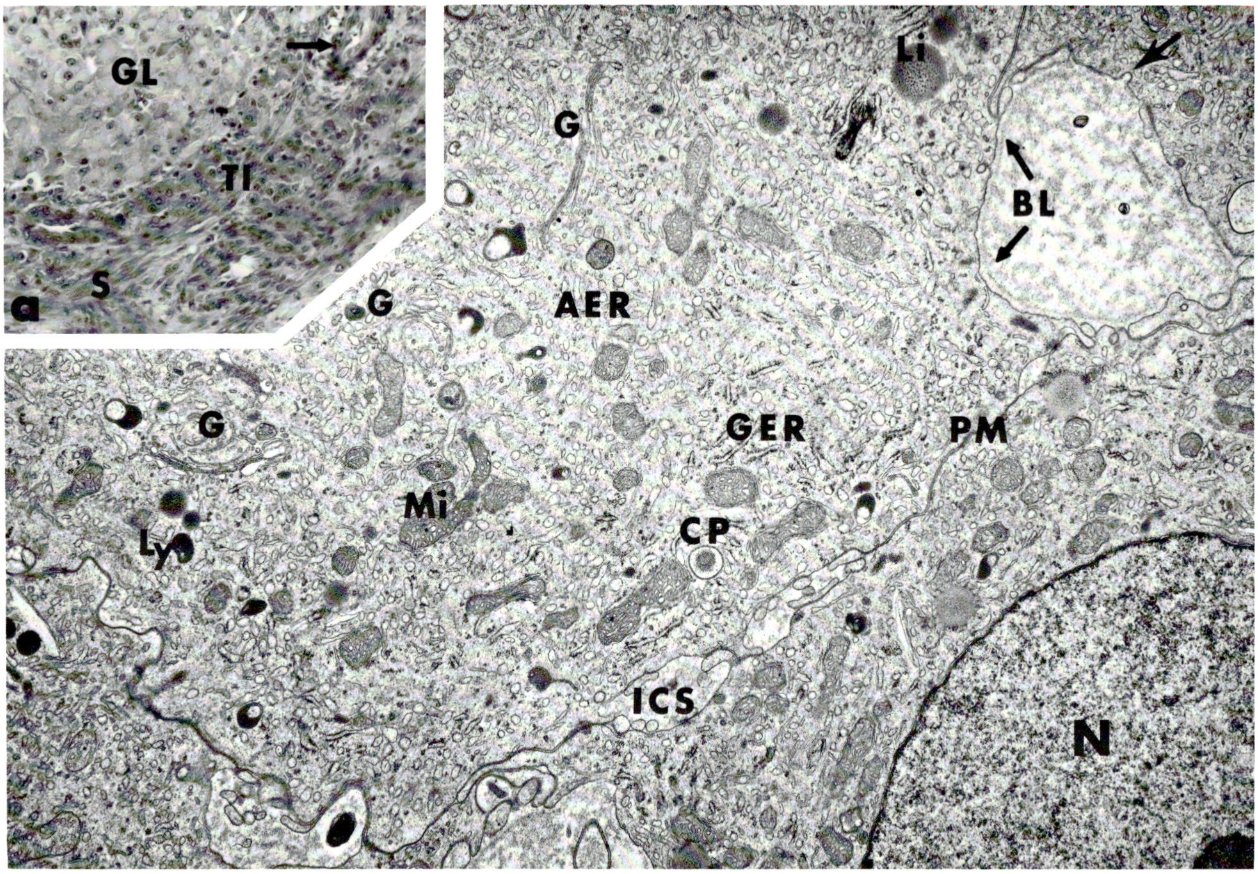

Figure 212a. *In the following vascularization phase* the corpus luteum contains well-developed granulosa lutein cells (GL), and the fibrovascular (arrow) stroma (S) from the theca interna (TI) reaches the central congulum. (H & E stain, × 30.)

Figure 212. *Ultrastructurally, in the vascularization stage,* typical granulosa lutein cells contain a profusion of agranular endoplasmic reticulum. By means of ultracytoenzymologic techniques, the AER has been shown to contain NAD-dependent 3-β-hydroxysteroid dehydrogenase and NADP-dependent glucose-6-phosphate dehydrogenase activity in a perilipidic and perimitochondrial location,[5] suggesting that the agranular endoplasmic reticulum is the site of steroidogenesis.[6] In addition, the luteinized cells acquire abundant mitochondria (Mi), providing a source of energy for hormonal biosynthesis, as well as Golgi (G), free and bound ribosomes (GER), and lipid droplets (Li),[4,6-9] these droplets being the site of storage of steroid hormone precursors such as cholesterol and its esters.[6] These ultrastructural features found in the granulosa lutein cells are characteristic of active steroidogenic cells in general, and the luteinized granulosal cells are believed to be the major source of progesterone production. Concomitantly with the penetration of the fibrovascular stroma, stellate, deeply acidophilic cells ("K cells")[10] appear in the theca and later in the granulosa cell layer. Contrary to earlier opinions, these cells lack both histochemical[11] and ultrastructural[4,6] evidence of active steroidogenic activity and are considered to be perivascular macrophages[6] or metabolically altered cells of thecal origin.[4] × 3600. N: nucleus of granulosa lutein cell; Ly: lysosomes; CP: intracytoplasmic spherical plasma membrane complexes (annular nexus); ICS: intercellular space; PM: plasma membrane; arrow: micropinocytic vesicle; BL: basal lamina. *From* T. Okagaki. Professor of Pathology, University of Minnesota, Department of Obstetrics and Gynecology, Box 395, Mayo Memorial Building, Minneapolis, Minn. 55455.

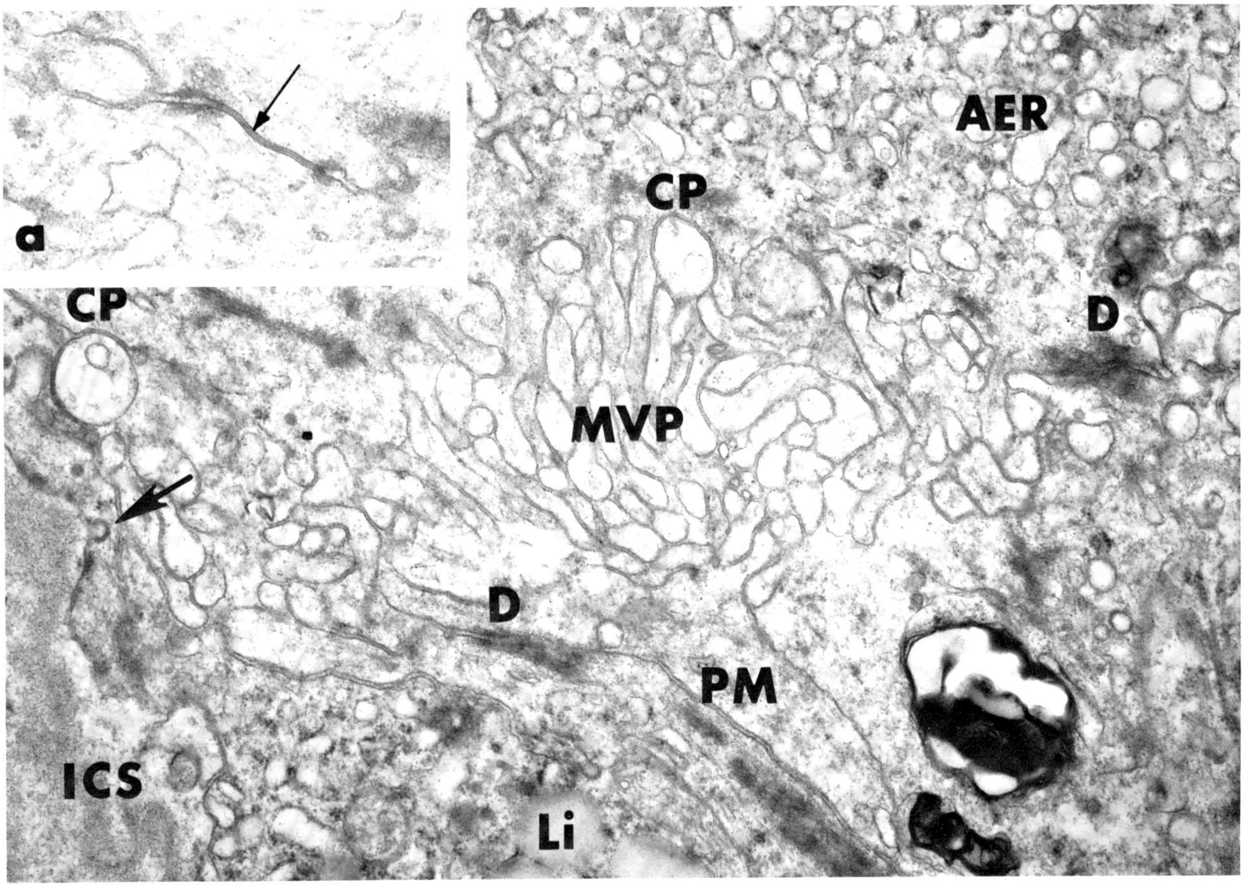

Figure 213. *In the third phase* (maturation) both the granulosa and theca lutein cells become larger, with prominent organellar content coinciding with the maximum serum progesterone levels,[6] and fibroblastic organization of the central coagulum begins. Characteristically, lutein cells have closely apposed plasma membranes (PM) reinforced by desmosomal (D) and pentalaminar tight junctional (nexus) complexes.[4,6,9] The most unusual feature of the luteinized granulosa cells are conspicuous intercellular and pericapillary, microvillous, cytoplasmic extensions (MVP),[4,6,9,12] which are thought to play a role in the transport of steroid hormones into the adjacent capillaries.[4,9,12] × 25,600. CP: folded, spherical plasma membrane complexes (annular nexus); AER: agranular endoplasmic reticulum; Li: lipid droplets; arrow: micropinocytic vesicle; ICS: intercellular space.

Figure 213a. *Granulosa lutein cell* with a pentalaminar tight junctional nexus (arrow). × 34,000.

REFERENCES (The corpus luteum—Figure 213a)

1. Bogumil, R. J., M. Ferin, J. Rootenberg, L. Speroff, and R. L. Vande Wiele. Mathematical studies of the human menstrual cycle. I. Formulation of a mathematical model. *J. Clin. Endocrinol Metab.* **35:** 126 (1972).
2. Arceo, R. B. and K. J. Ryan. Conversion of androst-4-ene-3,17-dione-4-^{14}C to estrogens by subcellular fractions of the human corpus luteum of the normal cycle. *Acta Endocrinol.* **56:** 225 (1967).
3. Savard, K., J. M. Marsh, and B. F. Rice. Gonadotropins and ovarian steroidogenesis. *Rec. Prog. Horm. Res.* **21:** 285 (1965).
4. Adams, E. C. and A. T. Hertig. Studies on the human corpus luteum. I. Observations on the ultrastructure of development and regression of the luteal cells during the menstrual cycle. *J. Cell Biol.* **41:** 696 (1969).
5. Laffargue, P., A. Chamlin, and L. Adéchy-Benkoel. Localization probable en microscopie éléctronique de la 3-β-hydroxystéroide déshydrogénase, de la glucose-6-phosphate déshydrogénase et de la NADH diaphorase dans le corps jaune ovarien de la femme. *J. Microsc.* **13:** 235 (1972).
6. Gillim, S. W., A. K. Christensen, and C. E. McLennan. Fine structure of the human menstrual corpus luteum at its stage of maximum secretory activity. *Am. J. Anat.* **126:** 409 (1969).
7. Green, J. A. and M. Maqueo. Ultrastructure of the human ovary. I. The luteal cell during the menstrual cycle. *Am. J. Obstet. Gynecol.* **92:** 946 (1965).
8. Tokida, A. Electron microscopic studies on the corpora lutea obtained from normal human ovaries. *Mie Med. J.* **15:** 27 (1965).
9. Crisp, T. M., D. A. Dessouky, and F. R. Denys. The fine structure of the human corpus luteum of early pregnancy and during the progestational phase of the menstrual cycle. *Am. J. Anat.* **127:** 37 (1970).
10. White, R. F., A. T. Hertig, J. Rock, and E. C. Adams. Histological and histochemical observations on the corpus luteum of human pregnancy with special reference to corpora lutea associated with early normal and abnormal ova. *Contrib. Embryol.* **34:** 55 (1951).
11. Feinberg, R. and R. B. Cohen. A comparative histochemical study of the ovarian stromal lipid band, stromal theca cell, and normal ovarian follicular apparatus. *Am. J. Obstet. Gynec.* **92:** 958 (1965).
12. Green, J. A., J. A. Gracilazo, and M. Maqueo. Ultrastructure of the human ovary. III. Canaliculi of the corpus luteum. *Am. J. Obstet. Gynecol.* **102:** 57 (1968).

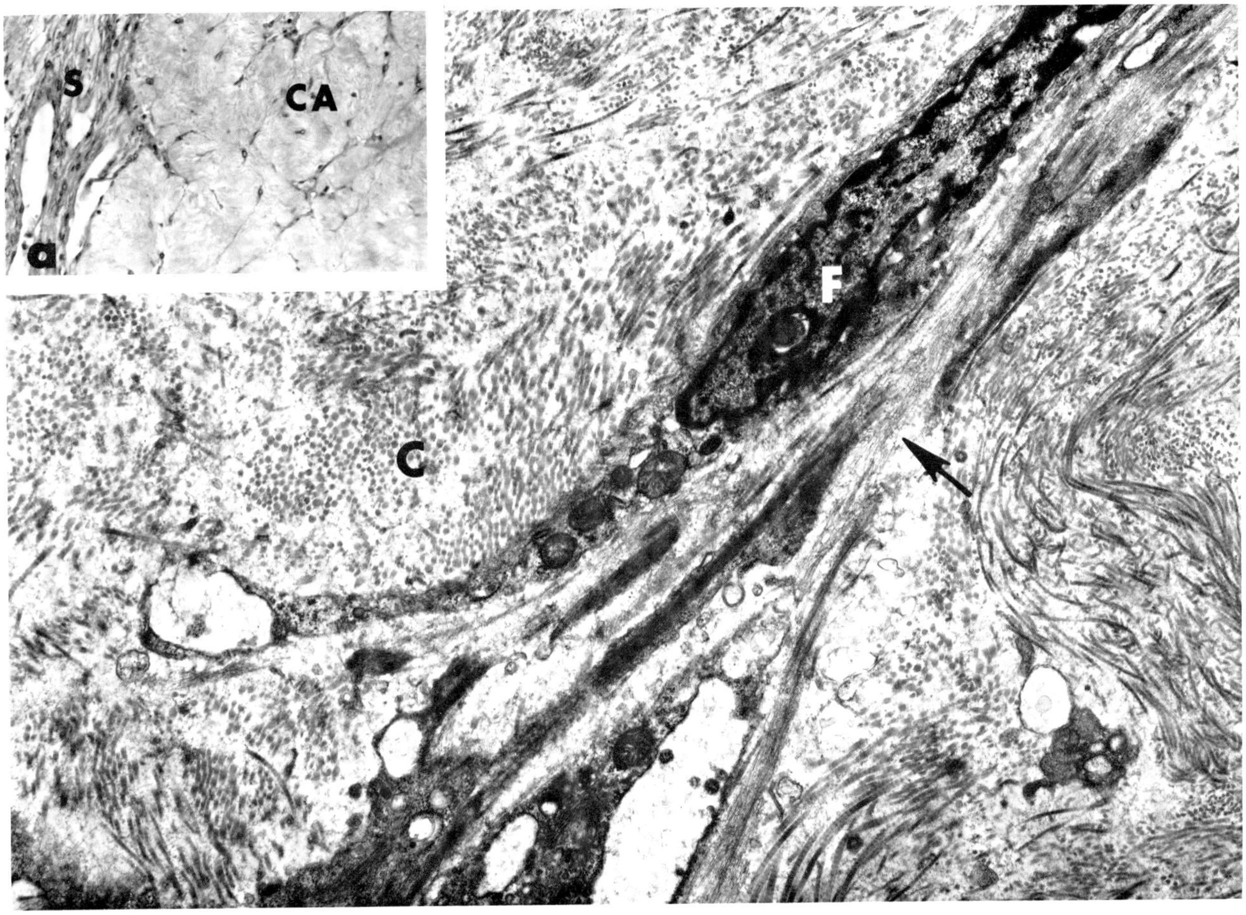

57

Corpus Albicans

If conception does not supervene, luteolysis (regression phase) occurs, with a decrease in the endoplasmic reticulum and ribosomes and an increase in cytolysosomes[1] and hydrolytic enzymes, accompanied by the collapse of the luteal body and its vascular skeleton.

Figure 214a. *Subsequently, a gradual invasion* of connective tissue occurs, resulting in the transformation of the corpus luteum into the hyalinized corpus albicans (CA). (H & E stain, × 30.) S: surrounding cellular stroma.

Figure 214. *Ultrastructurally, the corpus albicans* contains masses of collagen fibers (C) and degenerating fibroblasts (F), rich in precollagen fibers (arrow). × 9800.

58

Corpus Luteum of Gestation

The corpus luteum of gestation, although essentially similar in ultrastructure[2-6] the corpus luteum of menstruation, has certain distinctive features.[3,5-7] The gestational granulosa lutein cells have a larger cellular volume and are polyploid.[7] There is an increase in granular and agranular endoplasmic reticulum, numerous concentric whorls are formed, and the numbers of lysosomes, pleomorphic mitochondria, and homogeneous, globular (colloid) bodies increase.[4,6] These features are thought to be related to the high levels of chorionic gonadotropins that occur in early gestation.[3] In the theca lutein cells these changes are comparatively less conspicuous than in the granulosal cells, and the prominent, microvillous surface specialization characteristic of the granulosa lutein cells is uniformly lacking. Contrary to previous reports, no fine structural evidence of involutional changes is seen in either the early or the late (term) corpora lutea vera.[3,4,6]

REFERENCES (If conception does not supervene—Figure 215)

1. Adams, E. C. and A. T. Hertig. Studies on the human corpus luteum. I. Observations on the ultrastructure of development and regression of the luteal cells during the menstrual cycle. *J. Cell Biol.* **41:** 699 (1969).
2. Tokida, A. Electron microscopic studies on the corpora lutea obtained from normal human ovaries. *Mie Med. J.* **15:** 27 (1965).
3. Crisp, T. M., D. A. Dessouky, and F. R. Denys. The fine structure of the human corpus luteum of early pregnancy and during the progestational phase of the menstrual cycle. *Am. J. Anat.* **127:** 37 (1970).
4. Green, J. A., J. A. Carcilazo, and M. Maqueo. Ultrastructure of the human ovary. II. The luteal cell at term. *Am. J. Obstet. Gynecol.* **99:** 855 (1967).
5. Pedersen, P. H. and J. F. Larsen. The ultrastructure of the human granulosal lutein cell of the first trimester of gestation. *Acta Endocrinol.* **58:** 481 (1968).
6. Adams, E. C. and A. T. Hertig. Studies on the human corpus luteum. II. Observation on the ultrastructure of luteal cells during pregnancy. *J. Cell Biol.* **41:** 716 (1969).
7. Stangel, J. J., R. M. Richart, T. Okagaki, and G. Cottral. Nuclear DNA content of luteinized cells of the human ovary. *Am. J. Obstet. Gynecol.* **108:** 543 (1970).

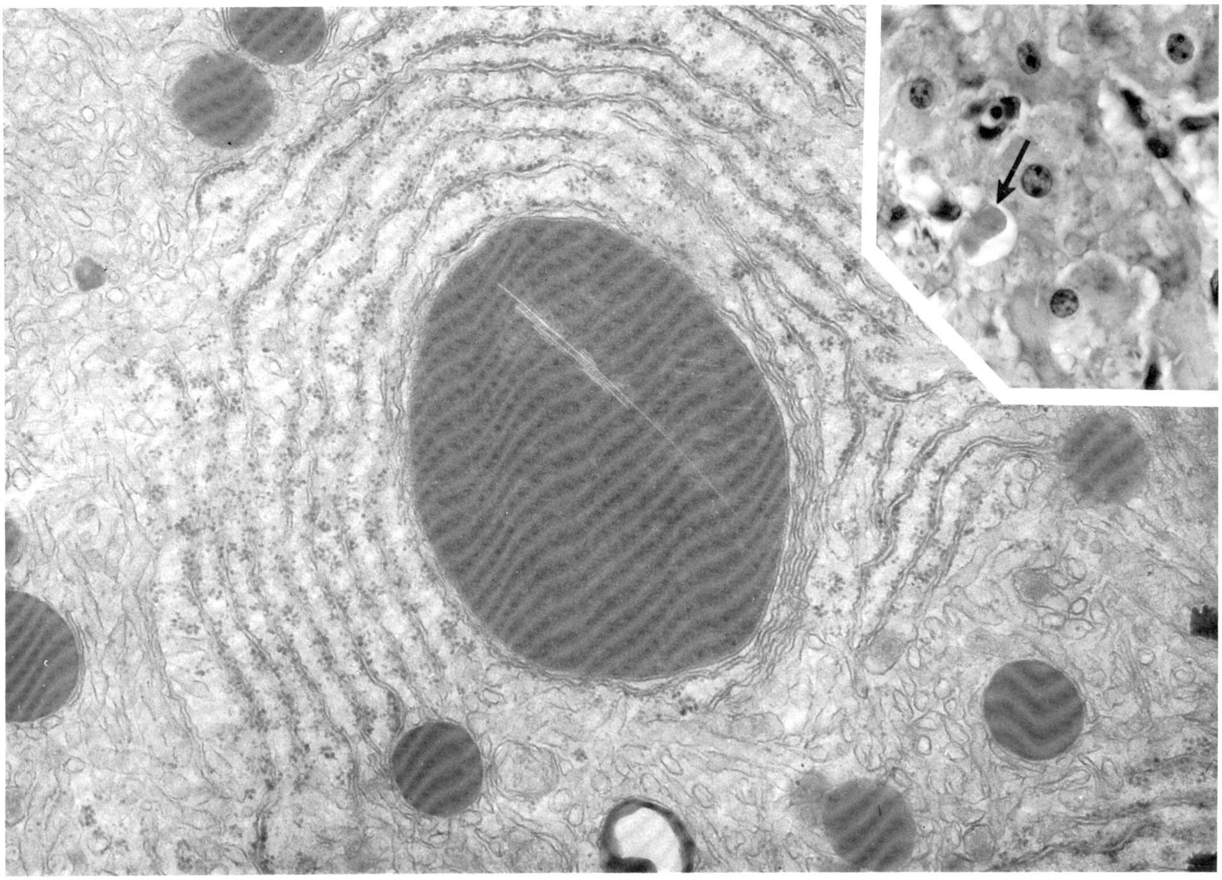

Figure 215a. *Corpus luteum of gestation (15th week of pregnancy).* Light photomicrograph illustrating a "colloid body" arrow) in a granulosa lutein cell. (H & E stain, × 120.)

Figure 215. *A hyaline (colloid) body* in a luteal cell from a 16-week pregnancy. Note needlelike crystals within the homogeneous, electron-opaque material. Some smaller hyaline bodies such as this one are surrounded by granular endoplasmic reticulum, but other, larger ones are not. × 22,000. *From* E. C. Adams and A. T. Hertig. Studies on the human corpus luteum. II. Observations on the ultrastructure of luteal cells during pregnancy. *J. Cell Biol.* **41:** 716–735 (1969).

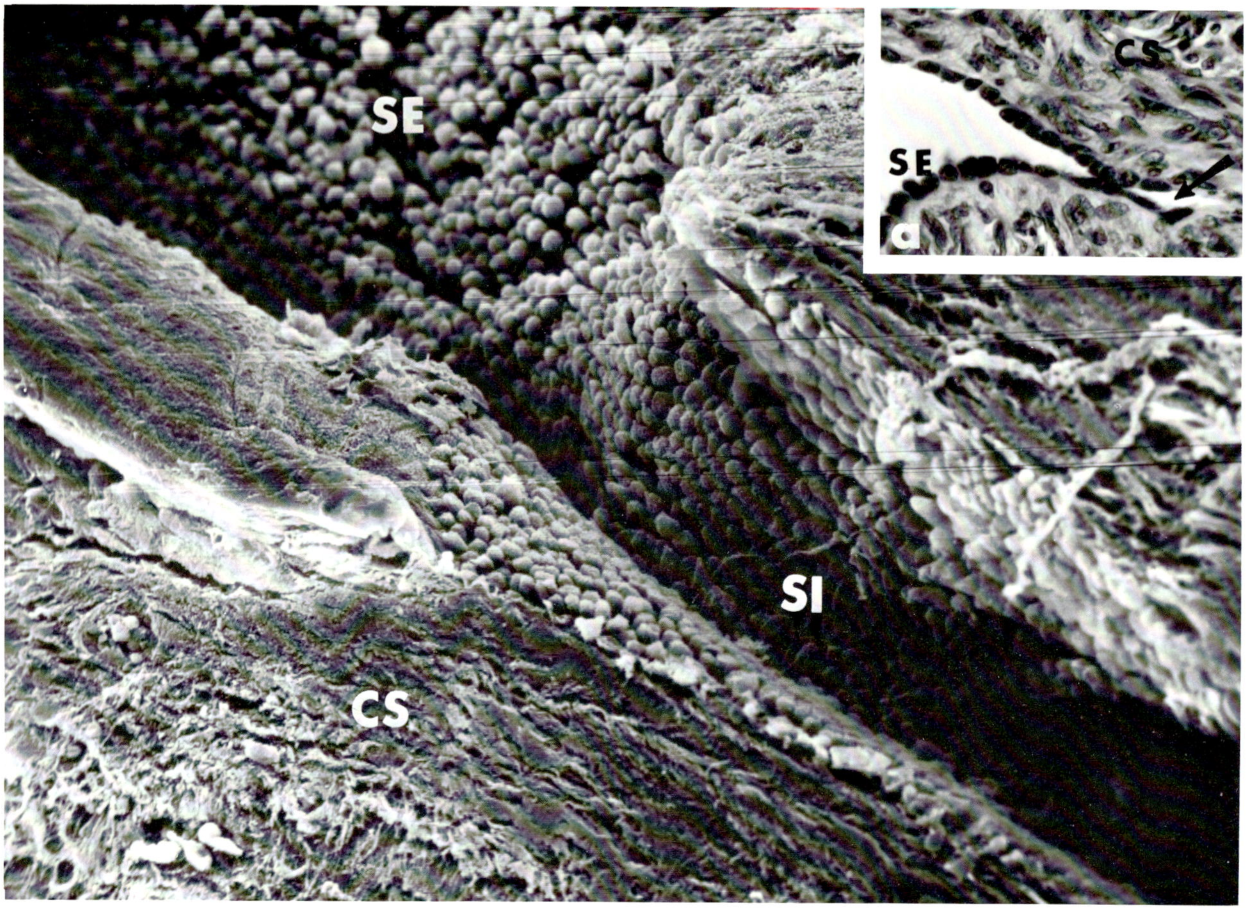

59

Surface Epithelium

Figure 216a. *Ovary from a 42-year-old woman.* The ovarian surface (SE), covered by a single layer of low cuboidal epithelium, often invaginates (arrow) into the cortical stroma (CS). (H & E stain, × 12.)

Figure 216. *Ovary from a 38-year-old woman.* With the scanning electron microscope the ovarian surface epithelium (SE) appears as a tightly packed, dome-shaped cell population with deep extensions (Si) into the cortical substance (CS). × 360.

The ovarian surface epithelium in man, rodents, and many other mammals consists of a flattened to cuboidal celomic layer of cells which, both histologically and ultrastructurally,[1-7] appears similar to extragonadal mesothelial membranes[8,9] and to embryonal mesothelium.[10] The ultrastructural features of ovarian surface epithelium are considered to be primarily related to active fluid and ion transport, occurring partly through intercellular spaces and partly through surface pinocytosis.

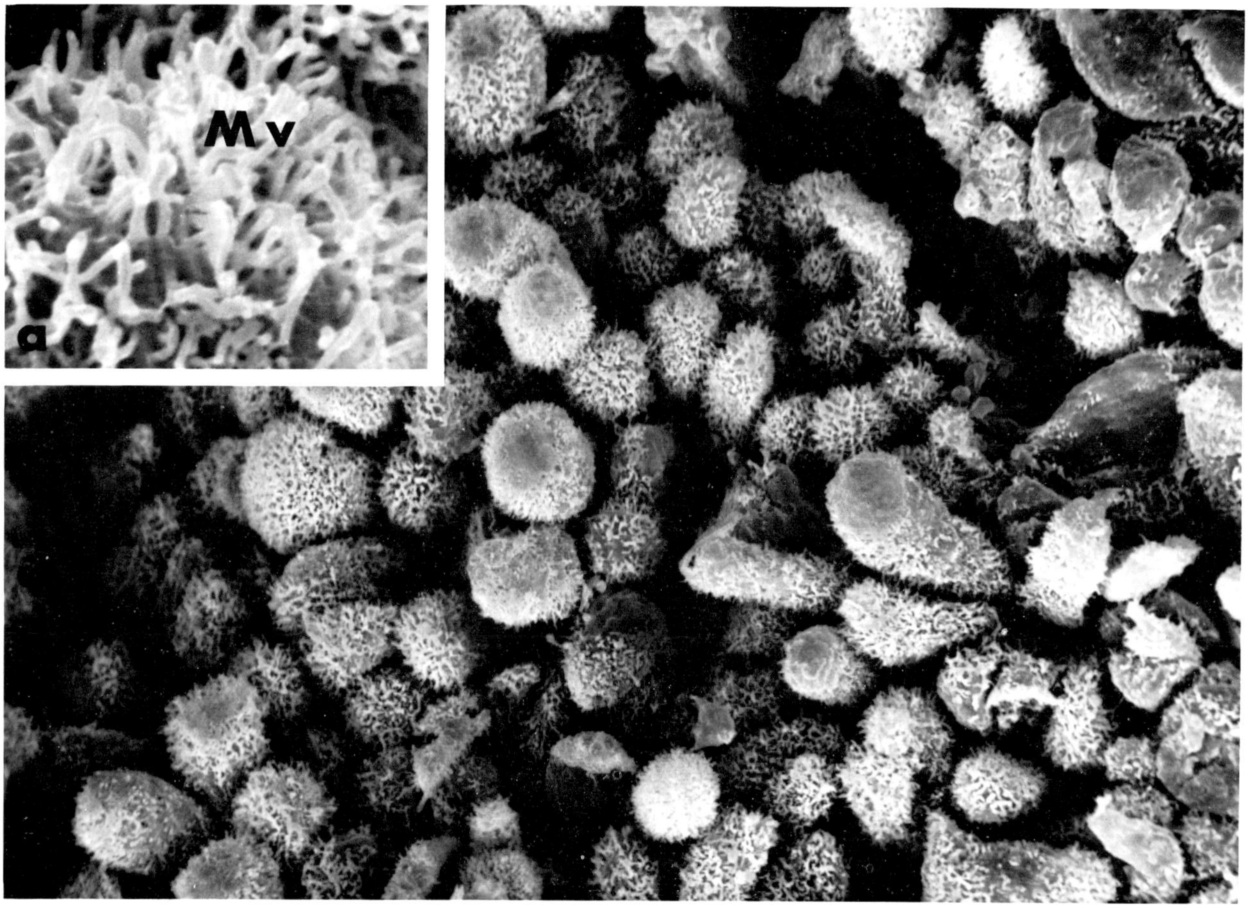

Figure 217. *Higher magnification of Figure 216.* The characteristic features of the ovarian celomic epithelium include the presence of dome-shaped apices covered by generally abundant, surface microvilli. × 2000.

Figure 217a. *Detailed view* of slender and often branching surface microvilli (Mv). × 12,000. *From* A. Ferenczy and R. M. Richart. Scanning electron microscopy of the human female genital tract. *N.Y. State J. Med.* (in press).

REFERENCES (The ovarian surface epithelium—Figure 217a)

1. Wischnitzer, S. The ultrastructure of the germinal epithelium of the mouse ovary. *J. Morphol.* **117:** 387 (1965).
2. Weakley, B. S. Differentiation of the surface epithelium of the hamster ovary. An electron microscopic study. *J. Anat.* **105:** 129 (1969).
3. Gondos, B. Ultrastructure of the germinal epithelium during oogenesis in the rabbit. *J. Exp. Zool.* **172:** 465 (1969).
4. Papadaki, L. and J. O. W. Beilby. The fine structure of the surface epithelium of the human ovary. *J. Cell Sci.* **8:** 445 (1971).
5. Ebe, T. and S. Kobayashi (Eds.). *Fine Structure of Human Cells and Tissues.* John Wiley & Sons, New York, 1972, pp. 210–211.
6. Motta, P., D. D. Cherney, and L. J. Didio. Scanning and transmission electron microscopy of the ovarian surface in mammals with special reference to ovulation. *J. Submicrosc. Cytol.* **3:** 85 (1971).
7. Ferenczy, A. and R. M. Richart. Scanning electron microscopy of the human female genital tract. *N.Y. State J. Med.* (in press).
8. Baradi, A. F. and J. Hope. Observations on ultrastructure of rabbit mesothelium. *Exp. Cell Res.* **34:** 33 (1964).
9. Stoebner, P., G. Miech, A. Sengel, and J. P. Witz. Notions d'ultrastructure pleurale. I. L'hyperplasie mésothéliale. *Presse Med.* **78:** 1179 (1970).
10. Hesseldahl, H. and J. F. Larsen. Ultrastructure of human yolk sac: endoderm, mesenchyme, tubules and mesothelium. *Am. J. Anat.* **126:** 315 (1969).

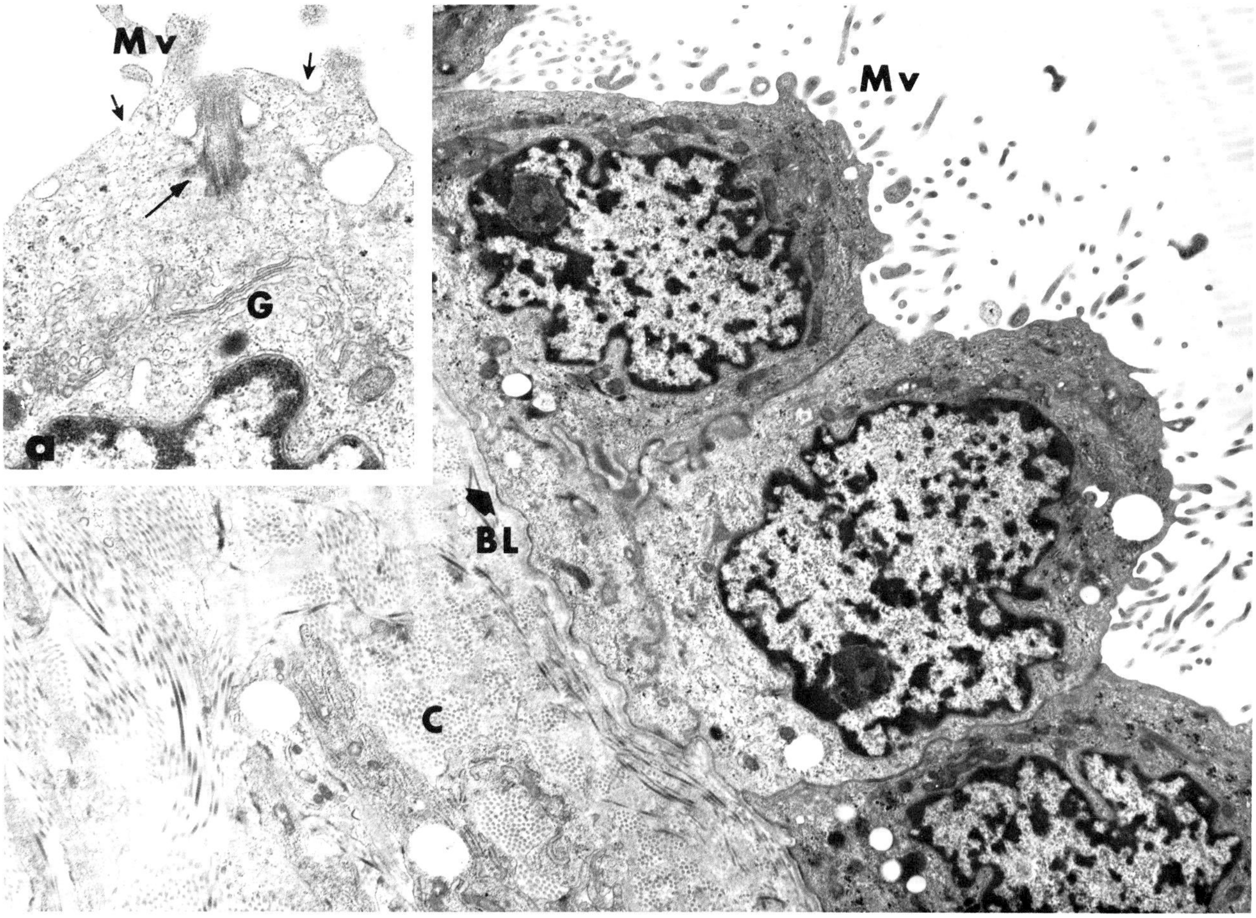

Figure 218. *Ovary from a 39-year-old woman.* The low cuboidal surface epithelium has numerous, often branching, microvilli (Mv), and the cytoplasm contains well-developed organelles in a perinuclear location. The nuclei have indented nuclear membranes and peripheral nucleoli. Lateral plasma membranes are straight or convoluted, reinforced by luminal junctional complexes and scattered desmosomes, but are occasionally widely separated, resulting in greatly dilated intercellular spaces. A well-defined basal lamina (BL) separates the cells from the underlying collagenous (C) albuginea. × 6400.

Figure 218a. *Ovary from a 33-year-old woman.* Surface microvilli (Mv) are associated with pinocytic vesicles (short arrows) and occasional single cilia.[1-3] Electron photomicrograph of a developing supranuclear cilium in close relationship with the Golgi (G). The ciliary basal body contains satellite processes (long arrow) and ciliary vesicles. × 22,000.

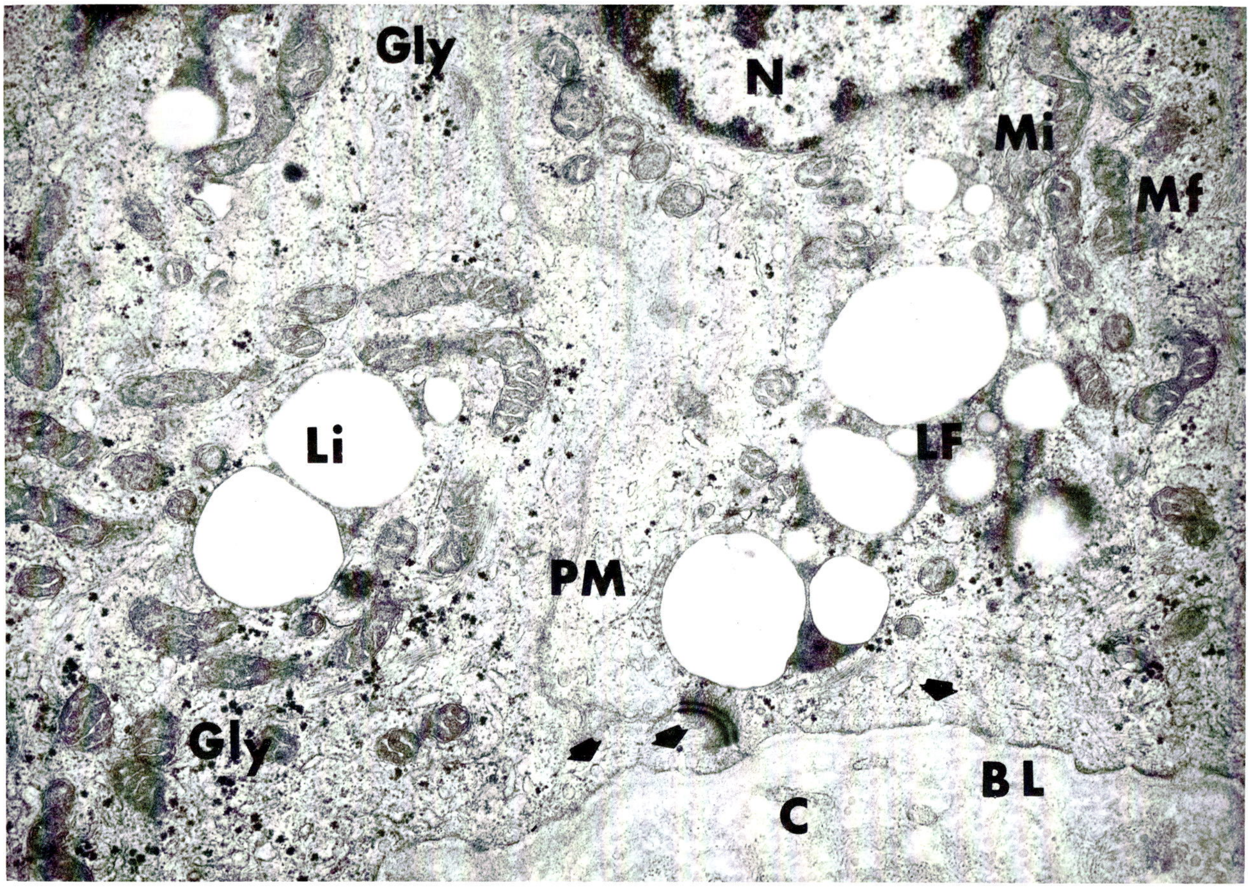

Figure 219. *Ovary from a 33-year-old woman.* Detailed view of the subnuclear (N) portion of the ovarian surface epithelium. The cytoplasm contains prominent aggregates of lipofuschin granules (LF), lipid droplets (Li), and mitochondria (Mi). Glycogen particles (Gly) and microfilaments (Mf) are scattered throughout, and the basal plasma membrane (PM) has rows of micropinocytic vesicles (arrows). The tightly apposed lateral plasma membranes (PM) are occasionally attached near the basal lamina (BL) by well-developed desmosomes. × 23,040. C: collagenous albuginae.

REFERENCES (Figures 218–219)

1. Weakley, B. S. Differentiation of the surface epithelium of the hamster ovary. An electron microscopic study. *J. Anat.* **105:** 129 (1969).
2. Motta, P., D. D. Cherney, and L. J. Didio. Scanning and transmission electron microscopy of the ovarian surface in mammals with special reference to ovulation. *J. Submicrosc. Cytol.* **3:** 85 (1971).
3. Papadaki, L. and J. O. W. Beilby. The fine structure of the surface epithelium of the human ovary. *J. Cell Sci.* **8:** 445 (1971).

60

Stroma

The ovarian stroma arises from the primitive urogenital mesenchyme during gonadal development and is composed of spindle-shaped, fibroblastlike cells with complex cytoplasmic processes.[1-4] The cytoplasmic matrix contains organelles for fibrillogenesis, and the cells form and secrete extracellular collagen. Unlike the fibroblasts of extragenital sites, however, ovarian stromal cells are sensitive to hormonal stimuli (gonadotropins) and give rise to both thecal and granulosal cells, either of which may become luteinized. The non-corpus luteum, luteinized stromal cells have abundant lipid droplets[1,3,4] and agranular endoplasmic reticulum, and are similar ultrastructurally to the luteinized thecal cells of the corpus luteum. These cells are capable of active steroid synthesis,[5,6] as are theca lutein cells. Cells[1,3,4] with abundant cytoplasm containing numerous lipid droplets, mitochondria, Golgi, and microfibrils are also seen and are considered to be intermediate forms between the unstimulated stromal spindly cells and the luteinized stromal cells.

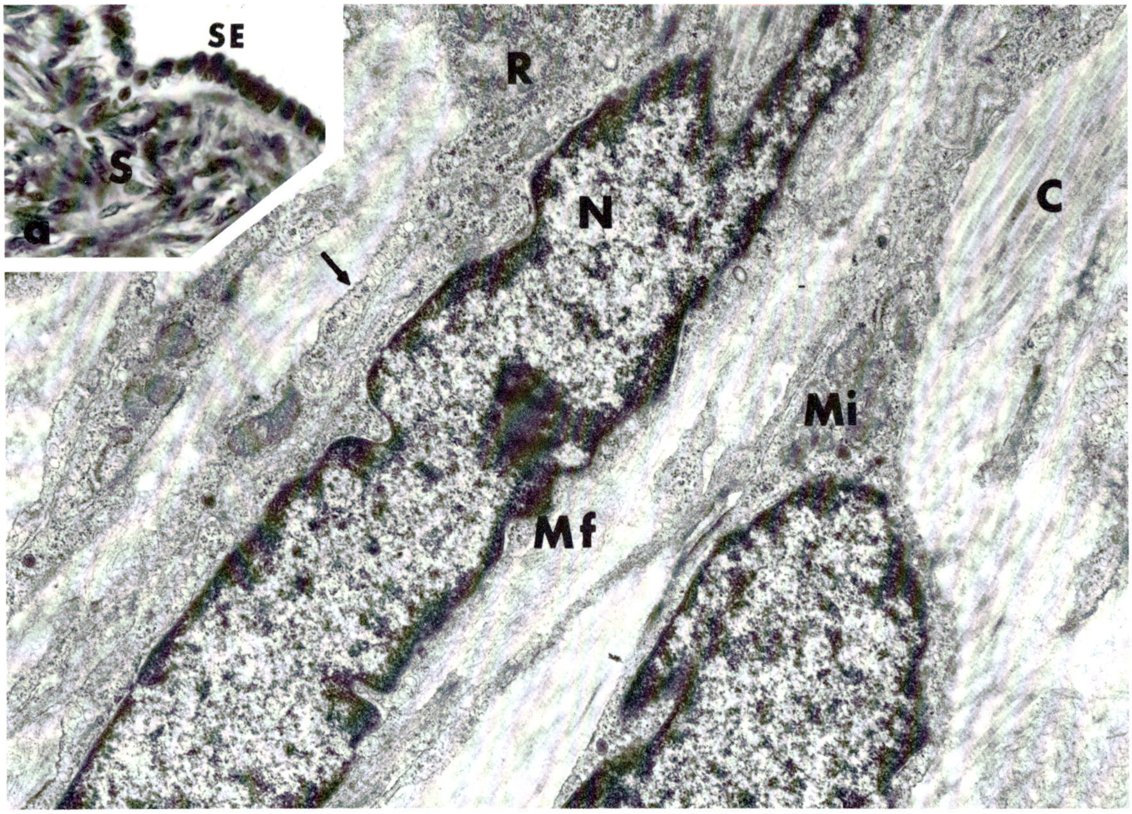

Figure 220a. *Ovarian stromal cells* (S) are spindle-shaped, fibroblastlike cells arranged in a haphazard fashion. (H & E stain, × 120.) SE: ovarian surface epithelium.

Figure 220. *Ultrastructurally,* the cells have narrow, cigar-shaped nuclei (N), and the slender cytoplasm is rich in free ribosomes (R) and microfilaments (Mf). Rows of micropinocytic vesicles (arrow) are found along the plasma membrane. Small clusters of mitochondria (Mi) provide the energy necessary for fibrillogenesis. × 15,600. C: extracellular collagen.

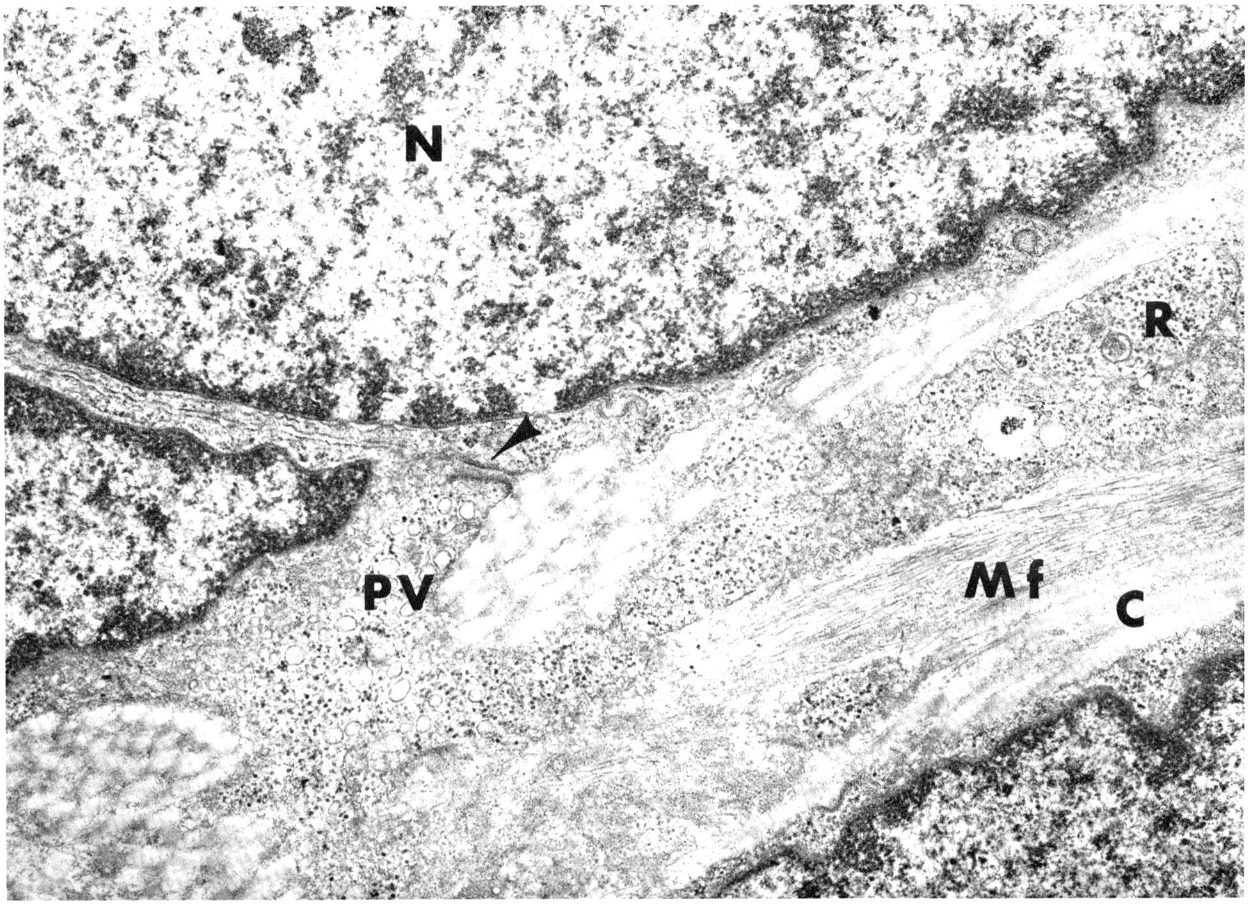

Figure 221. *In the ovary, as in other parts of the body,* the formation of collagen fibers (C) occurs extracellularly by the "polymerization" of tropocollagen fibrils (Mf), which are generated within the cells, concentrated at the periphery of the cytoplasm, and eventually deposited in the intercellular space. Note the close interrelationship between extracellular microfilamentous tropocollagen and cross-striated collagen fibers. × 25,600. N: nucleus; PV: micropinocytic vesicles; R: free ribosomes; arrow head: desmosomelike attachment between two stromal cells.

REFERENCES (The ovarian stroma–Figure 221)

1. Laffargue, P., L. Adechy-Benkoel, and C. Valette. Ultrastructure of the ovarian stroma. *Ann. Anat. Pathol. (Paris)* **13:** 381 (1968).
2. Kempson, R. L. Ultrastructure of ovarian stromal cell tumors. *Arch. Pathol.* **86:** 492 (1968).
3. Serment, H., P. Laffargue, and C. Vallette. The functional stroma of the menopausal ovary. *Presse Med.* **77:** 1653 (1969).
4. Amin, H. K., T. Okagaki, and R. M. Richart. Classification of fibroma and thecoma of the ovary. An ultrastructural study. *Cancer* **27:** 438 (1971).
5. Feinberg, R. and R. Cohen. A comparative histochemical study of the ovarian stromal lipid band, stromal theca cell, and normal ovarian follicular apparatus. *Am. J. Obstet. Gynecol.* **92:** 958 (1965).
6. Rice, B. F. and K. Savard. Steroid hormone formation in the human ovary. IV. Ovarian stromal compartment; formation of radio-active steroids from acetate 1-^{14}C and action of gonadotropins. *J. Clin. Endocrinol.* **26:** 593 (1966).

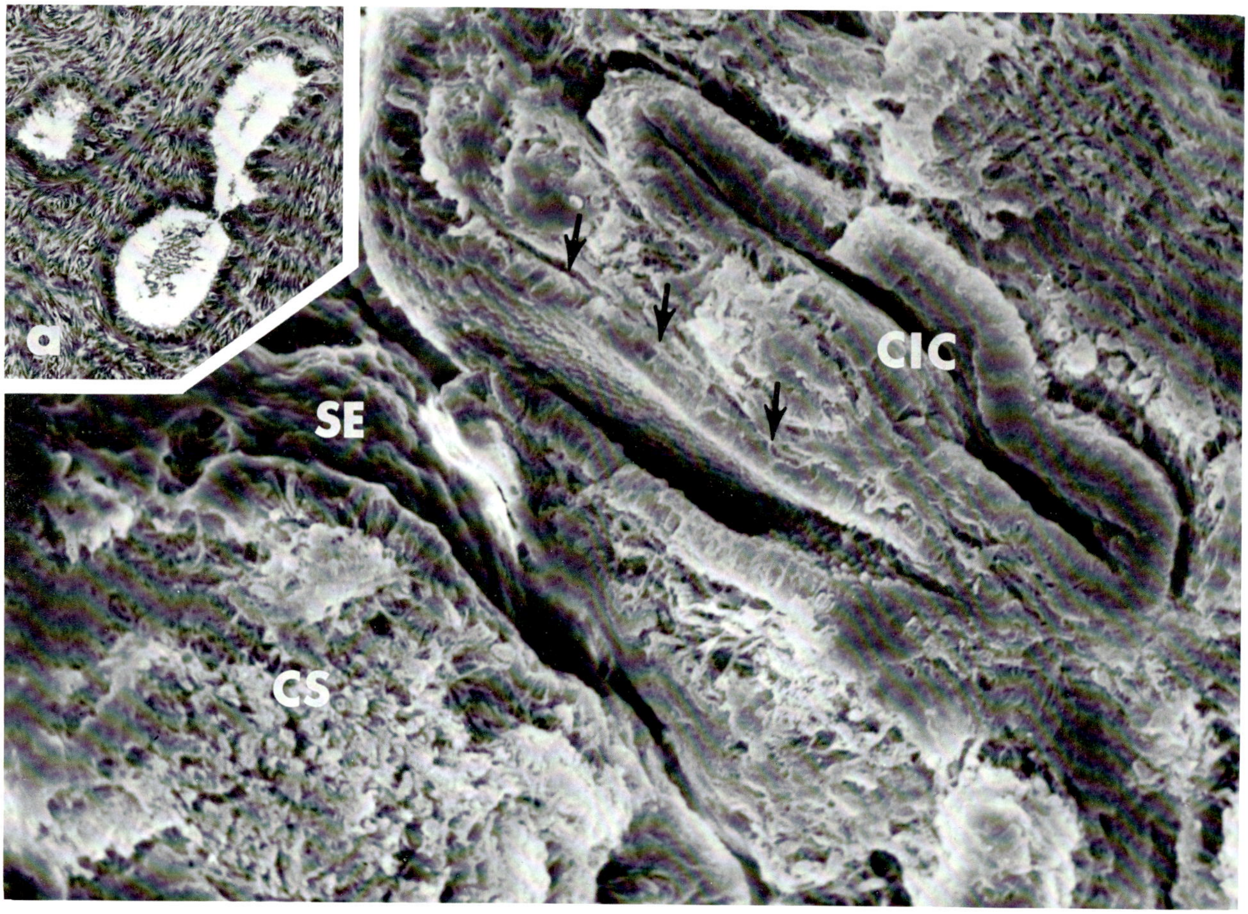

61

Cortical Inclusion Cysts

Benign and malignant serous neoplasms are the most commonly occurring ovarian tumors in aging women. The neoplasms are thought to arise by "tubal" metaplasia from celomic epithelium-derived *cortical inclusion cysts* or from exophytic epithelial sprouting of the ovarian surface.

Figure 222a. *Several cortical inclusion cysts* lined by numerous clear, ciliated cells embedded in a dense cellular stroma. (H & E stain, × 30.)

Figure 222. *Scanning electron micrograph of a cross-sectioned ovary* in which the surface epithelium (SE) contains several deep cortical (CS) invaginations (arrows). The separation of these infoldings from the surface epithelium presumably occurs by the proliferation of adjacent ovarian stroma, resulting in the development of cortical inclusion cysts (CIC). × 250.

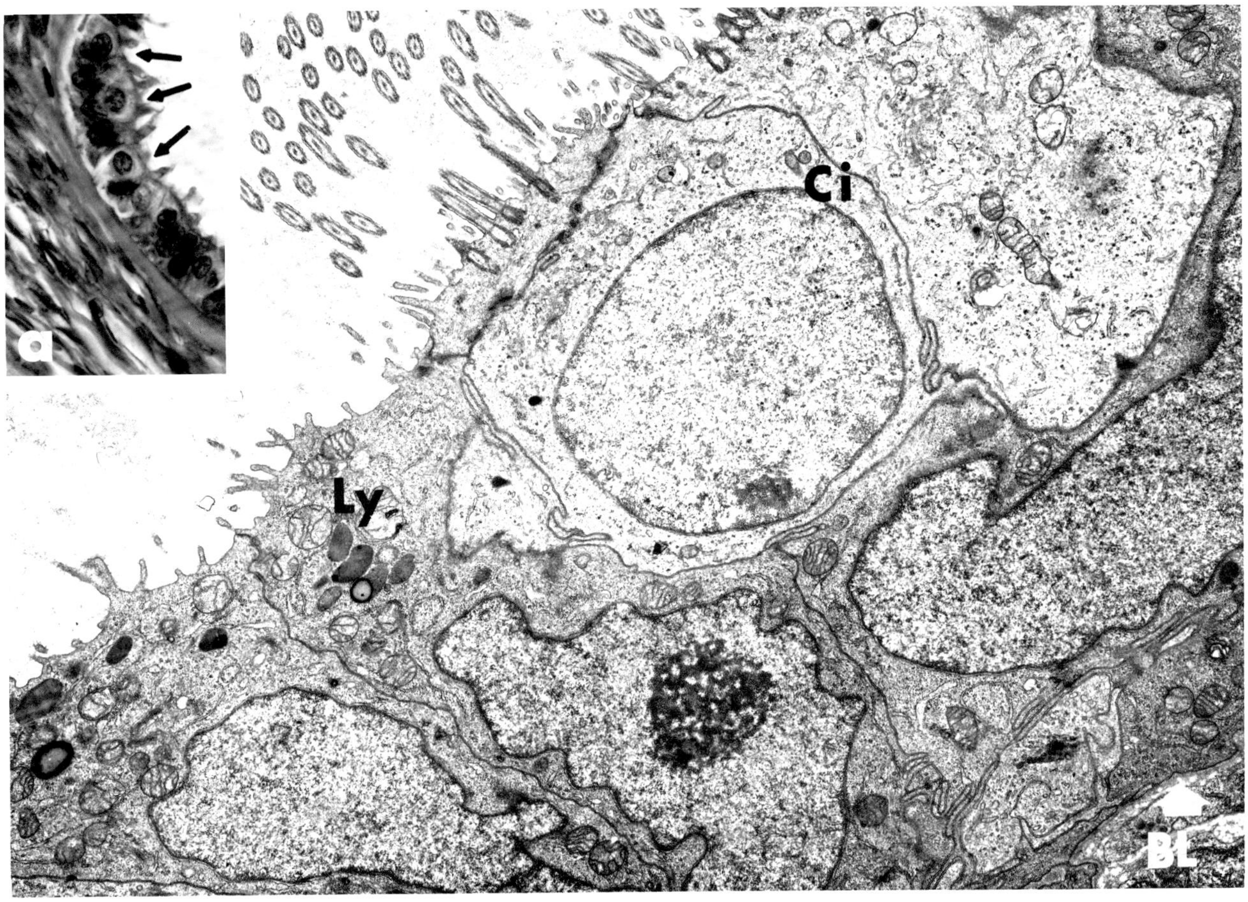

Figure 223a. *Light micrograph of the lining epithelium of a cortical inclusion cyst.* Numerous ciliated cells (arrows) with clear cytoplasm intermingle with nonciliated secretory and a few degenerating "peg" cells. This type of epithelium is identical to normal oviductal epithelium: hence the term "tubal" or "serous" metaplasia. (H & E stain, × 120.)

Figure 223. *The morphologic similarity* of cortical inclusion cyst epithelium and tubal mucosa is confirmed with the electron microscope. The pale appearance of ciliated cells (Ci) is due to the clear cytoplasmic matrix and to the relatively few cytoplasmic organelles. These cells are considered to be immature ciliated cells. Adjacent nonciliated cells have abundant organelles and clusters of supranuclear lysosomes (Ly). The luminal microvilli are well developed, with occasional branching, and the tightly apposed and convoluted lateral plasma membranes are attached by infrequent desmosomes. × 6400. BL: basal lamina.

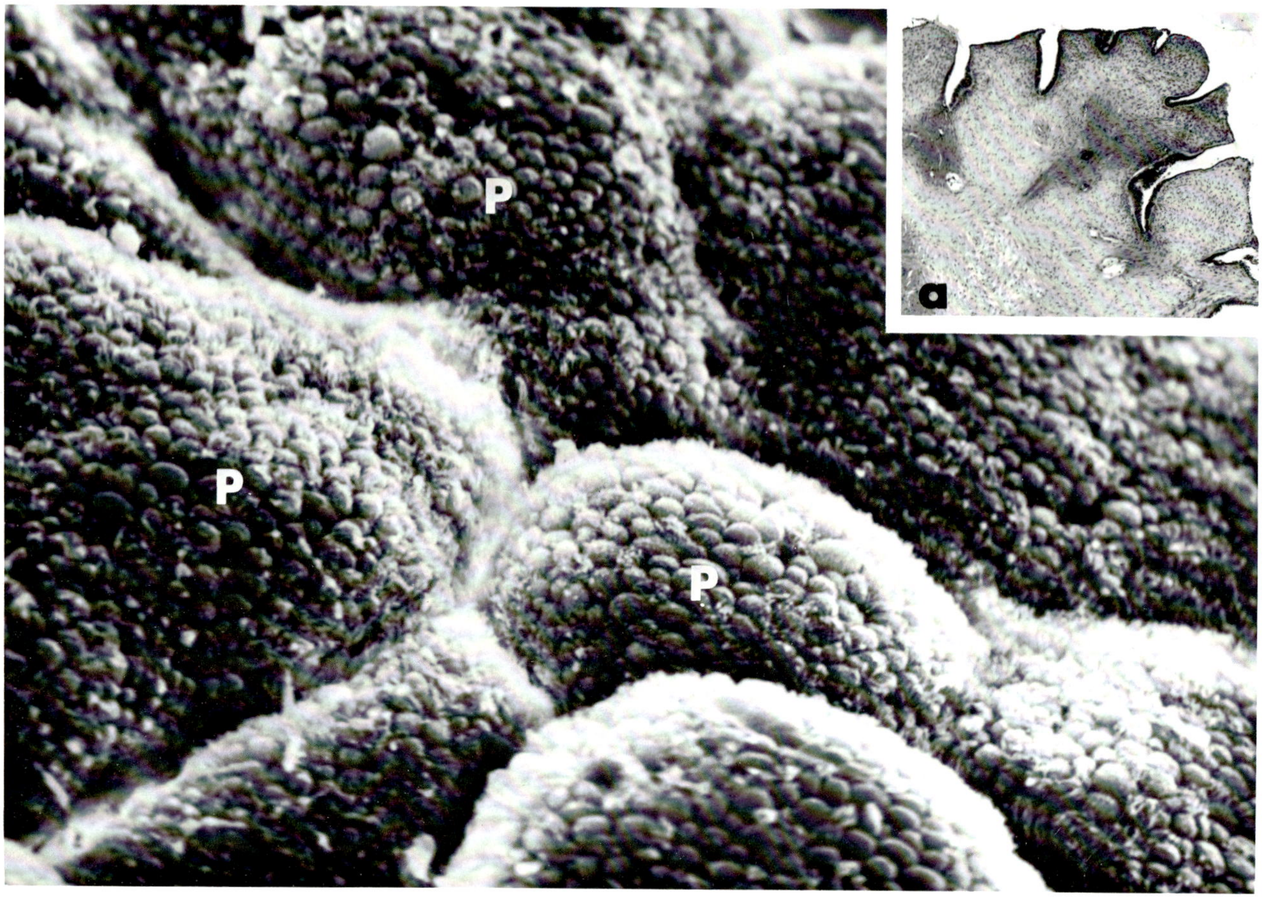

62

Serous Cystadenofibroma

Subsequent to the tubal metaplasia, the papillary and nonpapillary serous cystadenomas, cystadenofibromas, and surface papillomas are lined by a well-differentiated epithelium composed of ciliated and secretory cells, similar in surface topography[1] and fine structure[2,3] to those of normal oviductal mucosa.[4,5] The supporting stroma varies from a dense fibrocellular core in the surface papillomas and cystadenofibromas to a loose, myxoid connective tissue in the papillary cystadenomas. It may contain stromal lutein cells, and occasionally there are signs of hyperestrogenism.

Figure 224a. *Papillary, serous cystadenofibroma.* The blunt-ended papillae are lined by a tubal type of epithelium, and the hypocellular stroma is markedly desmoplastic. (H & E stain, × 12.)

Figure 224. *Papillary serous cystadenofibroma.* Topographic appearance of prominent club-shaped papillae (P). The lining epithelium has a cobblestone pattern and contains both ciliated and nonciliated cells. × 560.

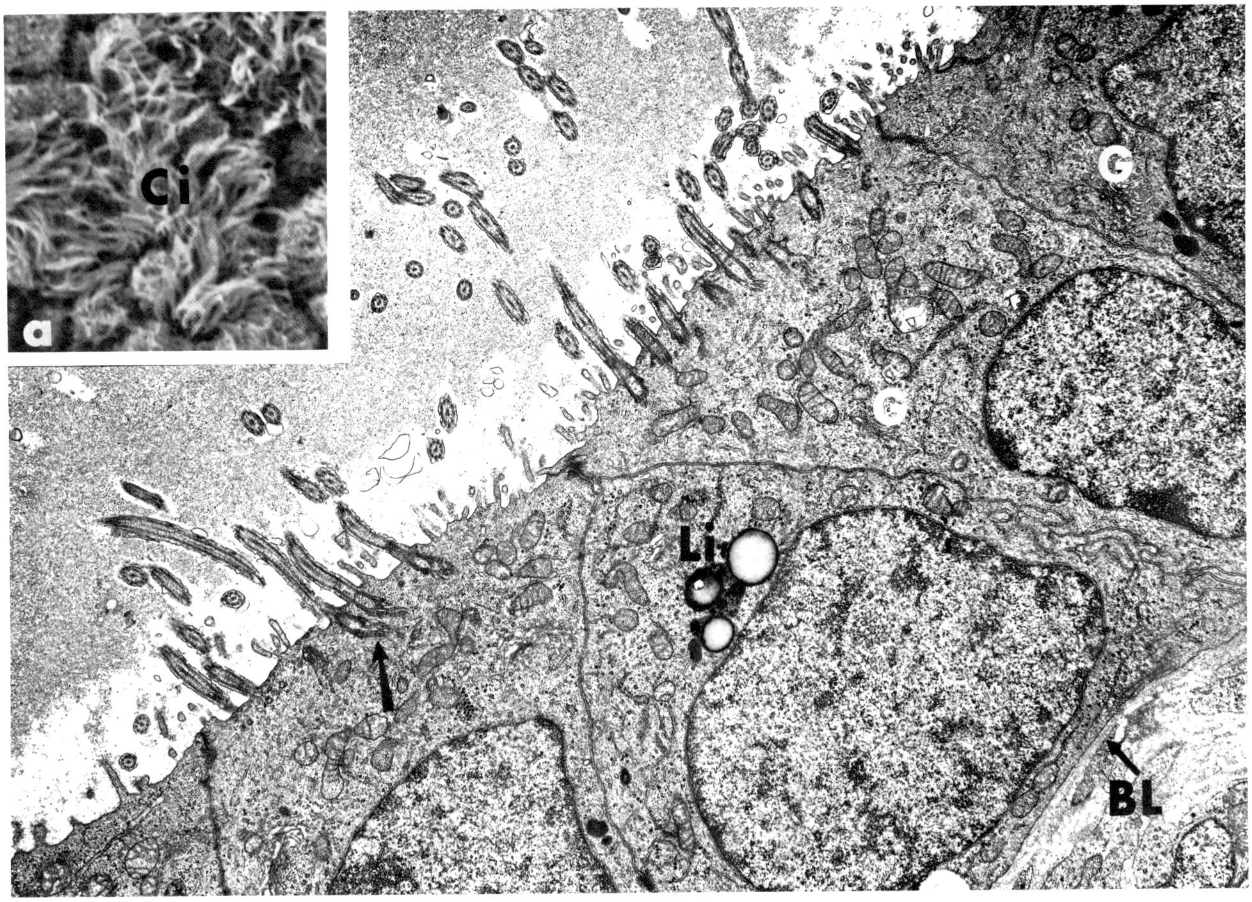

Figure 225a. *Higher magnification of Figure 224.* As is characteristic of a tubal type of epithelium, ciliated cells (Ci) are abundant and are arranged in clusters. × 2000.

Figure 225. *Papillary serous cystadenofibroma.* Both the ciliated and the nonciliated cells have similar cytoplasmic density and contain numerous supranuclear mitochondria, Golgi (G), free and bound ribosomes, and lipid droplets (Li). This type of ciliated cell with electron-dense cytoplasmic matrix is considered to be mature. Cross-striated ciliary rootlets (arrow) are often seen. × 6800. BL: basal lamina.

REFERENCES (Subsequent to the tubal metaplasia–Figure 225)

1. Ferenczy, A. and R. M. Richart. Scanning electron microscopy of the female genital tract. *N.Y. State J. Med.* (in press).
2. Zambernard, J., W. Blackburn, and D. Roberts. The reproductive system. In *Ultrastructural Aspects of Disease,* D. W. King (Ed.). Hoeber Medical Division, Harper & Row, New York, 1966, pp. 186–187.
3. Gondos, B. Electron microscopic study of papillary serous tumors of the ovary. *Cancer* **27:** 1455 (1971).
4. Overbeck, L. Ultrastructure of the Fallopian epithelium in the female menstrual cycle. *Arch. Gynaekol.* **207:** 165 (1969).
5. Ferenczy, A., R. M. Richart, F. Agate, Jr., M. L. Purkerson, and E. Dempsey. Scanning electron microscopy of the human Fallopian tube. *Science* **175:** 783 (1972).

63

Serous Cystadenocarcinoma

Figure 226a. *In low-grade (borderline) papillary serous cystadenocarcinomas,* delicate, multibranching papillae are formed, usually lined by a single-layered epithelium with the nuclear atypia seen in the presence of aneuploidy.[1,2] Ultrastructurally,[3,4] the lining epithelium retains its similarity to tubal epithelium, including the presence of ciliated cells,[3,4] although their numbers are reduced[3] in comparison to the oviduct or the benign serous neoplasms. (H & E stain, × 30.)

Figure 226. *Scanning electron micrograph of low-grade papillary serous cystadenocarcinoma.* Ciliated cells (Ci) are considerably reduced, and the characteristic clustering of such cells seen in the oviduct or in benign serous neoplasms is no longer evident. Cellular pleomorphism is minimal. × 3000. *From* A. Ferenczy and R. M. Richart. Scanning electron microscopy of the human female genital tract. *N. Y. State J. Med.* (in press).

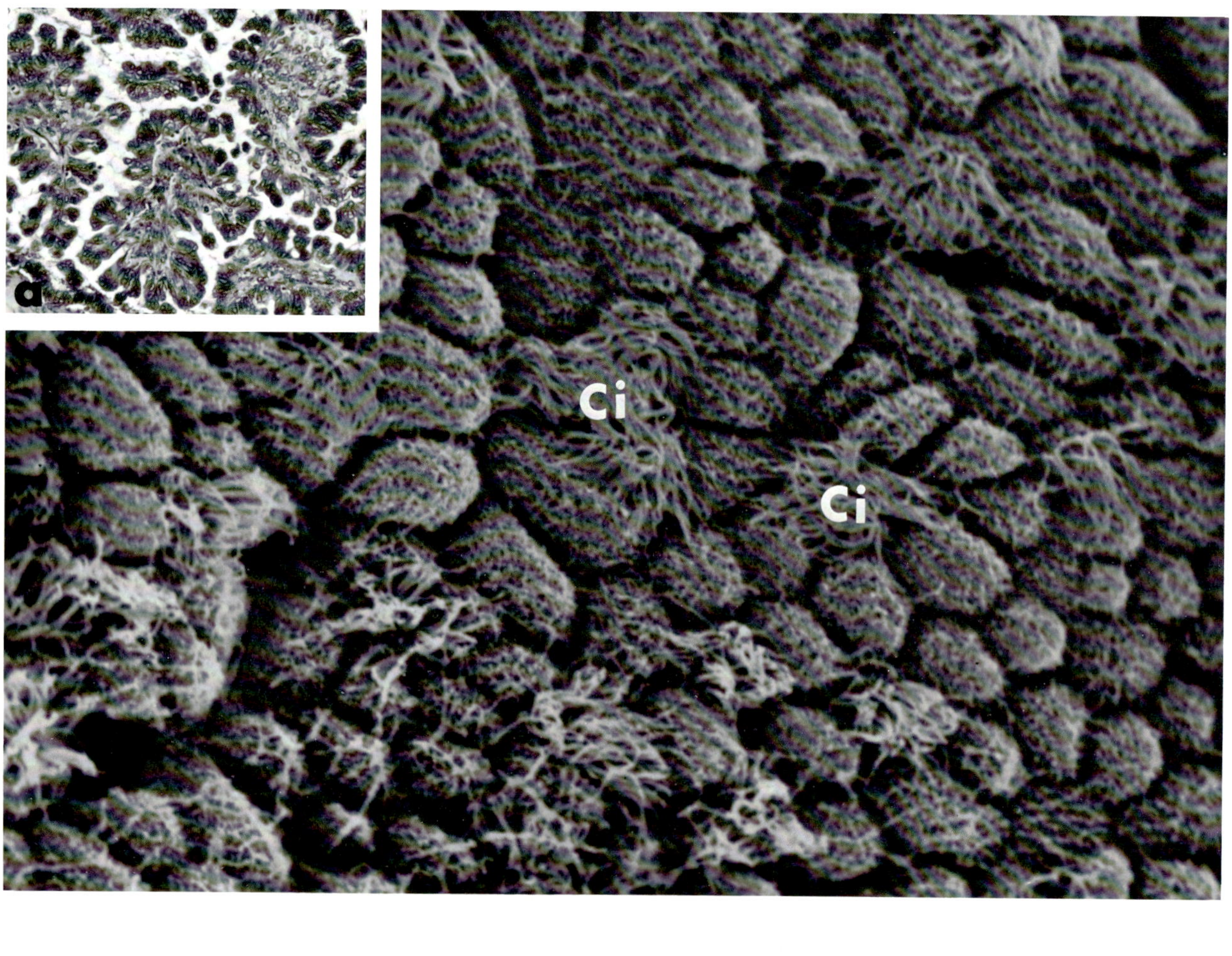

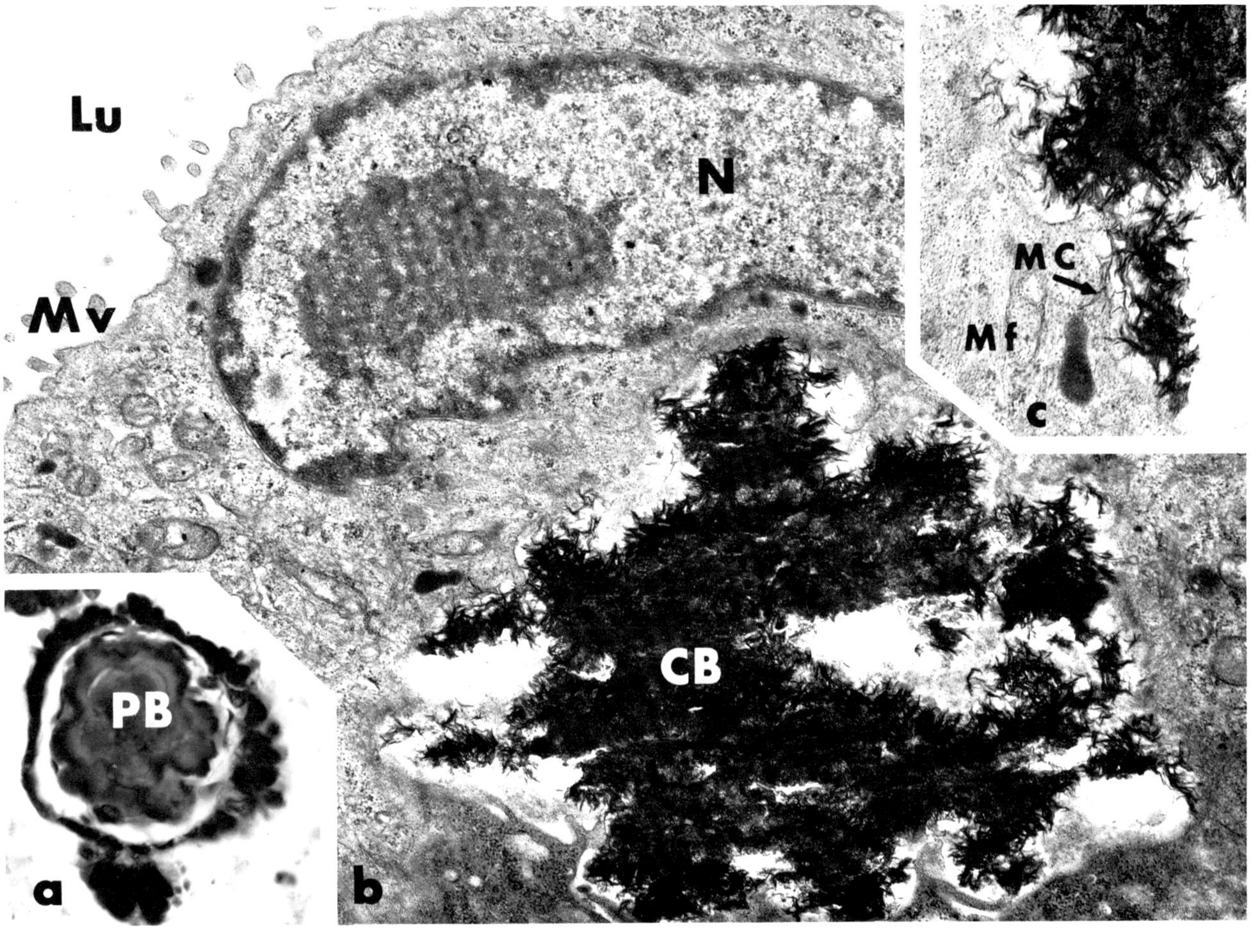

In *papillary serous ovarian neoplasms,* especially the low-grade variety, lamellated psammoma bodies are often numerous. The fine structural[5-7] and X-ray defraction studies[5] of psammoma bodies suggest that they are made of calcium apatite.[8] Their formation is a characteristic feature of papillary neoplasms in general, and the common morphologic denominator appears to be the conspicuous presence of intracytoplasmic filaments, which provide a matrix for a seeding site for mineralization. The intracellular calcification of cytoplasmic microfilaments is said to be preceded by focal cytoplasmic degeneration.

Figure 227a. *Low-grade papillary serous cystadenocarcinoma.* A large, lamellated psammoma body (PB) is seen surrounded by neoplastic cells. (H & E stain, × 90.)

Figure 227b. *Low-grade, papillary serous cystadenocarcinoma.* Transmission electron micrograph of a large subnuclear (N) intracytoplasmic calcific body (CB). × 12.500. Lu: neoplastic glandular lumen; Mv: luminal microvilli.

Figure 227c. *Detail of Figure 227b.* Numerous fine microfilaments (Mf) are seen at the periphery of the calcific body, mineralization of which results in the formation of microneedle crystals (MC) arranged in a haphazard pattern. Microcrystals are formed by the conglomeration of microneedle crystals. The coalescence of several calcific cells results in the formation of large psammoma bodies. Large calcified bodies found in the stroma either may originate in situ, by calcification of the interstitial collagen fibers, or may represent calcified neoplastic epithelium incorporated within the stroma. × 41,000.

REFERENCES (Figures 226a–227c)

1. Richart, R. M. and A. S. Ludwig, Jr. Alterations in chromosomes and DNA content in gynecologic neoplasms. *Am. J. Obstet. Gynecol.* **104:** 463 (1969).
2. Atkins, N. B. Modal DNA value and chromosome number in ovarian neoplasia. *Cancer* **27:** 1064 (1971).
3. Ferenczy, A. and R. M. Richart. Scanning electron microscopy of the human female genital tract. *N.Y. State J. Med.* (in press).
4. Gondos, B. Eletcron microscopic study of papillary serous tumors of the ovary. *Cancer* **27:** 1455 (1971).
5. Bennington, J. L., J. V. Smith, and D. Lagunoff. Calcification in psammoma bodies of the human meningioma. *Lab. Invest.* **22:** 241 (1970).
6. Nystrom, S. M. A study of supratentorial meningiomas, with special reference to gross and fine structure. *Acta Pathol. Microbiol. Scand. (Suppl.)* **176:** 1 (1965).
7. Hameed, K. and D. A. Morgan. Papillary adenocarcinoma of endometrium with psammoma bodies. Histology and fine structure. *Cancer* **29:** 1326 (1972).
8. Paegle, R. D. Ultrastructure of calcium deposits in arteriosclerotic human aortas. *J. Ultrastruct. Res.* **26:** 412 (1969).

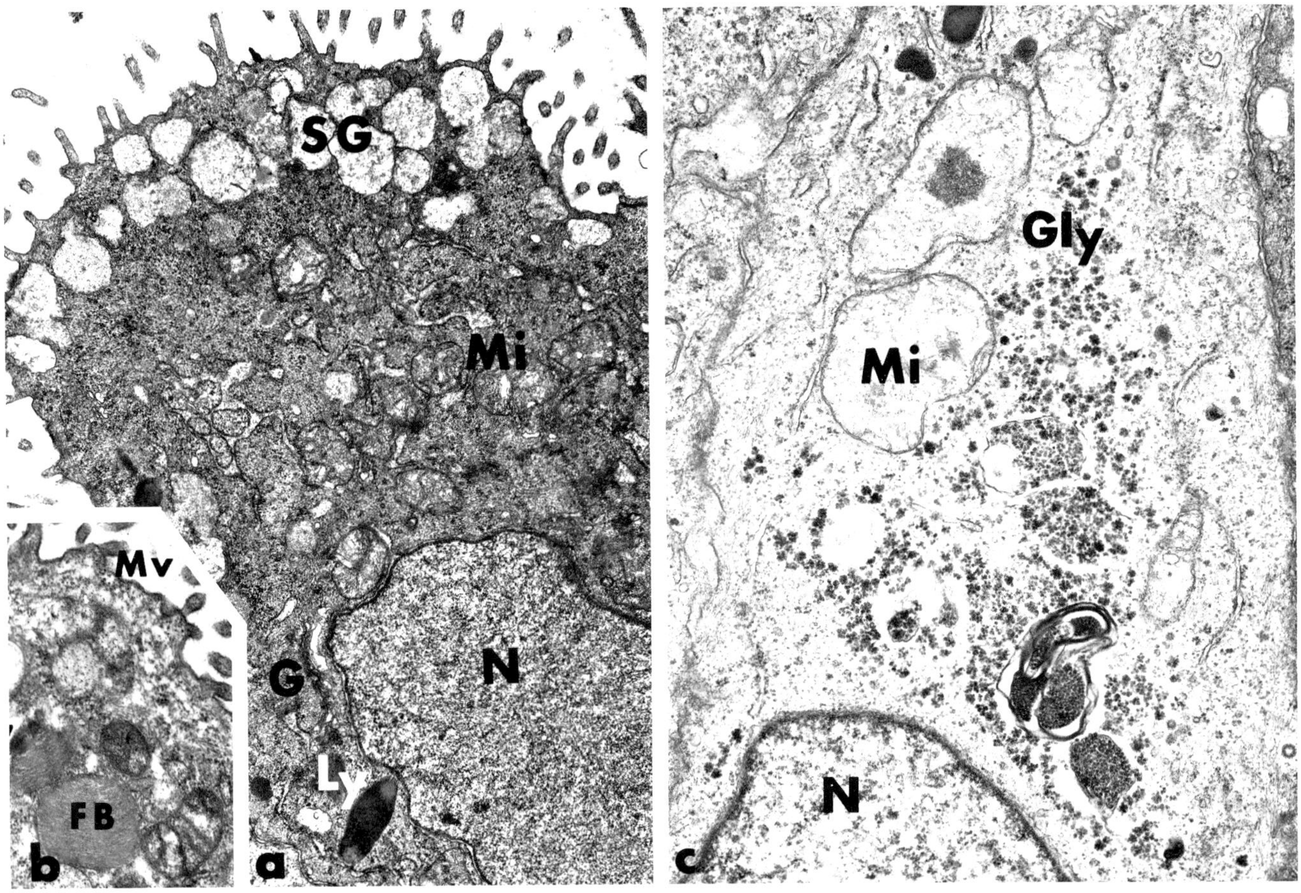

In well-differentiated papillary serous cystadenocarcinomas, ciliated and nonciliated tubal-type epithelial cells predominate, but other cells are also present. One type resembles the cells lining the endometrial glands,[1] and another, with apical, mucous-type secretory vacuoles,[1,2] is similar to those found in the endocervical type of epithelium. The latter cells may be the source of the occasional conspicuous acidic mucin production in serous-type neoplasms.[3]

Figure 228a. *Well-differentiated papillary serous cystadenocarcinoma.* A neoplastic cell contains an apical concentration of membrane-bound secretory granules (SG), which resemble those found in the mucus-secreting endocervical epithelium. The secretory granules with filamentous secretory material are associated with supranuclear (N) mitochondria (Mi), Golgi (G), and abundant free and bound ribosomes. × 12,600. Ly: lysosomes.

Figure 228b. *Well-differentiated papillary serous cystadenocarcinoma.* Occasionally, secretory granules are associated with membrane-bound fibrillar bodies (FB), another characteristic feature of mucus-secreting cells. × 18,500. Mv: luminal microvilli.

Figure 228c. *Well-differentiated papillary serous cystadenocarcinoma.* Endometrial-type neoplastic cells with conspicuous collections of supranuclear (N) glycogen particles (Gly), associated with mitochondria (Mi), free ribosomes, and granular endoplasmic reticulum, are evident. Note the presence of fine microfilaments near the lateral plasma membranes. × 23,040.

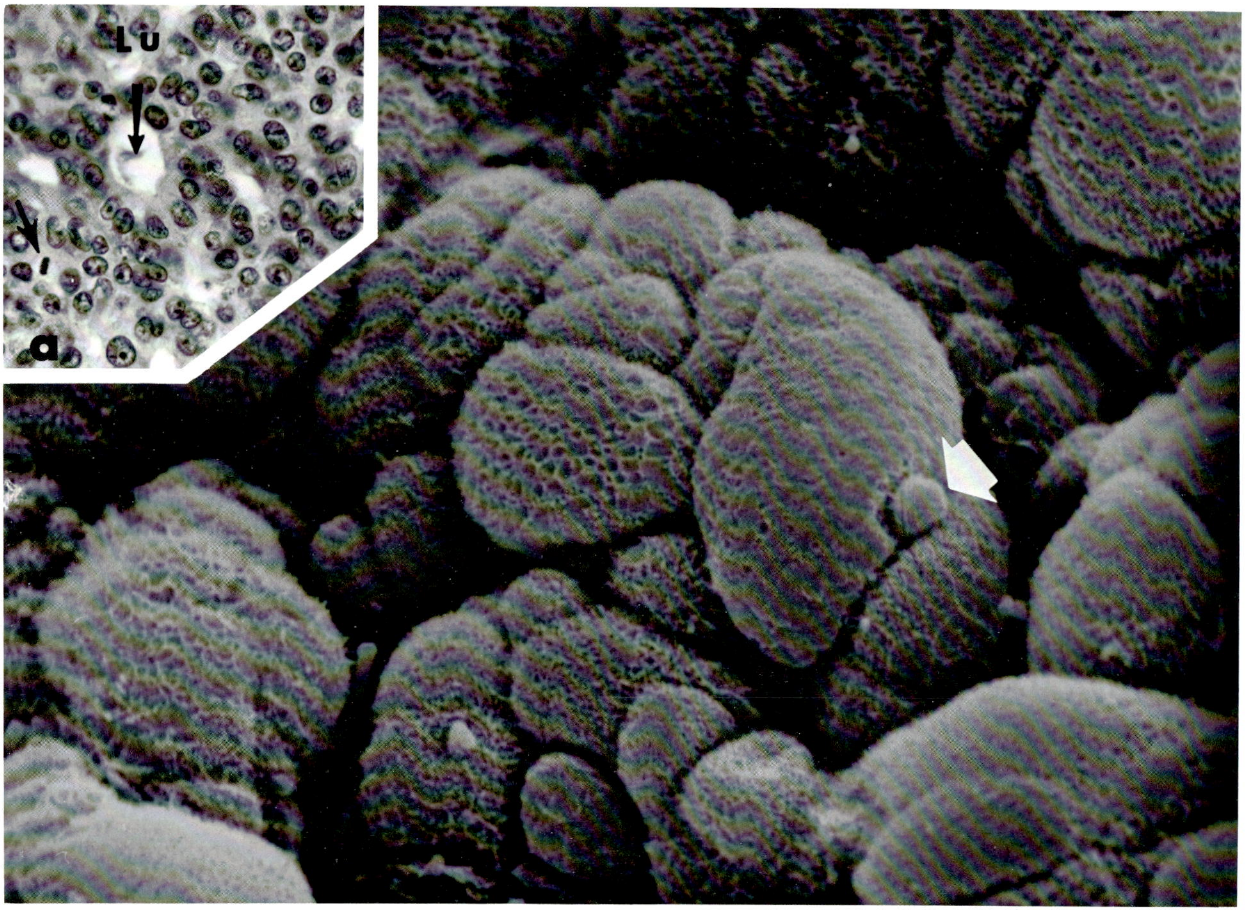

Figure 229a. *Poorly differentiated serous cystadenocarcinoma.* Although the bulk of the lesion consists of solid sheets of undifferentiated neoplastic cells, foci containing narrow or abortive glands (Lu) are occasionally seen, lined by highly atypical cells with prominent nuclei and nucleoli, and mitoses (short arrow) are common. (H & E stain, × 120.)

Figure 229. *Poorly differentiated serous cystadenocarcinoma.* Profound surface ultrastructural changes are observed in the poorly differentiated lesions, as indicated by marked cellular pleomorphism [cells varying from minute (arrow) to prominent giant cells], loss of cellular cohesion, and disorganization. Ciliated cells are uniformly lacking, and the surface microvillous processes appear to be agglutinated by the secretory material. × 1120. *From* A. Ferenczy and R. M. Richart. Scanning electron microscopy of the human female genital tract. *N.Y. State J. Med.* (in press).

REFERENCES (In well-differentiated papillary serous cystadenocarcinomas—Figure 229)

1. Roberts, D. K., R. B. Marshall, and J. T. Wharton. Ultrastructure of ovarian tumors. I. Papillary serous cystadenocarcinoma. *Cancer* **25:** 947 (1970).
2. Gondos, B. Electron microscopic study of papillary serous tumors of the ovary. *Cancer* **27:** 1455 (1971).
3. Scully, R. E. Recent progress in ovarian cancer. *Human Pathol.* **1:** 73 (1970.)

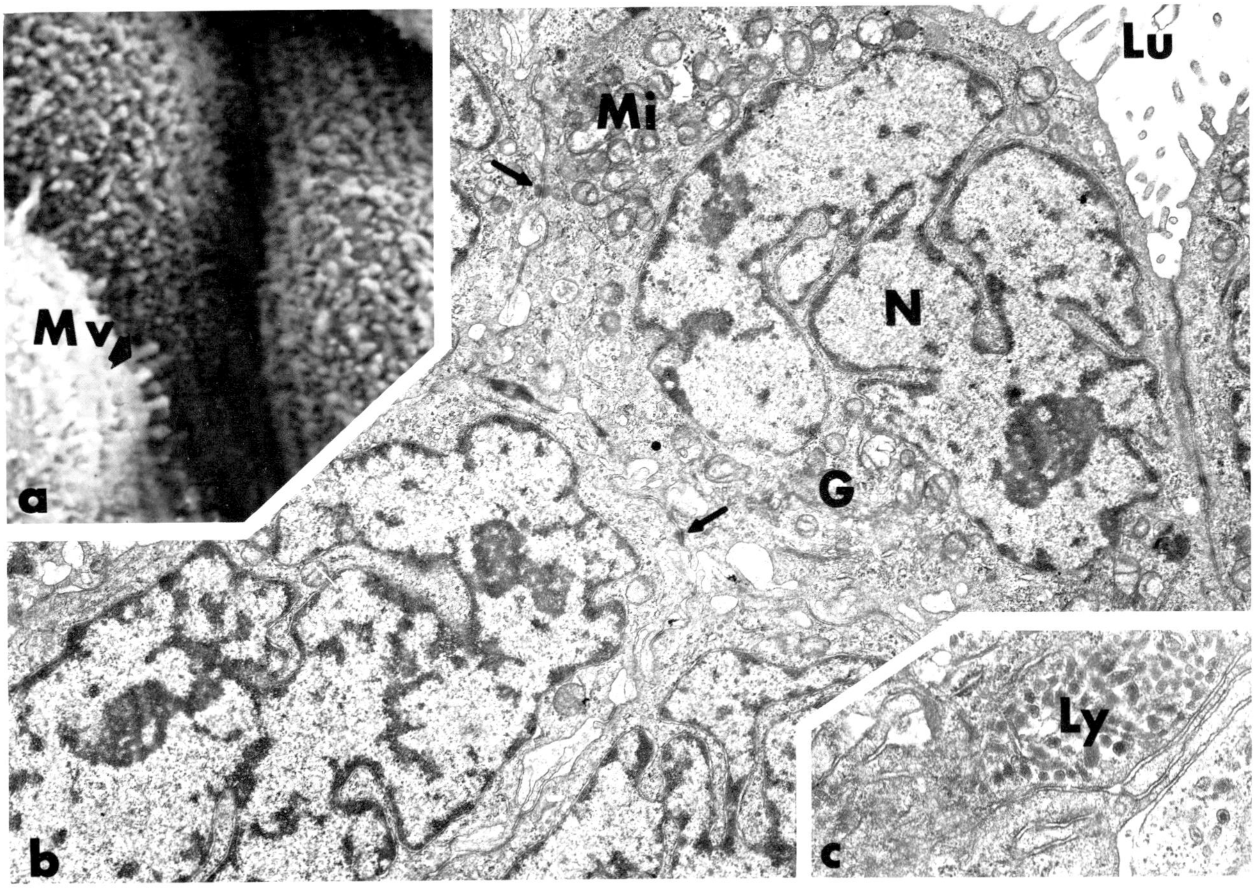

Figure 230a. *Poorly differentiated serous cystadenocarcinoma.* Higher-power view of the surface microvillous projections (Mv), which appear considerably shorter and fewer in the poorly differentiated neoplastic cells than in the benign or well-differentiated variety. × 4800.

Figure 230b. *In poorly differentiated serous cystadenocarcinoma,* profound intracellular structural changes include a progressive increase in the nucleo–cytoplasmic ratio, chromatin clumping associated with irregular nuclear (N) contour (cerebriform nuclear pattern), and anisonucleolosis. There are an increase in cytoplasmic organelles and a loss of desmosomal attachments. The highly convoluted lateral plasma membranes are attached by infrequent and poorly developed desmosomes (short arrows), and fine, interdigitating microvilli project into slightly dilated intercellular spaces. × 7800. Mi: mitochondria; G: Golgi; Lu: glandular lumen.

Figure 230c. *Poorly differentiated serous cystadenocarcinoma.* Electron micrograph of a large collection of membrane-bound lysosomes (Ly). These membrane-bound dense bodies seem to represent a characteristic intracellular element in epithelial cells of "serous nature," for they are often observed in normal and neoplastic[1] tubal epithelium as well as in benign and malignant serous ovarian neoplasms. × 23,600.

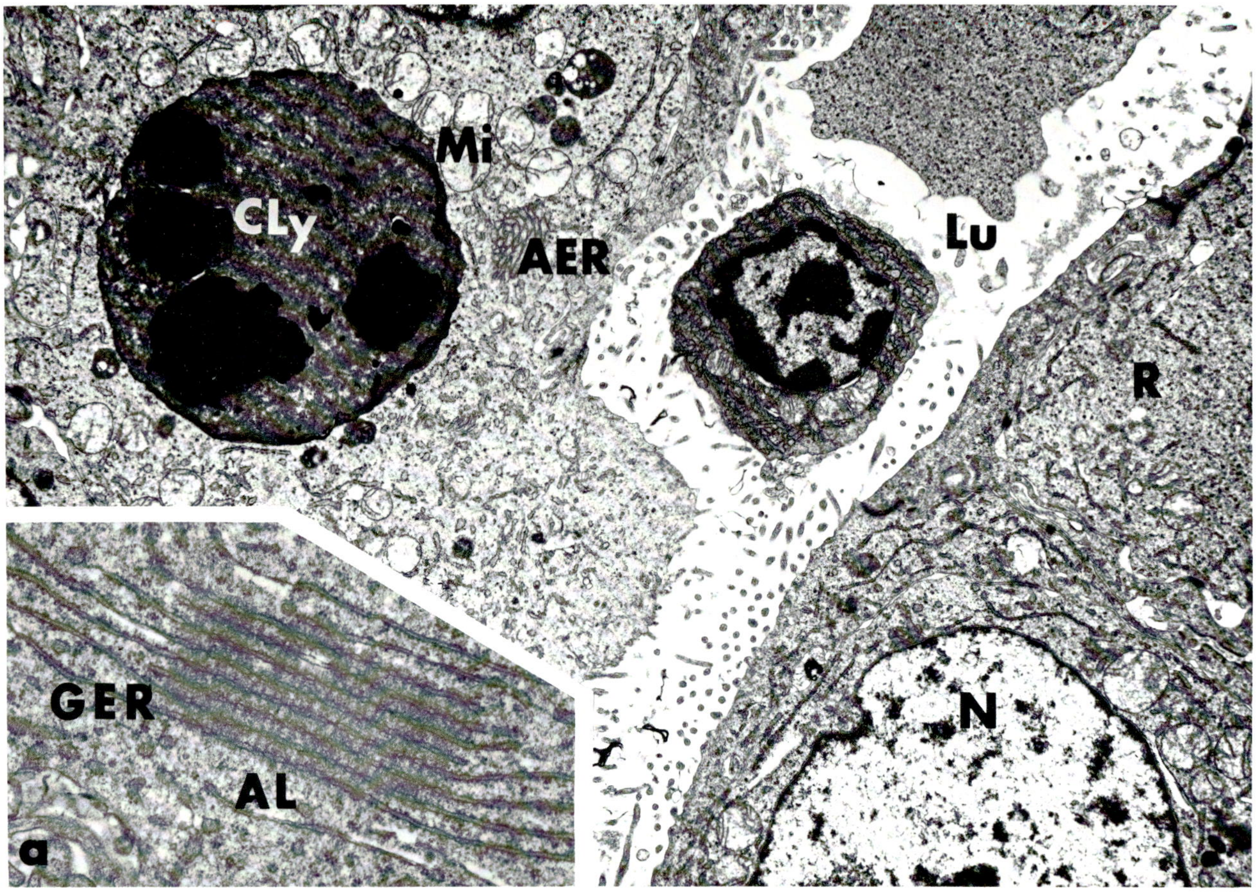

Figure 231. *Poorly differentiated serous cystadenocarcinoma.* With increasing dedifferentiation, focal or total cellular degeneration, accompanied by marked autophagic activity, as indicated by the appearance of prominent autophagic cytolysosomes (Cly), is observed. Cytoplasmic organelles such as mitochondria (Mi), granular and agranular endoplasmic reticulum (AER), and free ribosomes (R) are plentiful. × 5600. Lu: glandular lumen with a degenerated neoplastic cell and fragments of cytoplasmic substance; N: nucleus.

Figure 231a. *Poorly differentiated serous cystadenocarcinoma.* In addition to the abundant cytoplasmic organelles, structures resembling annulate lamellae (AL) are observed. These are made of parallel cisternae of granular endoplasmic reticulum (GER), interrupted by fine porelike diaphragms at regular intervals. The intermembranous space is occupied by finely granular electron-dense material. Similar structures, although most often composed of agranular endoplasmic reticulum, are found in a great variety of cells, such as primitive germ cells, steroidogenic cells, and highly malignant neoplastic cells, all of which are known to contain increased proliferating and metabolic potentials. × 20,600.

REFERENCE (Figures 230a–231a)

1. Ferenczy, A. and R. M. Richart. Unpublished data.

64

Mucinous Cystadenoma

Although *mucinous cystadenomas* are almost as common as their benign serous counterparts, malignant change occurs comparatively less often. The benign lesions are usually nonpapillary and are lined by tall columnar, mucus-secreting cells resembling endocervical epithelium[2] both histologically and ultrastructurally.[1] Numerous goblet cells, occasional argentaffin cells, and rare Paneth cells,[3] all of which are characteristic of intestinal-type epithelium, are seen. This intermixture of endocervical and intestinal epithelia has been noted in both transmission and scanning electron microscopy. Both types of epithelia contain abundant mucous secretions which are released into the cyst lumen. The resulting intracystic acid mucopolysaccharide (sulfomucin)-rich mucin has histochemical staining characteristics, enzyme content, and specific antigenecity[4,5] similar to those of intestinal mucin. These observations and the occasional (5%) association with benign cystic teratoma ("dermoid cyst") suggest that mucinous neoplasms are of germ cell origin. In this regard, Linder and Power,[6] in an electrophoretic-genetic study, found for the mucinous epithelium associated with a benign cystic teratoma a cell origin different from that of the other cells comprising the teratoma, although the study failed to establish whether the cell origin was of the germinal or the somatic type.

Despite the foregoing observations, the frequent finding of serous and endometrioid elements in mucinous lesions favors a metaplastic, rather than a teratomatous, origin for the vast majority of mucin-secreting ovarian growths. The lesions presumably arise via differentiation from the surface celomic epithelium, as described for the serous neoplasms. The observation that intestinal epithelium, with or without argentaffin and Paneth cells, may be found in inflamed or neoplastic urothelium and respiratory tract epithelium, and in endometrial adenocarcinoma, as well as in normal[7] and neoplastic[8] endocervical epithelium, suggests that intestinal epithelium may be generated from endodermal or a mesodermal epithelium. Thus it is difficult to know whether mucinous cystadenomas are derived from simplified teratomas, celomic epithelium, or both.

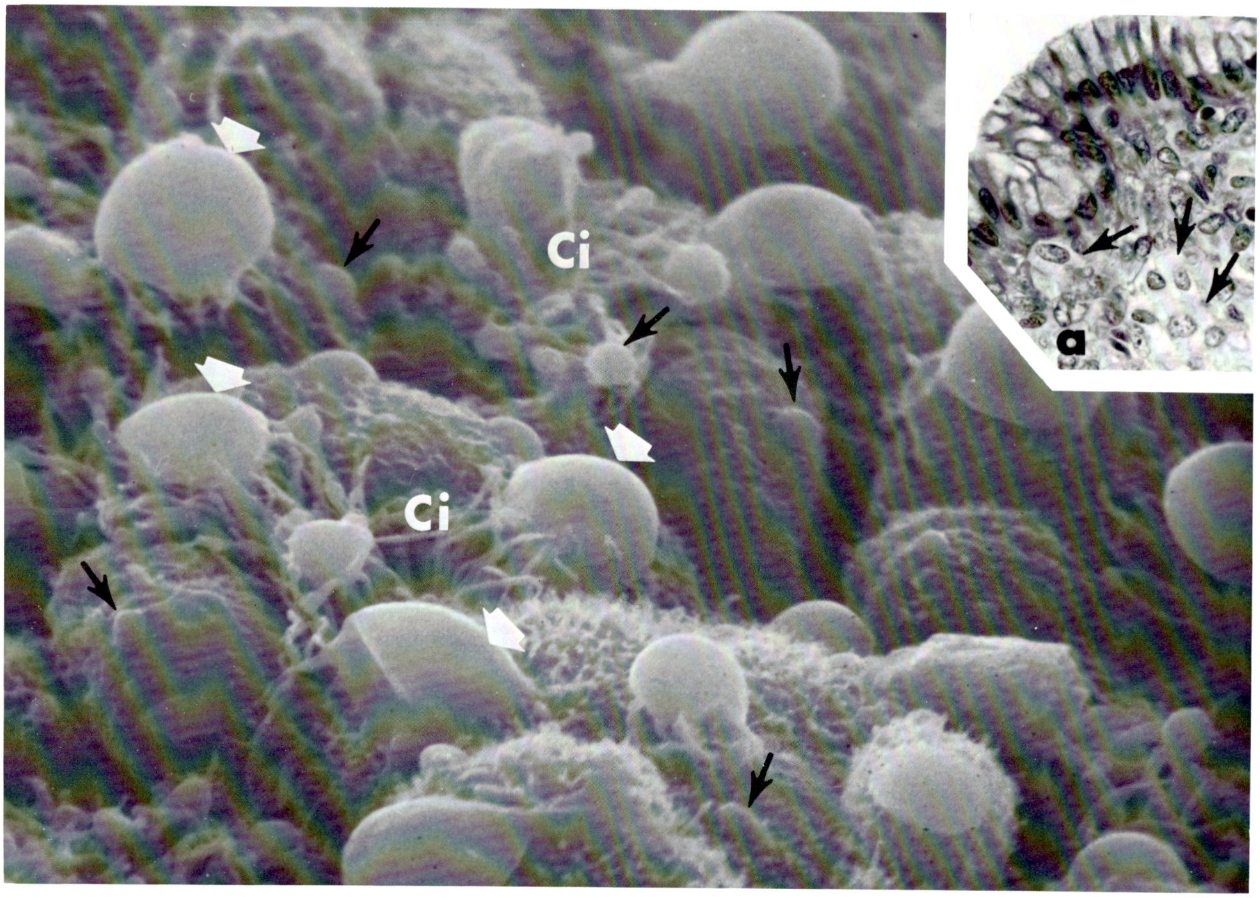

Figure 232a. *Nonpapillary mucinous cystadenoma* lined by tall columnar, mucus-secreting cells (picket-fence pattern) resembling endocervical epithelium. Occasionally, in both benign and malignant mucinous tumors, the stroma contains clusters of luteinized cells (arrows). These cells are thought to be responsible for the occasional androgenic or estrogenic manifestation associated with mucinous neoplasms.[9] (H & E stain, × 120.)

Figure 232. *Nonpapillary mucinous cystadenoma, endocervical type.* Occasional ciliated cells (Ci) intermingle with nonciliated, microvillous, secretory cells exhibiting different phases of apocrine secretion. The prominent surface cytoplasmic protuberances (white arrows), rich in secretory granules, result from the progressive enlargement of smaller bulgings (black arrows). × 4800. *From* A. Ferenczy and R. M. Richart. Scanning electron microscopy of the human genital tract. *N.Y. State J. Med.* (in press).

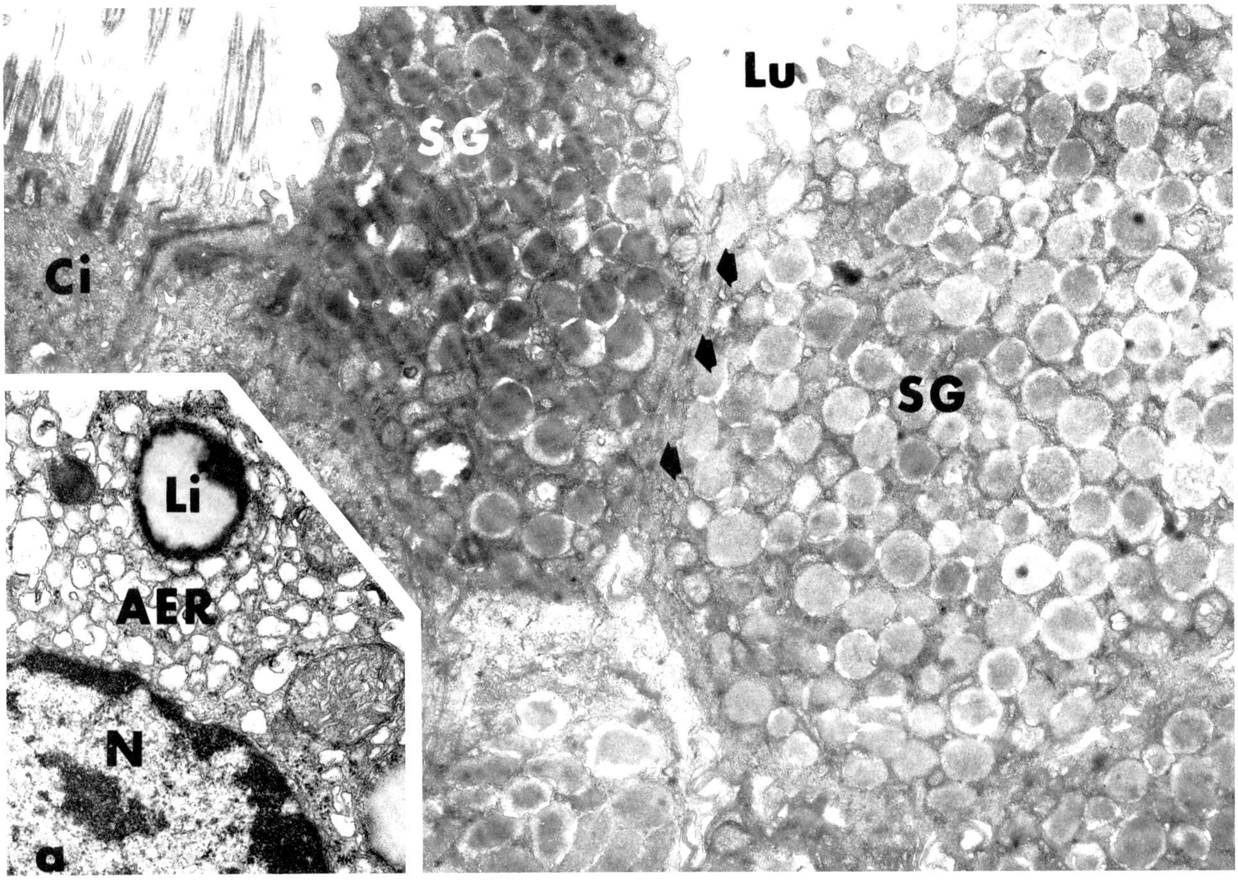

Figure 233. *Nonpapillary mucinous cystadenoma, endocervical type.* As in normal endocervical epithelium, in neoplastic ovarian mucinous cells the cytoplasm is packed with membrane-limited secretory granules (SG), and the apices are often seen protruding into the cyst's lumen (Lu). The different electron density of the secretory granule contents is due to fixation artifact. The luminal microvilli of both ciliated (Ci) and secretory cells are short and sparse, and the lateral plasma membranes are reinforced by luminal tight junctional complexes and desmosomes (arrows). × 5200.

Figure 233a. *Nonpapillary mucinous cystadenoma.* Transmission electron micrograph of luteinized stromal cells seen in Figure 232*a*. The abundant vesicular, agranular endoplasmic reticulum (AER), associated with lipid droplets (Li) and pleomorphic mitochondria with tubular cristae, represents an ultrastructural feature characteristic of active steroidogenic cells. × 6000. N: nucleus of stromal lutein cell.

REFERENCES (Although mucinous cystadenomas—Figure 233a)

1. Overbeck, L. The ultrastructure of pseudomucinous ovarian cystomas. *Z. Geburtsh. Gynaekol.* **168:** 1 (1967).
2. Philipp, E. and L. Overbeck. Die Ultrastruktur des Zervixepithels. *Z. Geburtsh. Gynaekol.* **171:** 159 (1969).
3. Scully, R. E. Germ cell tumors of the ovary. In *Progress in Gynecology,* S. H. Sturgis and M. L. Taymor (Eds.). Grune & Stratton, New York, 1970.
4. McNeil, C., J. N. Ladle, W. M. Helmick, E. Trentelman, and M. W. Wentz. An antiserum to ovarian mucinous cyst fluid with colon cancer specificity. *Cancer Res.* **29:** 1535 (1969).
5. Nairn, R. C., A. C. Wallace, and E. P. Guli. Intestinal antigenecity of ovarian mucinous cystadenomas. *Brit. J. Cancer* **25:** 276 (1971).
6. Linder, D. and J. Power. Further evidence for a post-meiotic origin of teratomas in the human female. *Ann. Hum. Genet.* **34:** 21 (1970).
7. Fox, H., B. Kazzaz, and F. A. Langley. Argyrophil and argentaffin cells in the female genital tract and in ovarian mucinous cysts. *J. Pathol. Bacteriol.* **88:** 479 (1964).
8. Azzopardi, J. G. and L. T. Hou. Intestinal metaplasia with argentaffin cells in cervical adenocarcinoma. *J. Pathol. Bacteriol.* **90:** 686 (1965).
9. Scully, R. E. Androgenic lesions of the ovary. In *The Ovary,* International Academy of Pathology Monograph, H. E. Grady and D. E. Smith (Eds). Williams & Wilkins, Baltimore, 1963, pp. 143–174.

65

Mucinous Cystadenocarcinomas

Figure 234a. *Low-grade (borderline) papillary mucinous cystadenocarcinomas* have complex papillae with secondary branching, and the nuclei are pleomorphic and have an aneuploid DNA content.[1] Mucus-filled goblet cells (arrows) are a common finding. (H & E stain, × 120.)

Figure 234. *Well-differentiated papillary mucinous cystadenocarcinoma.* Low-power scanning electron micrograph of the complex papillary tree, which is composed of large cylindrical structures (black arrows) giving rise to increasingly fine and branching secondary papillae (white arrows). × 200. *From* A. Ferenczy and R. M. Richart. Scanning electron microscopy of the human female genital tract. *N.Y. State J. Med.* (in press).

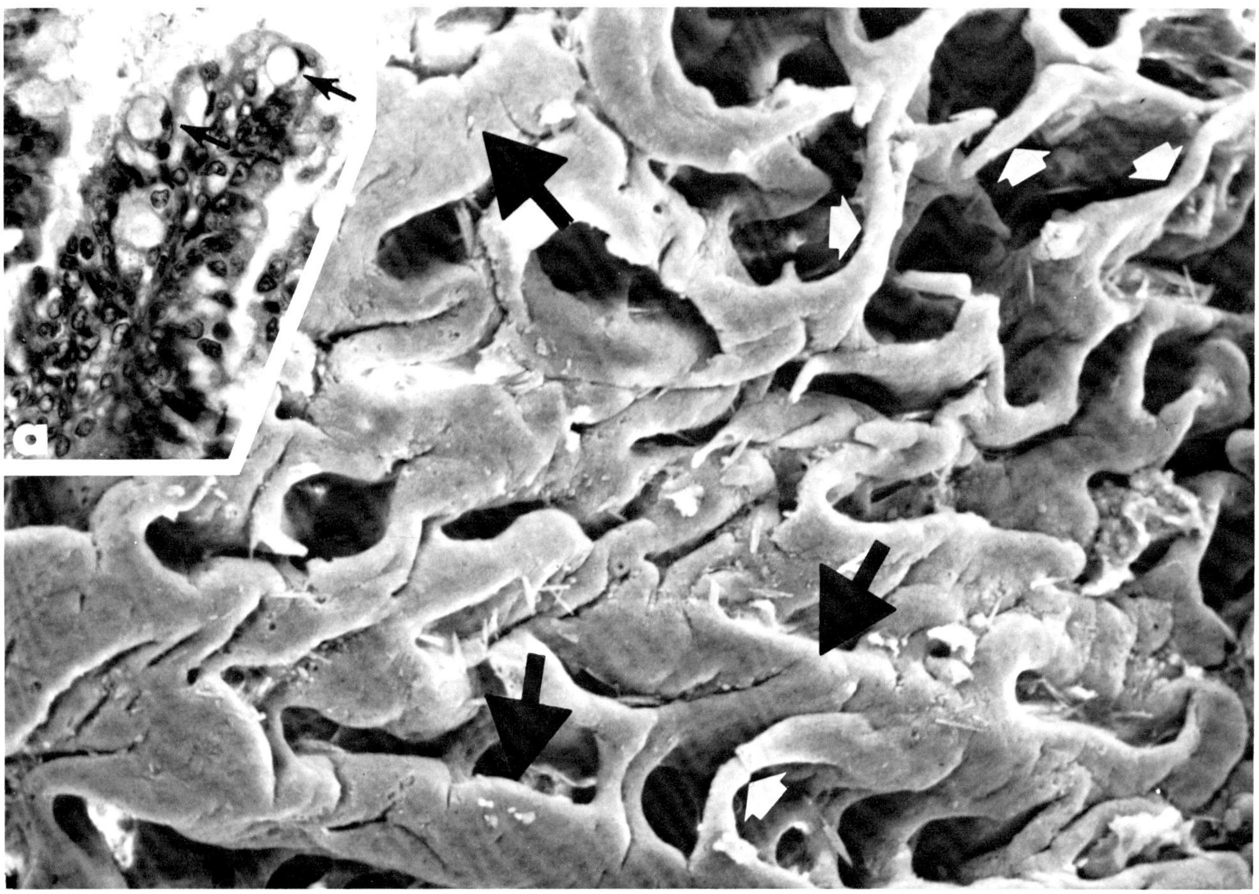

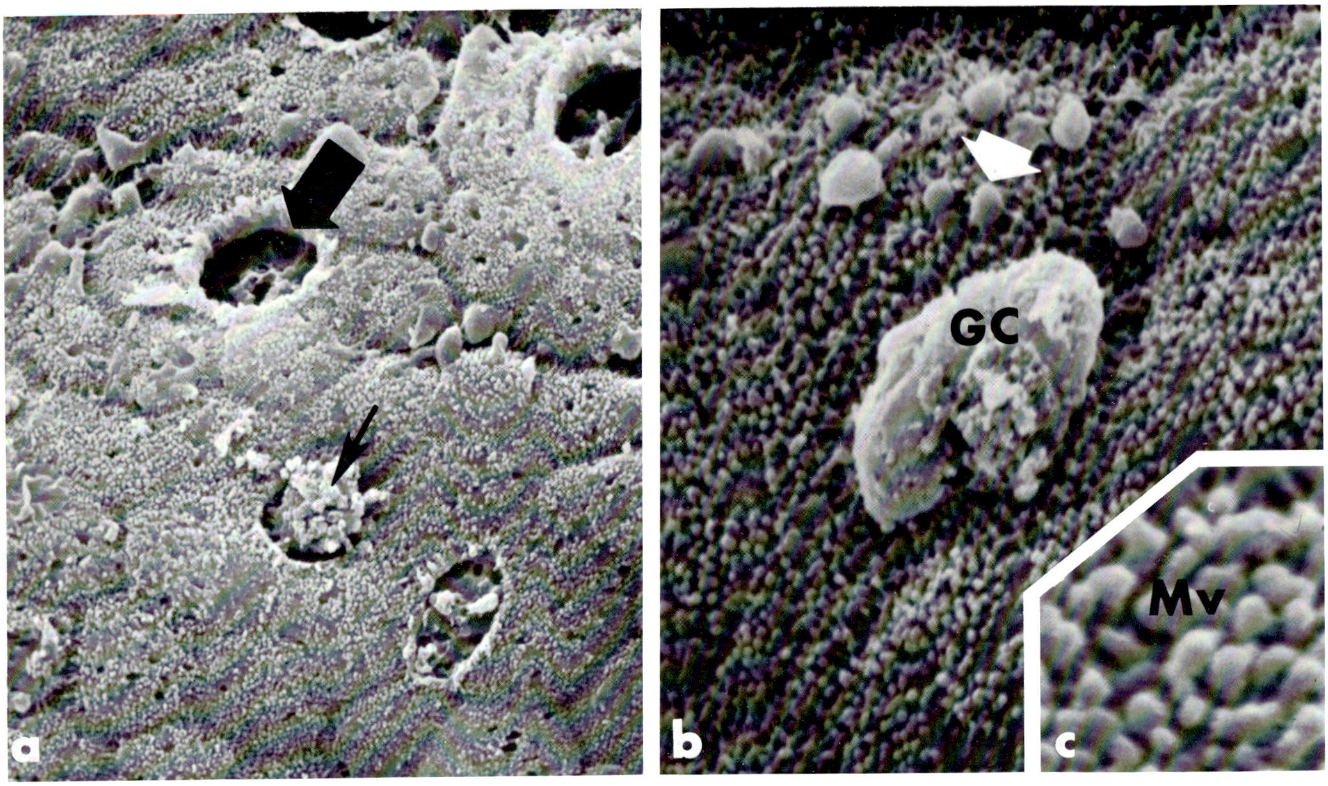

Figure 235a. *Well-differentiated papillary mucinous cystadenocarcinoma. Ultrastructurally, the epithelium in low-grade and well-differentiated papillary mucinous carcinomas* appears to be exclusively of the intestinal type, resembling, both stereoscopically[2,3] and fine structurally, normal colonic[4,5] epithelium. In the epithelium of normal colonic and ovarian mucinous cystadenocarcinoma the dominant cell type is the sulfomucin-filled goblet cell. Secretion occurs predominantly by apocrine expulsion of the supranuclear secretory contents (narrow arrow). Goblet cells that have emptied their granular secretory material resemble large cellular craters (large arrow). Nonsecretory, absorptive cells have a hexagonal outline and contain numerous secretory granules. × 2000. *From* A. Ferenczy and R. M. Richart. Scanning electron microscopy of the human female genital tract. *N.Y. State J. Med.* (in press).

Figure 235b. *Well-differentiated papillary mucinous cystadenocarcinoma.* A mature goblet cell (GC) has a prominent apical bulging, covered by a partially ruptured surface plasma membrane revealing its glandular mucous content. The adjacent microvillous cells contain scattered secretory granules (arrow). × 6000. *From* A. Ferenczy and R. M. Richart. Scanning electron microscopy of the human female genital tract. *N.Y. State J. Med.* (in press).

Figure 235c. *Well-differentiated papillary mucinous cystadenocarcinoma.* High-power view, illustrating the short, stubby, and broad-based surface microvillous processes (Mv) of nonsecretory cells. These resemble the "brush border" of normal colonic mucosa. × 20,000. *From* A. Ferenczy, and R. M. Richart. Scanning electron microscopy of the human female genital tract. *N.Y. State J. Med.* (in press).

REFERENCES (Figures 234a–235c)

1. Weiss, R. R., R. M. Richart, and T. Okagaki. DNA content of mucinous tumors of the ovary. *Am. J. Obstet. Gynecol.* **103:** 409 (1969).
2. Kavin, H., J. D. Eckert, G. Zuidema, R. E. Greasely, and D. G. Hamilton. Studies of human rectal mucosa by scanning electron microscopy. In *Annual SEM Symposia,* O. Johari (Ed.). IIT Research Institute, Chicago, 1970, p. 233.
3. Landboe-Christensen, E. and S. B. Parapat. The gastrointestinal mucosa in man, its surface architecture. Some observations by the scanning electron microscope. In *JEOL News,* Vol. 9, *JEOL Ltd., Tokyo,* 1972, pp. 12–15.
4. Pittman, F. E. and J. C. Pittman. An electron microscopic study of the epithelium of normal human sigmoid colonic mucosa. *Gut* **7:** 644 (1966).
5. Toner, P. G., K. E. Carr, and G. M. Wyburn. *The Digestion System: an Ultrastructural Atlas and Review.* Butterworth, London, 1971.

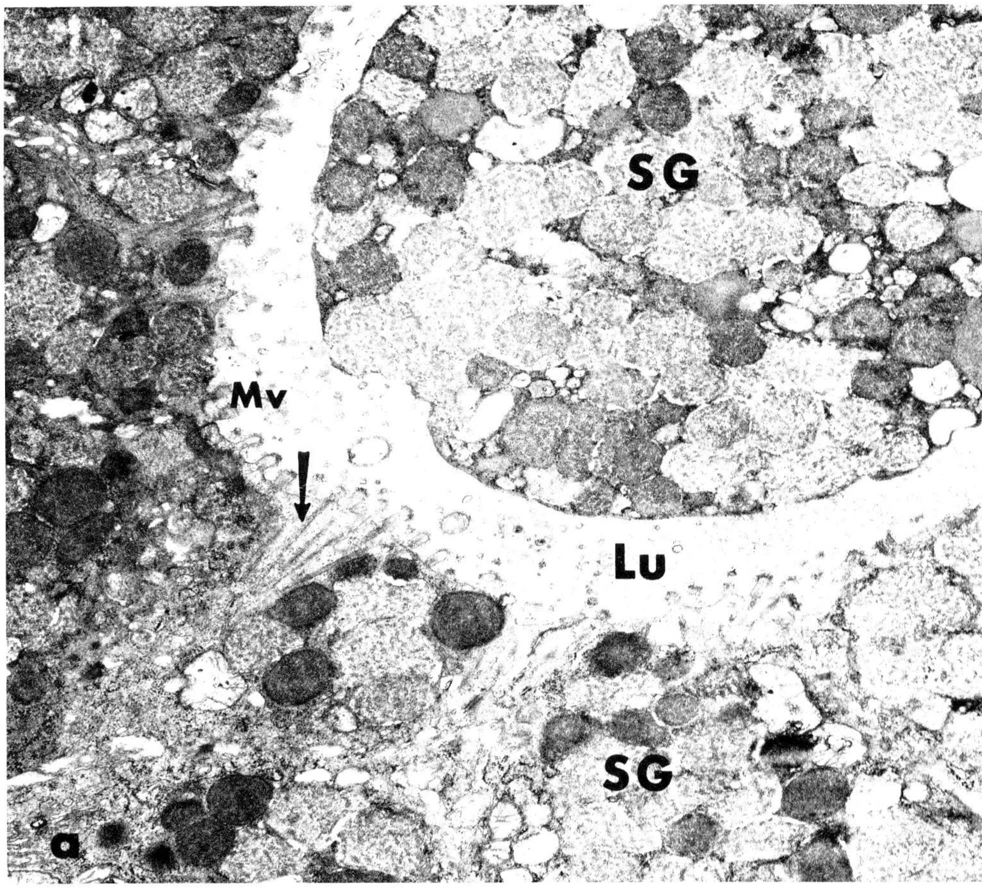

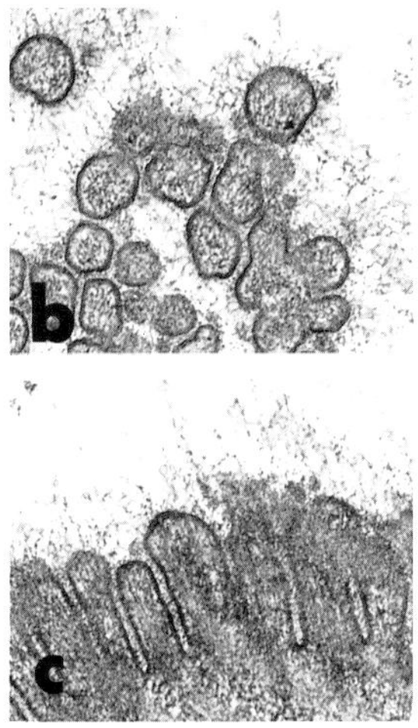

In normal colonic goblet cells, sulfated mucin synthesis has been shown by light[1] and electron microscopic[2] histochemistry to be initiated in the supranuclear Golgi, and both the production and discharge of secretory products seem to be continuous[1] processes. Similar secretory activity is observed in ovarian mucinous neoplasms.[3,4] In contrast to normal colonic mucosa, however, in both mucinous ovarian and colonic[5,6] neoplasms the surface microvilli are greatly altered and are irregular in size and distribution, and the terminal web, a characteristic feature of normal intestinal epithelium, is seldom seen.

Figure 236a. *Well-differentiated papillary mucinous cystadenocarcinoma.* The glandular lumen (Lu) contains most of a goblet cell's secretory content, delimited by an ill-defined plasma membrane. The lumen-lining cells are rich in coalescing secetory granules (SG) filled with filamentous material, and the luminal microvilli (Mv) appear short and irregular with occasional microfilamentous (arrow) extensions. × 6200.

Figures 236b and c. *Well-differentiated papillary mucinous cystadenocarcinoma.* Cross (*b*) and longitudinal (*c*) sections of surface microvilli. They appear short, often fused together, and are surrounded by fine, branching, filamentous material (glycocalyx). The microvillous processes are penetrated by abundant cytoplasmic microfilaments. × 30,000.

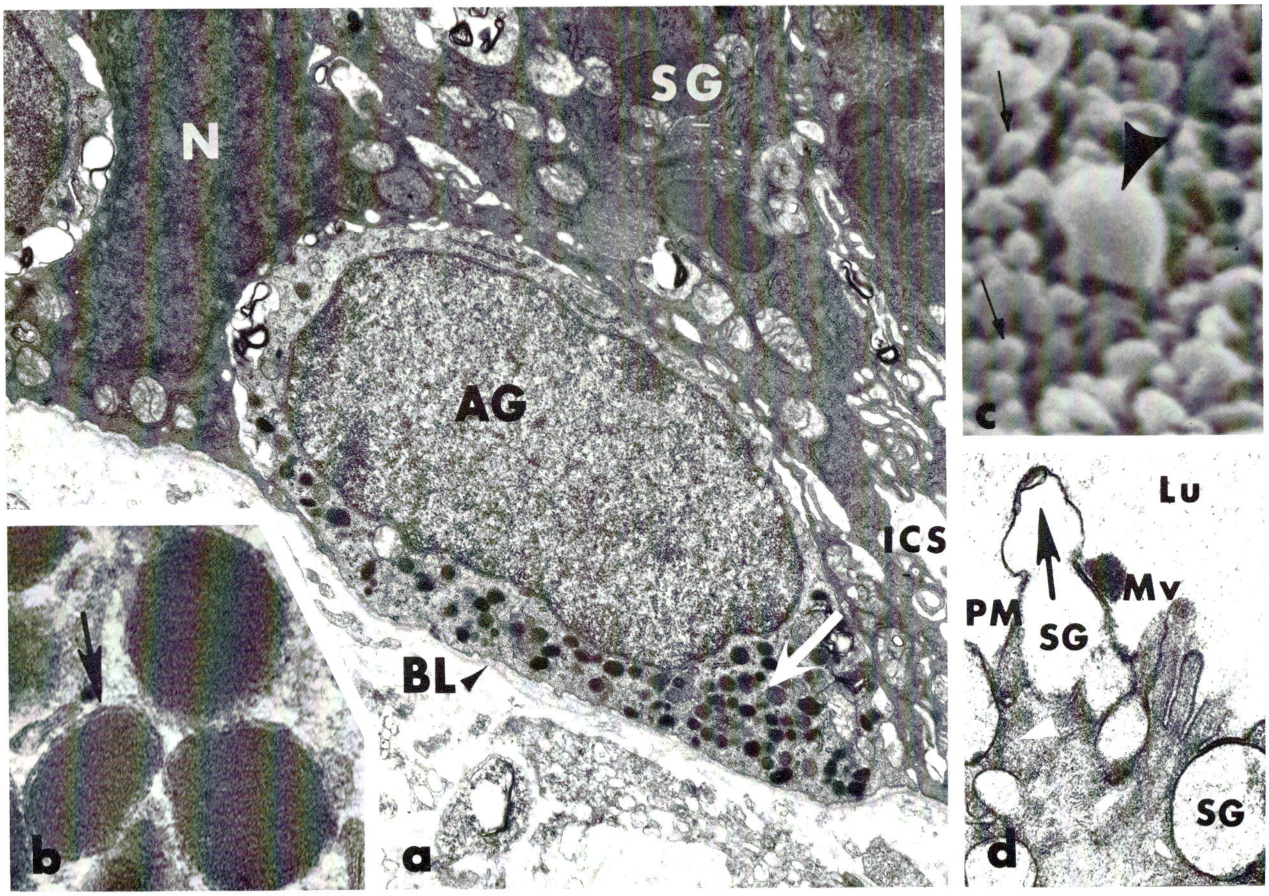

Figure 237a. *Well-differentiated papillary mucinous cystadenocarcinoma.* A basally located argentaffin cell (AG) with numerous pleomorphic secretory granules varying from 75 to 500 mμ in diameter (arrow) is seen surrounded by mucus (SG) containing goblet cells. × 7000. N: nucleus of a goblet cell; ICS: dilated intercellular spaces; BL: basal lamina.

Figure 237b. *Higher magnification of Figure 237a,* showing membrane-bound (arrow) secretory granules with uniform electron-dense matrix. Similar secretory granules are distinctive of carcinoid tumors of mid-gut derivation.[7] × 84,275.

Figure 237c. *Well-differentiated papillary mucinous cystadenocarcinoma.* In addition to apocrine secretion, secretion occasionally occurs by merocrine buddings of single secretory vacuoles (arrow head). Note the adjacent stubby microvilli (arrows). × 16,000.

Figure 237d. *Well-differentiated papillary mucinous cystadenocarcinoma.* Transmission electron microscopic appearance of merocrine secretion. A secretory granule (SG) protrudes (arrow) into the lumen (Lu) through the surface plasma membrane (PM). The adjacent microvilli (Mv) are compressed, and another secretory granule (SG, in lower right corner) is located just beneath the plasma membrane, ready to be expelled. × 20,000.

REFERENCES (In normal colonic goblet cells—Figure 237d)

1. Florey, H. The secretion of mucus and inflammation of mucous membranes. In *General Pathology,* H. Florey (Ed.). Lloyd-Luke, 1962, pp. 167–196.
2. Wetzel, M. G., B. K. Wetzel, and S. S. Spicer. Ultrastructural localization of acid mucosubstances in the mouse colon with iron containing stains. *J. Cell Biol.* **30:** 299 (1966).
3. Overbeck, L. The ultrastructure of pseudomucinous ovarian cystomas. *Z. Geburtsh. Gynaekol.* **168:** 1 (1967).
4. Kawase, T. and M. Hashimoto. Ultrastructural considerations on the histologic origin of ovarian mucinous cysts. *J. Jap. Obstet. Gynecol. Soc.* **23:** 77 (1971).
5. Fisher, E. R. and D. A. Sharkey. The ultrastructure of colonic polyps and cancer with special reference to the epithelial inclusion bodies of Leuchtenberger. *Cancer* **15:** 160 (1962).
6. Spjut, H. J. and M. N. Smith. A comparative electron microscopic study of human and rat colonic polyps and carcinomas. *Exp. Mol. Pathol.* **6:** 11 (1967).
7. Black, W. C. Enterochromaffin cell types and corresponding carcinoid tumors. *Lab. Invest.* **19:** 473 (1968).

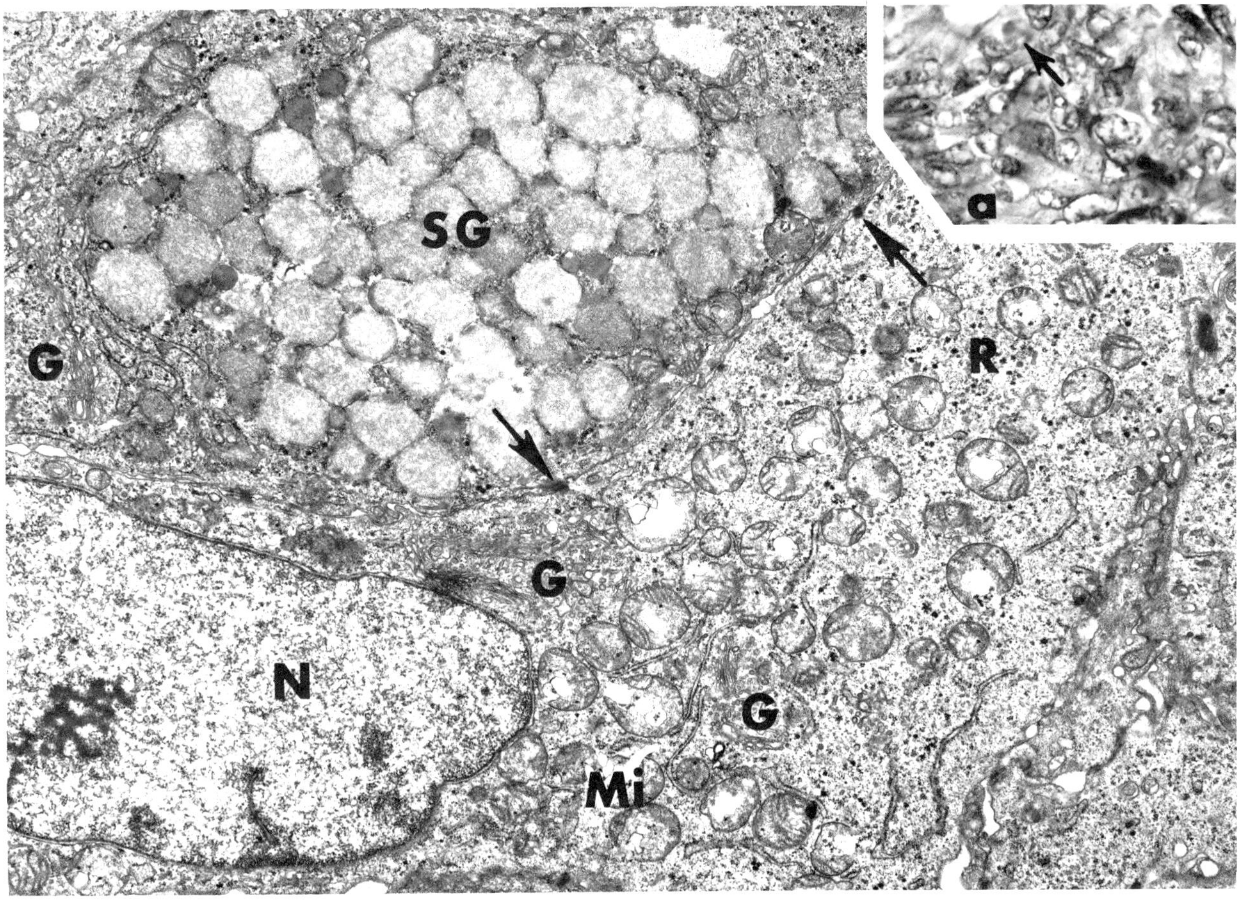

Figure 238a. *In moderately and poorly differentiated ovarian neoplasms,* as in their colonic counterparts, the production of mucus is reduced, paralleling the profound decrease of goblet cells (arrow) in the increasingly dedifferentiated lesions. Similarly, argentaffin cells are usually absent, and nuclear pleomorphism with prominent nucleolar substance predominates. Gland formation remains in an abortive stage. (H & E stain, × 120.)

Figure 238. *Moderately to poorly differentiated mucinous cystadenocarcinoma.* A poorly formed goblet cell has tightly packed secretory granules (SG), presumably formed by the adjacent Golgi (G). The neighboring cell contains abundant perinuclear (N) Golgi, mitochondria (Mi), free ribosomes (R), and parallel membranes of granular endoplasmic reticulum, all of which are needed for mucinogenesis. The lateral plasma membranes are convoluted, and desmosomal attachments (arrows) are infrequent. × 6000.

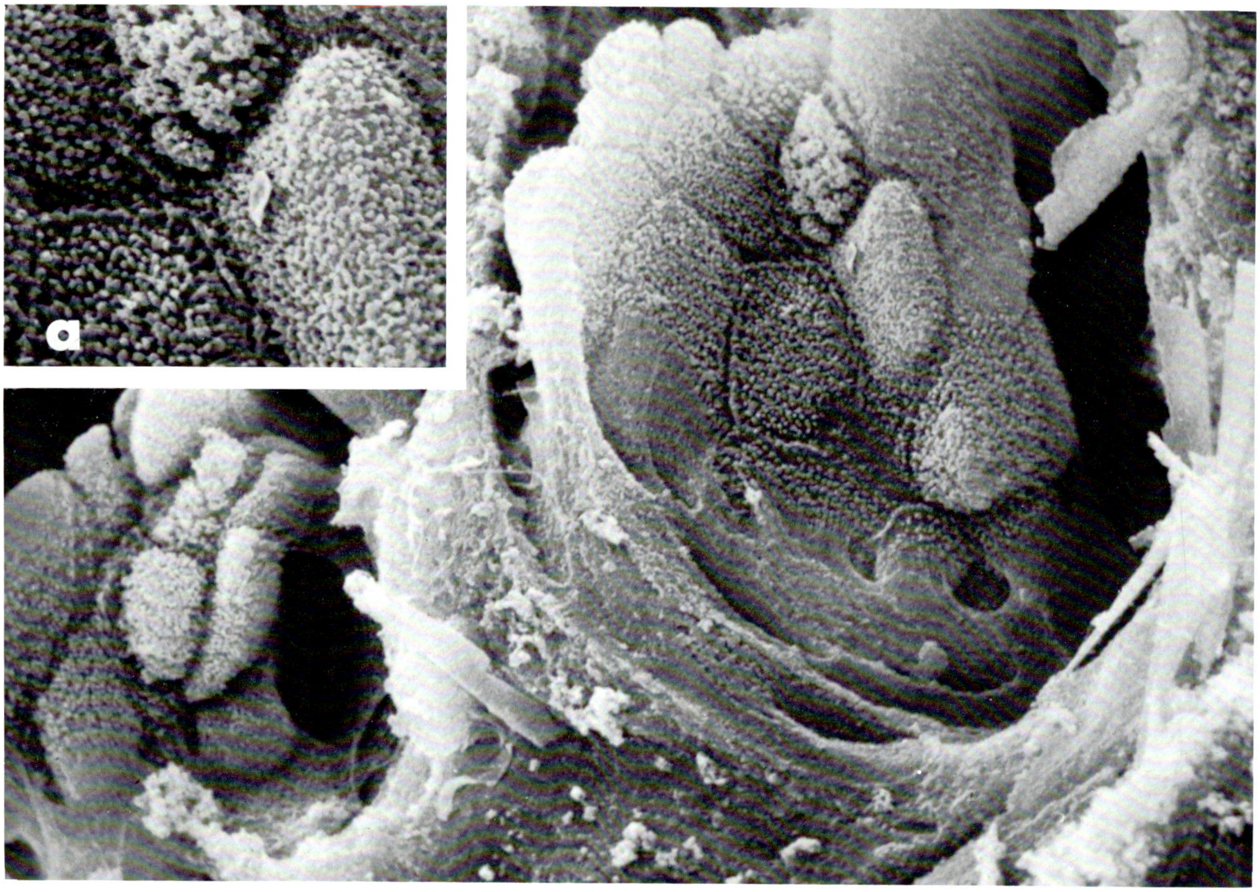

Figure 239. *Moderately to poorly differentiated mucinous cystadenocarcinoma.* Scanning electron micrograph of a blunt-ended papilla covered by large polyhedral cells devoid of goblet cells. Secretion, however, occurs, and the lower portion of the photograph is obscured by mucous material. × 1600.

Figure 239a. *Detail of Figure 239,* illustrating the abundant but short surface microvillous processes. The cells are attached by nodular tight junctional complexes. × 4800.

66

Endometrioid Carcinomas

Endometrioid carcinomas of the ovary represent the second most common primary ovarian malignancy[1] and are characterized by a proliferation of neoplastic glands, with or without squamous metaplasia which are identical histologically, histochemically,[1] and ultrastructurally to those of adenocarcinomas of endometrial origin. Although one-third of endometrioid carcinomas are associated with superficial adenocarcinoma of the endometrium,[1] suggesting the possibility of ovarian metastasis, it is generally believed that endometrioid tumors are primary lesions arising through the process of celomic metaplasia. This histogenetic origin is supported by their occasional occurrence within endometriotic cysts and by the presence of both serous and mucinous elements within endometrioid lesions. The relatively favorable prognosis of endometrial adenocarcinoma applies also to endometrioid tumors of the ovary, and these lesions have a comparatively better 5-year survival rate than serous carcinomas.

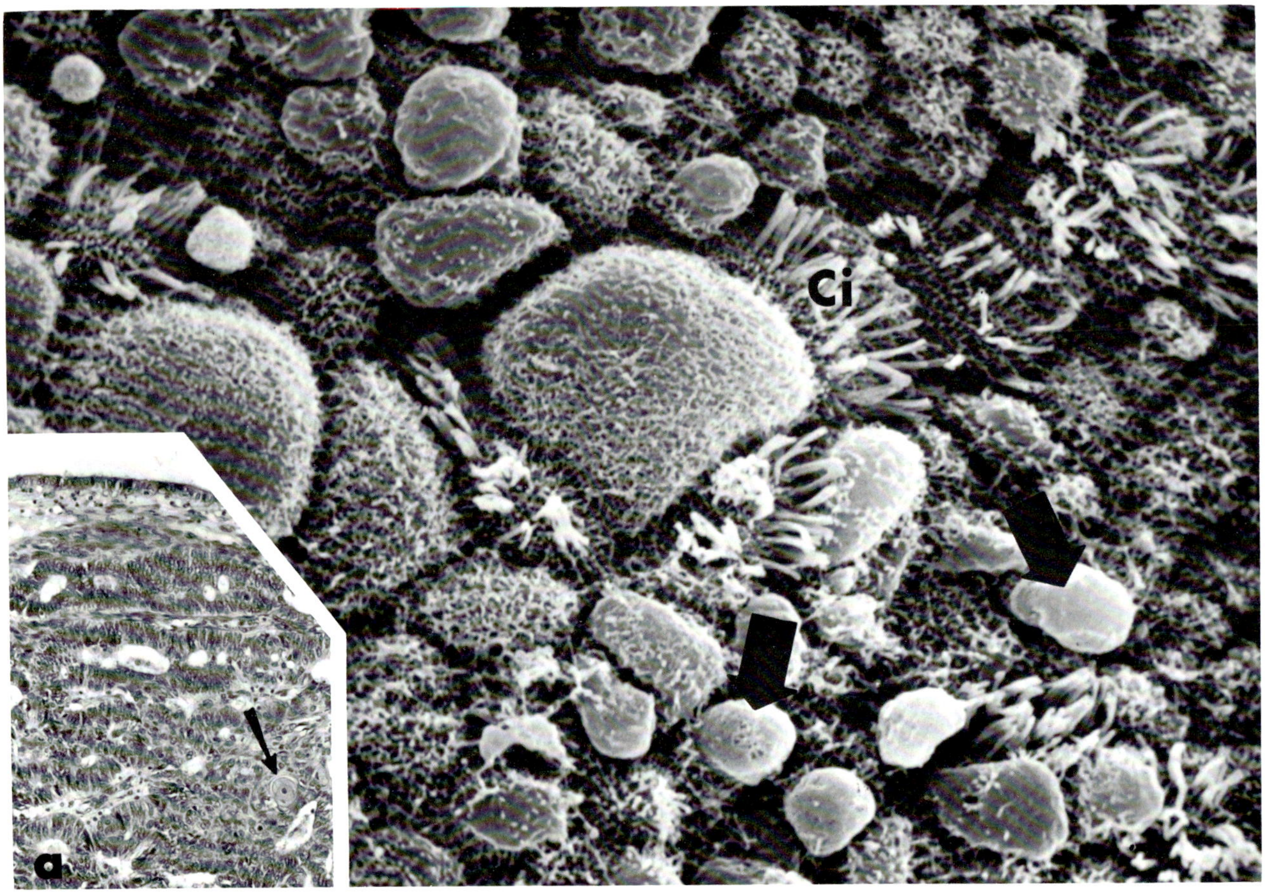

Figures 240a. *Moderately differentiated endometrioid carcinoma with squamous metaplasia (arrow) (adenoacanthoma).* Note the striking resemblance of the neoplastic glands to those of endometrial adenocarcinoma. (H & E stain, × 30.)

Figures 240. *Moderately differentiated endometrioid carcinoma with squamous metaplasia.* As in endometrial adenocarcinoma, in endometrioid carcinoma of the ovary occasional ciliated cells (Ci) are seen, and the nonciliated microvillous cells exhibit pleomorphism and degenerative changes (arrows). × 2240.

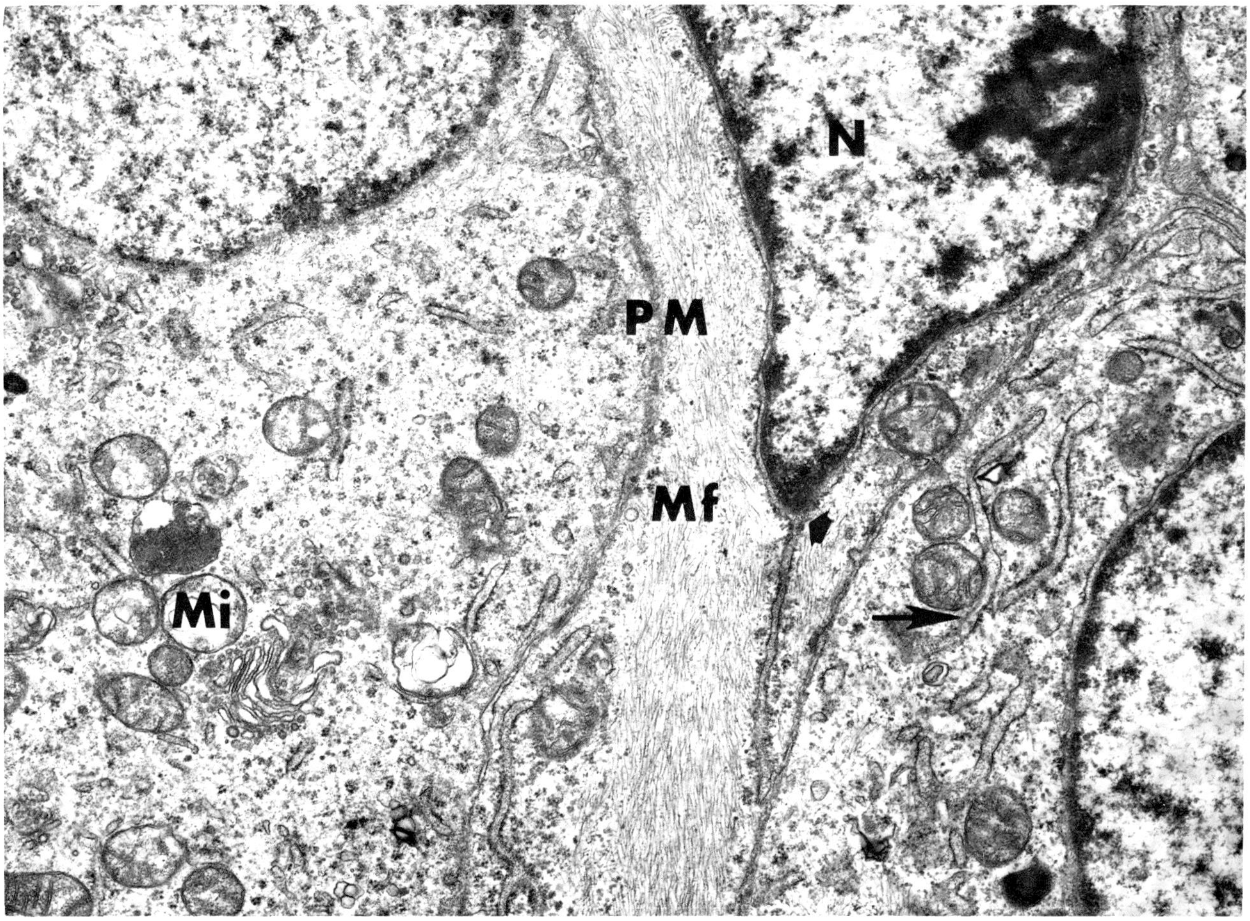

Figure 241. *Well-differentiated endometrioid carcinoma.* Many of the neoplastic glandular cells have conspicuous bundles of perinuclear (N) microfilaments (Mf). Mitochondria (Mi) are in close apposition (long arrow) with parallel membranes of granular endoplasmic reticulum and are occasionally in continuity with the nuclear membrane (short arrow). × 18,000. PM: plasma membrane.

REFERENCE (Endometrioid carcinomas–Figure 241)

1. Scully, R. E. Recent progress in ovarian cancer. *Human Pathol.* **1:** 73 (1970).

67

Clear Cell Adenocarcinoma

Figure 242a. *Clear cell adenocarcinoma* (mesonephroma, mesonephroid, or hypernephroid carcinoma) of the ovary may be a predominantly solid or cystic growth. It is composed of tubules with intraluminal secretions (arrow) and solid sheets of large epithelial cells with abundant, glycogen-rich, clear cytoplasm and "hobnail" cells with bulging, apical nuclei. (H & E stain, × 60.)

Figure 242. *Ultrastructurally,*[1] the epithelial clear cells contain pools of glycogen granules (Gly) associated with prominent lamellar endoplasmic reticulum (GER), mitochondria, and Golgi (G), features reflecting active biosynthetic activity. The luminal (Lu) plasma membrane has short, sparse microvilli, whereas the lateral plasma membranes are tightly apposed and highly convoluted. × 6100. Ly: lysosomes; N: nucleus; BL: basal lamina. *From* T. Okagaki. Professor of Pathology, University of Minnesota, Department of Obstetrics and Gynecology, Box 395, Mayo Memorial Building, Minneapolis, Minn. 55455.

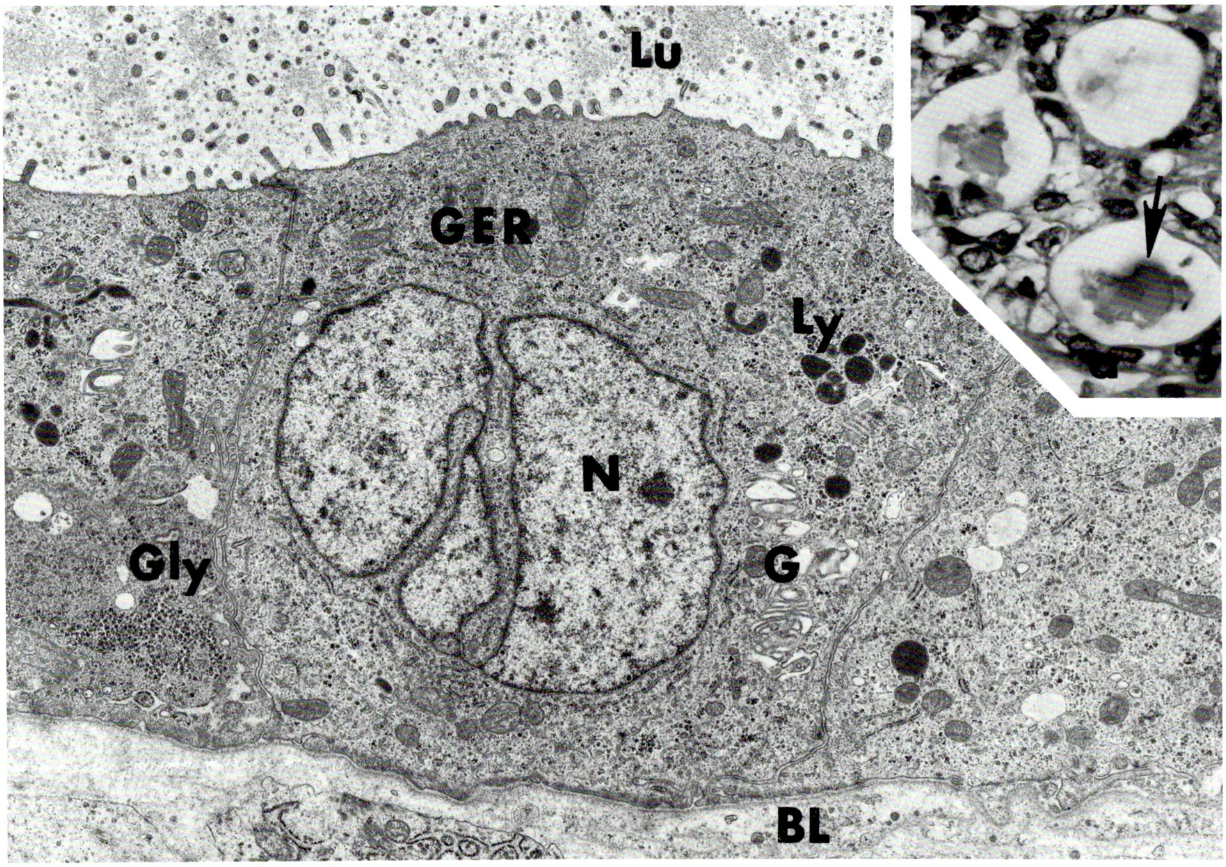

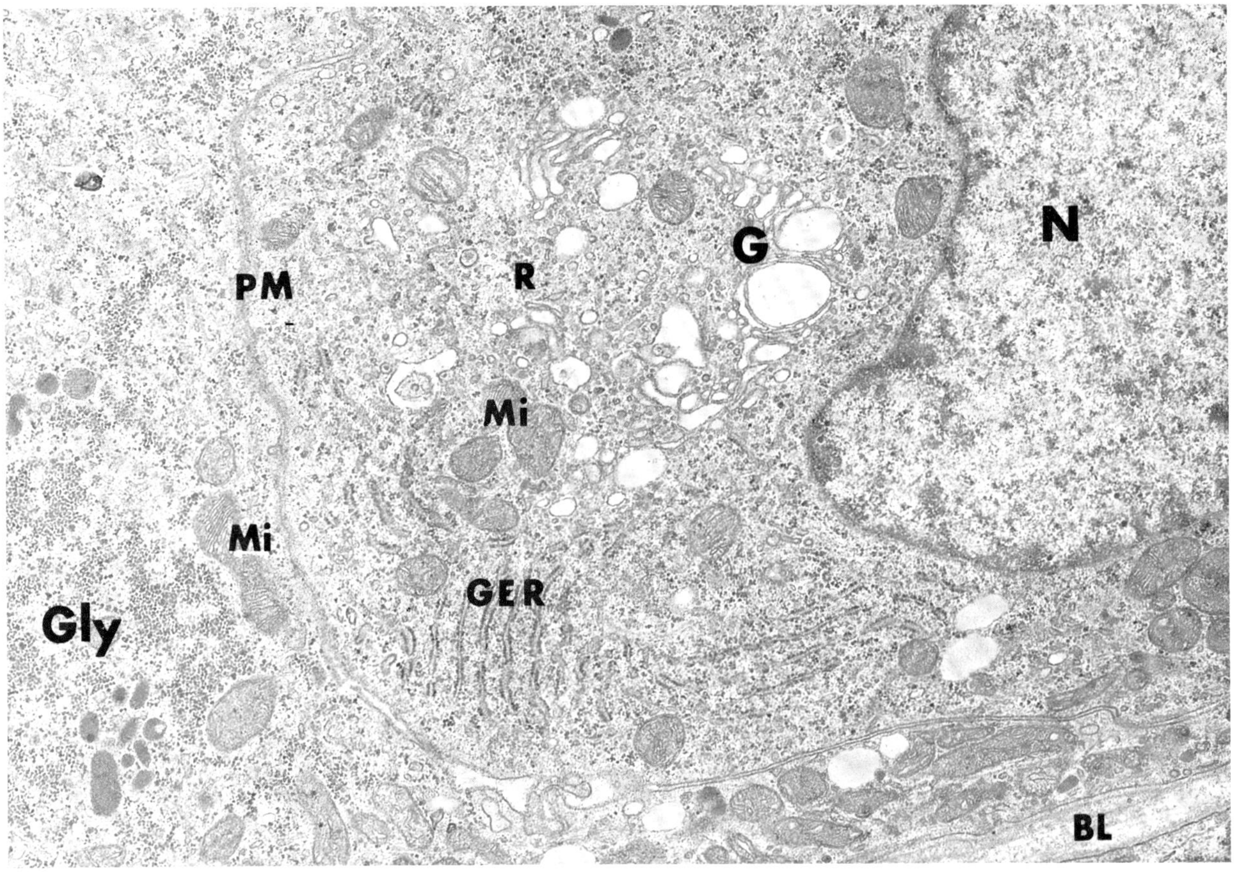

Figure 243. *Clear cell adenocarcinoma.* Note the prominent aggregates of glycogen particles (Gly) in close relationship with stacks of granular endoplasmic reticulum (GER), mitochondria (Mi), free ribosomes (R), and perinuclear (N) Golgi (G). A similar submicroscopic organization has been reported in clear cell carcinomas of endometrial,[2] cervical,[3] and vaginal[4] origin, suggesting that glycogen-rich, clear cell tumors of the female genital tract may have a common Müllerian[5,6] rather than mesonephric[7] or metanephric,[8] origin and may be related to endometrial epithelium. On the basis of the available histologic evidence,[5,6] clear cell adenocarcinoma in the ovary presumably arises by "endometrioid" metaplasia (endometriosis) from invaginated surface celomic epithelium and represents a morphologic variant of the more common ovarian endometrioid carcinoma. Although clear cell tumors of the reproductive tract are ultrastructurally similar to the mucopolysaccharide-synthesizing cells found in progesterone-treated hyperplastic[2] and neoplastic[9] endometria, there is no evidence to indicate endo- or exogenous progestational influence on the development of clear cell carcinoma. × 24,000. PM: plasma membrane; BL: basal lamina. *From* T. Okagaki, Professor of Pathology, University of Minnesota, Department of Obstetrics and Gynecology, Box 395, Mayo Memorial Building, Minneapolis, Minn. 55455.

REFERENCES (Figures 242a–243)

1. Okagaki, T. and R. M. Richart, "Mesonephroma ovarii (hypernephroid carcinoma)"light and ultrastructural study of a case. *Cancer* **26:** 453 (1970).
2. Rorat, E., R. Ferenczy, and R. M. Richart. The ultrastructure of clear cell adenocarcinoma of the endometrium. *Cancer* (in press).
3. Woyke, S., W. Damagala, and W. Olszewski. Mesonephroma of the uterine cervix: submicroscopic study and comparison with fine structure of endocervical adenocarcinoma. *Virchows Arch. Abt. Pathol. Anat.* **355:** 29 (1972).
4. Silverberg, S. G. and L. S. DeGiorgi. Clear cell carcinoma of the vagina. A clinical, pathologic and electron microscopic study. *Cancer* **29:** 1680 (1972).
5. Scully, R. E. and J. F. Barlow. "Mesonephroma" of ovary. Tumor of Müllerian nature related to the endometrioid carcinoma. *Cancer* **20:** 1405 (1967).
6. Scully, R. E. Recent progress in ovarian cancer. *Human Pathol.* **1:** 73 (1970).
7. Hertig, A. T. and H. Gore. Tumors of the female sex organs. Part 3. Tumors of the ovary and Fallopian tube. In *Atlas of Tumor Pathology*. Armed Forces Institute of Pathology, Washington, D.C., 1961, p. 124.
8. Novak, E. R. and J. D. Woodruff. Mesonephroma of the ovary—thirty-five cases from the Ovarian Tumor Registry of the American Gynecological Society. *Am. J. Obstet. Gynecol.* **77:** 632 (1959).
9. Hayakawa, K. Effects of dimethisterone on endometrial adenocarcinoma—electron microscopic study. *Acta Obstet. Gynaecol.* **16:** 285 (1969).

68

Brenner Tumor

The Brenner tumor is a relatively rare ovarian neoplasm, most commonly found in peri- or post menopausal women.[1,2] The lesion is usually a fibrous-appearing, solid growth, which, microscopically, consists of a fibromatous stroma containing epithelial islands that resemble both Walthard cell nests and urothelium. Mucinous cells of goblet type are frequently seen within cystic epithelial nests. Characteristically, the surrounding stroma has a fibrothecomatous appearance with foci or stromal lutein cells, which are presumably responsible for the occasional estrogenic stimulation of the endometrium associated with the neoplasm.

At an ultrastructural level,[3-9] the histological similarity between Brenner epithelium and the transitional-type epithelium of Walthard cell nests[8] and of the urinary tract[8] is confirmed. The common submicroscopic features include deep nuclear ingrooving, dilated intercellular spaces, and abundant agranular endoplasmic reticulum with conspicuous autophagic activity (autophagolysosomes) in the central, or luminal, cell layers. In the Brenner epithelium,[3,7-9] as in the Walthard cell nests,[8] central cellular degeneration associated with autolytic activity results in cyst formation, the cysts being lined by microvillous epithelial cells. The mucinous cells are presumably derived from the subjacent transitional cells.[4] Ultrastructurally, the nonepithelial portion of the Brenner tumor is completely separated from the epithelial nests by a well-developed basal lamina and is composed of cells varying from unremarkable, spindle-shaped stromal to plump, fully luteinized cells. It is similar in ultrastructure to a fibroma-thecoma.[10] Further morphologic evidence for a commonality between the Brenner tumor and urothelium is afforded by the so-called proliferating Brenner tumor.[11,12] This lesion closely resembles the low-grade papillary, transitional cell carcinoma of the urinary bladder and apparently represents an intermediate stage between the classical Brenner tumor and the rare malignant variety,[12] which is histologically similar to invasive transitional cell carcinoma of the urinary tract.

These morphologic observations, demonstration of the direct histologic continuity of the Brenner epithelium with the ovarian surface lining, and the tumor's principally cortical location, associated with surface infoldings, cortical inclusion cysts, and mucinous and serous neoplasms (structures considered to be derived from the ovarian surface epithelium), suggest that Brenner tumors arise from the ovarian celomic epithelium by transitional metaplasia. The genesis of the stromal component of the tumor and the question of whether it precedes or follows the formation of Brenner nests are not clear, although its presence may explain the rarity of this neoplasm in extraovarian sites.

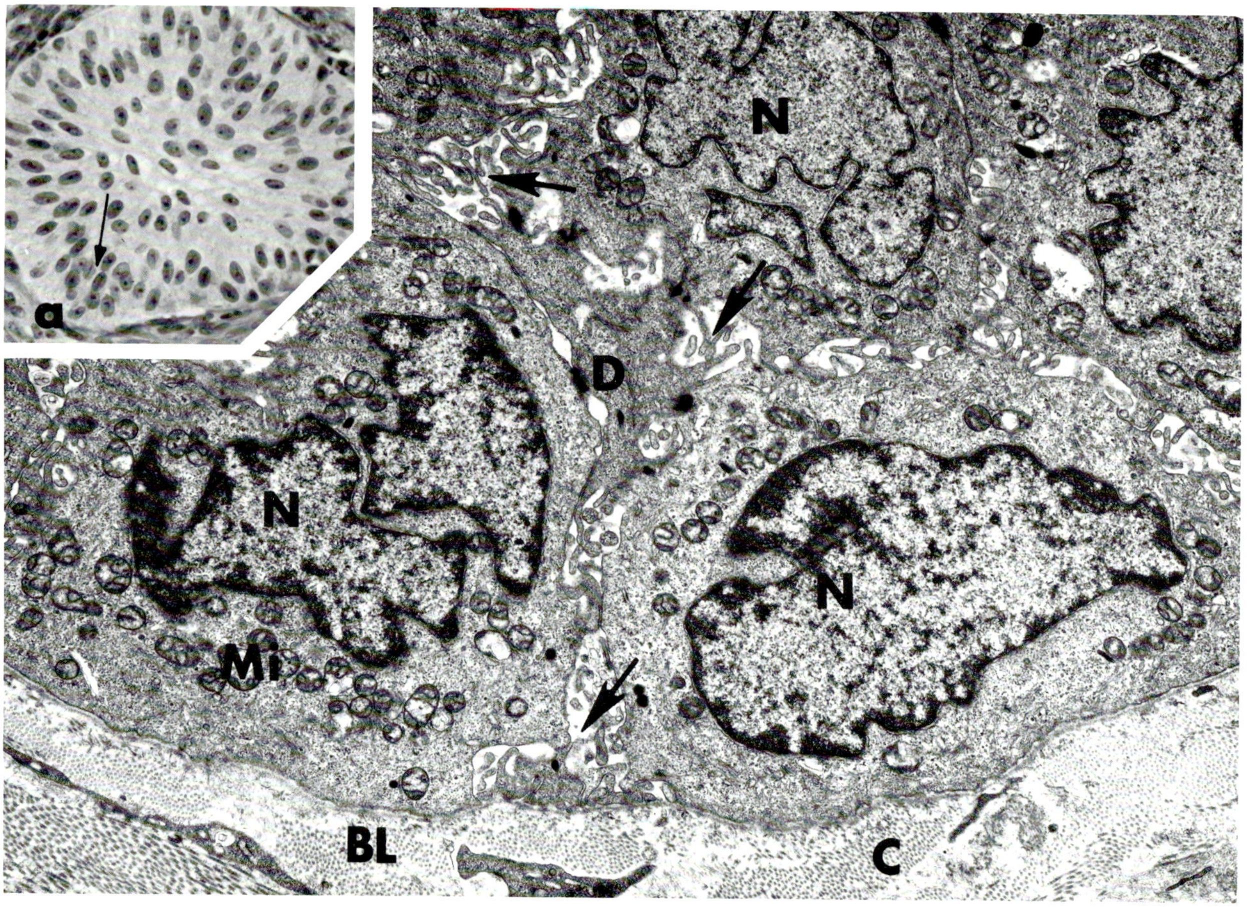

Figure 244a. *Brenner tumor.* Light micrograph of an island of Brenner epithelium, composed of stratified transitional-like cells in which the nuclei show the characteristic "coffee-bean" pattern (arrow). (H & E stain, × 18.)

Figure 244. *Electron micrograph of the basal portion of a Brenner nest.* The cells have highly indented nuclei (N) (the feature responsible for the histologic "coffee-bean" pattern), scant organelles in a perinuclear location, and dilated intercellular spaces with numerous interdigitating microvilli (arrows). The lateral plasma membranes are attached by occasional desmosomal (D) belts. The Brenner nests are separated by a well-defined basal lamina (BL) from the surrounding fibrothecomatous stroma (C). × 5800. Mi: mitochondria.

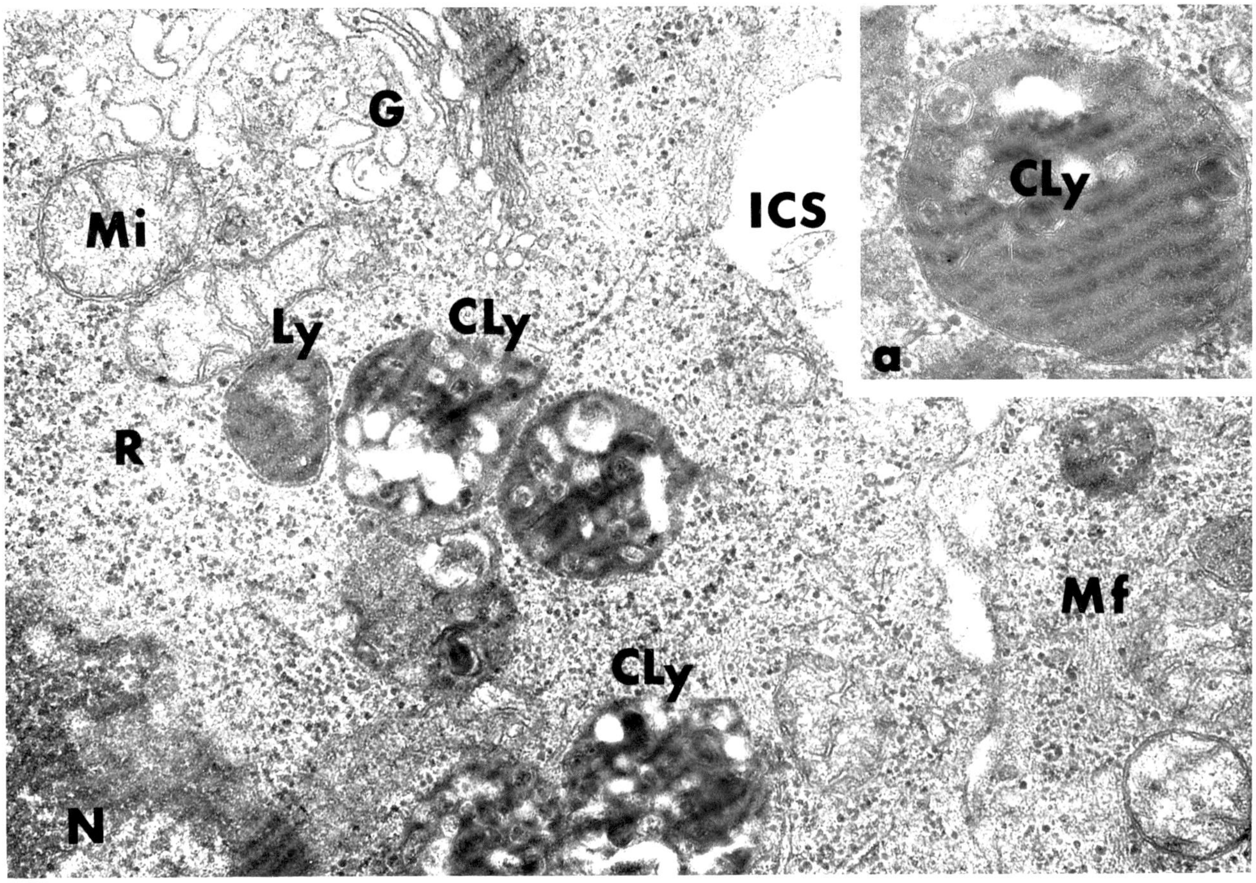

Figure 245. *Characteristic of cells of the central layer of solid or cystic Brenner nests* are numerous prominent autophagic cytolysosomes (CLy), and lysosomes (Ly) associated with well-developed Golgi (G), agranular endoplasmic reticulum, and ribosomes (R). × 32,000. N: nucleus; Mf: microfilaments; ICS: dilated intercellular space; Mi: mitochondria.

Figure 245a. *A membrane-bound giant cytolysosome* (CLy), filled with polyhedral lamellated inclusions and finely granular electron-dense material. × 40,000. *From* B. R. Bransilver, A. Ferenczy, and R. M. Richart. Brenner tumors and Walthard cell nests. A comparative ultrastructural study in preparation.

REFERENCES (The Brenner tumor–Figure 245a)

1. Ehrlich, C. E. and M. Roth. The Brenner tumor. A clinicopathologic study of 57 cases. *Cancer* **27:** 332 (1971).
2. Silverberg, S. G. Brenner tumor of the ovary. A clinicopathologic study of 60 tumors in 54 women. *Cancer* **28:** 588 (1971).
3. Philipp, E. and L. Overbeck. Zur Ultrastruktur des Brenner-Tumors. *Z. Geburtsh. Gynaekol.* **173:** 196 (1970).
4. Kawase, T. and M. Hashimoto. Ultrastructural considerations on the histologic origin of ovarian mucinous cysts. *J. Jap. Obstet. Gynecol. Soc.* **23:** 77 (1971).
5. Roth, L. M. Fine structure of the Brenner tumor. *Cancer* **27:** 1482 (1971).
6. Silverberg, S. G. and M. A. Willson. Ultrastructure of the Brenner tumor. *Am. J. Obstet Gynecol.* **112:** 91 (1972).
7. Hameed, K. Brenner tumor of the ovary with Leydig cell hyperplasia. *Cancer* **30:** 945 (1972).
8. Bransilver, B. R., A. Ferenczy, and R. M. Richart. Brenner tumors and Walthard cell nests. A comparative ultrastructural study (in preparation).
9. Merkow, L. P., H. Salazar, and M. Pardo. Human ovarian neoplasms, light and electron microscopic correlations. I. The Brenner tumor. *Obstet. Gynecol.* **40:** 667 (1972).
10. Amin, H. K., T. Okagaki, and R. M. Richart. Classification of fibroma and thecoma of the ovary. An ultrastructural study. *Cancer* **27:** 438 (1971).
11. Roth, L. M. and W. H. Sternberg. Proliferating Brenner tumors. *Cancer* **27:** 687 (1971).
12. Miles, P. A. and H. J. Norris. Proliferative and malignant Brenner tumors of the ovary. *Cancer* **30:** 174 (1972).

69

Benign Mesothelioma (Adenomatoid Tumor)

Benign ovarian mesothelioma (adenomatoid tumor) is a very rare neoplasm, found in the hilum or mesovarium, usually in close association with the celomic epithelium. Histologically, the lesion consists of a sponge-work of canalicular and glandlike spaces lined with dome-shaped, flattened to cuboidal cells, embedded in a fibrovascular stroma. Similar lesions are also found near, or in histologic continuity with, the serosal covering of the oviduct or posterior wall of the uterus. They also commonly occur in the epididymis and, occasionally, in extragenital locations.[1] Ultrastructural[1-4] and histochemical[5,6] studies support the postulate of Masson et al.[7] that the cells lining the glandlike spaces are derived from mesothelial[1,3,4] rather than endothelial, mesonephric,[8] or glandular epithelium and that the lesion arises from the ovarian celomic epithelium. The fine structural and histochemical characteristics common to genital mesotheliomas and ovarian, celomic,[9] and other extragenital mesothelial membranes[10] and mesothelioma[1] include abundant and branching microvilli with occasional single cilia, surface pinocytosis, widened intercellular spaces, and abundant intraglandular and extracellular acid mucopolysaccharide that is rich in hyaluronic acid.[5,6]

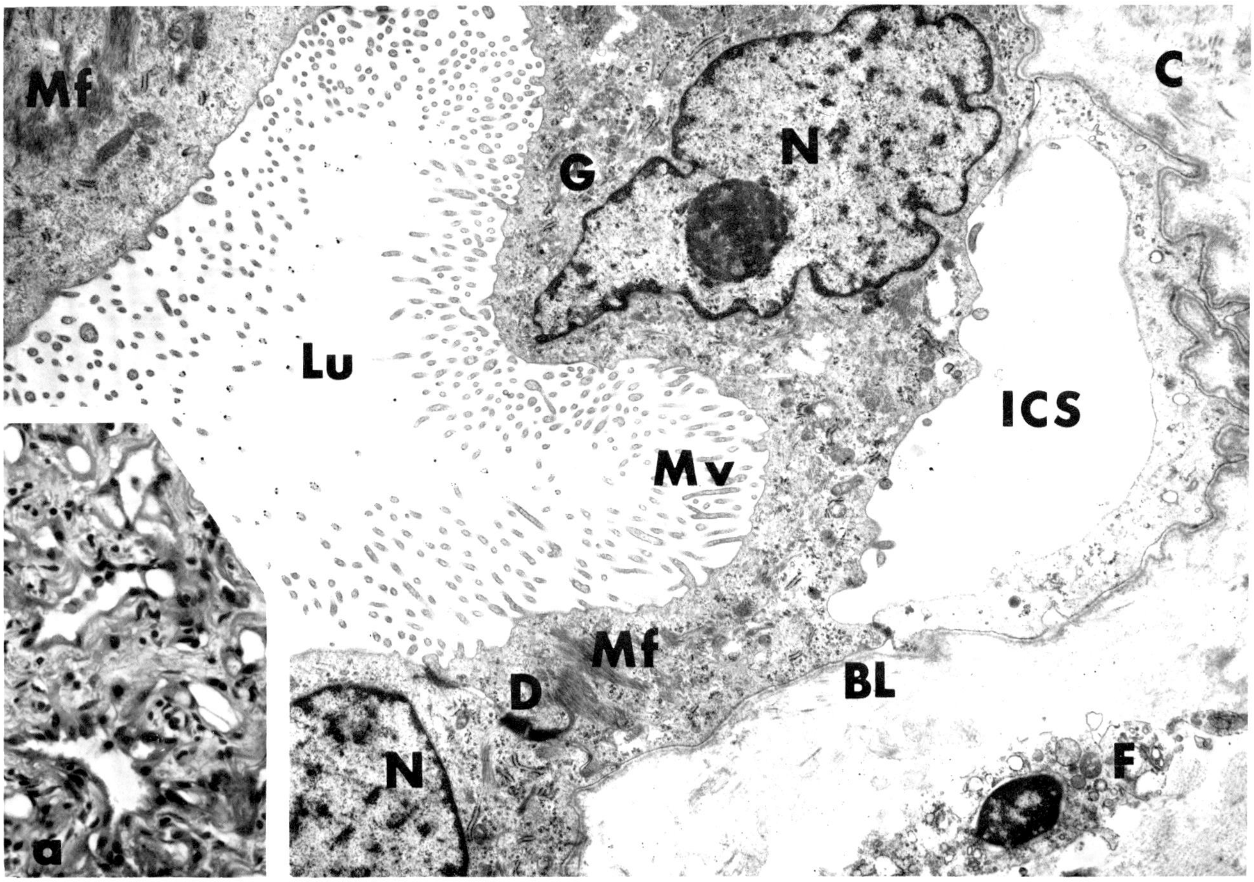

Figure 246a. *Benign ovarian mesothelioma.* The canaliculi are lined by dome-shaped, flattened cells surrounded by a fibrovascular stroma. There are several desquamated epithelial cells and lymphocytes in the lumina. (H & E stain, × 78.)

Figure 246. *Benign ovarian mesothelioma.* The lining cells have large nuclei (N) with prominent nucleoli, and the luminal plasma membrane is covered by abundant and often branching microvilli (Mv). The narrow cytoplasmic substance is relatively poor in cytoplasmic organelles and contains scattered bundles of microfilaments (Mf) which occasionally establish contact with desmosomal plaques (D). Note the widely dilated intercellular space (ICS), forming a secondary channel system. The collagenous (C) stroma is separated from the epithelial cells by a well-developed basal lamina (BL). × 6900. Lu: lumen; G: Golgi; F: degenerating fibroblast.

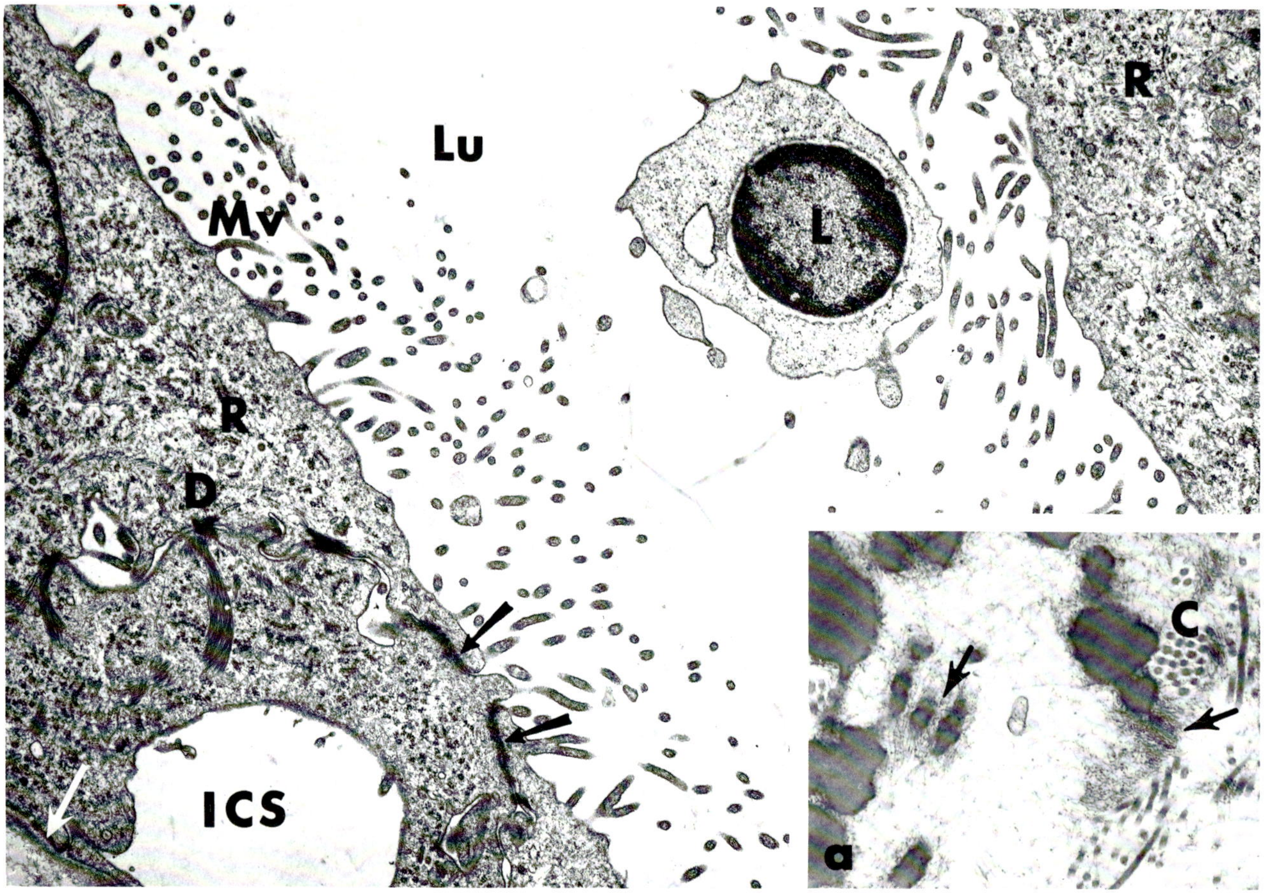

Figure 247. *Benign ovarian mesothelioma.* A lymphocyte (L) is seen in the central lumen. The intercellular spaces (ICS) are consistently separated from the central lumen (Lu) by tight junctional complexes (black arrow). The lateral plasma membranes are reinforced by well-developed tonofilament–desmosome complexes (D), and the predominant cytoplasmic organelles are free ribosomes (R). The white arrow indicates the delimiting basal lamina. × 8000. *From* A. Ferenczy, J. Fenoglio, and R. M. Richart. Observations on benign mesothelioma of the genital tract (adenomatoid tumor). A comparative ultrastructural study. *Cancer* **30:** 244–260 (1972).

Figure 247a. *Characteristic findings in benign ovarian mesothelioma* are masses of stromal homogeneous material associated with tropocollagen (arrows) and well-developed collagen fibers (C). × 25,000. *From* A. Ferenczy, J. Fenoglio, and R. M. Richart. Observations on benign mesothelioma of the genital tract (adenomatoid tumor). A comparative ultrastructural study. *Cancer* **30:** 244–260 (1972).

REFERENCES (Benign ovarian mesothelioma—Figure 247a)

1. Ferenczy, A., J. Fenoglio, and R. M. Richart. Observations on benign mesothelioma of the genital tract (adenomatoid tumor). A comparative ultrastructural study. *Cancer* **30:** 244 (1972).
2. Marcus, J. B. and J. A. Lynn. Ultrastructural comparison of an adenomatoid tumor, lymphangioma, hemangioma, and mesothelioma. *Cancer* **25:** 171 (1970).
3. MacKay, B., J. L. Bennington, and R. W. Skoglund. The adenomatoid tumor: fine structural evidence for a mesothelial origin. *Cancer* **27:** 109 (1971).
4. Salazar, H., A. Kanbour, and F. Burgess. Ultrastructure and observations on the histogenesis of mesotheliomas "adenomatoid tumors" of the female genital tract. *Cancer* **29:** 141 (1972).
5. Broth, G., W. K. Bullock, and J. Morrow. Epididymal tumors. I. Report of 15 new cases including review of literature. 2. Histochemical study of the so-called adenomatoid tumor. *J. Urol.* **100:** 530 (1968).
6. Castor, C. W. and B. Naylor. Characteristics of normal and malignant human mesothelial cells studied in vitro. *Lab. Invest.* **20:** 437 (1969).
7. Masson, P., J. L. Riopelle, and L. C. Simard. Le mésothéliome bénin de la sphère génitale. *Rev. Can. Biol.* **1:** 720 (1942).
8. Fresco, R. and M. Chang-Lo. Adenomatoid tumor of the testis, a mesonephric hamartoma. In *Proceedings EMSA, Twenty-Ninth Annual Meeting,* C. J. Arceneaux (Ed.). Claitors, Boston, 1971, pp. 318–319.
9. Wischnitzer, S. The ultrastructure of the germinal epithelium of the mouse ovary. *J. Morphol.* **117:** 387 (1965).
10. Stoebner, P., G. Miech, A. Sengel, and J. P. Witz. Notions d'ultrastructure pleurale. I. L'hyperplasie mésothéliale. *Presse Med.* **78:** 1179 (1970).

70

Fibroma-Thecomas

Fibroma-thecomas occur primarily in the postmenopausal age group and arise from normal or hyperplastic ovarian stroma. Clinical hyperestrinism has been reported in association with the fibroma-thecoma. Fibroma-thecomas, regardless of their degree of cellularity (thecoma) or collagenization (fibroma), contain admixtures of cell types forming a morphologic continuum,[1] similar to the continuous variation of ovarian cortical stromal cells.[1-4] Included are[1,5] spindle-shaped fibroblastlike cells associated with abundant collagen formation; polyhedral theca interna-type cells rich in organelles, which histochemically denote active estrogenic steroid synthesis;[6] and intermediate cells with increased organelles for fibrillogenesis. The ultrastructural studies cited support the view that the fibroma and thecoma are not separate entities but are variants of a single neoplasm best designated as fibroma-thecoma.[1]

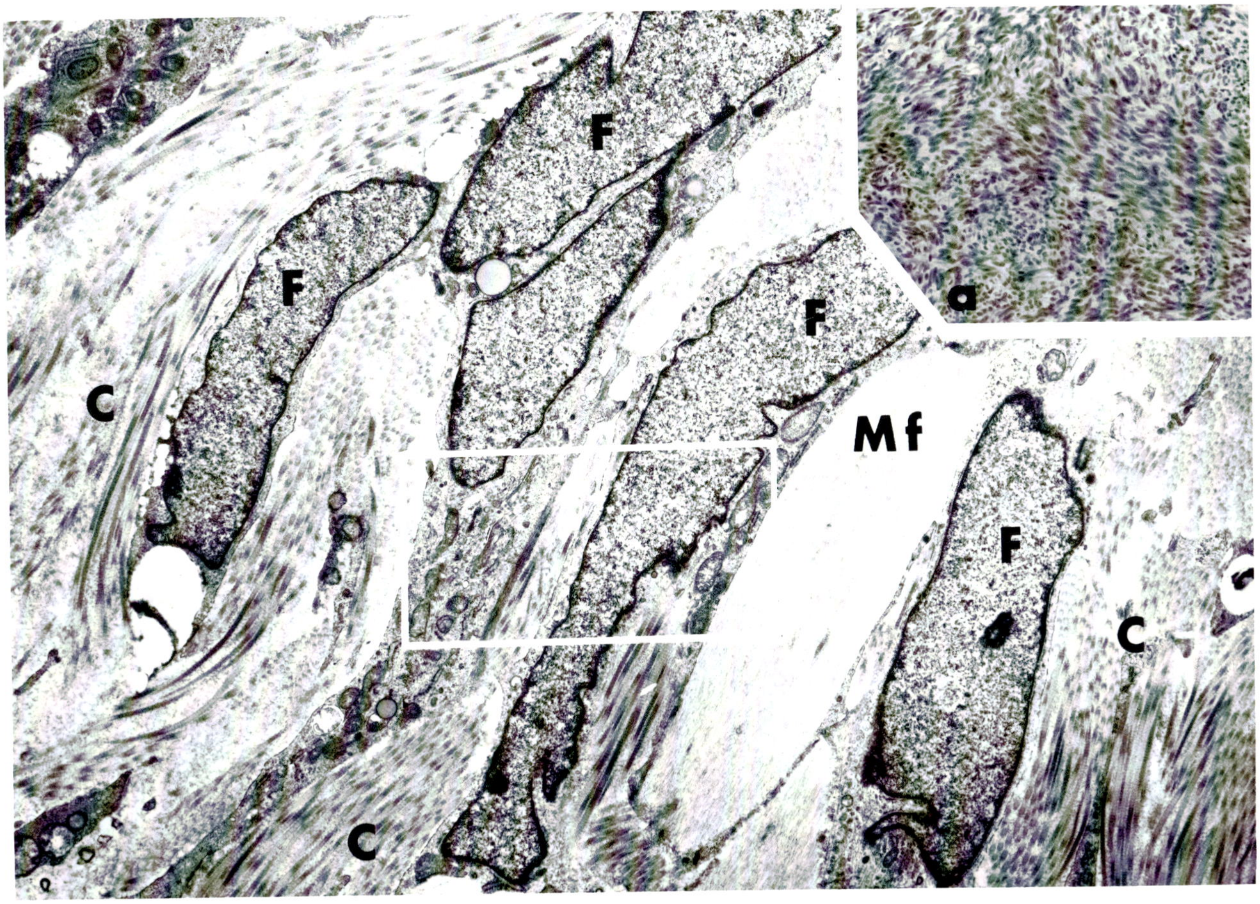

Figure 248a. *Fibroma-thecoma, fibroblastic type.* Spindle-shaped fibroblastlike cells are arranged in interlacing bundles. (H & E stain, × 30.)

Figure 248. *Ultrastructurally,* the cells (F) of fibroblastic fibroma-thecoma are indistinguishable from ordinary fibroblasts. The common features include elongated, spindle-shaped nuclei, scant cytoplasm, and conspicuous collagen (C) fiber production. × 5700. Mf: extracellular tropocollagen fibrils.

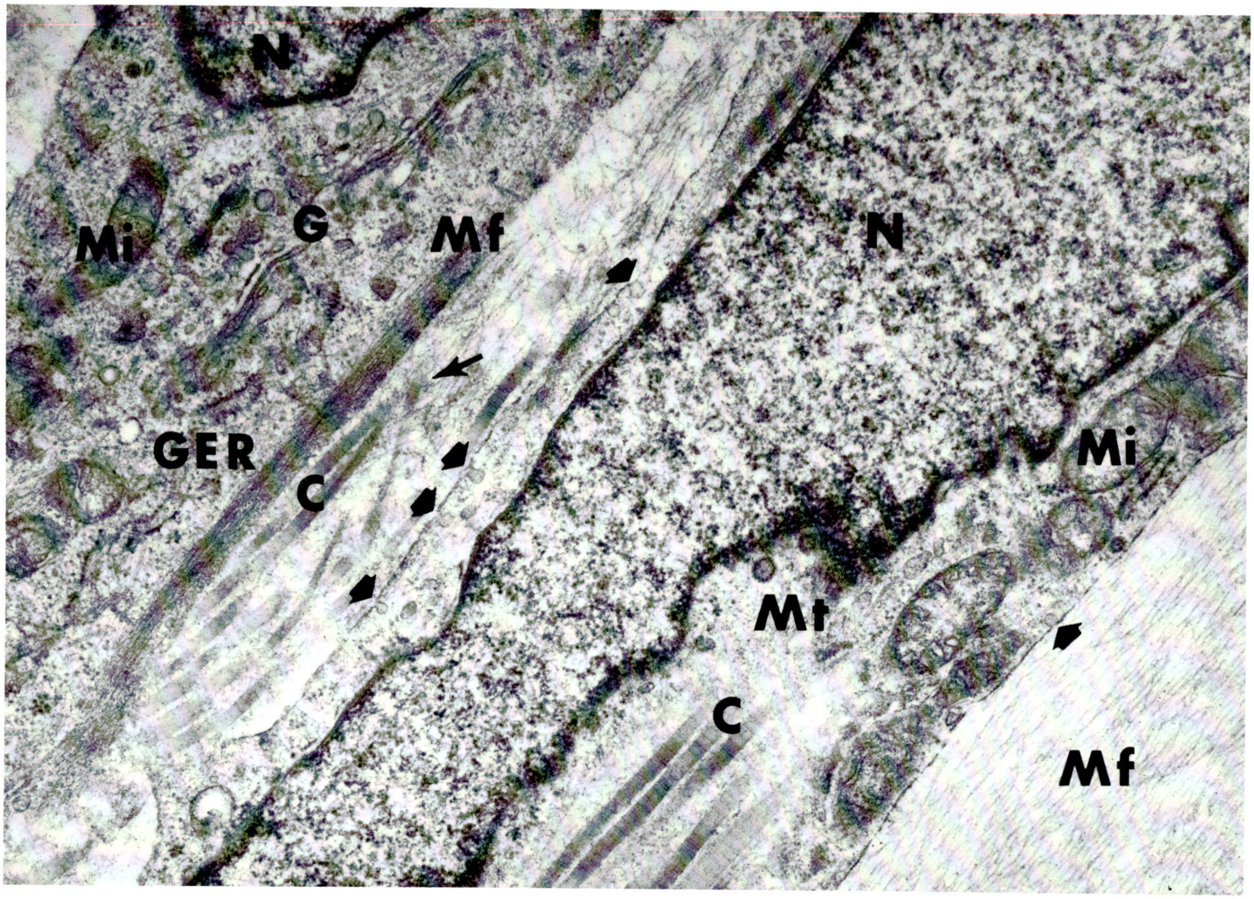

Figure 249. *Detail of Figure 248.* The formation of tropocollagen (50–150 Å thick) is initiated in the L-proline-containing granular endoplasmic reticulum (GER), transferred in the Golgi (G), and secreted into the extracellular space either by secretory vesicles or by shedding of the peripheral cytoplasmic substance rich in tropocollagen fibrils (Mf). Most of the active collagen synthesis takes place in the extracellular space by the polymerization of tropocollagen and cross-striated precollagen (350–550 Å thick) fibrils (long arrows), resulting in the formation of 1300- to 2000-Å-thick mature collagen fibers (C). Although the plasma membrane is often ill defined, rows of micropinocytic vesicles (short arrow) are present, especially at the site of active fibrillogenesis. × 23,600. N: nucleus; Mi: mitochondria; Mt: microtubules.

REFERENCES (Fibroma-thecomas–Figure 249)

1. Amin, H. K., T. Okagaki, and R. M. Richart. Classification of fibroma and thecoma of the ovary. An ultrastructural study. *Cancer* **27:** 438 (1971).
2. Laffargue, P., L. Adechy-Benkoel, and C. Valette. Ultrastructure du stroma ovarien. *Ann. Anat. Pathol.* **13:** 381 (1968).
3. Kempson, R. L.: Ultrastructure of ovarian stromal cell tumors, Sertoli-Leydig cell tumor and Lipid cell tumor. *Arch. Pathol.* **86:** 492 (1968).
4. Serment, A., P. Laffargue, and C. Vallette. Le stroma fonctionnel de l'ovaire ménopausique. *Presse Med.* **77:** 1653 (1969).
5. Toker, C. Theca cell tumor. An ultrastructural study. *Am. J. Obstet. Gynecol.* **100:** 779 (1968).
6. Lynn, J. A., H. H. Varon, W. B. Kingsley, and J. H. Martin. Ultrastructural and biochemical studies of estrogen secretory capacity of a "non-functional" ovarian neoplasm (dysgerminoma). *Am. J. Pathol.* **51:** 639 (1967).

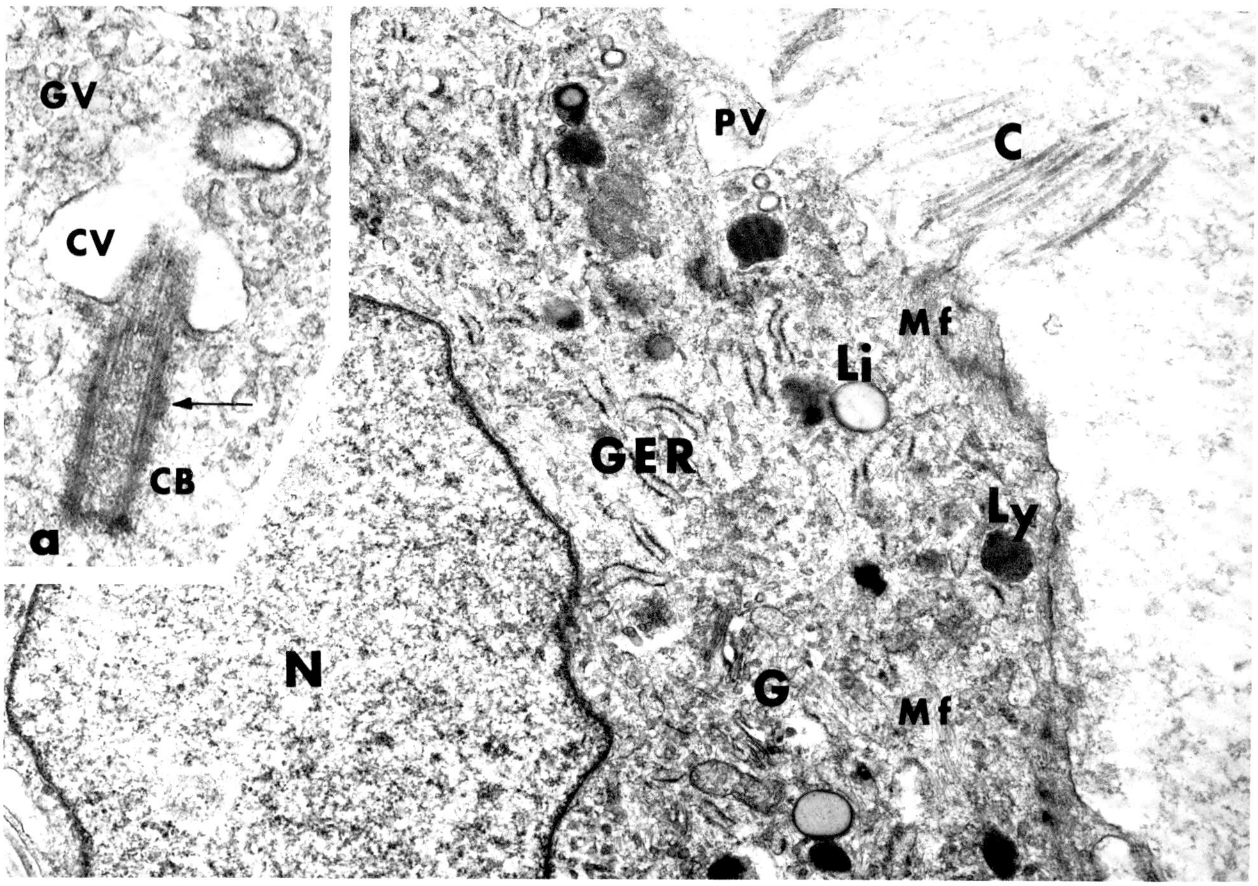

Figure 250. *Fibroma-thecoma with intermediate cell type.* This type of cell has a large, oval nucleus (N) and abundant cytoplasmic substance rich in granular endoplasmic reticulum (GER), free ribosomes, Golgi (G), membrane-bound lysosomes (Ly), and lipid droplets (Li). Microfilaments (Mf) are scattered throughout, with greater concentration near the plasma membrane. Pinocytic vesicles (PV) and plasma membrane infoldings are observed. × 16,900. **C:** extracellular collagen.

Figure 250a. *Electron micrograph,* illustrating a developing intracellular cilium. The basal body (CB) contains small satellite processes (arrow) and prominent ciliary vesicles (CV), surrounded by numerous Golgi vesicles (GV) . × 53,570.

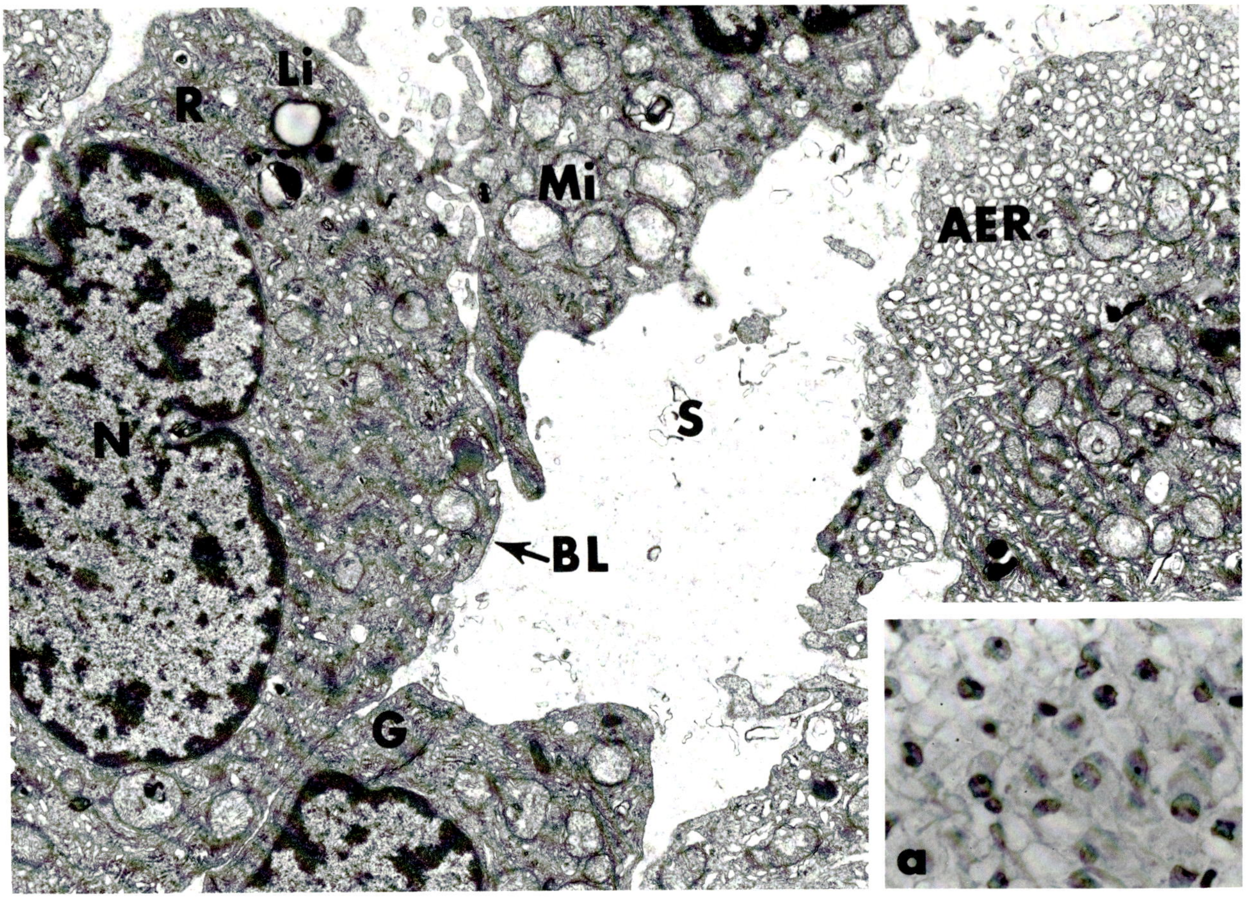

Figure 251a. *Thecoma (fibroma-thecoma, thecoma type).* The lesion is composed of tightly packed, large, luteinized cells with plump nuclei, resembling theca lutein cells. (H & E stain, × 120.)

Figure 251. *At the electron microscopic level,* the abundant cytoplasmic substance is filled with tubular and vesicular agranular endoplasmic reticulum (AER), pleomorphic mitochondria (Mi), Golgi (G), free ribosomes (R), and lipid droplets (Li). These features are characteristic of normal and neoplastic steroidogenic cells. There is incomplete basal lamina (BL) formation, and the stroma (S) is poor in collagen fibers. × 6800. N: nucleus.

71

Granulosa-Theca Cell Tumor

The granulosa-theca cell tumor is the most common feminizing neoplasm of the ovary. Histologically, various growth patterns are recognized, including microfollicular, macrofollicular, trabecular, and solid sarcomatoid types. In all types, nests of granulosa cells are interspersed with fibrothecomatous elements, the latter varying from spindle-shaped fibroblastlike cells to luteinized theca cells. Ultrastructurally, benign[1-4] and malignant[5] granulosa cells are similar to nonluteinized, normal granulosa cells except for increased nuclear size. The common cytoplasmic elements include granular and agranular endoplasmic reticulum, lipid droplets, microfilamentous aggregates, and annular nexuses.[1] In contrast to the Δ-4,3-keto pathway for steroid synthesis, which is present in normal luteinized granulosa cells, in-vitro tumor biosynthetic studies[1] have suggested that in neoplastic granulosa cells steroid synthesis occurs by the Δ-3-β-hydroxy pathway, resulting in the production of androstendione[1] and estrogens.[6] The cells of the thecal portion of the granulosa-theca cell tumor are identical ultrastructurally to those occurring in a pure fibroma-thecoma.

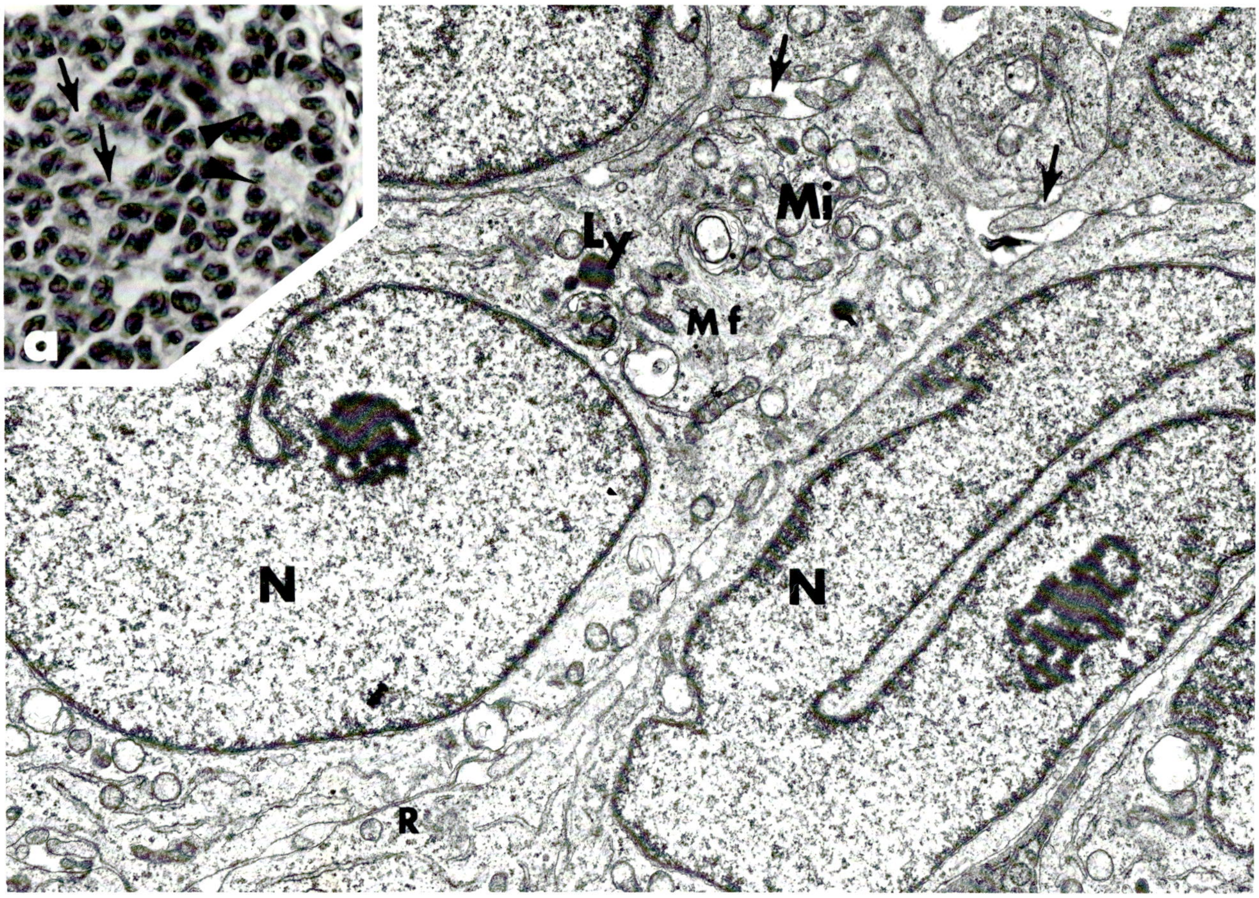

Figure 252a. *Microfollicular granulosa-theca cell tumor.* Epithelial cells with indistinct cytoplasm form rosettelike structures (arrows) containing vacuolated fluid referred to as the Call-Exner bodies. Note the oval, "coffee-bean" nuclear appearance (arrows), a characteristic feature of both normal and neoplastic granulosa cells. (H & E stain, × 120.)

Figure 252. *The frequently deep indentation of the nuclear membrane* of neoplastic granulosa cells is correlated with the characteristic light microscopic "coffee-bean" nuclear appearance.[4] The cytoplasm contains clusters of small mitochondria (Mi), free and bound ribosomes (R), lysosomes (Ly), and microfilaments (Mf). Microvillous cytoplasmic processes (arrows) protrude into slightly dilated intercellular spaces. × 66,900. N: nucleus.

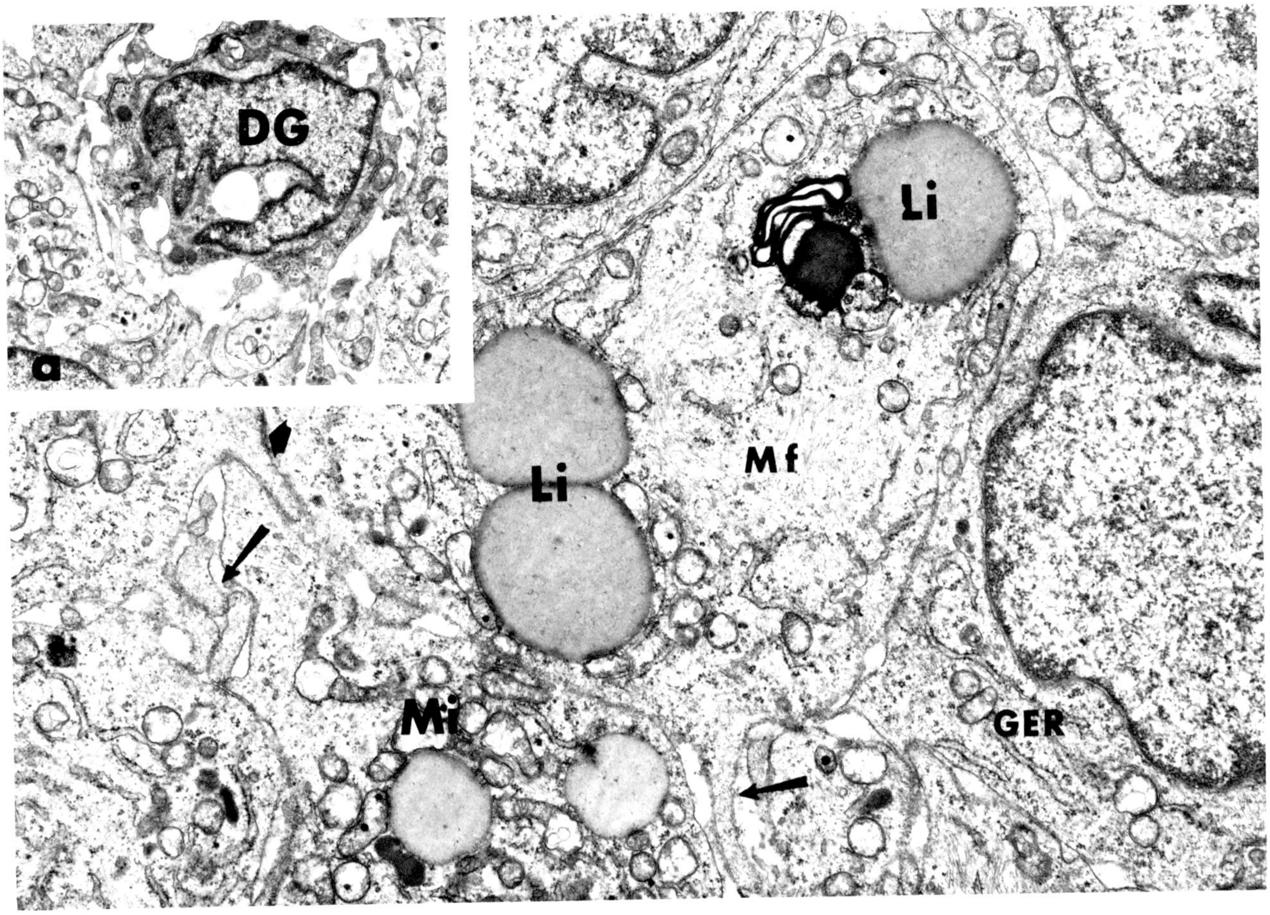

Figure 253. *Granulosa-theca cell tumor.* Several neoplastic granulosa cells contain abundant lipid droplets (Li) and mitochondria (Mi), associated with parallel membranes of granular endoplasmic reticulum (GER). Microfilaments (Mf) are distributed throughout the cytoplasm. The tightly apposed plasma membranes are infrequently attached by small, poorly developed desmosomal belts (short arrow). Note the well-developed configuration of interdigitating microvilli (long arrows). × 20,600.

Figure 253a. *Call-Exner bodies* in the granulosa-theca cell tumor, as in the normal follicle, are formed by cellular dissolution[1,3] and frequently contain intracystic degenerating granulosa cells (DG). The lining cells are often separated from the cystic cavity by a basal lamina. × 6300.

REFERENCES (The granulosa-theca cell tumor—Figure 253a)

1. MacAulay, M. A., I. Welicky, and R. A. Schulz. Ultrastructure of a biosynthetically active granulosa cell tumor. *Lab. Invest.* **17:** 562 (1967).
2. Toker, C. Ultrastructure of a granulosa cell tumor. *Am. J. Obstet. Gynecol.* **100:** 388 (1968).
3. Gondos, B. and S. A. Monroe. Cystic granulosa cell tumor with massive hemoperitoneum. Light and electron microscopic study. *Obstet. Gynecol.* **38:** 683 (1971).
4. Bransilver, B. R., A. Ferenczy, and R. M. Richart. Brenner tumors and Walthad cell nests. A comparative ultrastructural study (in preparation).
5. Gondos, B. Ultrastructure of a metastatic granulosa-theca cell tumor. *Cancer* **24:** 954 (1969).
6. Kase, N. Steroid synthesis in abnormal ovaries. II. Granulosa cell tumor. *Am. J. Obstet. Gynecol.* **90:** 1262 (1964).

72
Arrhenoblastoma

Sertoli-Leydig cell tumors (arrhenoblastoma), the most common virilizing ovarian neoplasms, are composed of Sertoli and Leydig cells (which resemble their testicular counterparts) in varying degrees of differentiation and growth patterns. In well-differentiated lesions, Sertoli cells line narrow tubules resembling fetal testes; in the intermediate form trabecular cords resembling primitive sex cords predominate; and in poorly differentiated lesions there is a sarcomatoid appearance. Mature Leydig cells, which occasionally contain Reinke's crystals, are abundant in the intermediate and sarcomatoid forms, the lesions most commonly associated with virilization, and uncommon in the well-differentiated form. Virilization is due to androgen production[1] by the neoplastic Leydig cells. In-vitro biosynthetic studies[2] and analysis of venous blood draining the neoplasms have shown that both testosterone[2] and androstendione[3] are synthesized, suggesting the existence of a Δ-5,3-β-ol-dehydrogenase steroid pathway similar to that which operates in the testis.

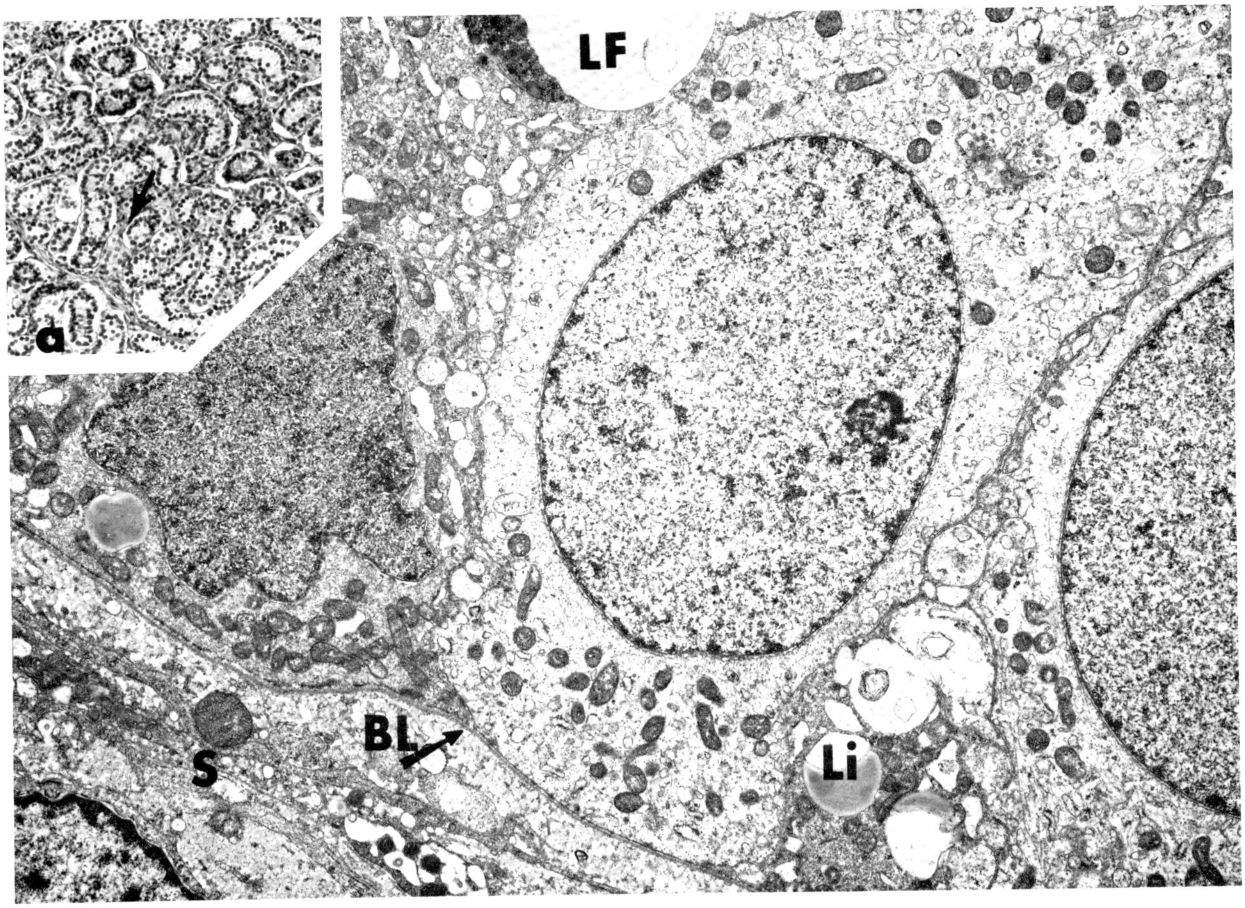

Figure 254a. *Well-differentiated Sertoli-Leydig cell tumor.* The narrow, lumenless tubules resemble fetal seminiferous tubules, and in the intertubular space are clusters of Leydig cells (arrow). (H & E stain, × 30.)

Figure 254. *Ultrastructurally,* in the well-differentiated lesions, the tubular epithelial cells resemble fetal,[4,5] rather than adult normal[6,7] or neoplastic,[8] testicular Sertoli cells. There are a well-developed vesicular granular endoplasmic reticulum, relatively scant mitochondria, and prominent lipid (Li) and lipofuschin (LF) granules. The abundant agranular endoplasmic reticulum observed in neoplastic Sertoli cells[8] is not found in the tubular epithelial cells. Several dark cells with electron-dense cytoplasm and dilated endoplasmic reticulum represent degenerating Sertoli cells. In the tubular form the epithelial cells are separated from the stroma (S) by a basal lamina (BL), whereas in the intermediate type cords of cells often lack a delimiting boundary membrane and the cells are said to resemble granulosa rather than Sertoli cells.[9] × 7600.

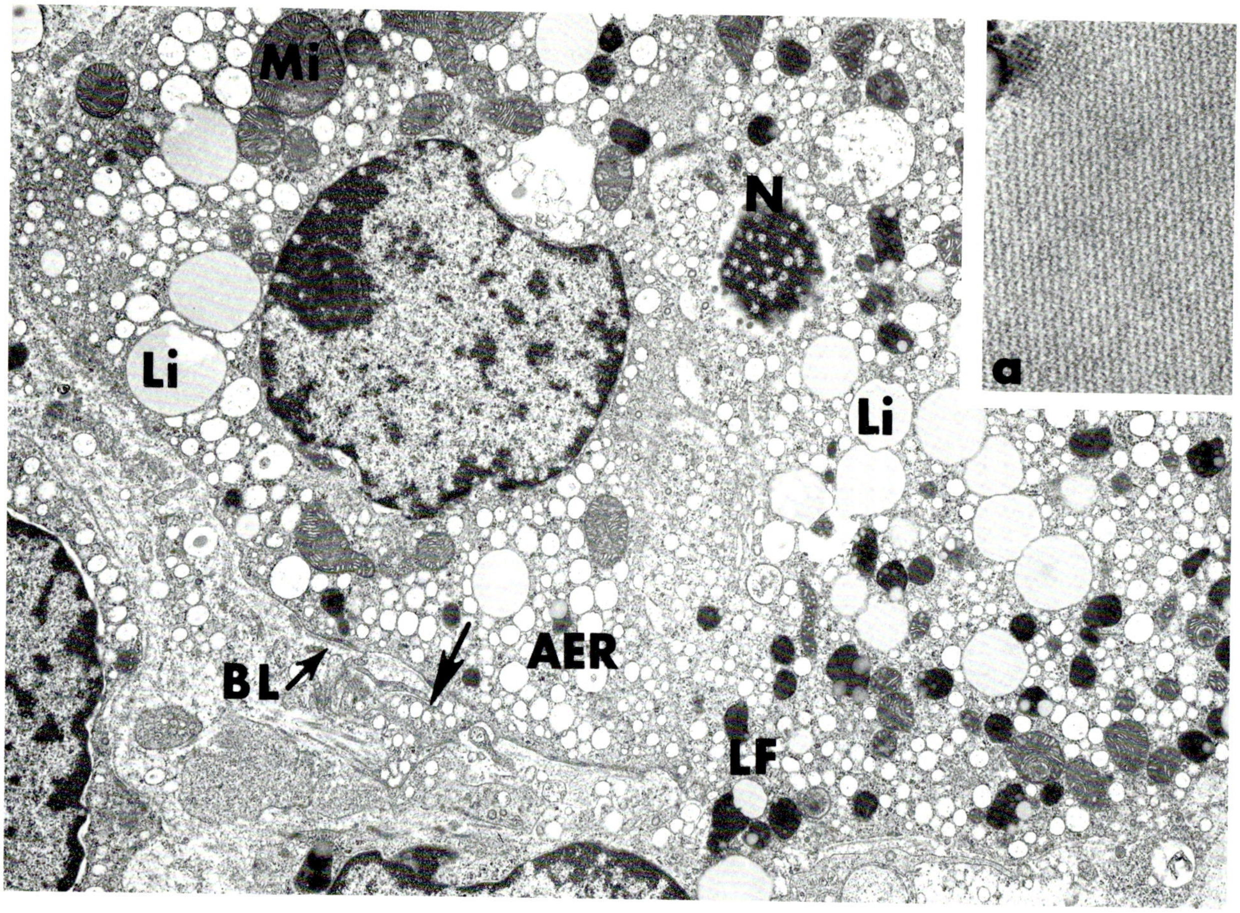

Figure 255. *The neoplastic Leydig cells*[9-11] have a fine structure identical to that of similar cells found in hilus[12] and lipid cell[10,13] tumors and in the normal testis,[7] including abundant vesicular agranular endoplasmic reticulum (AER), mitochondria with tubular cristae (Mi), lipid (Li), and, occasionally, crystals of Reinke and their presumed precursor elements.[11] A fine, but often interrupted, basal lamina (BL) is present, and numerous cytoplasmic processes (arrow) with vesicular agranular endoplasmic reticulum extend into the collagenous stroma. × 6800. N: transected edge of the nucleus with nuclear pores; Lf: lipofuschin granules.

Figure 255a. *High-power view of a crystal of Reinke,* composed of tightly packed hexagonal microtubules, alternating with parallel intertubular spaces. × 60,000.

REFERENCES (Sertoli-Leydig cell tumors—Figure 255a)

1. Scully, R. E. Androgenic lesions of the ovary. In *The Ovary*, H. E. Grady and D. E. Smith (Eds.). International Academy of Pathology Monograph, Williams & Wilkins, Baltimore, 1963, pp. 143–174.
2. Savard, K., M. Gut, R. I. Dorfman, J. L. Gabrilove, and L. J. Soffer. Formation of androgens by human arrhenoblastoma tissue in vitro. *J. Clin. Endocrinol Metab.* **21:** 165 (1961).
3. Wiest, W. G., J. Zander, and E. G. Holmstrom. Metabolism of progesterone-4-C^{14} by an arrhenoblastoma. *J. Clin. Endocrinol. Metab.* **19:** 297 (1959).
4. Gondos, B. and C. Hobel. Ultrastructure of germ cell development in the human fetal testis. *Z. Zellforsch. Mikrosk. Anat.* **119:** 1 (1971).
5. Ferenczy, A. and R. M. Richart. The fine structure of the gonads in the complete form of testicular feminization syndrome. *Am. J. Obstet. Gynecol.* **113:** 399 (1972).
6. Bawa, S. R. Fine structure of the Sertoli cell of the human testis. *J. Ultrastruct. Res.* **9:** 459 (1963).
7. Burgos, M. H., R. Vitale-Calpe, and A. Aoki. Fine structure of the testis and its functional significance. In *The Testis*, A. D. Johnson, W. R. Gomes, and M. L. Vandemark (Eds.). Academic Press, New York, 1970, pp. 551–577.
8. Able, M. E. and J. C. Lee. Ultrastructure of a Sertoli cell adenoma of the testis. *Cancer* **23:** 481 (1969).
9. Jensen, A. B., and R. E. Fechner. Ultrastructure of an intermediate Sertoli-Leydig cell tumor. A histogenetic misnomer. *Lab. Invest.* **21:** 527 (1969).
10. Kempson, R. L. Ultrastructure of ovarian stromal cell tumors. *Arch. Pathol.* **86:** 492 (1968).
11. Berendsen, P. B., E. B. Smith, M. R. Abell, and R. B. Taffe. Fine structure of Leydig cells from an arrhenoblastoma of the ovary. *Am. J. Obstet. Gynecol.* **103:** 192 (1969).
12. Merkow, L. P., M. Slifkin, H. F. Acevedo, M. Pardo, and W. V. Greenberg. Ultrastructure of an interstitial (hilar) cell tumor of the ovary. *Obstet. Gynecol.* **37:** 845 (1971).
13. Koss, L. G., E. O. Rothschild, M. Fleisher, and J. E. Francis, Jr. Masculinizing tumor of the ovary, apparently with adrenocortical activity. A histologic, ultrastructural, and biochemical study. *Cancer* **23:** 1245 (1969).

73
Hilus Cell Tumors

Hilus cell tumors are rare neoplasms, occurring most commonly in elderly women. They are usually associated with virilization, although occasionally feminization is observed. Characteristically, in patients with hilus cell tumors, the urinary 17-ketosteroids and gonadotropins are within normal levels. The virilization accompanying the tumor is due to increased levels of testosterone. This hormone, which is found in high concentrations in the ovarian and peripheral veins and urine,[1] results from the conversion of the androsterone secreted by the neoplastic[2] or hyperplastic hilus cells[1] or hyperplastic stromal lutein cells.[3] Similar ultrastructural and biochemical findings occur in Reinke's crystal-free lipid cell (or lipoid) tumors of the ovary,[4] and it is difficult to draw a sharp distinction between the various cell types, either microscopically or clinically.

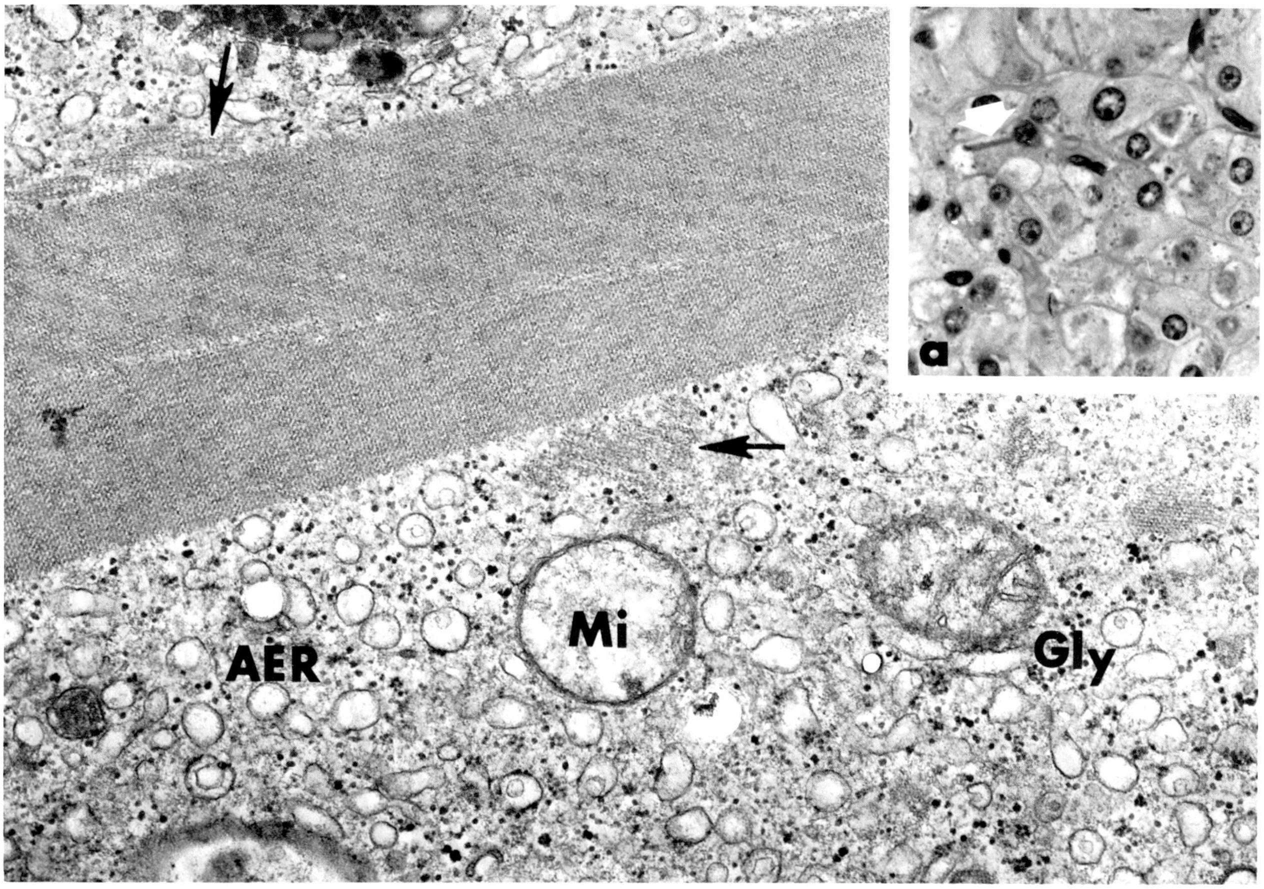

Figure 256a. *Histologically,* the hilus cell tumor is composed of sheets of large polyhedral cells with an eosinophilic, granular cytoplasm, and some cells contain lipochrome pigment and rod-shaped Reinke's crystals (arrow). The identification of the latter is considered to be pathognomonic of the hilus cell tumor[5] and to indicate benignancy. H & E stain, × 120.)

Figure 256. *At the ultrastructural level,* neoplastic hilus cells[6-8] are identical fine structurally to normal[9] and hyperplastic[1,10] hilus cells, as well as normal ovarian lipid cells and neoplastic testicular Leydig cells.[11,12] All these cell types contain abundant tubular and vesicular endoplasmic reticulum (AER), pleomorphic mitochondria (Mi), well-developed Golgi, glycogen granules (Gly), lipid-containing lysosomes (lipochrome pigment), and crystals of Reinke.[7,8,10] Presumably, the only distinctive feature between normal or neoplastic ovarian hilus cells and their testicular counterparts is the presence of a Barr body in the former, indicating their female histogenetic derivation.[8] Crystals of Reinke are protein-containing[13] intracytoplasmic and intranuclear inclusions that are composed of units of six 300-Å-wide hexagonal microtubules (separated from each other by a 150-Å-wide intertubular space) surrounding one central microtubule.[8] The ultrastructural organization and dimensions of the microtubules of mature Reinke's crystals closely resemble those of the hexagonal microtubular rosettes or "elementary" tubular inclusions[8] (arrows), which may represent precursors or intermediary elements of crystal development. In view of the ultrastructural characteristics of Reinke's inclusions, the term crystal, rather than crystalloid, should be used. Although the precise significance of Reinke's crystals as related to cellular metabolic activities is presently unknown, similar structures[8] are seen in the sexual antebrachial organ of a prosimian primate (*Lemur catta*), as well as in virus infected or chemically treated cells and several human neoplastic cells. × 30,500.

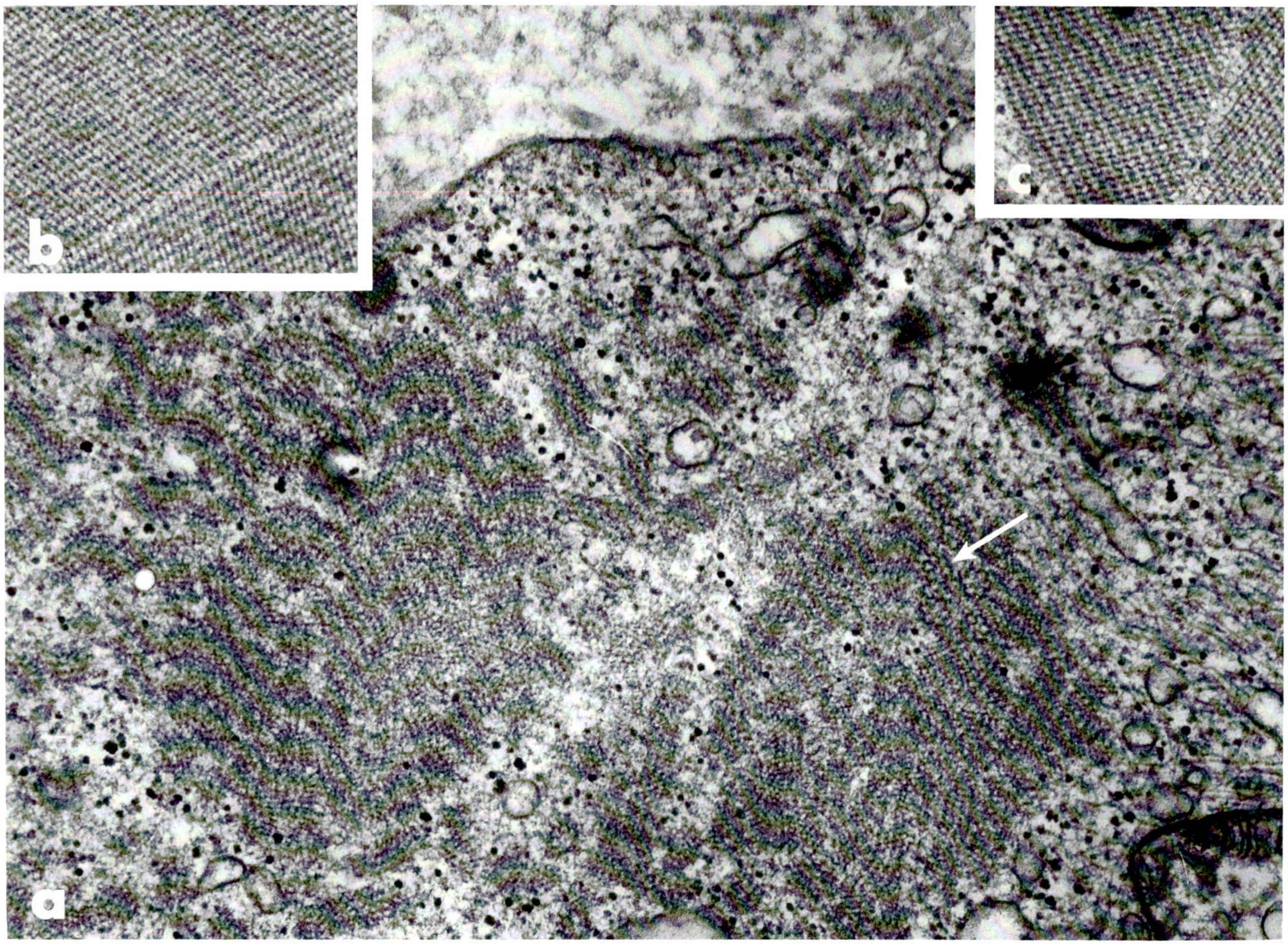

Figure 257a. *Neoplastic hilus cell* with intracytoplasmic, elementary, tubular inclusions, seen in both longitudinal and transverse planes of section. Note the characteristic rosette-like arrangement of six hexagonal microtubules surrounding one central tubule (arrow), forming an elementary tubular inclusion. × 31,500.

Figure 257b. *Hilus cell tumor.* Longitudinal section of a crystal of Reinke, illustrating the parallel organization of microtubules and the alternating intertubular spaces. × 60,750.

Figure 257c. *Hilus cell tumor. Reinke's crystal.* In this plane of section the characteristic hexagonal outlines of individual microtubules are evident. × 60,750.

REFERENCES (Hilus cell tumors–Figure 257c)

1. Novak, D. F., S. C. Lauchlan, J. C. McCawley, and C. Faiman. Virilization during pregnancy. *Am. J. Med.* **49:** 281 (1970).
2. Green, J. A. and M. Maqueo. Histopathology and ultrastructure of an ovarian hilar cell tumor. *Am. J. Obstet. Gynecol.* **96:** 478 (1966).
3. Bardin, C. W., M. B. Lipsett, J. H. Edgcomb, and J. R. Marshall. Studies of testosterone metabolism in a patient with masculinization due to stromal hyperthecosis. *New Engl. J. Med.* **277:** 399 (1967).
4. Koss, L. G., E. O. Rotschild, M. Fleisher, and J. E. Francis, Jr. Masculinizing tumor of the ovary, apparently with adrenocortical activity. A histologic, ultrastructural and biochemical study. *Cancer* **23:** 1245 (1969).
5. Boivin, Y. and R. M. Richart. Hilus cell tumors of the ovary. A review with a report of 3 new cases. *Cancer* **18:** 231 (1965).
6. Jensen, A. B. and R. E. Fechner. Ultrastructure of an intermediate Sertoli-Leydig cell tumor. A histogenetic misnomer. *Lab. Invest.* **21:** 527 (1969).
7. Berendsen, P. B., E. B. Smith, M. R. Abell, and R. B. Jaffe. Fine structure of Leydig cells from an arrhenoblastoma of the ovary. *Am. J. Obstet. Gynecol.* **103:** 192 (1969).
8. Merkow, L. P., M. Slifkin, H. F. Acevedo, M. Pardo, and W. V. Greenberg. Ultrastructure of an interstitial (hilar) cell tumor of the ovary. *Obstet. Gynecol.* **37:** 845 (1971).
9. Kempson, R. L. Ultrastructure of ovarian stromal cell tumors. Sertoli-Leydig cell tumor and lipid cell tumor. *Arch. Pathol.* **86:** 492 (1968).
10. Hameed, K. Brenner tumor of the ovary with Leydig cell hyperplasia. A histologic and ultrastructural study. *Cancer* **30:** 945 (1972).
11. Pierce, G. B., Jr. Ultrastructure of human testicular tumors. *Cancer* **19:** 1963 (1966).
12. Dadoune, J. P., P. Galian, A. Steg, P. Ganter, and R. Abelanet. Leydig-cell adenoma of the testis. A histological, ultrastructural, histoenzymatic and biochemical study of a case. *Arch. Anat. Pathol. (Paris)* **15:** 322 (1967).
13. Janko, A. B. and E. C. Sandberg. Histochemical evidence for the protein nature of the Reinke crystalloid. *Obstet. Gynecol.* **35:** 493 (1970).

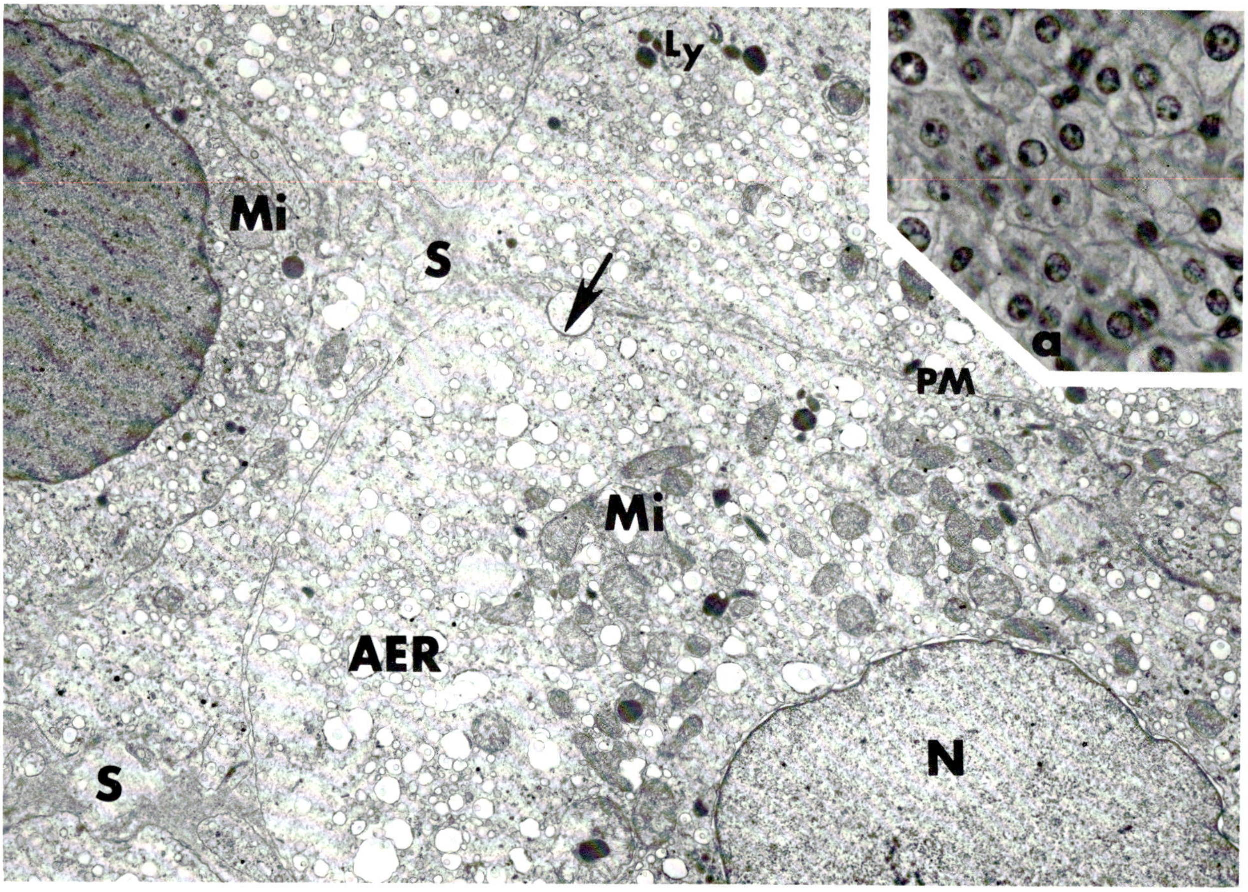

74

Luteoma of Pregnancy

The luteoma of pregnancy[1] is a reversible, chorionic gonadotropin-dependent, lutein cell hyperplasia rather than a true neoplasm, in which an increased production of androstenedione[2,3] may result in masculinization of both the mother and her infant. A morphologically and biochemically similar neoplastic lesion encountered rarely in postmenopausal women[4] may occur spontaneously[5] and can be produced experimentally[6] in mice.

Figure 258a. *Luteoma of pregnancy.* The lesion consists of large acidophilic luteinized cells with granular cytoplasm and tightly apposed plasma membranes producing a "honeycomb" pattern. (H & E stain, × 120.)

Figure 258. *Ultrastructurally,* the cells of the luteoma of pregnancy[7] and of transplantable mouse luteoma[5] contain abundant agranular endoplasmic reticulum (AER), Golgi, tubular mitochondrial cristae (Mi), and, characteristically, scant lipid.[7] In contrast to the rodent luteoma,[5] however, the luteoma of pregnancy contains cells that are often attached by straight and annular tight junctional nexuses (arrow), as are both granulosa and theca lutein cells of the corpus luteum (see **Corpus Luteum**), but uniformly lack the prominent microvillous plasma membrane specializations of granulosa lutein cells. These fine structural and biochemical characteristics suggest that luteoma of pregnancy derives from luteinized theca or stroma cells, rather than from granulosa lutein cells, of the ovary. The luteoma of the postmenopausal period has not been studied ultrastructurally. × 6600. Ly: lysosome; PM: plasma membranes are smooth and devoid of microvillous projections; S: stroma with electron-dense amorphous material;; N: nucleus.

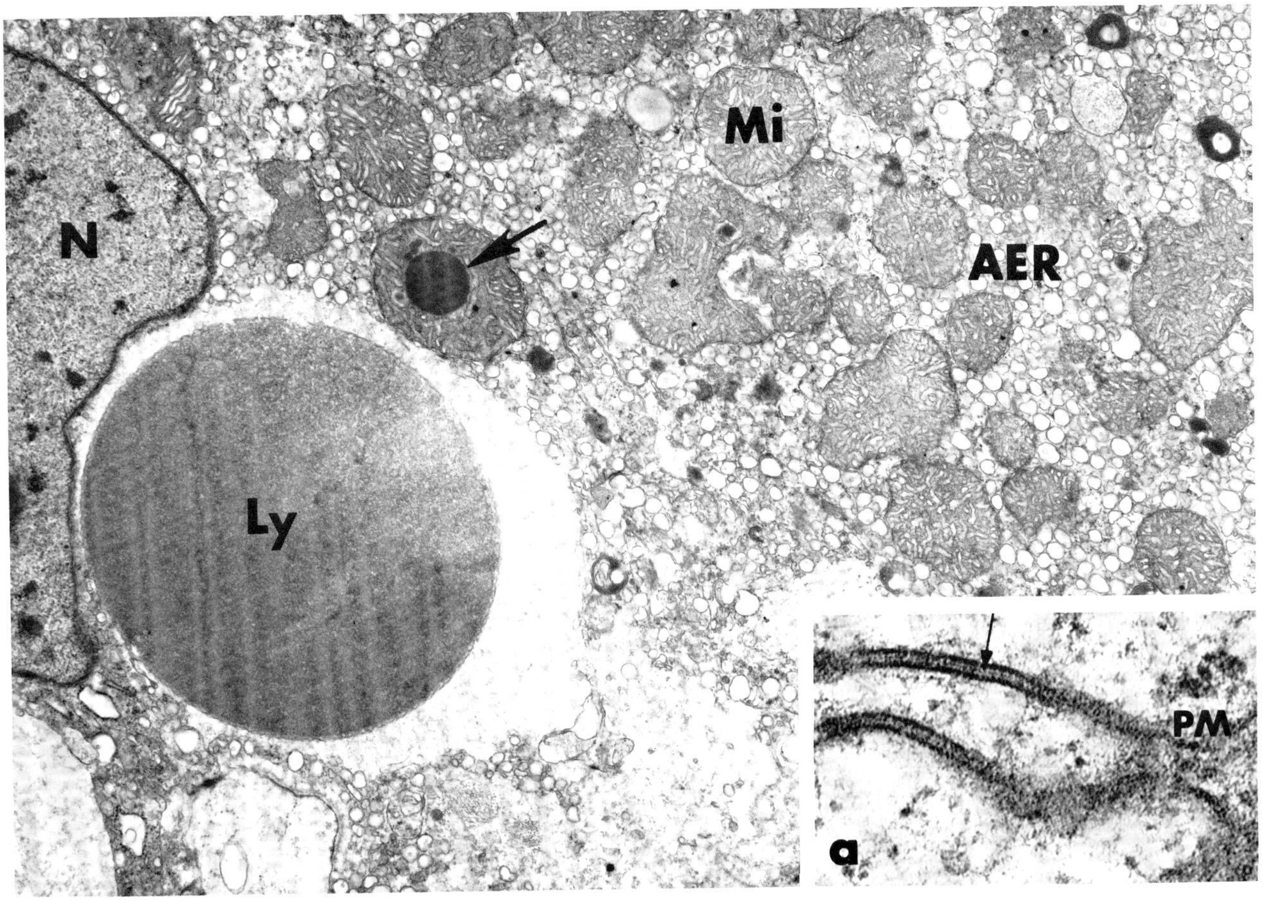

Figure 259. *Luteoma of pregnancy.* Higher magnification of pleomorphic mitochondria (Mi) with tubular cristae and electron-dense granules. The agranular endoplasmic reticulum (AER) is vesicular because of fixation artifact. There is a perinuclear (N) membrane-bound giant lysosome (Ly) with amorphous content, resembling the "colloid" bodies observed in granular lutein cells of the gestational corpus luteum (see **Corpus Luteum of Gestation**). × 12,600.

Figure 259a. *Detailed view of two pentalaminar tight junctional complexes (nexuses),* one of which contains a central core (arrow). The distance between the two thick membranes is approximately 20 to 40 Å. × 60,000. PM: plasma membrane.

REFERENCES (The luteoma of pregnancy—Figure 259a)

1. Sternberg, W. H. and D. L. Barclay. Luteoma of pregnancy. *Am. J. Obstet Gynecol.* **95:** 165 (1966).
2. Rice, B. F., D. L. Barclay, and W. H. Sternberg. Luteoma of pregnancy: steroidogenic and morphologic considerations. *Am. J. Obstet. Gynecol.* **104:** 871 (1969).
3. Rice, B. F., H. B. Woody, D. L. Barclay, and W. H. Sternberg. Virilizing luteoma of pregnancy: specific sterol and steroid hormone content. *J. Steroid Biochem.* **2:** 183 (1971).
4. Scully, R. E. Stromal luteoma of the ovary. A distinctive type of lipoid-cell tumor. *Cancer* **17:** 769 (1964).
5. Roth, L. M., W. H. Sternberg, R. A. Huseby, A. A. MacPhee, F. E. Cole, and B. F. Rice. Transplantable luteoma of the mouse. An ultrastructural and biochemical study. *Lab. Invest.* **27:** 115 (1972).
6. Furth, J. and H. Sobel. Transplantable luteoma in mice and associated secondary changes. *Cancer Res.* **7:** 246 (1947).
7. Krause, D. E. and V. A. Stembridge. Luteomas of pregnancy. *Am. J. Obstet. Gynecol.* **95:** 192 (1966).

75

Dysgerminoma

The dysgerminoma is a relatively rare, highly radiosensitive, malignant neoplasm occurring in children and young adults and, occasionally, in dysgenetic gonads.

Like the primitive germ cells, the dysgerminoma cells are alkaline phosphatase-positive,[2] and ultrastructural studies of both ovarian[1,3,4] and testicular[5,6] dysgerminomas confirm their resemblance to primitive germ cells,[3-5] primordial ovocytes,[1] spermatogonia,[5] and spermatocytes.[4,6] In the spermatocytic seminoma type of germinoma, intercellular bridges and the chromosomal configuration of the meiotic prophase are indicative of a considerable degree of maturation.[6]

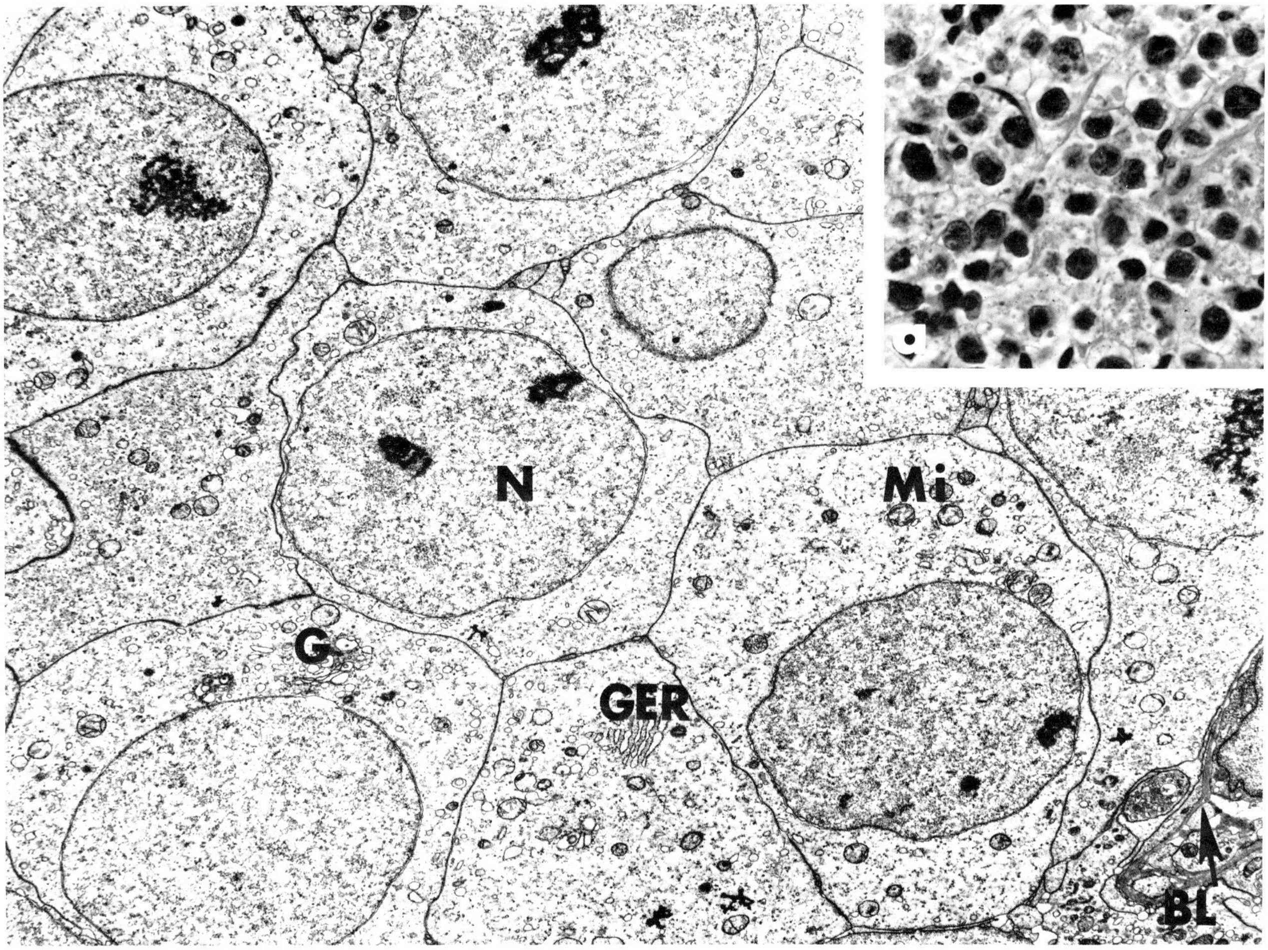

Figure 260a. *The cells of the dysgerminoma* are identical, chemically and histologically, to those of the testicular seminoma. Both consist, in their most common growth pattern, of sheets or large cords of uniform, round, malignant cells resembling the undifferentiated germ cells of the early embryonal gonads and separated by fibrous septae. Characteristically, the fibrous septae contain a chronic inflammatory infiltrate and foreign body-type, giant-cell, granulomatous foci. Occasionally, ultrastructurally and biochemically active, steroidogenic, luteinized, stromal cells are observed.[1] As in seminomas of the testis, teratomatous or choriocarcinomatous elements are sometimes present. (H & E stain, × 120.)

Figure 260. *Dysgerminoma of the ovary.* The immature neoplastic germ cells have tightly apposed plasma membranes. The prominent nuclei (N) contain one or more nucleoli, and the pale cytoplasmic substance has few organelles. A well-developed basal lamina (BL) separates the epithelial nest from the stroma. × 5000. Mi: mitochondria; GER: granular endoplasmic reticulum; G: Golgi; BL: basal lamina. *From* L. Overbeck and E. Philipp. Die Ultrastruktur des Disgerminoms im Ovar. Zugleich eim Beitrag zur Histogenese des Tumors. *Z. Geburtsh. Gynaekol.* **170:** 125–136 (1969).

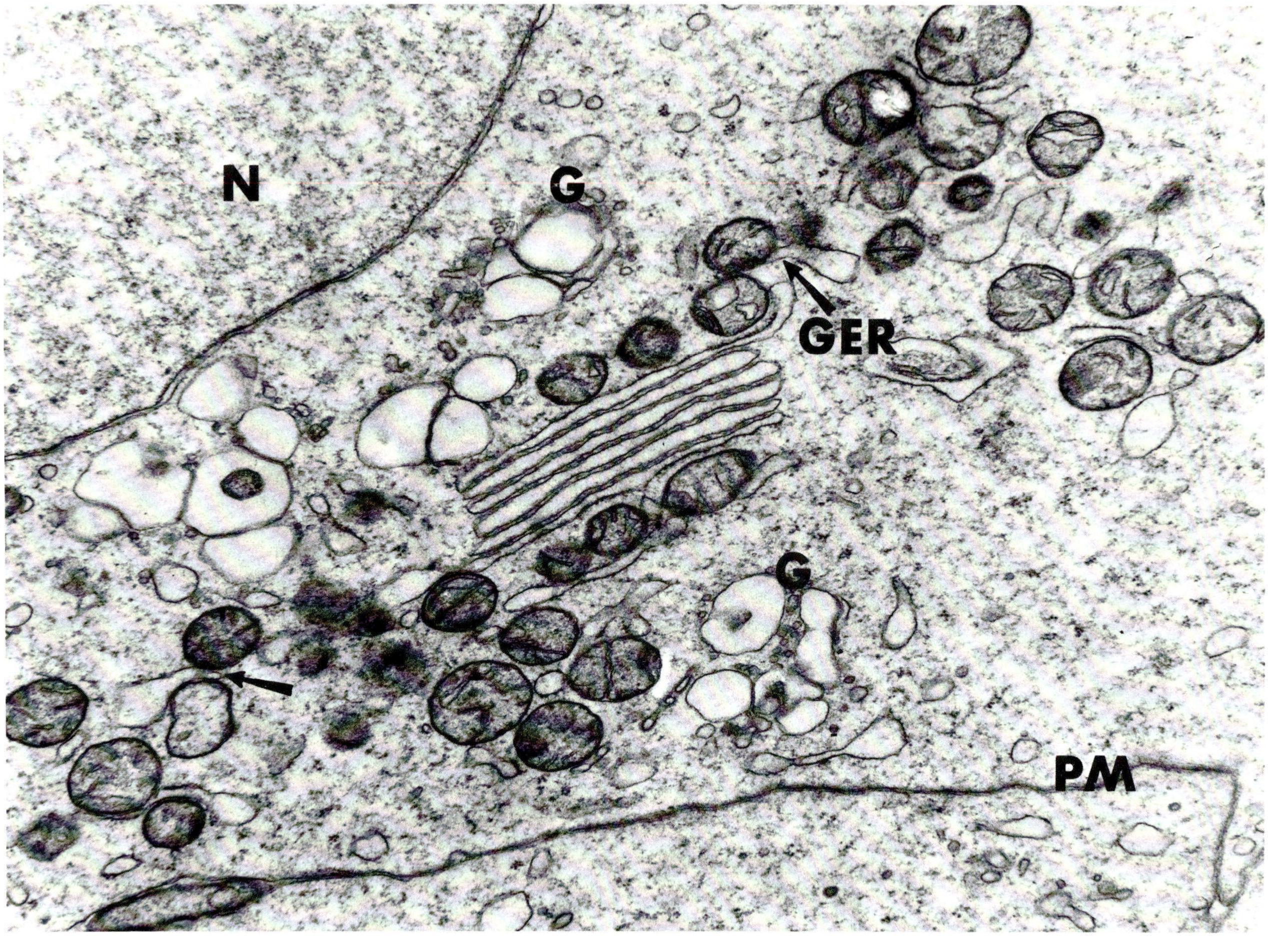

Figure 261. *Dysgerminoma cell* exhibiting cytoplasmic differentiation. The membranes of the Golgi (G) and the finely granular endoplasmic reticulum (GER) are in close relationship. The latter are occasionally in contact with mitochondria (arrows) and have a parallel configuration. × 27,000. PM: plasma membrane; N: nucleus. *From* L. Overbeck and E. Philipp. Die Ultrastruktur des Disgerminoms im Ovar. Zugleich eim Beitrag zur Histogenese des Tumors. *Z. Geburtsh. Gynaekol.* **170:** 125–136 (1969).

REFERENCES (Figures 260a–261)

1. Lynn, R. A., H. H. Varon, W. B. Kingsley, and T. H. Martin. Ultrastructural and biochemical studies of estrogen secretory capacity of a "nonfunctional" ovarian neoplasm (dysgerminoma). *Am. J. Pathol.* **51:** 639 (1967).
2. McKay, D. G., A. T. Hertig, E. C. Adams, and S. Danzinger. Histochemical observations on germ cells of human embryos. *Anat. Res.* **117:** 201 (1953).
3. Overbeck, L. and E. Philipp. Die Ultrastruktur des Disgerminoms im Ovar. Zugleich eim Beitrag zur Histogenese des Tumors. *Z. Geburtsh. Gynaekol.* **170:** 125 (1969).
4. Kay, S., S. G. Silverberg, and P. F. Schatzki. Ultrastructure of an ovarian dysgerminoma: report of a case featuring neurosecretory-type granules in stromal cells. *Am. J. Clin. Pathol.* **58:** 458 (1972).
5. Pierce, G. B., Jr. Ultrastructure of human testicular tumors. *Cancer* **19:** 1963 (1966).
6. Rosai, J., K. Khodadoust, and I. Silber. Spermatocytic seminoma. II. Ultrastructural study. *Cancer* **24:** 103 (1969).

76

Embryonal Carcinoma

Embryonal carcinoma is a rare, highly aggressive, ovarian neoplasm occurring most commonly in the first two decades of life. Histologically, the lesion is composed of solid masses of malignant, poorly differentiated, embryonal cells with pleomorphic nuclei and abundant, amphophilic, syncytial-like cytoplasm. Ultrastructurally, poorly differentiated embryonal carcinoma cells have a general cytoplasmic simplicity except for prominent collections of polyribosomes.[1] Although the plasma membranes occasionally contain desmosomal attachments, the formation of a basal lamina appears generally incomplete and abortive.[1]

Embryonal carcinoma should be distinguished from neoplasms containing the so-called Schiller-Duval, glomeruluslike bodies, which consist of intraglandular epithelial projections with central blood vessel and perivascular mesenchyme. These structures were originally interpreted as primitive mesonephric glomeruli[2] (Schiller's mesonephroma ovarii), but more recently their close resemblance to the endodermal sinus of Duval of the rodent's yolk sac has been stressed.[3] Although such a structure is not found in the human embryo, the concept that the "endodermal sinus tumor"[3] or yolk-sac carcinoma[4] represents a neoplastic entity that should be distinguished from embryonal carcinoma seems, with few exceptions,[5] to be generally accepted. This distinction is based on experimental teratogenetic studies[5-9] which have shown that yolk-sac carcinoma occurs as a result of the differentiation of embryonal carcinoma into extraembryonic yolk-sac elements and mesenchyme. A further basis is found in clinical studies that have shown that, at least for testicular yolk-sac tumors, the survival rates[4] are age related. A similar correlation has not been established for ovarian yolk-sac carcinomas.[10] The germ cell, histogenetic origin of ovarian embryonal carcinoma and teratocarcinoma, as well as yolk-sac tumors, is indirectly supported by experimental[6-8] and electron microscopic studies[9] which have shown that murine testicular, embryonal carcinomas are derived from primordial germ cells[8,9] and that embryonal cancer cells are multipotential stem cells giving rise to teratocarcinoma,[6-8] choriocarcinoma, and yolk-sac, or vitelline, carcinoma,[4] each neoplastic cell type representing, respectively, a terminal stage of differentiation. The immunoelectrophoretic demonstration that both normal human yolk sac[11] and vitelline carcinoma[12] produce α-fetoprotein lends additional support to the thesis that the endodermal sinus tumor is composed of malignant germ cells which have differentiated in the direction of yolk sac.

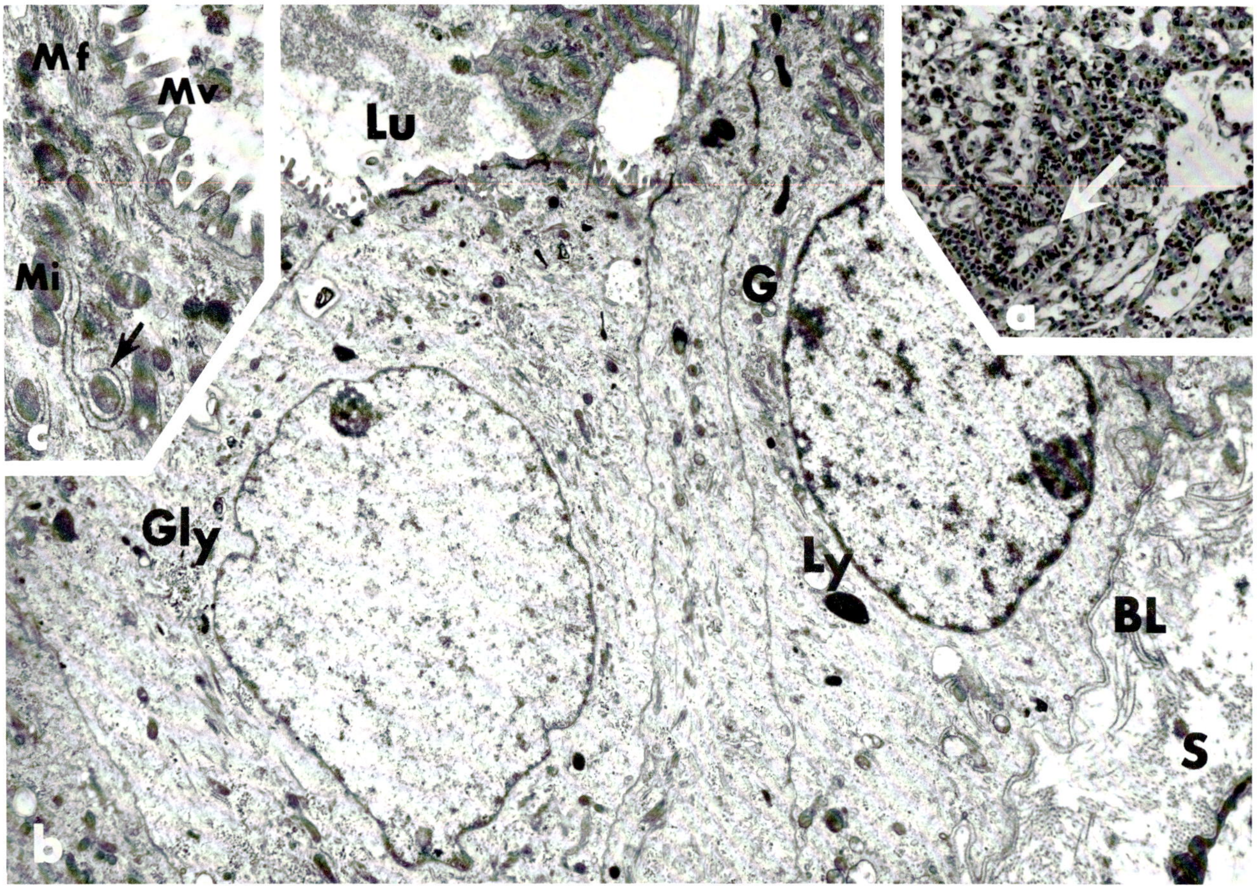

Figure 262a. *The better- and well-differentiated regions of embryonal carcinoma* contain lacunar and glandular spaces (arrow) lined by primitive epithelial cells. Characteristically, the lesion contains numerous intra- and extracellular eosinophilic, globoid, hyaline bodies throughout. (H & E stain, × 30.)

Figure 262b. *Well-differentiated embryonal adenocarcinoma* cells have luminal microvilli and sparse cytoplasmic organelles, but cytoplasmic filaments and glycogen particles (Gly) are comparatively abundant. Tightly apposed, lateral plasma membranes are reinforced by luminal tight junctional complexes and a small number of poorly developed desmosomes, and the glands are invested by a well-defined basal lamina (BL). Essentially similar findings have been reported in well-differentiated human testicular embryonal carcinoma and teratocarcinoma.[1] × 5600. Lu: glandular lumen; G: Golgi; Ly: lysosomes; S: collagenous stroma.

Figure 262c. *Higher-power view of Figure 262b.* The luminal microvilli (Mv) are short and irregular, and the cytoplasm contains small mitochondria (Mi) encircled by membranes of granular endoplasmic reticulum (arrow). × 30,400. Mf: microfilaments.

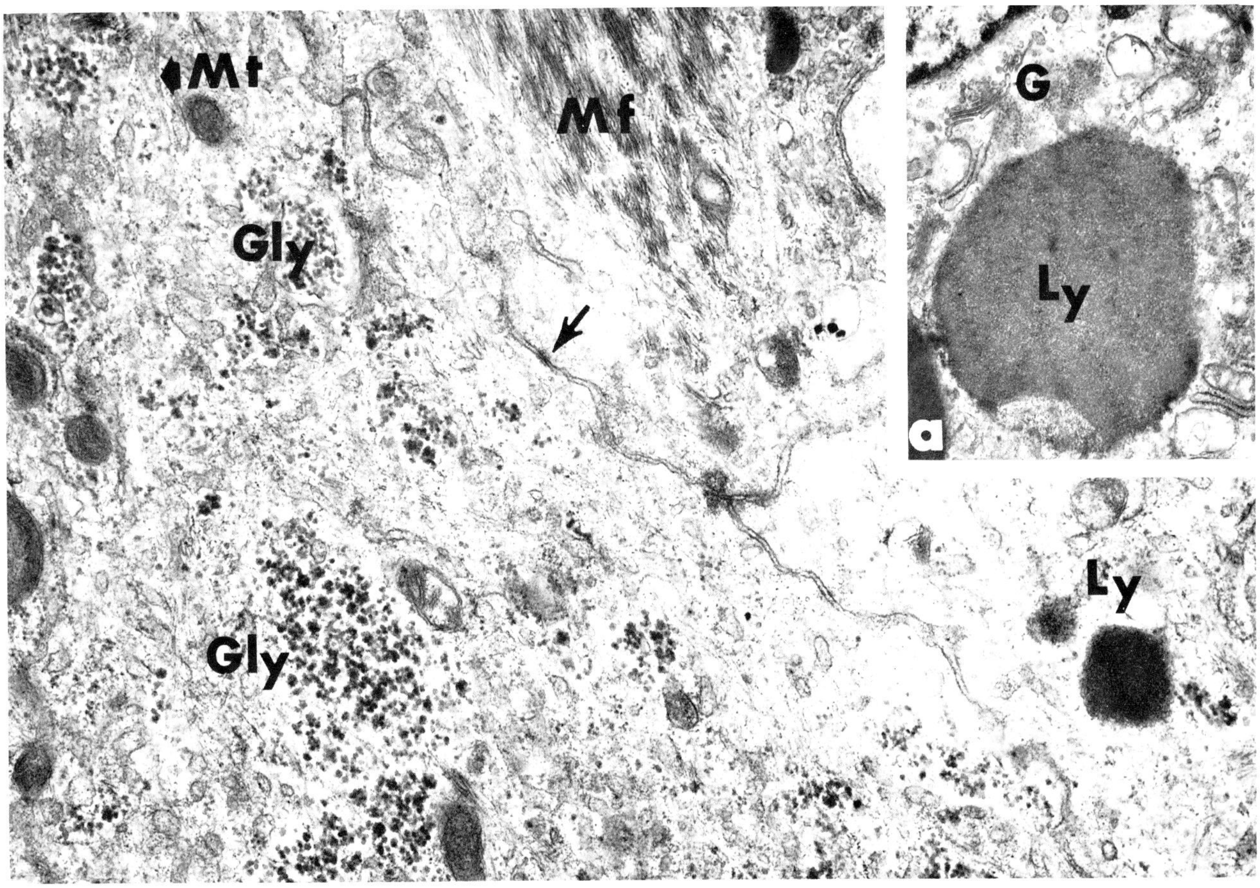

Figure 263. *Well-differentiated embryonal carcinoma cells* with abundant glycogen granules (Gly) and bundles of undifferentiated microfilaments (Mf). Poorly developed plasma membrane attachments (arrow) are infrequently encountered. × 25,600. Mt: microtubule; Ly: lysosome.

Figure 263a. *Well-differentiated embryonal carcinoma.* The prominent intracellular, membrane-bound bodies (Ly) with amorphous contents probably correspond to the eosinophilic globoid elements seen histologically. × 25,600. G: Golgi.

REFERENCES (Embryonal carcinoma–Figure 263a)

1. Pierce, G. B. Ultrastructure of human testicular tumors. *Cancer* **19:** 1963 (1966).
2. Schiller, W. Mesonephroma ovarii. *Am. J. Cancer* **35:** 1 (1939).
3. Teilum, G. Classification of endodermal sinus tumor (mesoblastoma vitellinum) and so-called "embryonal carcinoma" of the ovary. *Acta Pathol. Microbiol. Scand.* **64:** 407 (1965).
4. Pierce, G. B., W. K. Bullock, and R. W. Huntington. Yolk sac tumors of the testis. *Cancer* **25:** 644 (1970).
5. Norris, H. J., G. P. Bagley, and H. B. Taylor. Carcinoma of the infant vagina. *Arch. Pathol.* **90:** 473 (1970).
6. Pierce, G. B., F. J. Dixon, and E. L. Verney. Teratocarcinogenic and tissue forming potentialities of the cell types comprising neoplastic embryoid bodies. *Lab. Invest.* **9:** 583 (1960).
7. Kleinsmith, L. J. and G. B. Pierce, Jr. Multipotentiality of single embryonal carcinoma cells. *Cancer Res.* **24:** 1544 (1964).
8. Stevens, L. C. Origin of testicular teratomas from primordial germ cells in mice. *J. Natl. Cancer Inst.* **38:** 549 (1967).
9. Pierce, G. B., L. C. Stevens, and P. K. Nakane. Ultrastructural analysis of the early development of teratocarcinoma. *J. Natl. Cancer Inst.* **39:** 755 (1967).
10. Huntington, R. W. and W. K. Bullock. Yolk sac tumors of the ovary. *Cancer* **25:** 1357 (1970).
11. Gitlin, D. and A. Perricelli. Synthesis of serum albumin, prealbumin, alpha-fetoprotein, alpha-1-antitrypsin and transferrin by the human yolk sac. *Nature* **228:** 995 (1970).
12. Ballas, M. Yolk sac carcinoma of the ovary with alphafetoprotein in serum and ascitic fluid demonstrated by immunoosmophoresis. *Am. J. Clin. Pathol.* **57:** 511 (1972).

77

Benign Cystic Teratoma (Dermoid Cyst)

The benign cystic teratoma (dermoid cyst), one of the most common benign ovarian neoplasms, is composed of one or more histologically mature tissues of ectodermic, endodermic, or mesodermic origin. These tissues include skin and its appendages, primarily concentrated in the hillock, or pedicle, of Von Rokitansky, glial tissue, and intestinal and bronchial elements, as well as teeth, eye, and thyroid tissues. When the thyroid tissue is predominant, the lesion is referred to as a "struma ovarii," which often has the histological appearance of a nontoxic nodular goiter. Occasionally, malignant transformation, especially squamous cell carcinoma and carcinoid tumors,[1] generally of the mid-gut type with typical carcinoid syndrome, is encountered.

It is generally accepted that benign cystic teratomas are of germ cell origin and represent the final stage of teratomatous differentiation. They probably arise through a parthenogenetic (autofertilization without fecundation) mechanism. In ovarian benign cystic teratomas there are invariably a normal diploid chromosome number and typical female sex chromatin.[4] Recent electrophoretic and genetic studies[5,6] of benign cystic teratomas from women heterozygous for 6-phosphogluconate and glucose-6-phosphate dehydrogenase have suggested that the neoplasms arise from a single germ cell of post-meiotic origin, as indicated by the frequent loss within the neoplasm of genes which are present in the host. The data indicate that the benign cystic teratomas may arise from fusion of two haploid cell nuclei following either meiosis I or II,[6] supporting the concept that ovarian teratomas, like their testicular counterparts, have a parthenogenetic origin. Despite the chaotic and disorganized arrangements of various elements, transmission[2,3] and scanning electron microscopic examinations reveal an organization that is typical of the corresponding normal adult tissue.

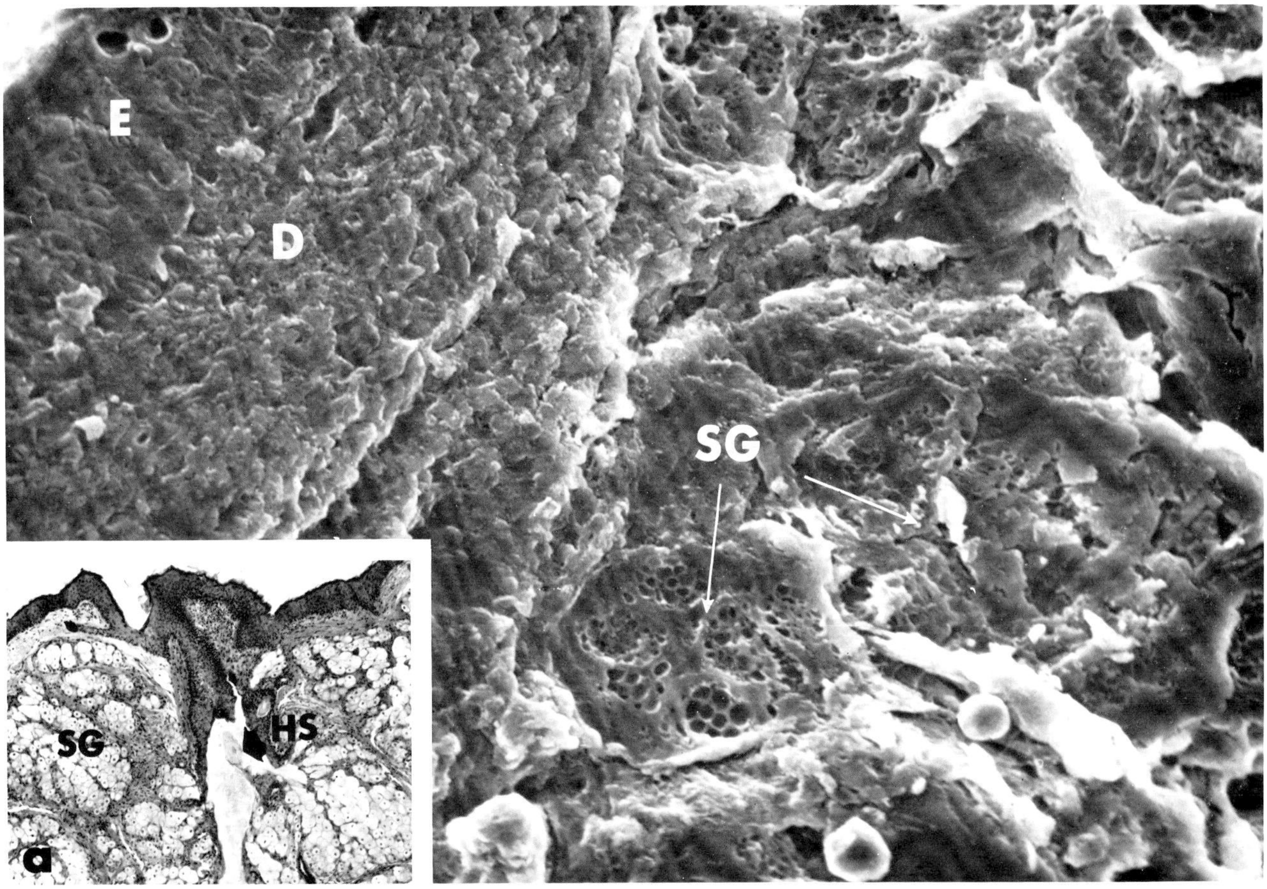

Figure 264a. *Histologic section through the polyp of Von Rokitansky,* which characteristically is covered by keratinizing, squamous, stratified epithelium. The underlying stroma contains prominent lobules of sebaceous glands (SG), associated with hair follicles and hair shafts (HS). (H & E stain, × 10.)

Figure 264. *Stereoscopic view of Figure 264a,* illustrating confluent lobules of sebaceous glands (SG) in which the cells have a honeycomb appearance, a pattern due to compression artifact (specimen prepared by freeze-drying technique). × 480. E: epidermis; D: dermis.

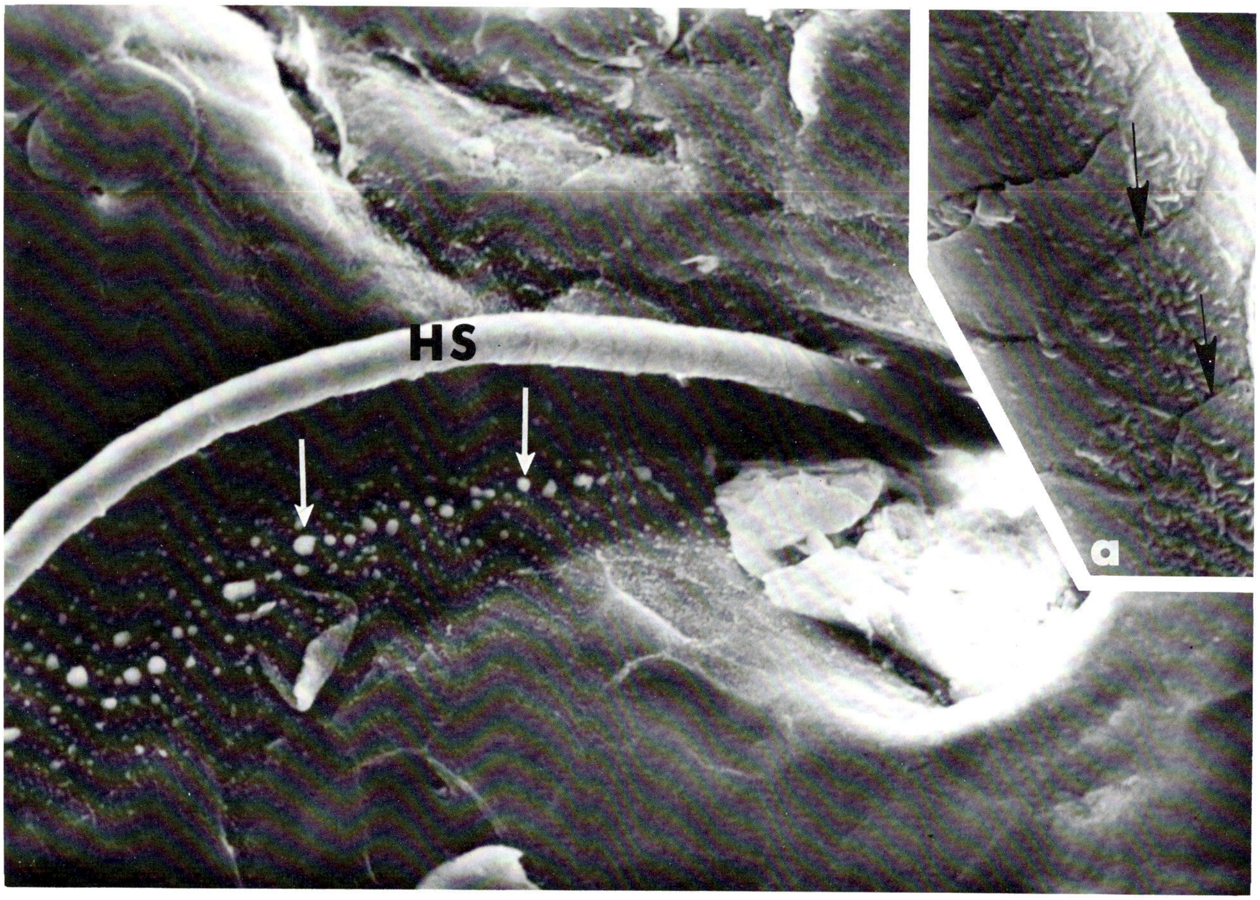

Figure 265. *Scanning electron microscopic appearance* of the epidermal lining of Von Rokitansky's polyp. The large epidermal cells have a polyhedral contour, and the protruding hair shaft (HS) is associated with abundant sebaceous secretions (arrows). × 480.

Figure 265a. *Higher magnification* of the hair shaft, covered by well-developed epicuticles (arrows). × 2400.

REFERENCES (The benign cystic teratoma–Figure 265a)

1. Toker, C. Ovarian carcinoid. A light and electron microscopic study. *Am. J. Obstet. Gynecol.* **103:** 1019 (1969).
2. Luse, S. A. and T. Vietti. Ovarian teratoma. Ultrastructure and neural component. *Cancer* **21:** 38 (1968).
3. Hardman, J. M., S. S. Schochet, J. H. Libcke, and K. M. Earle. Rosenthal fibers in ovarian teratomas. *Arch. Pathol.* **93:** 448 (1972).
4. Corfman, P. A. and R. M. Richart. Chromosome number and morphology of benign ovarian cystic teratomas. *New Engl. J. Med.* **271:** 1241 (1964).
5. Linder, D. Gene loss in human teratomas. *Proc. Natl. Acad. Sci. U. S.* **63:** 699 (1969).
6. Linder, D. and J. Power. Further evidence for postmeiotic origin of teratomas in the human female. *Ann. Hum. Genet. (London)* **34:** 21 (1970).

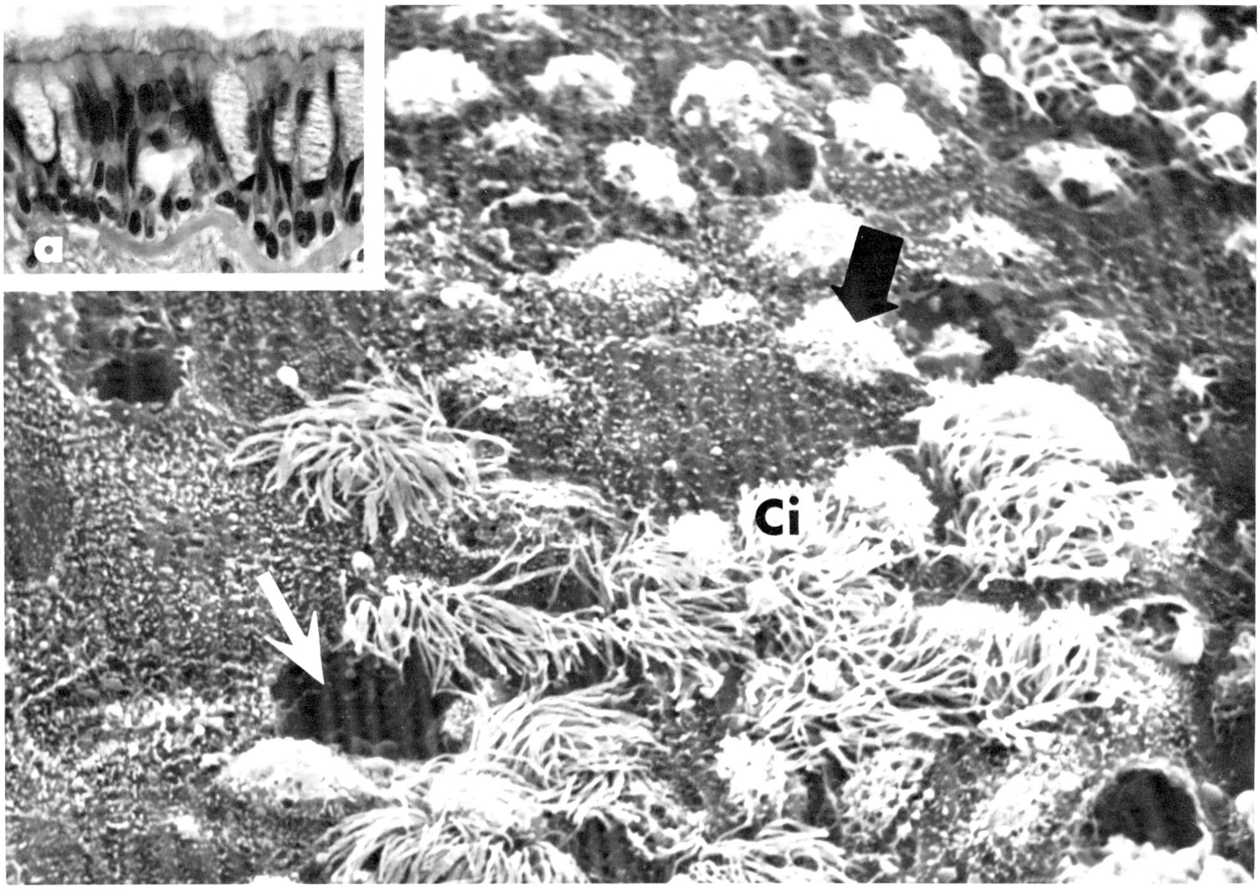

Figure 266a. *Benign cystic teratoma.* Histologic appearance of ciliated pseudostratified columnar epithelium with mucus-filled goblet cells, similar in all respects to the normal respiratory epithelium. (H & E stain, × 120.)

Figure 266. *With the scanning electron microscope,* the ciliated cells (Ci) are found to be arranged in clusters and the nonciliated cells have an abundant microvillous covering. The goblet cells, before secretion, are recognized by their bulging and granular secretory material (black arrow), whereas others, after secretion, resemble empty cellular craters (white arrow). × 1600.

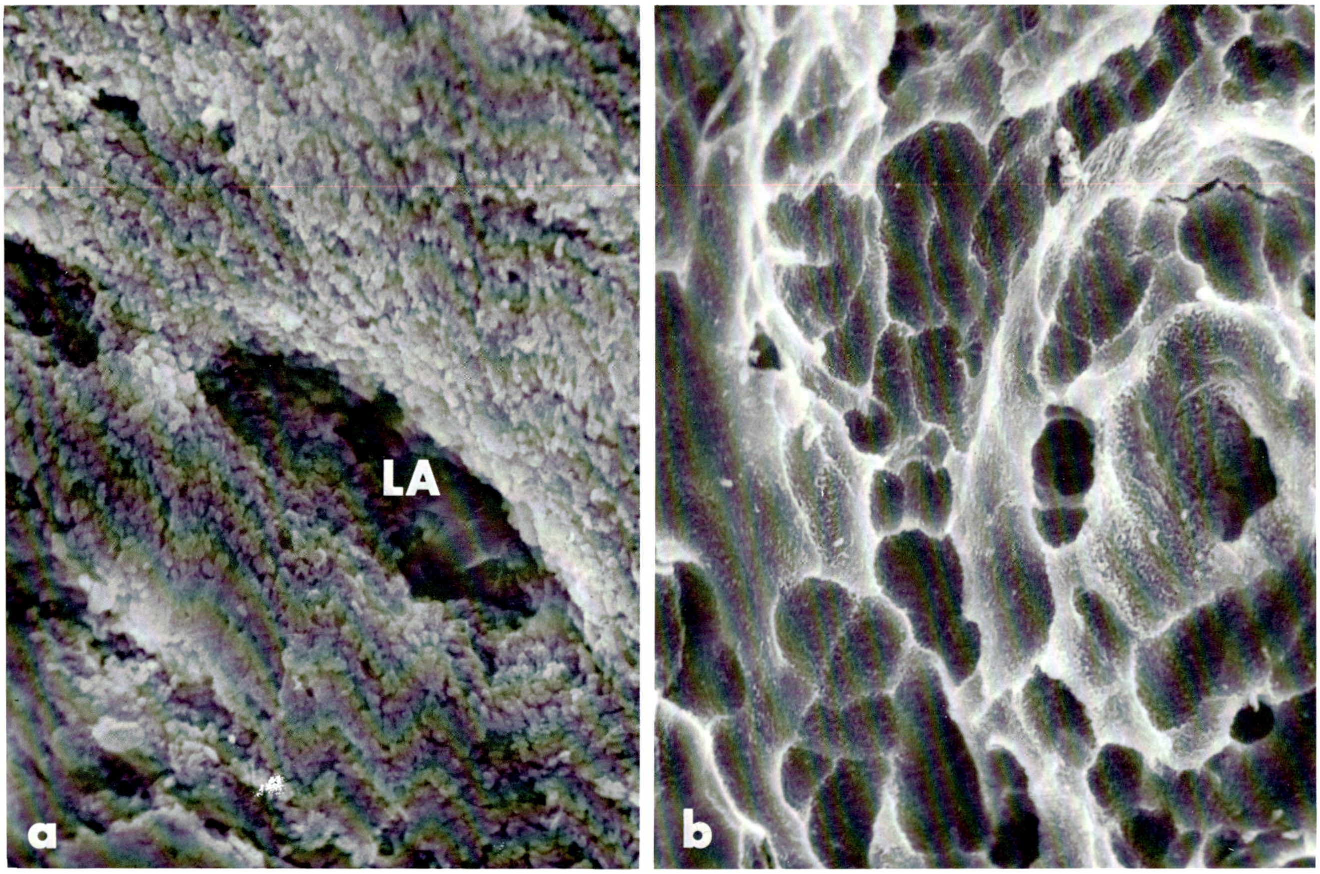

Figure 267a. *Benign cystic teratoma.* Scanning electron microscopy of a malformed teratomatous tooth, illustrating the dental cement which covers the root of the teeth and contains spindle-shaped lacunae (LA) of cementocytes. × 1120.

Figure 267b. *Benign cystic teratoma.* Note the irregular lacunar configuration of dental enamel in a malformed teratomatous tooth. × 960.

78

Testicular Feminization Syndrome (Gonadal Dysgenesis)

The testicular feminization syndrome (TFS) is a familial, inherited form of male pseudohermaphroditism, transmitted as a sex-linked recessive or as a male-limited, autosomal dominant gene.[1] The individuals have a female phenotype, possessing a normal male genetic constitution; although the external genitalia are those of a woman, the gonads are found to be aspermic testes in undescended or ectopic locations, and the internal reproductive tract is absent. Although the gonads produce androgens in the normal fashion, there is androgen insensitivity at a target cell level, which is thought to be responsible for the lack of androgenic characteristics. The precise etiologic factor of the conditions is not known, but it is currently believed that target cell refractoriness is not related to 5-α-reductase inactivity, since conversion of dihydrotestosterone from extracellular testosterone occurs normally. It is likely that the primary abnormality in testicular feminization syndrome is related to the deficiency of cytosol androgen receptors in target cells, which results in the noninducibility of structural gene products and thus in the androgen insensitivity of testicular feminization.[2] A similar genetic disturbance with no demonstrable specific androgen receptors has been reported in the X-linked testicular feminization syndrome of mice, rats, and cattle.[2,3]

In both man and animals, the absence of the masculinizing factor (which normally promotes a male phenotype) precludes the development of mesonephric duct derivatives and the urogenital sinus differentiates in a female direction. The formation of the Müllerian duct is inhibited, probably by a second morphogenetic factor, which presumably remains functional in male-destined TFS individuals.[4] The occurrence of female sex characteristics at the time of puberty is accounted for by the peripheral conversion of testicular androgens into estrogens.

The relatively poor cytoplasmic development of Sertoli cells, the occurrence of immature Leydig cells,[5-8] the uniform absence of Reinke's crystals,[8] and the lack of peritubular fibrosis in the complete form of TFS gonads[5-9] represent features in common with those of normal fetal,[10,11] rather than of pubertal or postpubertal, testes.[11] Additional support for the gonads being fetal,[7,8] rather than immature[6] or undescended-like,[5] is afforded by the exclusive presence of early fetal spermatogonia. The failure of further spermatogonial development and the presence of ovarian stroma[8] reflect an impairment of testicular differentiation and development during early fetal life.[8] The multinodular pattern of TFS gonads, with scattered spermatogonia and intertubular Leydig cells, which is consistent with Sertoli cell hyperplasia[6,8] rather than tubular adenomas, is a pattern likely to be related to the abnormal location of the gonads, for similar tubular organization has been observed in undescended testes in otherwise normal males.[12]

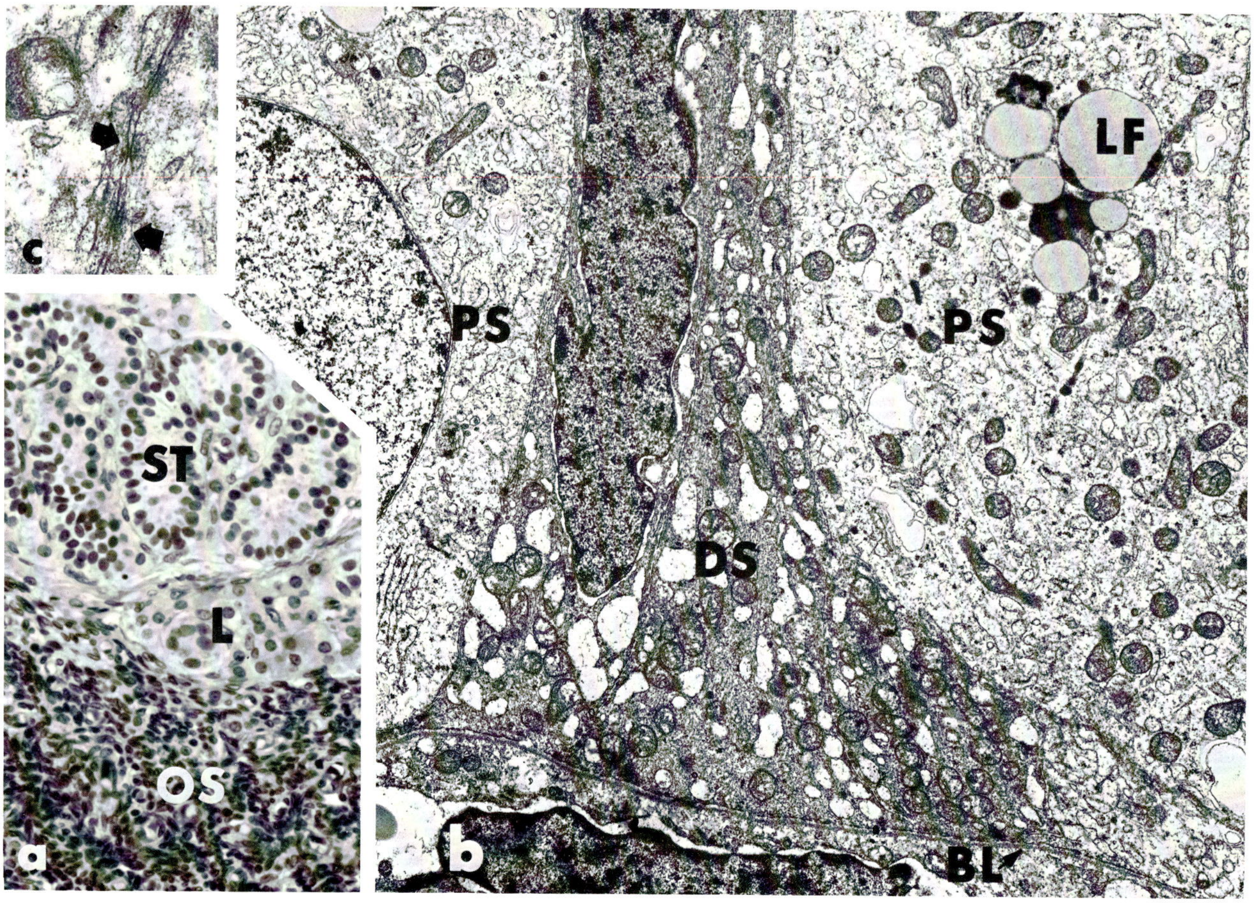

Figure 268a. *Histologically,* the gonads are multinodular, composed of lumenless seminiferous tubules (ST) devoid of spermatogenetic activity and peritubular fibrosis or hyalinization. Most of the cells lining the tubules are pale and triangular with oval nuclei resembling immature Sertoli cells, whereas others appear as dark, compressed cells with pyknotic nuclei, interpreted as degenerated Sertoli cells. Large collections of Leydig cells (L), identical to normal adult Leydig cells, are scattered through the intertubular space, and foci of ovarianlike stroma (OS) are occasionally seen in the periphery of the gonads. (H & E stain, × 290.) *From* A. Ferenczy and R. M. Richart. The fine structure of the gonads in the complete form of testicular feminization syndrome. *Am. J. Obstet. Gynecol.* **113:** 399–409 (1972).

Figure 268b. *The dark Sertoli cells* (DS) have an electron-dense cytoplasm with degenerative cytoplasmic processes, and the endoplasmic reticulum is markedly dilated. The nuclei have a spindle-shaped contour with peripheral condensation of nuclear chromatin. The large, triangular Sertoli cells have a pale (PS) to dark cytoplasmic matrix and round, centrally located nuclei with smooth envelopes. The cytoplasm contains a variable number of organelles, including vesicular, granular endoplasmic reticulum, mitochondria, and Golgi. Lipid and lipofuchsin (LF) granules, microfilaments, and microtubules are seen. Filamentous crystalloids of Charcot-Boltcher are absent. The tubular lining membrane appears indistinguishable from that of normal testicular tissue, and there is no evidence of abnormal fibrillogenesis by intertubular fibroblasts. × 5000. BL: basal lamina. *From* A. Ferenczy, and R. M. Richart. The fine structure of the gonads in the complete form of testicular feminization syndrome. *Am. J. Obstet. Gynecol.* **113:** 399–409 (1972).

Figure 268c. *The plasma membranes* are reinforced by infrequent zonula occludens and zonula adherens (arrows). × 35,000. *From* A. Ferenczy and R. M. Richart. The fine structure of the gonads in the complete form of testicular feminization syndrome. *Am. J. Obstet. Gynecol.* **113:** 399–409 (1972).

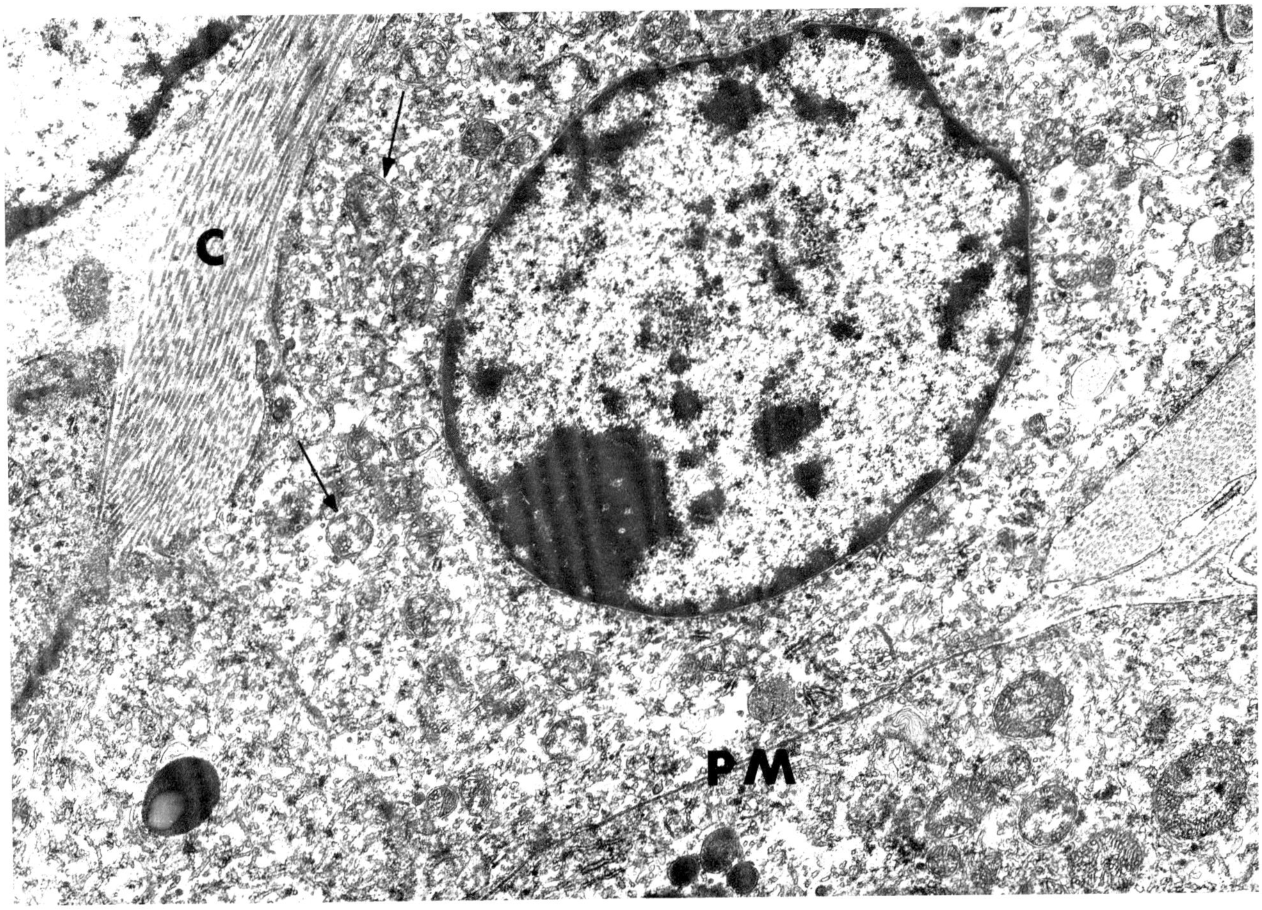

Figure 269. *Occasionally Leydig cells* have a fusiform contour and smooth plasma membranes (PM), and the cytoplasm is packed with tubular, agranular endoplasmic reticulum. Mitochondria are poorly developed (arrow). × 10,000. C: intercellular collagen. *From* A. Ferenczy and R. M. Richart. The fine structure of the gonads in the complete form of testicular feminization syndrome. *Am. J. Obstet. Gynecol.* **113:** 399–409 (1972).

REFERENCES (The testicular feminization syndrome—Figure 269)

1. Boczkowski, K. Genetical studies in testicular feminization syndrome. *J. Med. Genet.* **5:** 181 (1968).
2. Bullock, L. P. and C. W. Bardin. Androgen receptors in testicular feminization. *J. Clin. Endocrinol. Metab.* **35:** 935 (1972).
3. Dofuku, R., U. Tettenborn, and S. Ohno. Testotserone—"Regulon" in the mouse kidney. *Nature New Biol.* **232:** 5 (1971).
4. Turner, C. D. Special mechanisms in anomalies of sex differentiation. *Am. J. Obstet. Gynecol.* **90:** 1028 (1964).
5. Perez-Palacios, G., K. G. Lamont, A. E. Perez, R. B. Jaffe, and G. B. Pierce. De novo formation and metabolism of steroid hormones in feminizing testes. Biochemical and ultrastructural studies. *J. Clin. Endocrinol. Metab.* **29:** 786 (1969).
6. Gordon, G. B., L. R. Miller and K. G. Bensch. Electron microscopic observations of the gonad in the testicular feminization syndrome. *Lab. Invest.* **13:** 152 (1964).
7. Damjanov, I., P. Drobnjak, and V. Grizelj. Testicular feminization with immature Leydig cells—an ultrastructural demonstration. *Am. J. Obstet. Gynecol.* **110:** 594 (1971).
8. Ferenczy, A. and R. M. Richart. The fine structure of the gonads in the complete form of testicular feminization syndrome. *Am. J. Obstet. Gynecol.* **113:** 399 (1972).
9. Smith, B. D., C. R. Leeson, R. G. Bunge, and W. R. Anderson. Microscopic appearance of the gonads in postpubertal testicular feminization. *Invest. Urol.* **5:** 73 (1967).
10. Pelliniemi, L. J. Fine structure of germ cords in human fetal testis. In *Morphological Aspects of Andrology*, A. F. Holstein and E. Horstman (Eds.). Vol. 7, Grosse Verlag, Berlin, 1970, p. 5.
11. Leeson, C. R. An electron microscopic study of the cryptorchid and scrotal human testes, with special reference to pubertal maturation. *Invest. Urol.* **3:** 498 (1966).
12. Collins, D. H. and T. Symington. Sertoli-Cell tumour. *Brit. J. Urol.* **36** (Suppl.): 52 (1964).

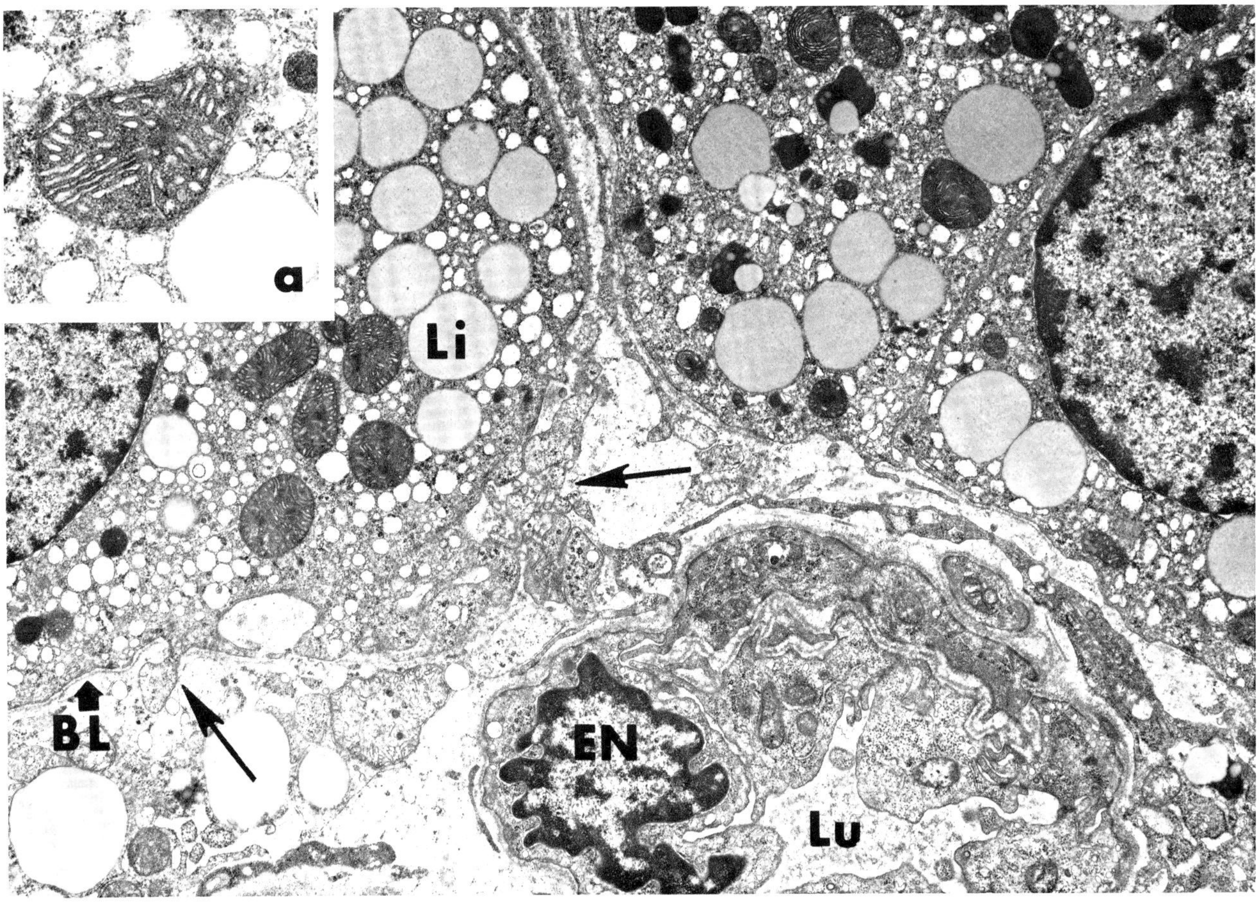

Figure 270. *The Leydig cells* contain the organellar contents necessary for the synthesis of sex steroids, including abundant vesicular, agranular endoplasmic reticulum, pleomorphic mitochondria with lamellated cristae, Golgi, free ribosomes, lipid droplets (Li), and lipofuchsin granules. Reinke's crystals or their microtubular precursors are uniformly absent. The free plasma membranes are enveloped by well-defined, but often interrupted, basal lamina (BL), and numerous cytoplasmic processes (arrows), especially pronounced near capillaries, are seen. × 6200. EN: capillary endothelium; Lu: capillary lumen. *From* A. Ferenczy and R. M. Richart. The fine structure of the gonads in the complete form of testicular feminization syndrome. *Am. J. Obstet. Gynecol.* **113:** 399–409 (1972).

Figure 270a. *Mitochondrion* with lamellated cristae. × 23,000. *From* A. Ferenczy and R. M. Richart. The fine structure of the gonads in the complete form of testicular feminization syndrome. *Am. J. Obstet. Gynecol.* **113:** 399–409 (1972).

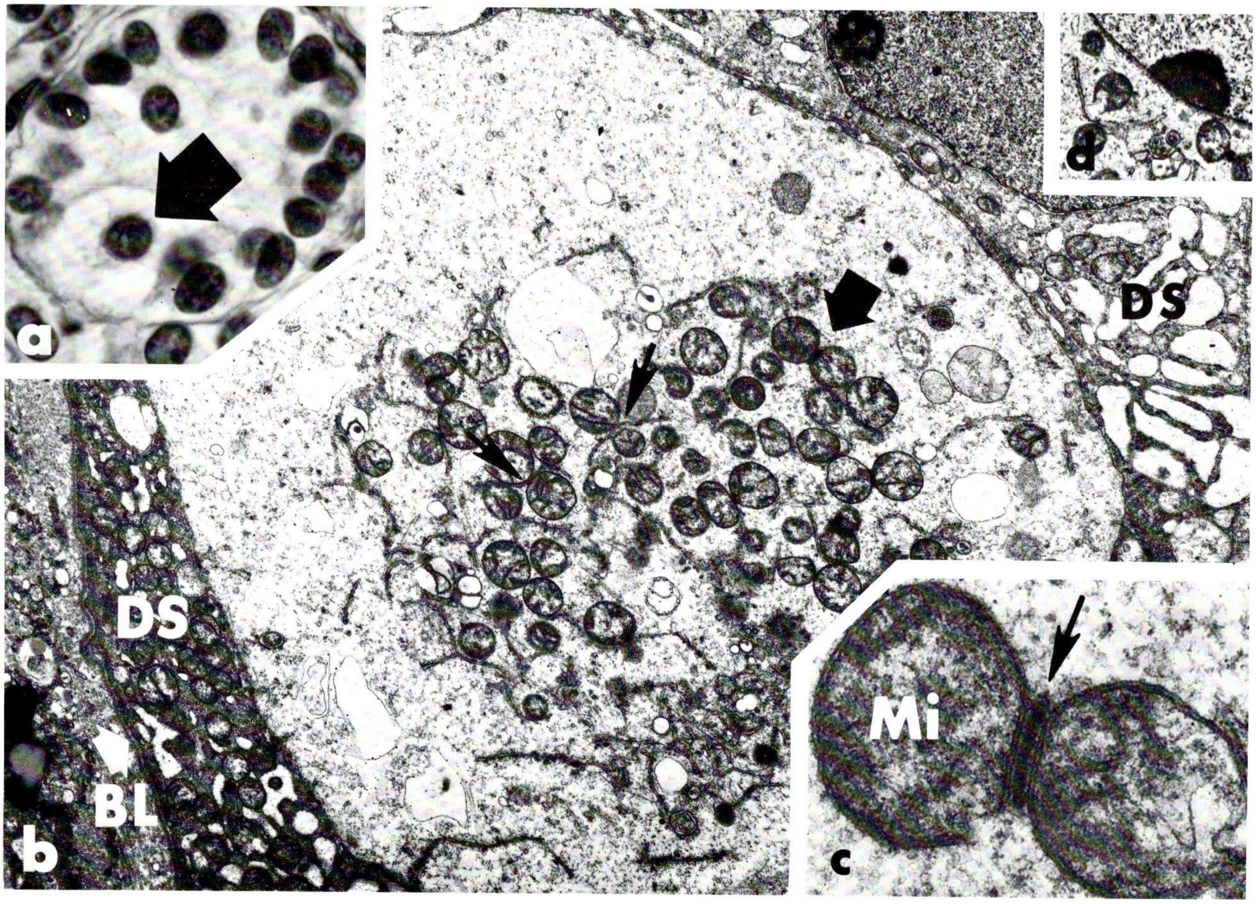

Figure 271a. *Several seminiferous tubules* contain single spermatogonia (arrow) with large amounts of pale cytoplasm located on the tubular basal lamina. (H & E stain, × 400.) *From* A. Ferenczy and R. M. Richart. The fine structure of the gonads in the complete form of testicular feminization syndrome. *Am. J. Obstet. Gynecol.* **113:** 399–409 (1972).

Figure 271b. *Most of the germ cells* are completely surrounded by degenerated Sertoli cells (DS), and the clear cytoplasm contains a central concentration of mitochondria, often interconnected by parallel membranes of granular endoplasmic reticulum (narrow arrows) and occasionally by "intermitochondrial cement" (large arrow). Intercellular bridges between adjacent germ cells, mitoses, and spermatocytes are uniformly absent. × 9000. BL: basal lamina. *From* A. Ferenczy and R. M. Richart. The fine structure of the gonads in the complete form of testicular feminization syndrome. *Am. J. Obstet. Gynec.* **113:** 399–409 (1972).

Figure 271c. *High magnification* of "intermitochondrial cement" (arrow). × 48,000. Mi: mitochondria. *From* A. Ferenczy and R. M. Richart. The fine structure of the gonads in the complete form of testicular feminization syndrome. *Am. J. Obstet. Gynecol.* **113:** 399–409 (1972).

Figure 271d. *Most of the germ cells* have compact, dome-shaped nucleoli in close contact with the nuclear membrane. × 12,000. *From* A. Ferenczy and R. M. Richart. The fine structure of the gonads in the complete form of testicular feminization syndrome. *Am. J. Obstet. Gynecol.* **113:** 399–409 (1972).

PLACENTA

Soon after implantation, the epithelium of the human placenta[1] is organized into cyto- and syncytiotrophoblastic compartments, which form a metabolically complex cell system with multiple functions of synthesis, secretion, and transport.

During the early stages of placental morphogenesis (13th–21st days), intervillous spaces are formed by the coalescence of lacunae in the primitive syncytium, followed by the formation of primary (cyto- and syncytiotrophoblast), secondary (ingrowth of fetal connective tissue), and tertiary (vascularized villous core) chorionic villi. After endometrial vascular invasion by the syncytiotrophoblast of the primary villi, the vascular system of the tertiary villous core develops contact with the embryonal vascular system, and a maternal–placental–fetal circulation is established.

The prominent nonvillous, cytotrophoblastic cell columns (anchoring villi) of early gestation attach the terminal chorionic villi to the decidua and form a portion of the trophoblastic shell. In the cell islands, the cytotrophoblast labels heavily with ^{3}H-thymidine,[2-5] numerous mitoses are seen, and there is increased glycolytic enzyme activity,[6-8] all related to the production of the trophoblast, which covers the extending chorionic villi. The cytotrophoblast is the generative compartment for the mature syncytiotrophoblast, and the cell types intermediary between the two can be readily identified.[5,9-11]

REFERENCES

1. Hertig, A. T. *Human Trophoblast.* Charles C Thomas, Springfield, Ill., 1968.
2. Richart, R. M. Studies of placental morphogenesis. I. Radioautographic studies of human placenta utilizing tritiated thymidine. *Proc. Soc. Exp. Biol. Med.* **106:** 829 (1961).
3. Pierce, G. B., Jr. and A. R. Midgely, Jr. The origin and function of human syncytiotrophoblast giant cells. *Am. J. Pathol.* **43:** 153 (1963).
4. Tao, T. W. and A. T. Hertig. Viability and differentiation of human trophoblast in organ culture. *Am. J. Anat.* **116:** 315 (1965).
5. Okudaira, Y., T. Hashimoto, N. Hamanaka, and S. Yoshinare. Electron microscopic study on the trophoblastic cell column of human placenta. *J. Electronmicrosc. (Tokyo)* **20:** 93 (1971).
6. Kaufmann, P. Observations on the Langerhans cells in the human placenta. *Z. Zellforsch.* **128:** 283 (1972).
7. Stark, J. and P. Kaufmann. Polypous syncytioplasma protrusions and regressive changes in the villous trophoblast of the human placenta. *Arch. Gynaekol.* **212:** 51 (1972).
8. Kaufmann, P. and J. Stark. Enzyme-histochemical studies on mature placental villi. I. Differentiation and degeneration of the trophoblast. *Histochimie* **29:** 65 (1972).
9. Boyd, J. D. and W. J. Hamilton. Development and structure of the human placenta from the end of the 3rd month of gestation. *J. Obstet. Gynaecol. Brit. Commonw.* **74:** 161 (1967).
10. Wynn, R. M. Cytotrophoblastic specialization. An ultrastructural study of the human placenta. *Am. J. Obstet. Gynecol.* **114:** 339 (1972).
11. Okudaira, Y., S. Suzuki, M. Okudaira, T. Hashimoto, and K. Hayakawa. Electron microscopic observations on the formation of syncytiotrophoblast from cytotrophoblast. *J. Electronmicrosc. (Tokyo)* **17:** 47 (1968).

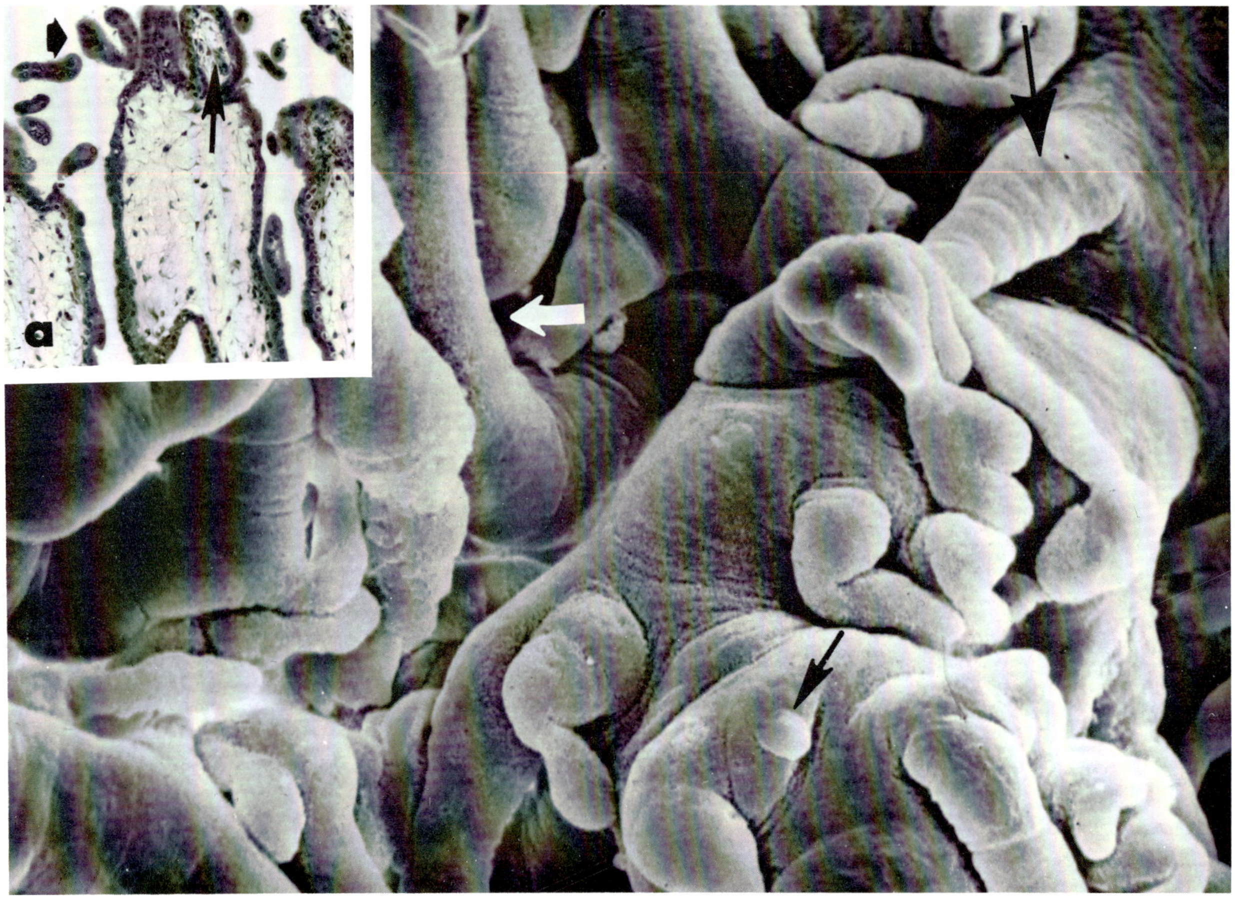

79

Immature Placenta

The immature chorionic villi (8–12th weeks) are covered by an outer syncytial and an inner cytotrophoblastic (Langerhans) cell layer.

Figure 272a. *Histologically, the immature chorionic villi* are large with a loose, myxoid villous core. The covering trophoblastic membrane contains numerous trophoblastic buddings, varying from fingerlike syncytial extensions (short arrow) to larger trophoblastic villous sprouts (long arrow). (H & E stain, × 30.)

Figure 272. *The terminal (white arrow) or free chorionic villi* in immature placentas appear as voluminous cylinders, with a complex interlacing pattern giving rise to a multitude of trophoblastic sprouts[1] or buds varying from minute (small arrow) to large, cylindrical villous structures (long arrow). These syncytiotrophoblastic protrusions[2,3] are believed to be developing chorionic villi,[4,5] and their abundance in early[1,3] gestation is a reflection of the active trophoblastic growth of this stage. Note the wide intervillous spaces and the short, noninterdigitating trophoblastic villosity. × 320. *From* A. Ferenczy and R. M. Richart. Scanning electron microscopic study of normal and molar trophoblast. *Gynecol. Oncol.* **1:** 95–110 (1972).

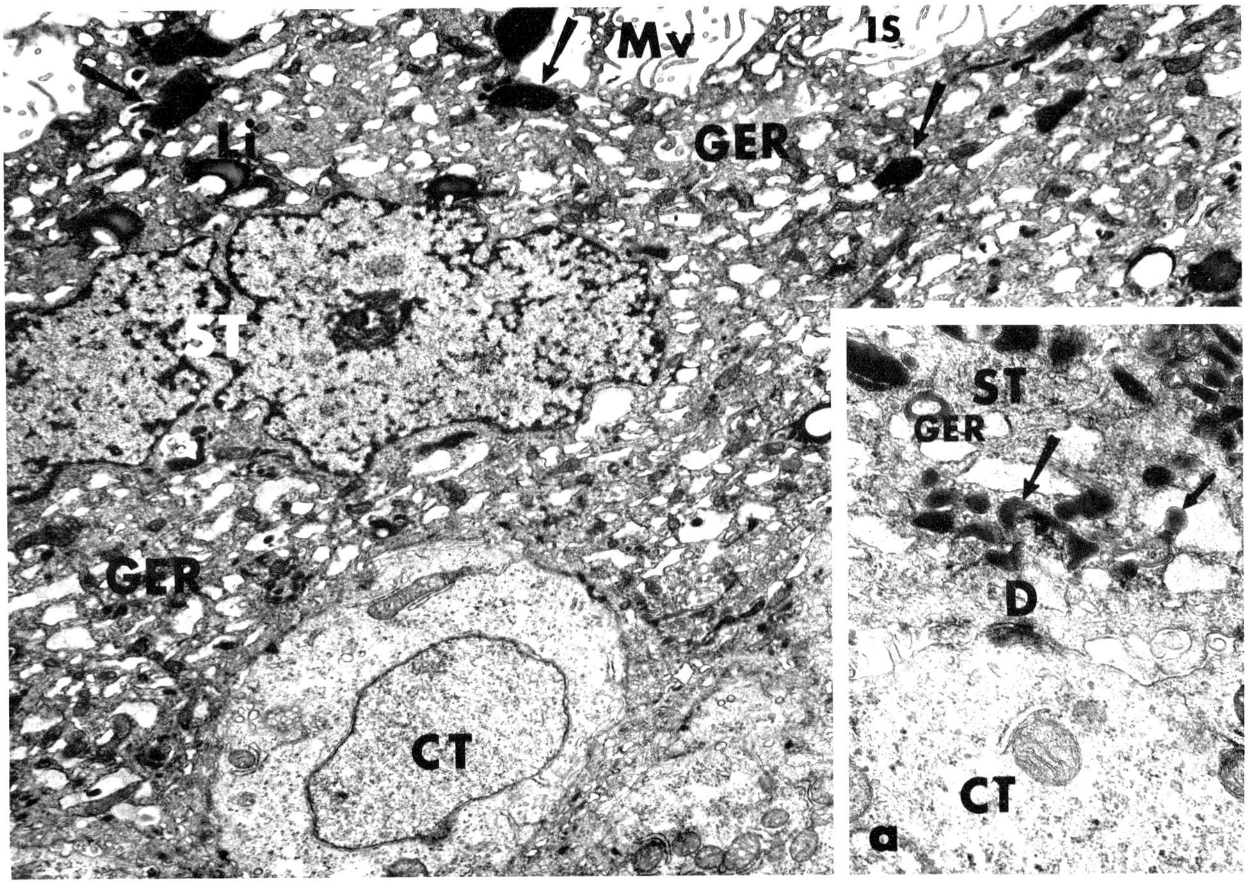

Figure 273. *Immature placenta (8–12th weeks).* Ultrastructurally, the syncytiotrophoblast (ST) does not have dividing cell membranes, and the nuclei are spaced at more or less regular intervals. The mid-portion of the cytoplasm ("secretory zone")[3] is filled with abundant, dilated granular endoplasmic reticulum (GER), associated with free ribosomes, mitochondria, lipid droplets (Li), glycogen, and lysosomes (arrows). [3,4,6,7] This richly equipped organellar system, although ultrastructurally different from steroidogenic cells, is oriented toward the elaboration of steroids, hormones, steroid precursors, and proteins. The role of the syncytium as the primary placental source of hormone production has been established by immunohistochemical studies using immunofluorescent antibody techniques. These studies have localized human chorionic gonadotropin[8,9] (HCG) and human placental lactogen (HPL), or chorionic somatomammotropin,[10,11] in the syncytiotrophoblast. Furthermore, transmission electron microscopic studies using enzyme-labeled antibody techniques[12] have demonstrated that HCG is associated with the granular endoplasmic reticulum and occasionally with the Golgi. In addition to the elaboration of protein hormones, the syncytium possesses a variety of enzymes contributing to the production of steroid hormones,[13] principally progesterone,[14] estrogens, and, in smaller quantities, cortisone and aldosterone.[14] × 5600. Mv: microvilli; IS: intervillous space; CT: cytotrophoblast.

Figure 273a. *Immature placenta.* While syncytial cells (ST) are unique to the human body in that they form an uninterrupted cytoplasmic substance (syncytium), the basal plasma membranes contain desmosomal attachments (D) to the underlying cytotrophoblast (CT). The cytotrophoblastic cells have a light cytoplasmic matrix and few organelles (except free ribosomes) and represent the trophoblastic "germinal" layer, as discussed previously.[15–17] There is a close interrelationship between the granular endoplasmic reticulum (GER) and membrane bound dense bodies (long arrow), one of which protrudes into a dilated granular cisterna (small arrow). × 24,040.

REFERENCES (Figures 272–273a)

1 Ferenczy, A. and R. M. Richart. Scanning electron microscopic study of normal and molar trophoblast. *Gynecol. Oncol.* **1:** 95 (1972).

2. Lister, U. M. Ultrastructure of the early human placenta. *J. Obstet. Gynaecol. Brit. Commonw.* **71:** 21 (1964).

3. Dempsey, E. W. and S. A. Luse. Regional specializations in the syncytial trophoblast of early human placentas. *J. Anat.* **108:** 545 (1971).

4. Boyd, J. D. and W. J. Hamilton. Development and structure of the human placenta from the end of the 3rd month of gestation. *J. Obstet. Gynaecol. Brit. Commonw.* **74:** 161 (1967).

5. Aladjem, S. Morphopathology of the human placental villi and the fetal outcome (a study by phase-contrast microscopy). *J. Obstet. Gynaecol. Brit. Commonw.* **75:** 1237 (1968).

6. Wislocki, G. B. and E. W. Dempsey. Electron microscopy of the human placenta. *Anat. Rec.* **123:** 133 (1955).

7. Tighe, J. R., P. R. Garrod, and R. C. Curran. The trophoblast of the human chorionic villus. *J. Pathol. Bacteriol.* **93:** 559 (1967).

8. Midgley, A. R., Jr. and G. B. Pierce, Jr. Immunohistochemical localization of human chorionic gonadotropin. *J. Exp. Med.* **115:** 289 (1962).

9. Dreskin, R. B., S. S. Spicer, and W. B. Greene. Ultrastructural localization of chorionic gonadotropin in human term placenta. *J. Histochem. Cytochem.* **18:** 862 (1970).

10. Grumbach, M. M. and S. L. Kaplan. On the placental origin and purification of chorionic "growth hormone—prolactin" and its immunoassay in pregnancy. *Trans. N. Y. Acad. Sci.* **27:** 189 (1970).

11. Beck, J. S. Time of appearance of human placental lactogen in the embryo. *New Engl. J. Med* **283:** 189 (1970)

12. Hamanaka, N., O. Tanizawa, T. Hashimoto, S. Yoshinare, and Y. Okudaira. Electron microscopic study on the localization of human chorionic gonadotropin (HCG) in the chorionic tissue by enzyme-labeled antibody technique. *J. Electronmicrosc. (Tokyo)* **20:** 128 (1970).

13. Benirschke, K. and S. G. Driscoll. *The Pathology of the Human Placenta,* Springer-Verlag, New York, 1967, pp. 431–456.

14. Villee, D. B. Development of endocrine function in the human placenta and fetus. *New Engl. J. Med.* **281:** 473, 533 (1969).

15. Kaufmann, P. Observations on the Langhans cells in the human placenta. *Z. Zellforsch.* **128:** 283 (1972).

16. Stark, J. and P. Kaufmann. Polypous syncytioplasma protrusions and regressive changes in the villous trophoblast of the human placenta. *Arch. Gynaekol.* **212:** 51 (1972).

17. Kaufmann, P. and J. Stark. Enzyme-histochemical studies on mature human placental villi. I. Differentiation and degeneration of the trophoblast. *Histochimie* **29:** 65 (1972).

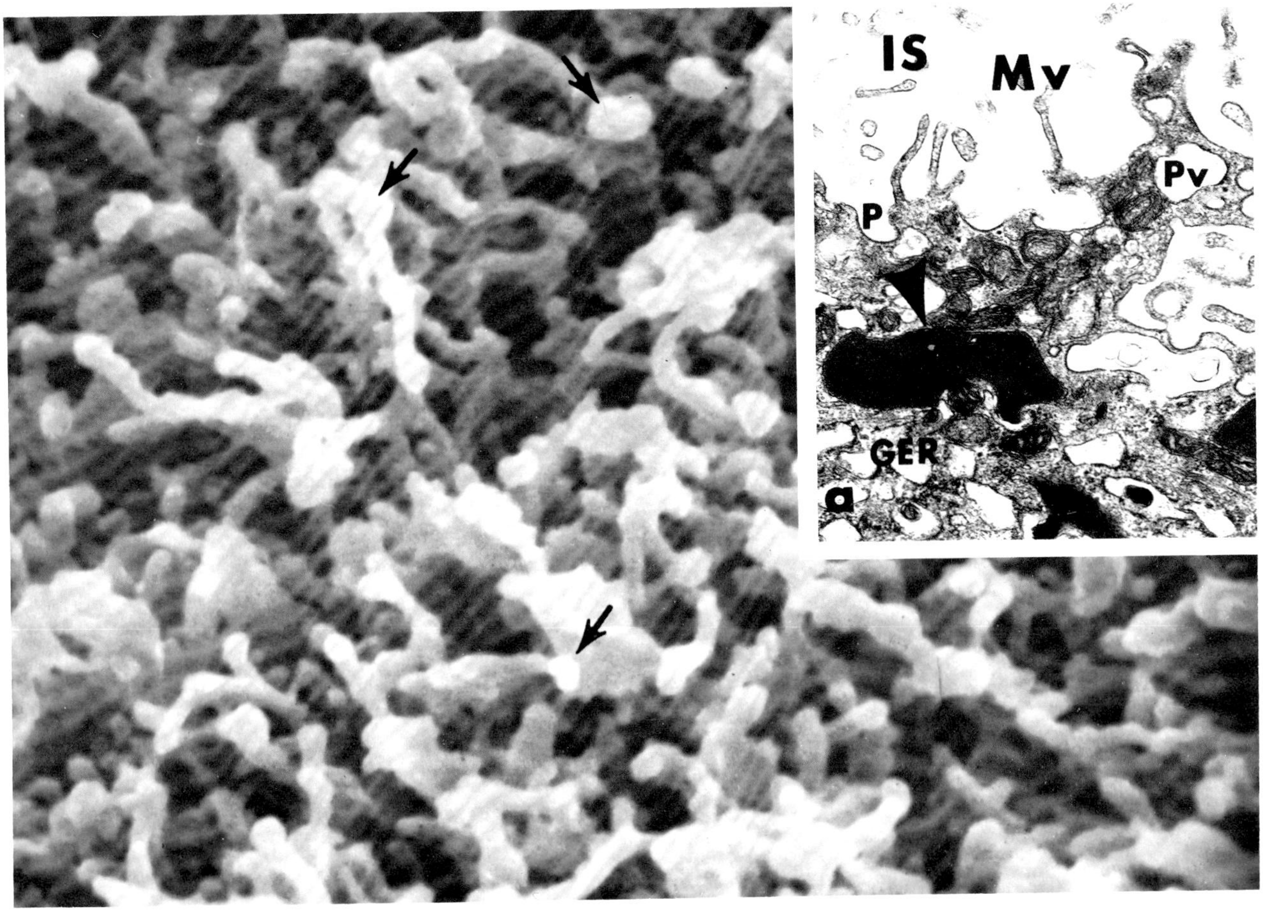

Figure 274. *Immature placenta (8–12 weeks).* The free surface of the syncytium contains a profusion of microvilli which,[1-5] although of varying length, shape, and number, are generally well developed. There are numerous microvillous promontories (arrows),[5] and considerable interbranching and many bulbous apices are obvious with the scanning electron microscope.[5,6] × 20,000. *From* A. Ferenczy and R. M. Richart. Scanning electron microscopic study of normal and molar trophoblast. *Gynecol. Oncol.* **1:** 95–110 (1972).

Figure 274a. *The conspicuous, microvillous (Mv) surface of* the immature placenta and its associated pinocytic activity (P and Pv) provide a mechanism for the high level of absorptive function[1-5,7,8] related to active fluid and ion transport that occurs in the immature placenta. In addition, the incorporation of ferritin[9] and iron particles[10] into apical vesicles suggests a phagocytic capacity of the syncytial cells. × 23,040. IS: intervillous space; arrow head: large, membrane-bound lysosome with amorphous dense material; GER: granular endoplasmic reticulum.

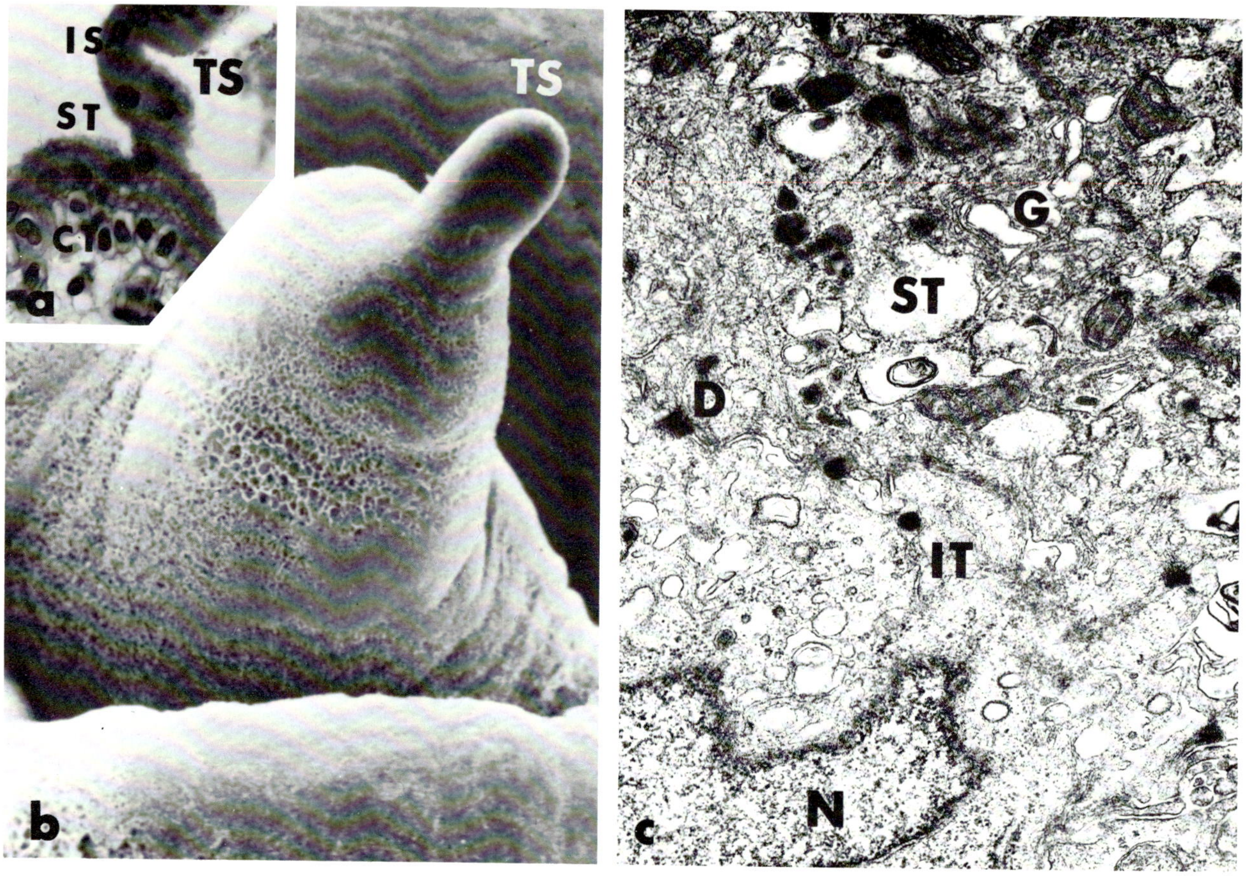

Figure 275a. *Immature placenta.* A slender trophoblastic extension (TS) composed entirely of multinucleated syncytiotrophoblasts projects into the intervillous space (IS). The chorionic villus has a well-developed syncytial (ST) and cytotrophoblastic (CT) layer. (H & E stain, × 75.)

Figure 275b. *Scanning electron micrograph,* illustrating the development of a new chorionic villus which is initiated by the apical proliferation and extension of the trophoblast (TS). × 560. *From* A. Ferenczy and R. M. Richart. Scanning electron microscopic study of normal and molar trophoblast. *Gynecol. Oncol.* **1**: 95–110 (1972).

Figure 275c. *The cells intermediate* (IT) between the syncytiotrophoblast (ST) and the cytotrophoblast have comparatively more abundant organelles, especially granular endoplasmic reticulum, than occur in the cytotrophoblast, but less than in the syncytial cells.[4] Similar cells are also seen in the placentas of subhuman primates[11] and in trophoblastic neoplasms.[11,12] × 23,040. G: Golgi in syncytial cell; D: desmosomal attachments between the intermediate and the syncytial cell; N: nucleus of intermediate cell.

REFERENCES (Figures 274–275c)

1. Wislocki, G. B. and E. W. Dempsey. Electron microscopy of the human placenta. *Anat. Rec.* **123:** 133 (1955).
2. Lister, U. M. Ultrastructure of the early human placenta. *J. Obstet. Gynaecol. Brit. Commonw.* **71:** 21 (1964).
3. Boyd, J. D. and W. J. Hamilton. Development and structure of the human placenta from the end of the 3rd month of gestation. *J. Obstet. Gynaecol. Brit. Commonw.* **74:** 161 (1967).
4. Tighe, J. R., P. R. Garrod, and R. C. Curran. The trophoblast of the human chorionic villus. *J. Pathol. Bacteriol.* **93:** 559 (1967).
5. Dempsey, E. W. and S. A. Luse. Regional specializations in the syncytial trophoblast of early human placentas. *J. Anat.* **108:** 545 (1971).
6. Ferenczy, A. and R. M. Richart. Scanning electron microscopic study of normal and molar trophoblast. *Gynecol. Oncol.* **1:** 95 (1972).
7. Schiebler, T. H. and P. Kaufmann. Uber die Gliederung der menschlichen Plazenta. *Z. Zellforsch.* **102:** 242 (1969).
8. Ashley, C. A. Study of the human placenta with the electron microscope. Functional implications of a canal system in the trophoblast. *Arch. Pathol.* **80:** 377 (1965).
9. Muir, A. R. On the phagocytosis of iron-dextran by the human plasmoditrophoblast. *J. Obstet. Gynaecol. Brit. Commonw.* **73:** 966 (1966).
10. Pierce, G. B., Jr. A. R. Midgley, Jr., and T. F. Beals. An ultrastructural study of differentiation and maturation of trophoblast of the monkey. *Lab. Invest.* **13:** 451 (1964).
11. Midgley, A. R., Jr. and G. B. Pierce, Jr. Immunohistochemical localization of human chorionic gonadotropin. *J. Exp. Med.* **115:** 289, 1962.
12. Wynn, R. M. and J. Davies. Ultrastructure of hydatidiform mole: correlative electron microscopic and functional aspects. *Am. J. Obstet. Gynecol.* **90:** 293 (1964).

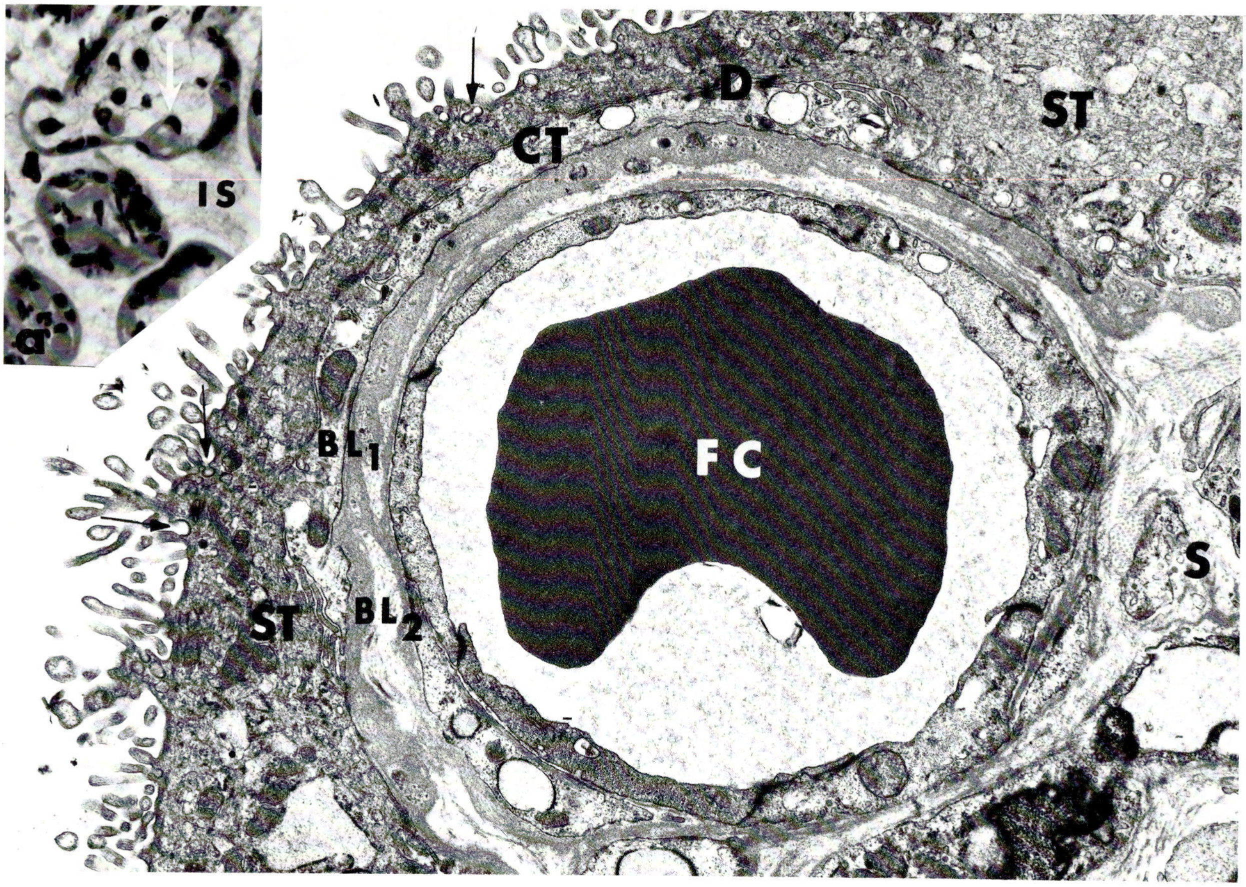

80

Mature Placenta

The chorionic villi are smaller at term than in early gestation[1] and are covered by a thinner trophoblastic layer in which the number of cytotrophoblastic cells is considerably reduced.[2]

Figure 276a. *Placenta at term.* The thin trophoblastic envelope of the mature chorionic villi is often closely associated with small capillaries (arrow), at which point the syncytial membrane is extremely thin and protrudes into the intervillous (IS) space. (H & E stain, × 120.)

Figure 276. *Placenta at term.* Although there is no change in general cytoplasmic organization with trophoblastic maturation, cellular specialization tends to occur in localized regions of the villus.[3-5] The electron micrograph illustrates a thin zone composed principally of syncytial cells (ST) with a predominantly absorptive function [microvilli, pinocytosis (arrows), phagocytosis, and lysosomal activity]. Characteristically, the fetal capillaries (FC) are concentrated beneath the thinner zone,[2] an anatomical relationship that would facilitate the rapid diffusion of oxygen and carbon dioxide between the maternal and fetal vessels.[5] Note the close relationship between the trophoblastic (BL_1) and endothelial (BL_2) basal laminae. A fetal red blood cell with irregular contour is seen within the capillary (FC). A narrow cytotrophoblastic process (CT) is interposed between the basal lamina (BL_1) and the overlying syncytiotrophoblast (ST). × 12,600. D: desmosomal attachment between cytotrophoblast and syncytiotrophoblast; S: villous stroma.

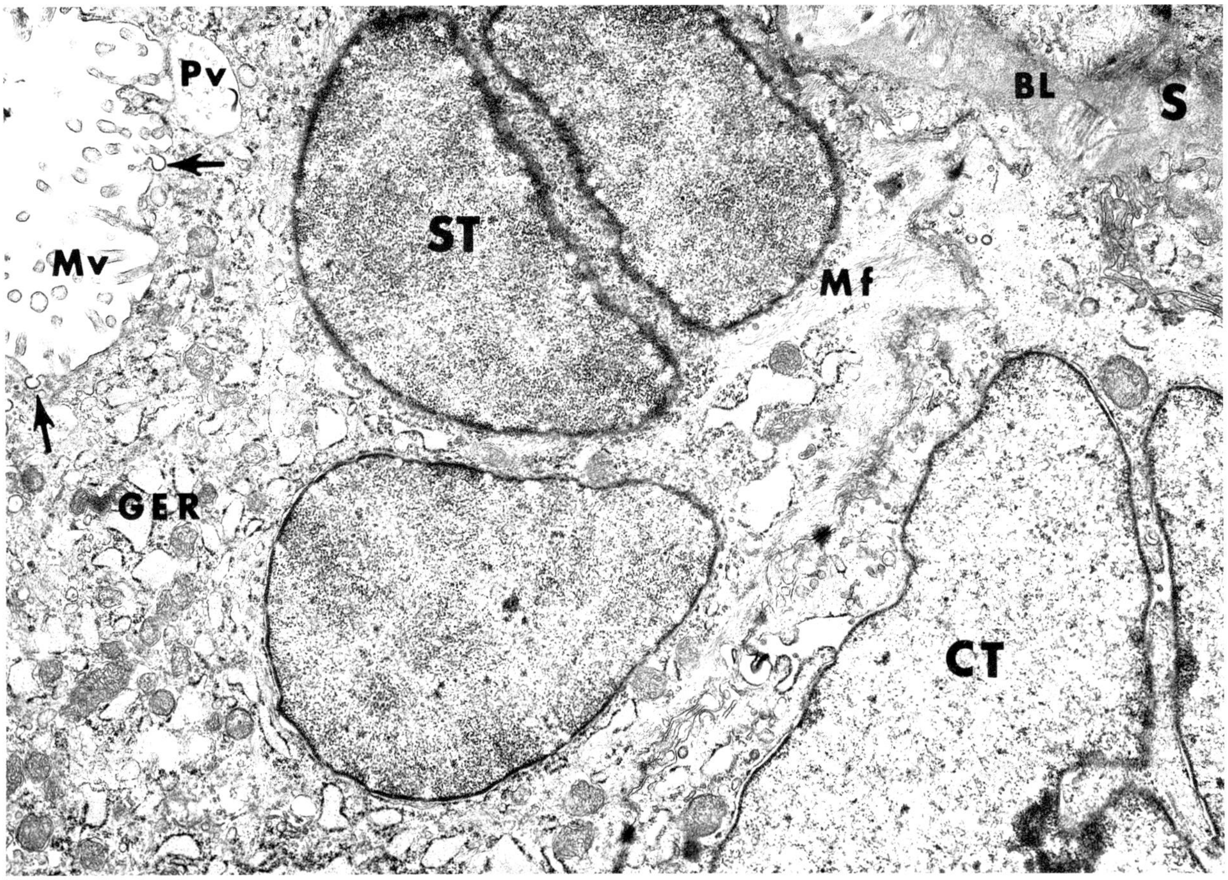

Figure 277. *Placenta at term.* Electron micrograph of a thick zone composed of syncytiotrophoblast (ST) and cytotrophoblast (CT) containing abundant granular endoplasmic reticulum (GER), free ribosomes, and mitochondria,[5] presumably involved principally in protein synthesis. Bundles of microfilaments (Mf) with a greater concentration near the syncytiocytotrophoblastic junction are seen in the syncytial cells. The syncytial surface plasma membrane contains several pinocytic invaginations (arrows) and large vesicles (Pv) of endocytic nature. In addition to surface microvilli (Mv), interdigitating microvillous processes are found between the syncytiotrophoblast and cytotrophoblast. × 20,600. BL: trophoblastic basal lamina. S: villous stroma.

REFERENCES (The chorionic villi–Figure 277)

1. Ferenczy, A. and R. M. Richart. Scanning electron microscopic study of normal and molar trophoblast. *Gynecol. Oncol.* **1:** 95 (1972).
2. Kaufmann, P. Observations on the Langhans cells in the human placenta. *Z. Zellforsch.* **128:** 283 (1972).
3. Rhodin, J. A. and J. Terzakis. The ultrastructure of the human full-term placenta. *J. Ultrastruct. Res.* **6:** 88 (1962).
4. Enders, A. C. A comparative study of the fine structure of the trophoblast in several hemochorial placentas. *Am. J. Anat.* **116:** 29 (1965).
5. Burgos, M. H. and E. M. Rodriguez. Specialized zones in the trophoblast of the human term placenta. *Am. J. Obstet. Gynecol.* **96:** 342 (1966).

Figure 278. *Placenta at term.* The terminal chorionic villi of full-term placenta appear as branching and interlacing solid cylinders of uniform and considerably smaller size than in the immature placenta. Although a few trophoblastic sprouts (TS) are present,[1] most are small, and others are cordlike (arrow). In the term placenta, the intervillous space (IS) is more regular than in the immature placenta and resembles a series of labyrinthine channels × 600. *From* A. Ferenczy and R. M. Richart. Scanning electron microscopic study of normal and molar trophoblast. *Gynecol. Oncol.* **1:** 95–110 (1972).

Figure 278a. *Detail of Figure 278.* Note the broad-based bulbous and syncytial cordlike configurations of the trophoblastic sprouts. × 2000. *From* A. Ferenczy and R. M. Richart. Scanning electron microscopic study of normal and molar trophoblast. *Gynecol Oncol.* **1:** 95–110 (1972).

REFERENCE (Figures 278 and 278a)

1. Ferenczy, A. and R. M. Richart. Scanning electron microscopic study of normal and molar trophoblast. *Gynecol. Oncol.* **1:** 95 (1972).

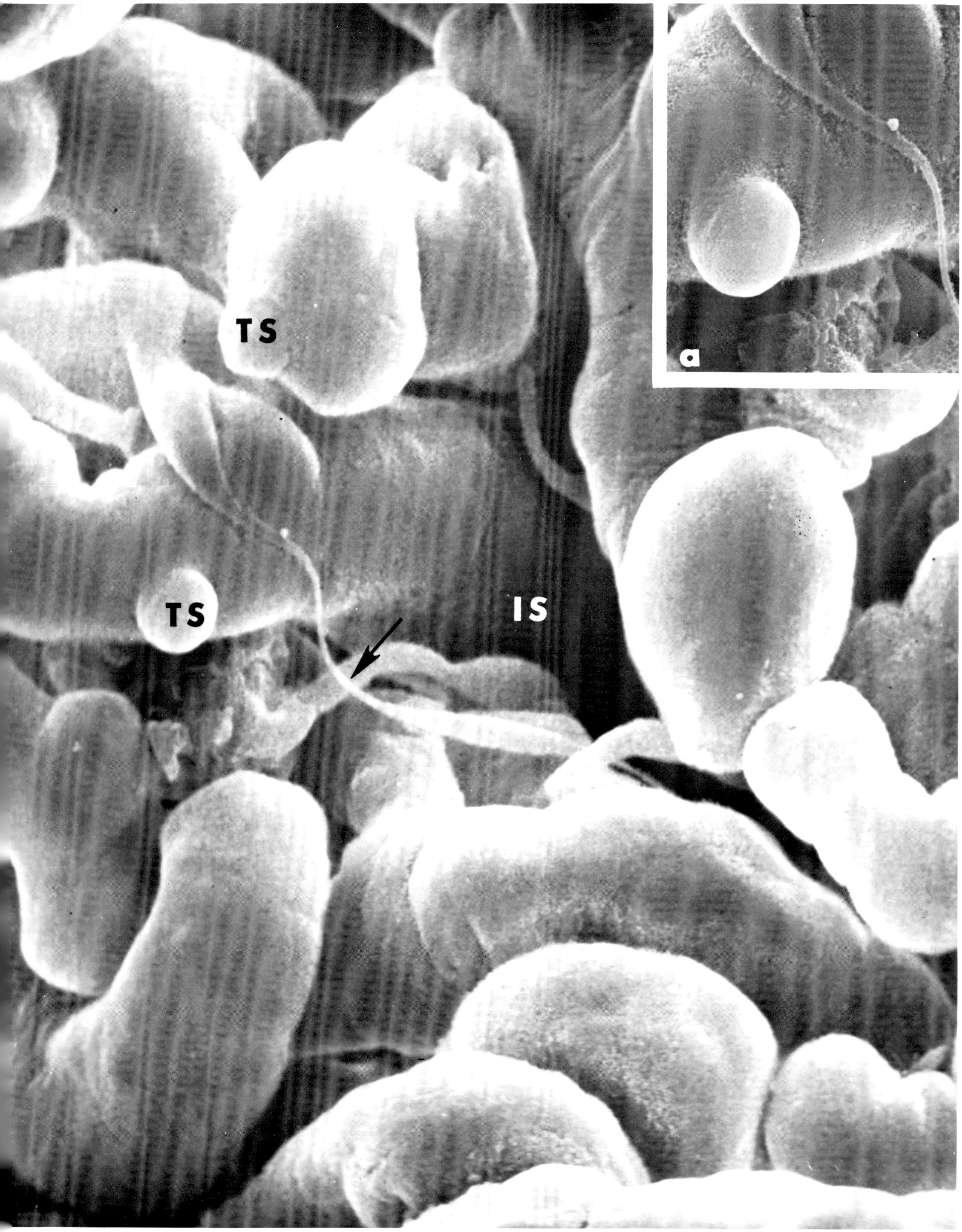
TS
TS
IS
a

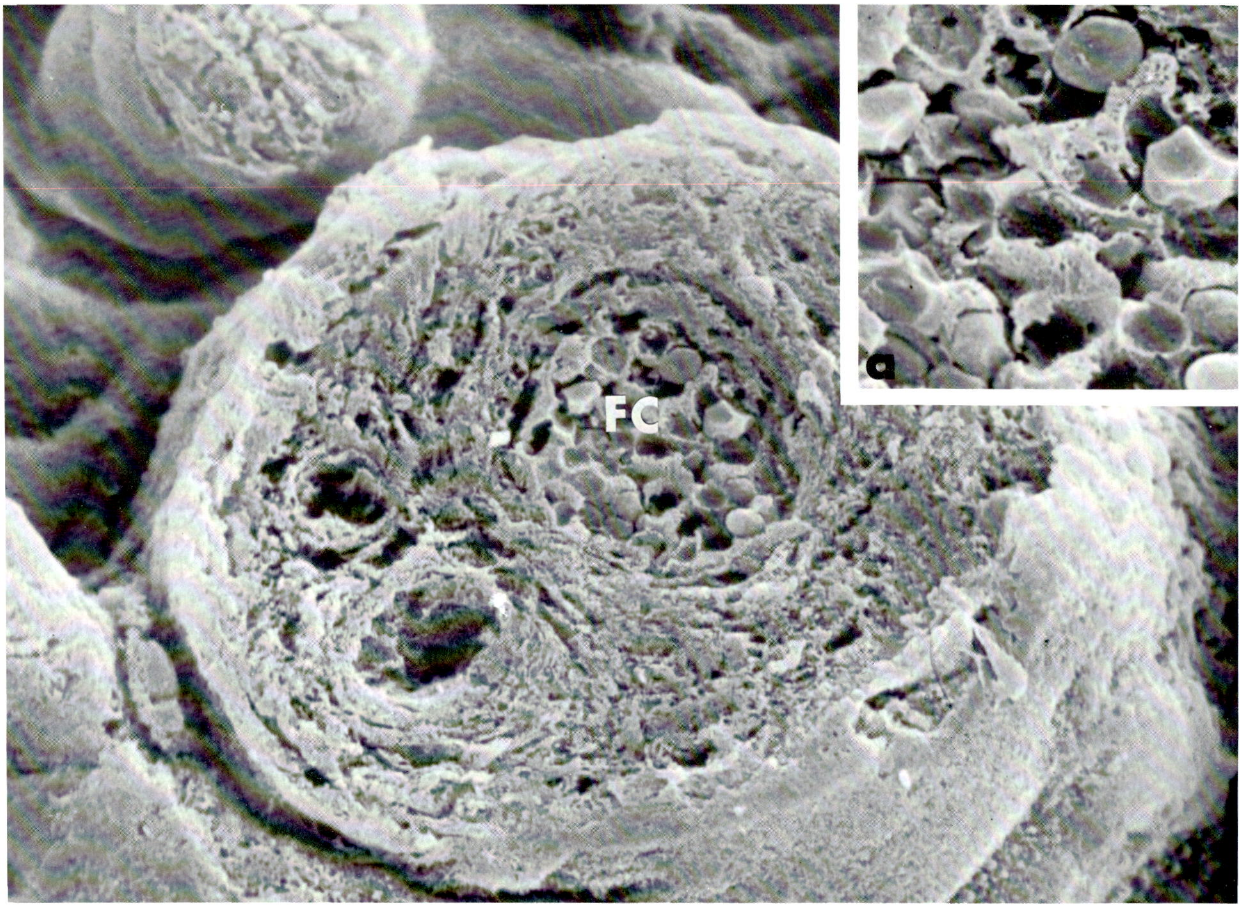

Figure 279. *Placenta at term.* Scanning electron micrograph of a cross-sectioned free villus, in which the connective tissue core contains a loose network of collagen fibers, capillaries (FC), fibroblasts with slender cytoplasmic processes, and the so-called Hofbauer cells. These cells are thought to be derived from the chorionic mesenchyme, and their ultrastructure, hydrolytic enzyme content, and phagocytic capability indicate a histiocytic nature related to phagocytosis.[1-3] Another cellular component, probably of maternal origin,[4] is found in the decidual floor and placental septa and is referred to as the "X-cell." These polygonal, mononuclear cells are commonly associated with protein synthesis[5] and are mitotically active.[6] It was not possible to demonstrate either human chorionic gonadotropin or human placental lactogen in them, and their function is unknown. × 800.

Figure 279a. *Higher magnification of fetal red blood cells.* Their polyhedral surface pattern is due to compression artifact (specimen prepared by freeze-drying technique). × 1600.

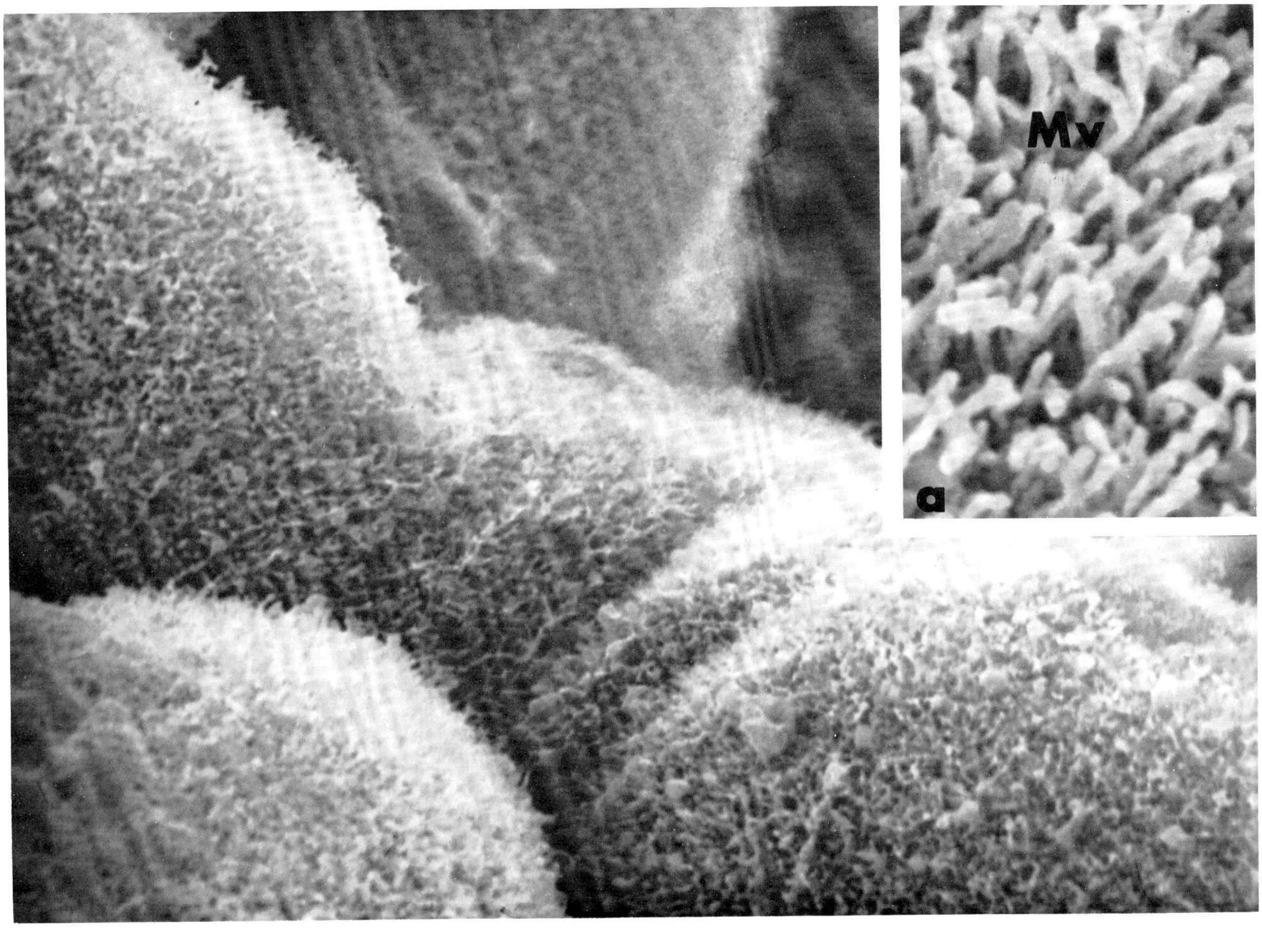

Figure 280. *Placenta at term.* The syncytial surface of the mature chorionic villi is covered by a profusion of hairlike, microvillous projections with occasional, bulbous microvillous apices. × 8000.

Figure 280a. *Higher magnification of the surface syncytial microvilli* (Mv), which are shorter,[1,7,8] and the microvillous interbranching, and apical promontories, which are comparatively less conspicuous,[9] than those in their immature counterparts. × 20,000.

REFERENCES (Figures 279–280a)

1. Wislocki, G. B. and E. W. Dempsey. Electron microscopy of the human placenta. *Anat. Rec.* **123:** 133 (1955).
2. Wynn, R. M. Derivation and ultrastructure of the so-called Hofbauer cell. *Am. J. Obstet. Gynecol.* **97:** 235 (1967).
3. Fox, H. and N. F. Kharkongor. Morphology and enzyme histochemistry of cells derived from placental villi in tissue culture. *J. Pathol.* **101:** 267 (1970).
4. Benirschke, K. and S. G. Driscoll. *The Pathology of the Human Placenta.* Springer, New York, 1967, pp. 203–215.
5. Ruffalo, R., K. Benirschke, H. I. Covington, and A. B. Munro. Electron microscopic study of the "X-cells" in septal cysts of the human placenta. *Am. J. Obstet. Gynecol.* **99:** 1147 (1967).
6. Kim, C. K. and K. Benirschke. Autoradiographic study of the "X" cells in the human placenta. *Am. J. Obstet. Gynecol.* **109:** 96 (1971).
7. Tighe, J. R., P. R. Garrod, and R. C. Curran. The trophoblast of the human chorionic villus *J. Pathol. Bacteriol.* **93:** 559 (1967).
8. Dempsey, E. W. and S. A. Luse. Regional specializations in the syncytial trophoblast of early human placentas. *J. Anat.* **108:** 545 (1971).
9. Ferenczy, A. and R. M. Richart. Scanning electron microscopic study of normal and molar trophoblast. *Gynecol. Oncol.* **1:** 95 (1972).

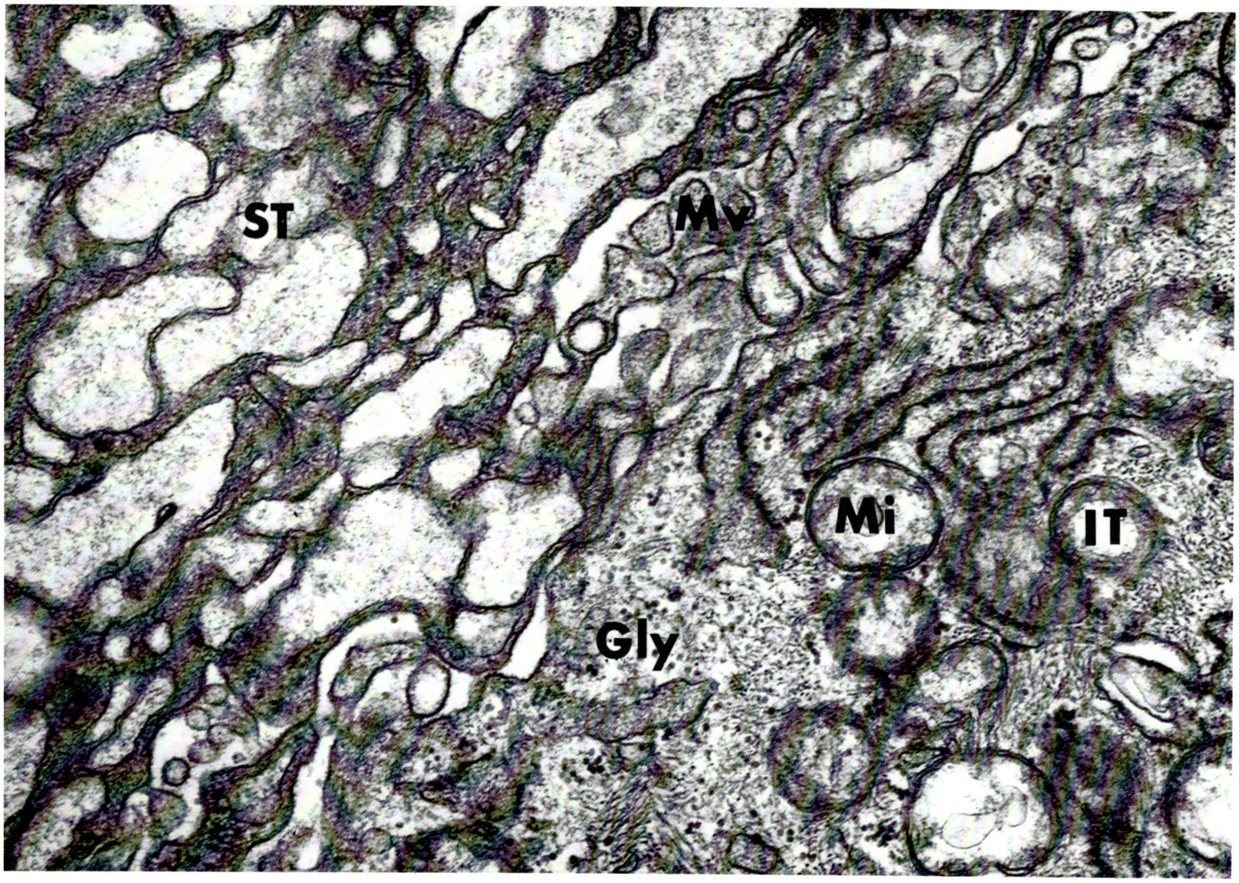

Figure 281. *Placenta at term.* Cellular detail of a syncytial cell (ST) and a rare intermediary trophoblast (IT). The syncytial cell has a prominent channel-like system of endoplasmic reticulum with a finely granular content and an indistinct microvillous (Mv) plasma membrane. The adjacent intermediary (IT) cell contains clusters of mitochondria (Mi), cisternae of granular endoplasmic reticulum, glycogen particles (Gly), and abundant microfilaments. The organellar content of this cell type is considerably better developed than that of the cytotrophoblast, but less conspicuous than that of the syncytial cell. × 35,000.

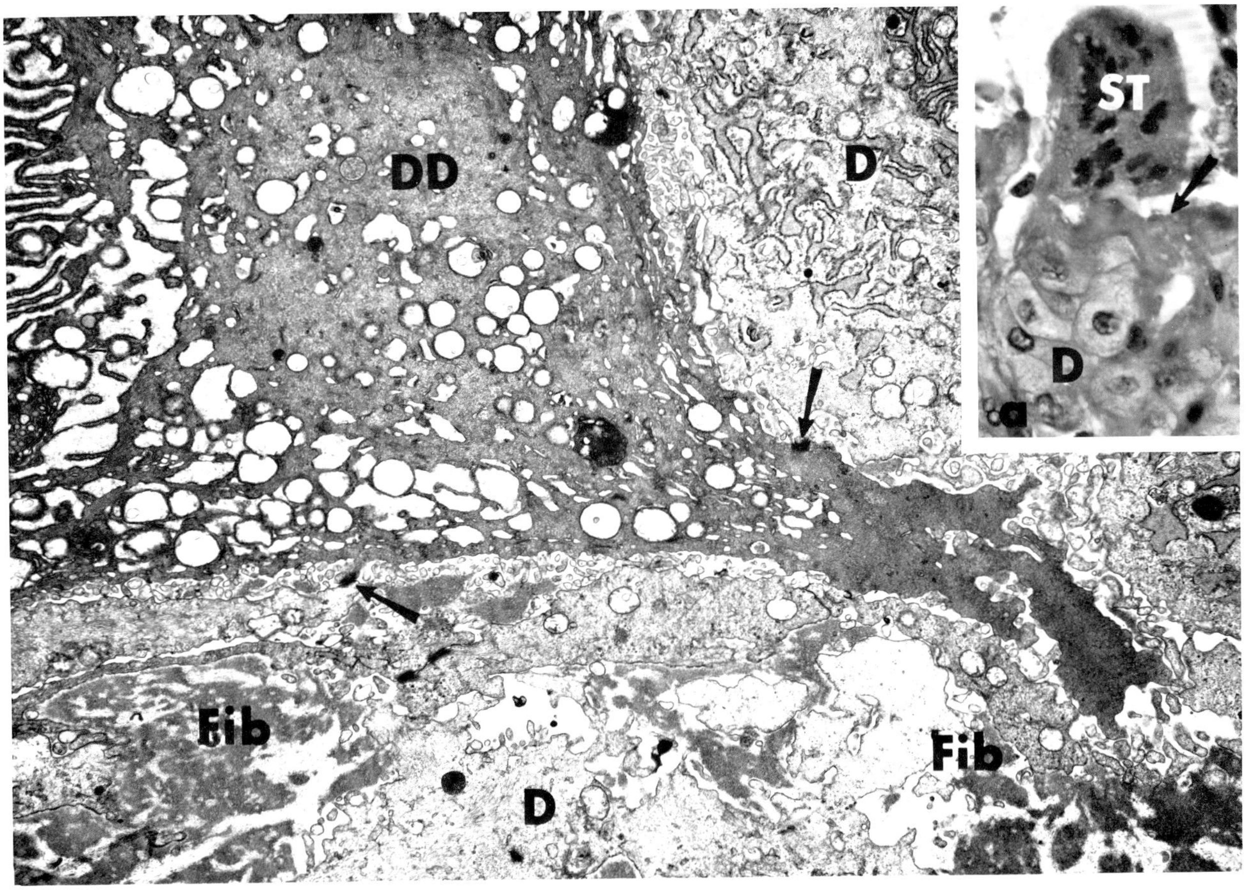

Figure 282a. *Light micrograph* illustrating the deciduotrophoblastic junction. Between the compact decidua (D) and syncytiotrophoblast (ST) is a well-defined band (arrow) of fibrinoid material, referred to as Nitabuch's striae. (H & E stain, × 120.)

Figure 282. *In the deciduotrophoblastic junctional zone* (Nitabuch's striae) the adjacent decidual (D) and syncytial cells undergo degeneration and are separated by a discontinuous[1] intercellular fibrillar (fibrin) and amorphous fibrinoid material.[1-4] In this electron micrograph the fibrinoid (Fib) is associated with a degenerating decidual cell (DD), which still contains several desmosomal attachments (arrows) to the adjacent decidual cells. Note the prominent microvillous plasma membranes of decidual cells near and at the deciduotrophoblastic junctional zone. × 6800.

REFERENCES (Figures 281–282)

1. Wynn, R. M. Cytotrophoblastic specialization. An ultrastructural study of the human placenta. *Am. J. Obstet. Gynecol.* **114:** 339 (1972).
2. Okudaira, Y., T. Hashimoto, N. Hamanaka, and S. Yoshinare. Electron microscopic study on the trophoblastic cell column of human placenta. *J. Electronmicrosc. (Tokyo)* **20:** 93 (1971).
3. Wynn, R. M. Noncellular components of the placenta. *Am. J. Obstet. Gynecol.* **103:** 723 (1969).
4. Dempsey, E. W., R. A. Lessey, and S. A. Luse. Electron microscopic observations on fibrinoid and histiotroph in the junctional zone and villi of the human placenta. *Am. J. Anat.* **128:** 463 (1970).

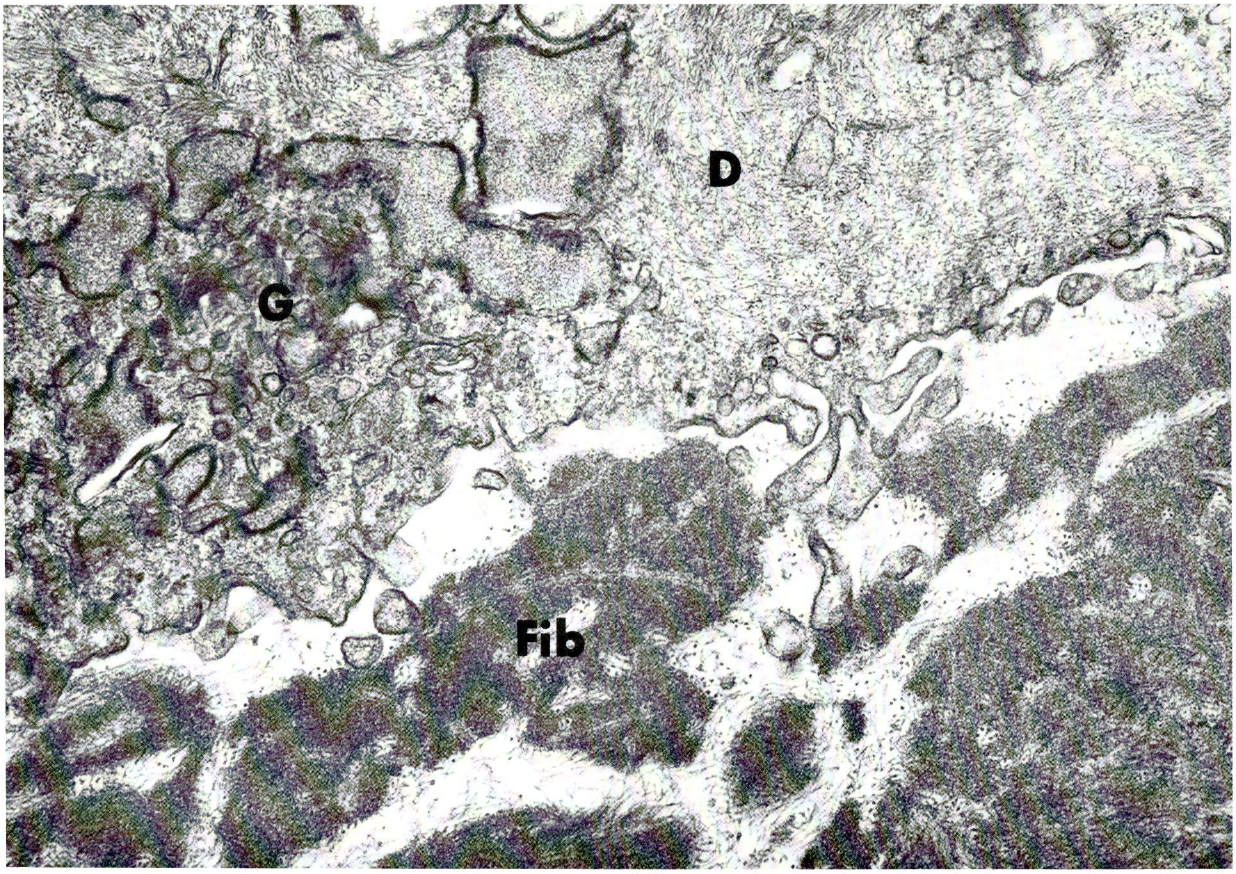

Figure 283. *Higher magnification* of the deciduotrophoblastic fibrinoid (Fib). Note the dense fibrillar nature of the fibrinoid, composed of approximately 300- to 450-Å-thick fibrils with shallow cross striations. The adjacent decidua (D) is rich in cytoplasmic microfibrils, dilated cisternae of granular endoplasmic reticulum, and Golgi (G) with abundant peripheral vesicles. Although the precise origin and nature of junctional fibrin and fibrinoid remain obscure, they are likely to occur as a result of deciduotrophoblastic degeneration or to represent precipitated acid mucopolysaccharides from the intercellular matrix.[1] Histochemical and ultrastructural studies indicate that fibrinoid is closely related to fibrin, differing from it only in the proportion of polysaccharides and in alterations in its fibrillar structure.[1,2] Deciduotrophoblastic junctional zone infarcts caused by maternal thrombi[3,4] may also contribute to the occurrence of fibrinoid.

Although the noncellular fibrinoid in the junctional zone most probably plays a role in the control of trophoblastic invasiveness,[1,5] its immunologic function as an antigenic barrier is not likely, since histocompatibility antigens are not expressed by trophoblastic tissue, whether fibrinoid is present or not.[6] Tryptophane-rich surface sialomucins[7] (glycocalyces), rather than deciduotrophoblastic fibrinoid, have been suggested as the primary antigen barrier, and probably act by creating strong electronegative charges on the surface of otherwise immunocompetent syncytial cells,[8-10] which would prevent contact with electronegative maternal lymphocytes by steric hindrance, thus eliminating access to trophoblastic antigens. × 35,000.

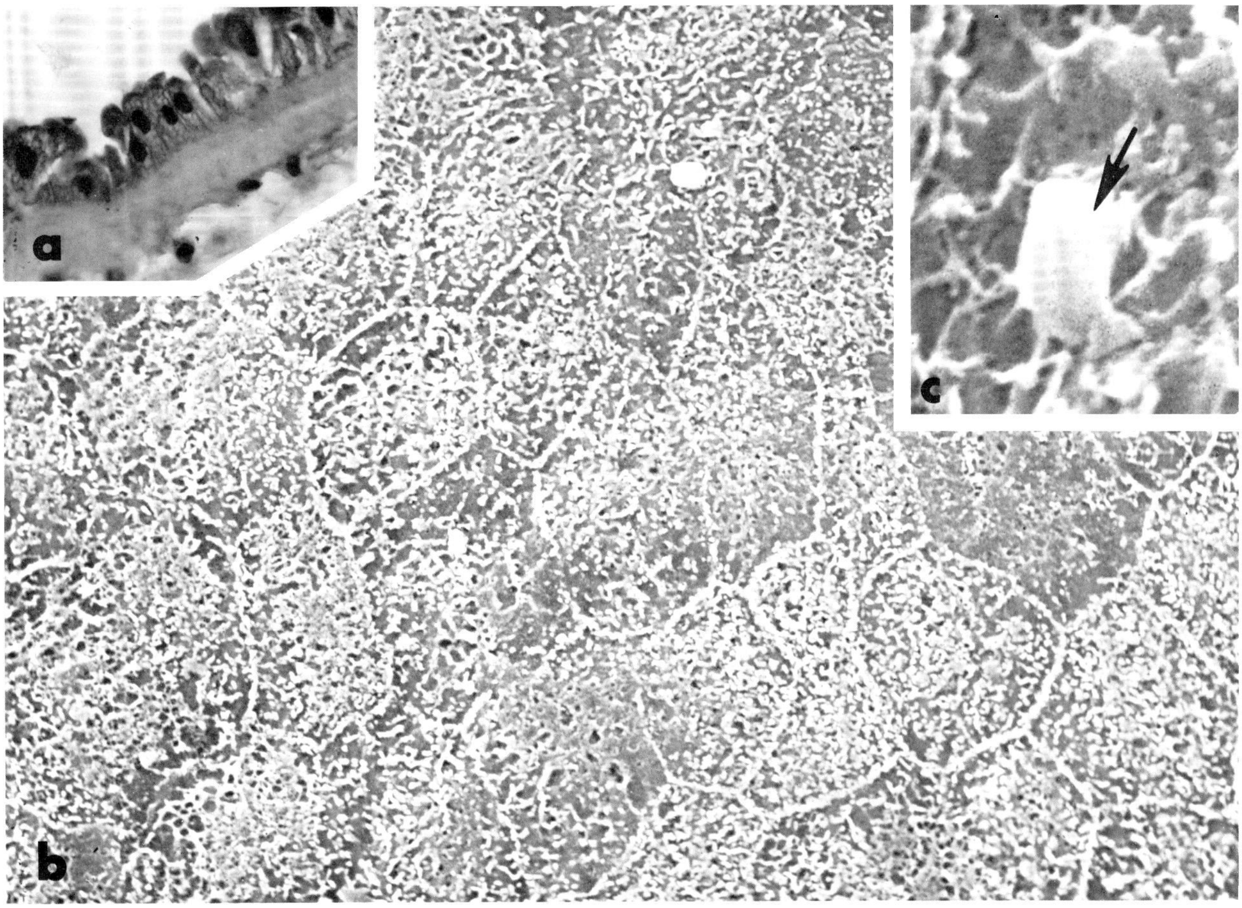

81

Amnion

The ultrastructural morphologic characteristics[11-14] of the amnion include surface microvilli,[11-13] which are increased in number and arborization toward the end of gestation, and dilated intercellular spaces, related to the transport of amniotic fluid (absorption).[11,13]

Figure 284a. *Amnion at term.* The epithelial cells of the amnion vary from club-shaped, tall columnar to flat or cuboidal cells. The cells contain numerous cytoplasmic vacuoles, which at the ultrastructural level correspond to secretory vacuoles. A well-developed basal lamina separates the cells from the underlying stroma. (H & E stain, × 120.)

Figure 284b. *Topographically,* the amnionic epithelial cells have a penta- to hexagonal contour, and the surface plasma membrane is covered by abundant partly agglutinated microvilli. × 1800.

Figure 284c. *Higher magnification* of an apical cytoplasmic protuberance (arrow), suggesting that, in addition to the absorptive function of amniotic cells, apocrine secretion may also take place. × 8000.

REFERENCES (Figures 283–284c)

1. Wynn, R. M. Noncellular components of the placenta. *Am. J. Obstet. Gynecol.* **103:** 723 (1969).
2. Wynn, R. M. Cytotrophoblastic specialization. An ultrastructural study of the human placenta. *Am. J. Obstet. Gynecol.* **114:** 339 (1972).
3. Okudaira, Y., S. Suzuki, M. Okudaira, T. Hashimoto, and K. Hayakawa. Electron microscopic observations on the formation of syncytiotrophoblast from cytotrophoblast. *J. Electronmicrosc. (Tokyo)* **17:** 47 (1968).
4. Dempsey, E. W., R. A. Lessey, and S. A. Luse. Electron microscopic observations on fibrinoid and histiotroph in the junctional zone and villi of the human placenta. *Am. J. Anat.* **128:** 463 (1970).
5. Wynn, R. M. Fetomaternal cellular relations in the human basal plate: an ultrastructural study of the placenta. *Am. J. Obstet. Gynecol.* **97:** 832 (1967).
6. Simmons, R. L., V. Cruse, and D. G. McKay. The immunologic problem of pregnancy. II. Ultrastructure of isogenic and allogeneic trophoblastic transplants. *Am. J. Obstet. Gynecol.* **97:** 218 (1967).
7. Kirby, D. R., W. D. Billington, and S. Bradbury. Antigen barrier of the mouse placenta. *Nature (London)* **204:** 548 (1964).
8. Currie, G. A., W. Van Doorninck, and K. D. Bagshawe. Effect of neuraminidase on the immunogenicity of early mouse trophoblast. *Nature (London)* **219:** 191 (1968).
9. Douthwaite, R. M. and G. I. Urbach. In vitro antigenicity of trophoblasts. *Am. J. Obstet. Gynecol.* **109:** 1023 (1971).
10. Beer, A. E., R. E. Billingham, and S. L. Yang. Further evidence concerning the autoantigenic status of the trophoblast. *J. Exp. Med.* **135:** 1177 (1972).
11. Thomas, C. E. The ultrastructure of human amnion epithelium. *J. Ultrastruct. Res.* **13:** 65 (1965).
12. Hoyes, A. D. Fine structure of human amniotic epithelium in early pregnancy. *J. Obstet. Gynaecol. Brit. Commonw.* **75:** 949 (1968).
13. Wynn, R. M. and G. L. French. Comparative ultrastructure of the mammalian amnion. *Obstet. Gynecol.* **31:** 759 (1968).
14. Bergstrom, S. Surface ultrastructure of human amnion and chorion in early pregnancy. A scanning and electron microscope study. *Obstet. Gynecol.* **38:** 513 (1971).

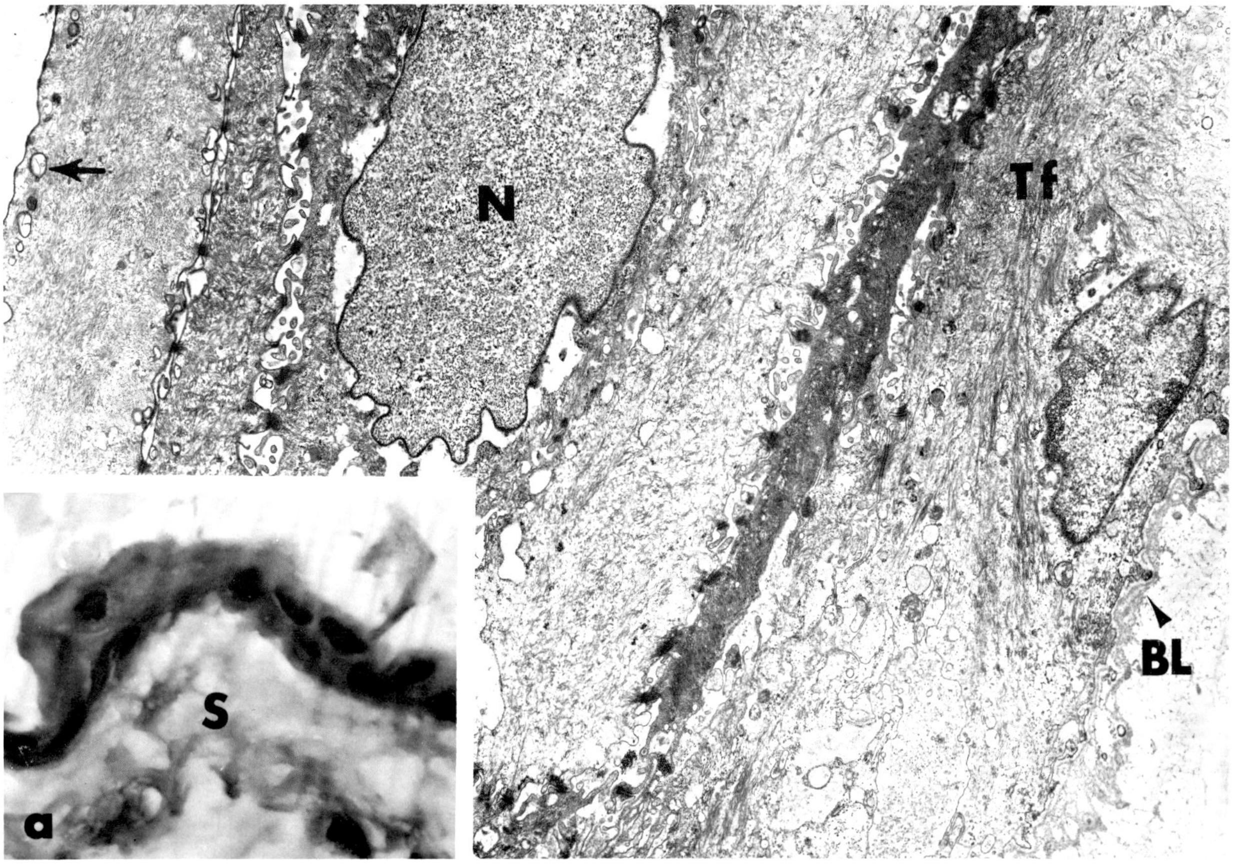

82

Umbilical Cord

Figure 285a. *The epithelium covering the umbilical cord* at term consists of a thin membrane of squamous, stratified cells devoid of surface keratinization. (H & E stain, × 150.) S: myxoid stroma of Warthin's jelly.

Figure 285. *Ultrastructurally,* the epithelium is composed of a basal, germinative layer; an intermediate stratum of one or two cell layers, rich in cytoplasmic tonofilaments (Tf) and dilated vesicular endoplasmic reticulum; and a superficial layer of flattened cells packed with fine tonofibrils. Beneath the surface plasma membrane of the superficial cells are numerous pinocytic vesicles (arrow). Intracytoplasmic glycogen, a prominent finding in the covering epithelium of the cord as well as in the fetal skin of early gestation,[1,2] is scant at term. As in other stratified squamous epithelia, cellular integrity is maintained by abundant tonofilament–desmosome complexes, although these are comparatively less well developed in the amnion than in the adult squamous or epidermal membranes. × 7200. N: nucleus; BL: basal lamina with convoluted contour.

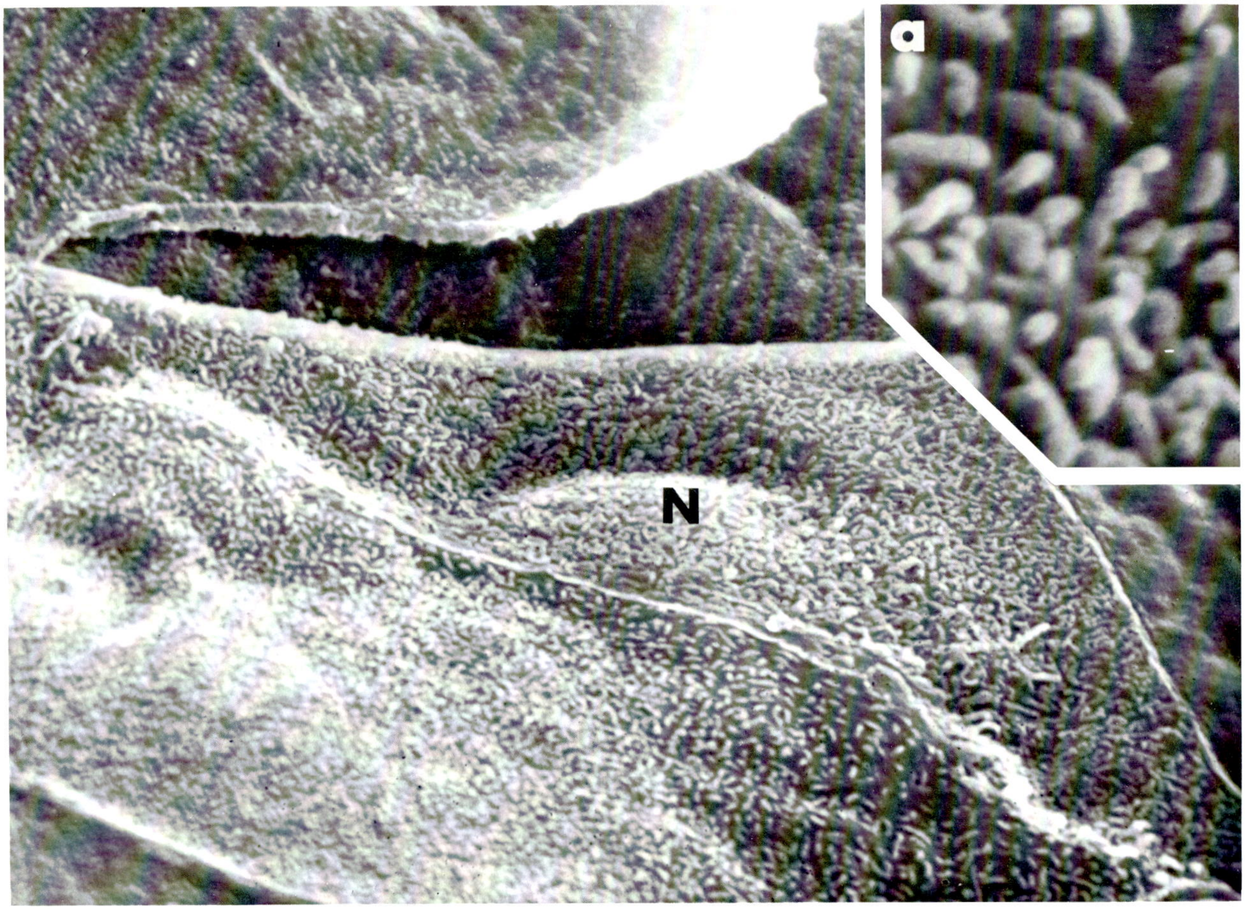

Figure 286. *With the scanning electron microscope* the most superficial cells of the mature umbilical cord appear as large polyhedral cells with an occasional bulging nucleus (N). The surface plasma membrane is covered by numerous microvilli. There is no ultrastructural evidence of keratinization under normal conditions, and the organellar contents (pinocytic vesicles) and the microvillous surface specialization indicate that the epithelial lining of the umbilical cord has an absorptive function. × 2560.

Figure 286a. *Higher magnification* of the stubby, broad-based microvillous projections. × 16,000.

REFERENCES (Figures 285–286a)

1. Breathnach, A. S. and L. M. Wyllie. Fine structure of cells forming the surface layer of the epidermis in human fetuses at fourteen and twelve weeks. *J. Invest. Dermatol.* **45:** 179 (1965).
2. Hoyes, A. D. Ultrastructure of the cells of the amniotic fluid. *J. Obstet. Gynaecol. Brit. Commonw.* **75:** 164 (1968).

83

Preeclampsia-Eclampsia (Toxemia)

Preeclampsia-eclampsia (toxemia) is a disease unique to pregnant women; it does not occur in animals. Clinically, edema, proteinuria, and hypertension occurs, most commonly in the last gestational trimester. Although vascular alterations may be found in the brain, liver, and lungs, the renal glomeruli are the principal site of toxemic lesions.

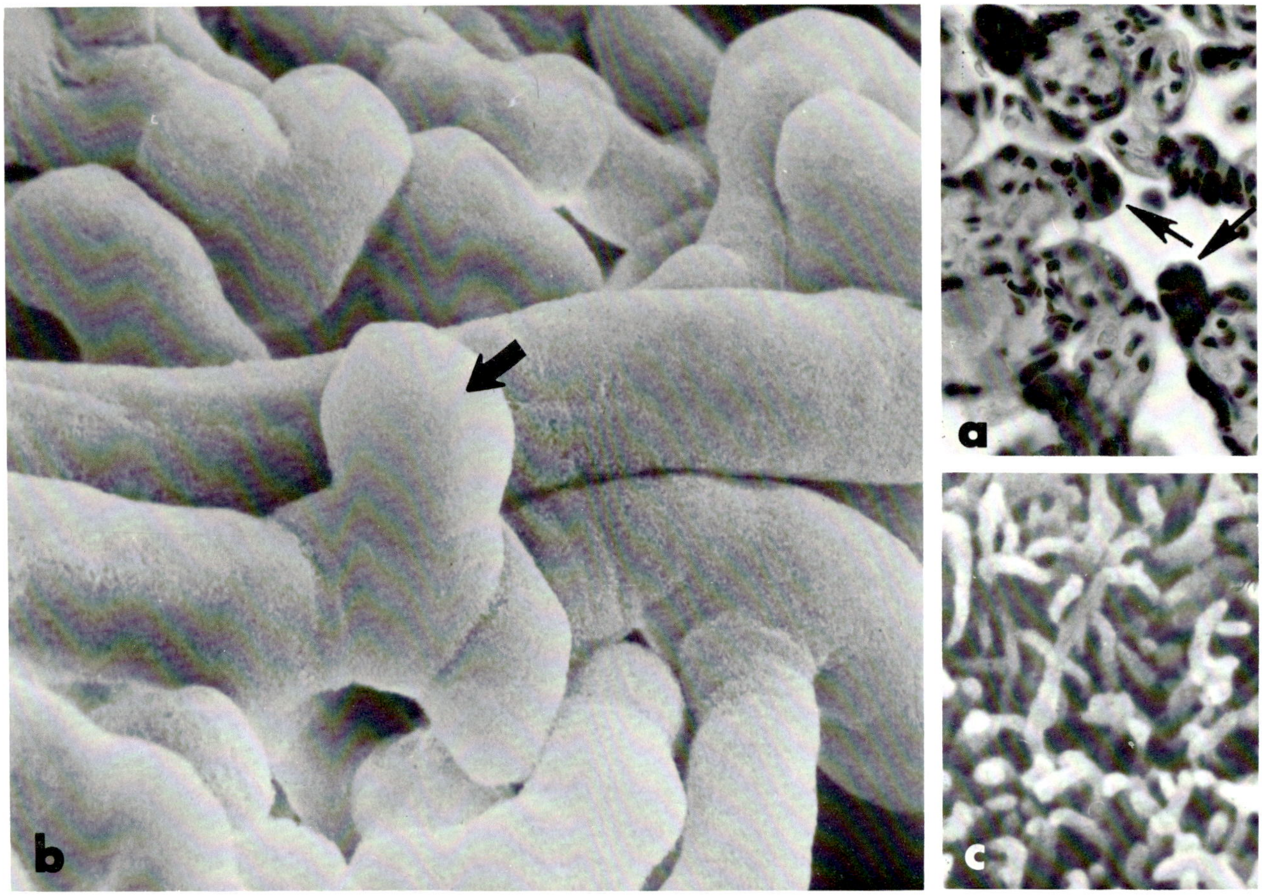

Figure 287a. *Placenta. The changes that occur in the pre-eclamptic placenta* include syncytial degeneration, with clumping of nuclei or syncytial knots (arrows), placental infarcts, fibrosis of villous stroma, increased vascular fibrin deposits, and endovascular sclerosis. In preeclamptic toxemia cytotrophoblastic hyperplasia, with increased reaction products of glycolytic enzymes,[1] may be regarded as a compensatory or reactive trophoblastic proliferation due to ischemic degeneration of syncytiotrophoblast. Similar cytotrophoblastic hyperplasia can be produced in trophoblastic organ cultures[2] under conditions of relative hypoxia. Transmission[3] electron microscopic observations, however, have not confirmed the light microscopic observations, probably because of sampling artifact. (H & E stain, × 120.)

Figure 287b. *Placenta. At the scanning electron microscopic level,* the chorionic villi appear as narrow cylinders containing numerous prominent club-shaped syncytial protrusions (arrow), which probably correspond to the syncytial knots seen with the light microscope. Because of the small volume and complexly interlacing pattern of the chorionic villi, the intervillous space is reduced to slitlike labyrinthine channels. × 4000.

Figure 287c. *Placenta. Although several villi have degenerative changes* with loss of syncytial microvillous processes, most of the chorionic villi and syncytial knots contain abundant surface microvillosity with occasional interbranching and bulbous promontories, consistent with an active absorptive and secretory function. × 16,000.

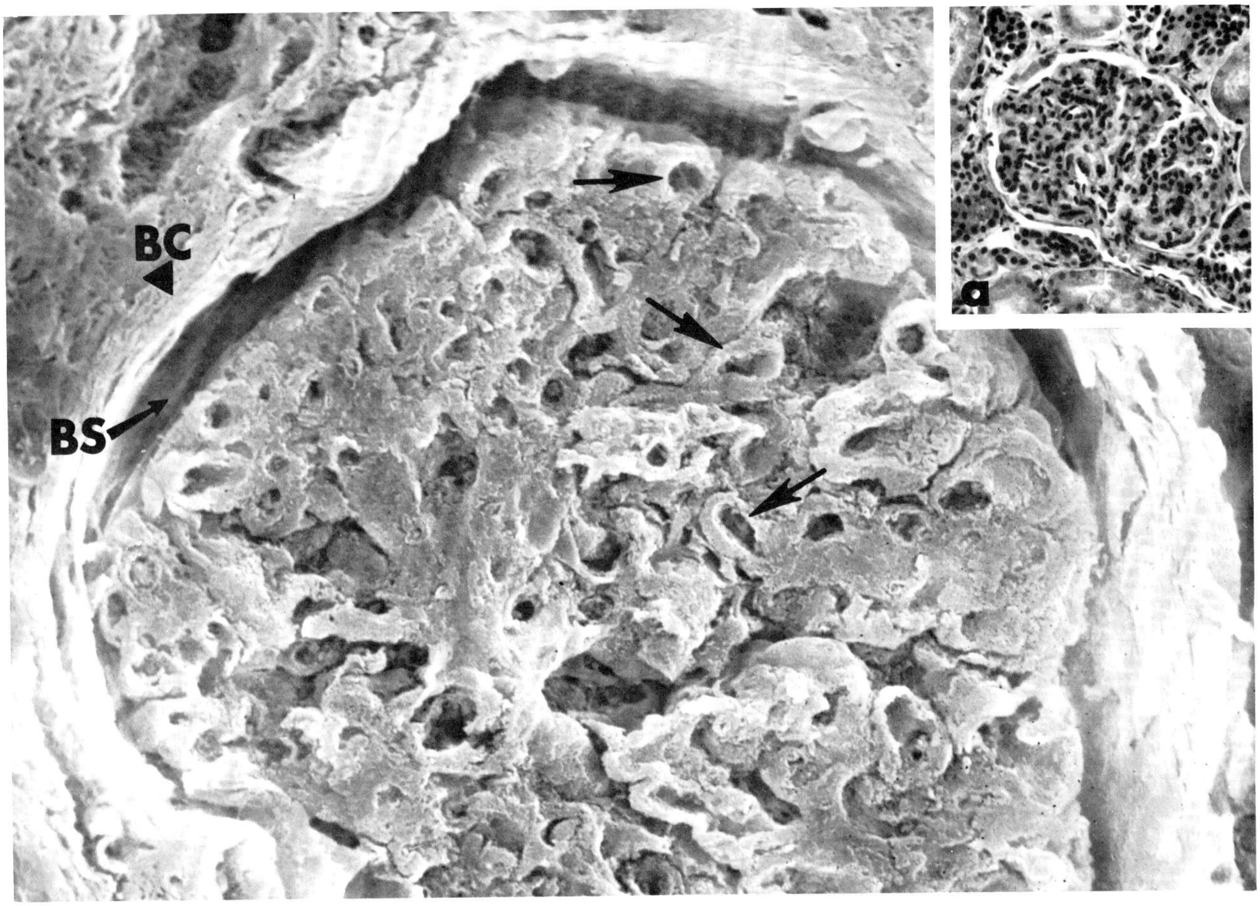

Figure 288a. *Kidney. Preeclampsia-eclampsia. Histologically* all of the glomeruli are affected, although the individual glomerulus may be diffusely or focally involved. In the affected glomeruli an increase in intercapillary mesangial cells and swelling of endothelial cells occur. Another[4,5] feature in renal toxemia, although inconsistently described, is hyperplasia and hypertrophy of the juxtaglomerular cells, providing a basis for the increased secretion of renin,[4,5] which may be involved in the afferent arteriolar vasospasm that seems to be at least partly responsible for toxemic hypertension. (H & E stain, × 48.)

Figure 288. *Kidney. Scanning electron microscopy of an eclamptic glomerulus.* There is glomerular enlargement, as well as considerable reduction of Bowman's space (BS). Note the thickened "wire-loop" appearance of the glomerular capillaries (arrows), a pattern due principally to the swelling of endothelial cells. [Specimen obtained at autopsy from a 36-year-old toxemic woman, who suddenly developed convulsions and coma (36th week of gestation) and died 3 days after admission.] × 960.

REFERENCES (Figures 287a–288)

1. Kaufmann, P. Observations on the Langerhans cells in the human placenta. *Z. Zellforsch.* **128:** 283 (1972).
2. Fox, H. Effect of hypoxia on trophoblast in organ culture. A morphologic and autoradiographic study. *Am. J. Obstet. Gynecol.* **107:** 1058 (1970).
3. Zacks, S. I. and A. S. Blazer. Chorionic villi in normal pregnancy, preeclamptic toxemia, erythroblastosis, and diabetes mellitus. *Obstet. Gynecol.* **22:** 149 (1963).
4. Altcheck, A., N. L. Albright, and S. C. Sommers. The renal pathology of toxemia of pregnancy. *Obstet. Gynecol.* **31:** 595 (1968).
5. Fisher, E. R., V. Pardo, R. Paul, and T. T. Hayashi. Ultrastructural studies in hypertension. *Am. J. Pathol.* **55:** 109 (1969).

84

Kidney in Preeclampsia-Eclampsia (Toxemia)

In addition to an increase in intercapillary mesangial cells and the swelling of endothelial cells, ultrastructurally[1-8] granular, fibrillar, and basal laminalike deposits are found within the endothelial cells and in a subendothelial location. Similar deposits within the lumina of glomerular capillaries[5,8] contain fibrin and/or fibrinogen derivatives[9] virtually devoid of immunoglobulins or complement, suggesting a nonimmunologic, hematogenous derivation. In the light of the phagocytic capability of glomerular endothelial cells and their morphologic characteristics, it is possible that the fibrin-derived deposits are incorporated by the endothelium from the capillary lumen.[5,8] The renal lesions are not pathognomonic for gestational toxemia, however, since identical glomerular changes are reported in abruptio placentae[8] (see Figures 291 and 292), systemic lupus erythematosus,[5] and other renal disorders not associated with pregnancy.[7] Most of these morphologic changes resolve in the postpartum period,[6] but some apparently persist over several years.[3]

The pathogenesis of preeclampsia and its associated glomerular lesions is still a matter for discussion. One school of investigators favors the possibility of "functional disorders" of renal vasculature,[7] but others believe that disseminated intravascular coagulation,[5,8] secondary to the release of deciduotrophoblastic thromboplastin, is the responsible factor. In this case, the glomerular lesions would be secondary to deposited fibrin or its derivatives. Evidence for the intravascular coagulation theory is provided by the experimental injection of thromboplastin in rabbits[10] and the production of structurally similar[5] "toxemiclike" glomerular deposits. Further support is afforded by the presence of clotting abnormalities, high serum fibrin levels, high serum fibrin degradation products, and the presence of disseminated fibrin deposits in postmortem studies of eclamptics.

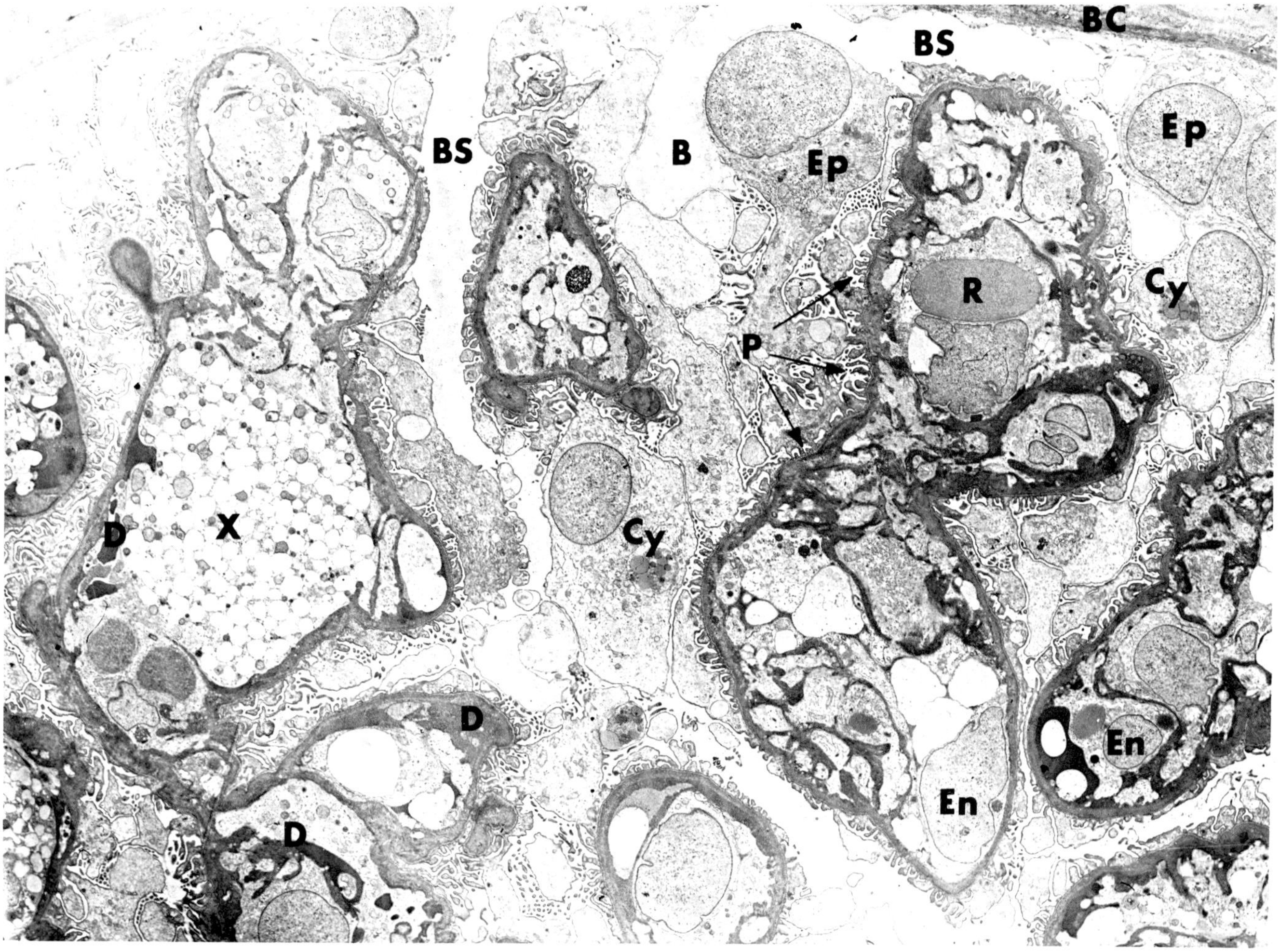

Figure 289. *Preeclampsia.* Low-magnification view of several peripheral capillary loops. Bowman's capsule (BC) and Bowman's space (BS) are at the upper right. The epithelial cells (Ep) contain several cytosomes (Cy). Large, pale cytoplasmic blebs (B) are preparative artifacts. Note the many intact epithelial pedicels (P). The capillary lumina are nearly obliterated; only one erythrocyte (R) is clearly seen. Numerous swollen processes of endothelial and mesangial cells are surrounded by deposit material (D). A cell (X) of unknown identity is laden with multitudinous vacuoles, most of which presumably contained lipid. × 2500. EN: endothelial nuclei. *From* G. C. Faith, and B. F. Trump. The glomerular capillary wall in human kidney disease: acute glomerulonephritis, systemic lupus erythematosus, and preeclampsia-eclampsia. Comparative electron microscopic observations and a review. *Lab. Invest.* **15:** 1682–1718 (1966).

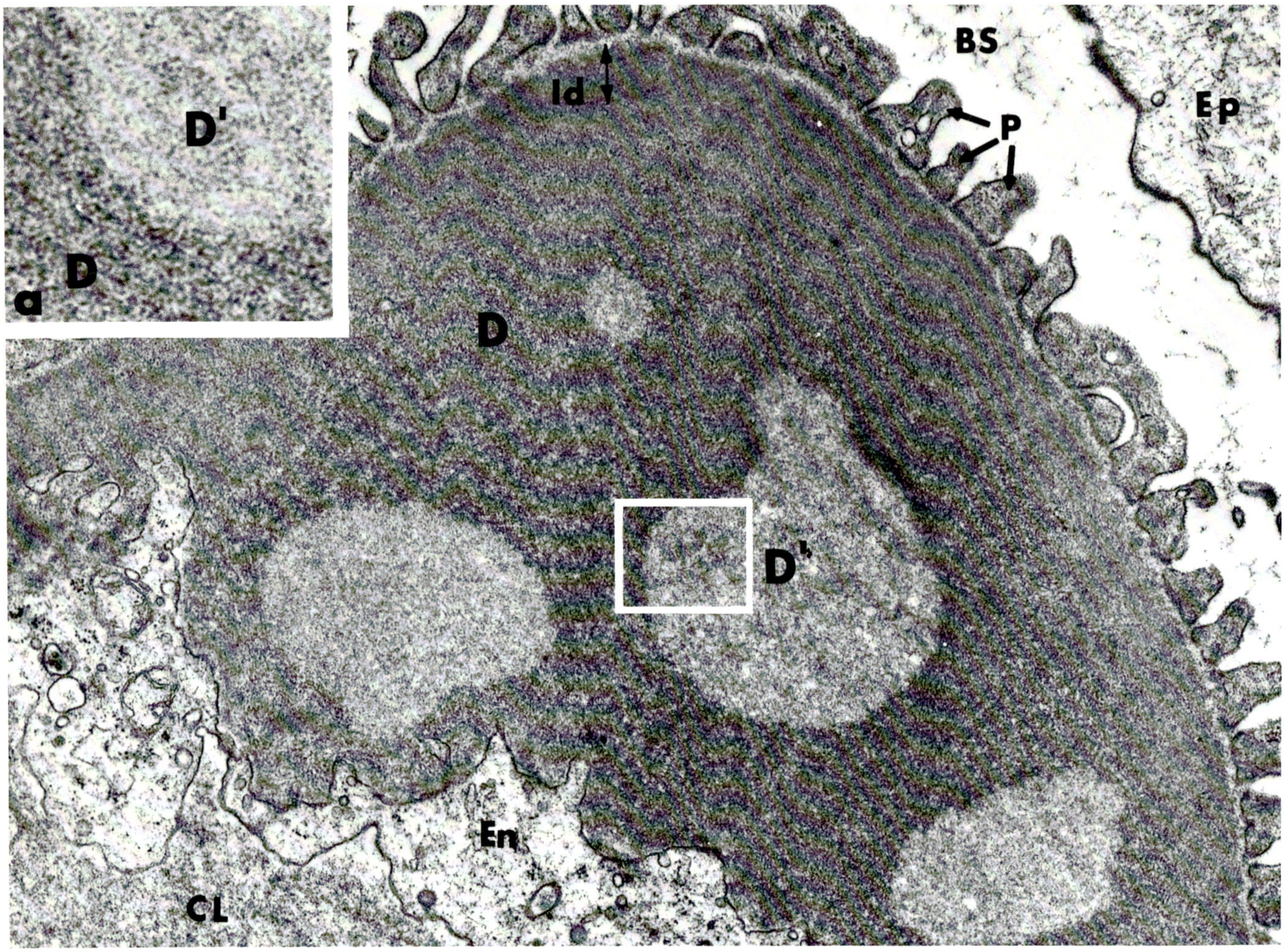

Figure 290. *Preeclampsia.* This portion of a glomerular capillary wall shows flocculent deposits interposed between endothelium (En) and a scarcely demarcated lamina densa (ld). Note the two density patterns (D and D′) within the deposit. The approximate outlines of the lamina densa are indicated by the parallel lines. An abundance of fine particulate material is seen in the capillary lumen (CL). Distinct pedicels (P) of the epithelial cells (Ep) are present in this area. × 19,000. BS: Bowman's space. *From* G. C. Faith and B. F. Trump. The glomerular capillary wall in human kidney disease: acute glomerulonephritis, systemic lupus erythematosus, and preeclampsia-eclampsia. Comparative electron microscopic observations and a review. *Lab. Invest.* **15:** 1682–1718 (1966).

Figure 290a. *Higher magnification* of the deposited material of Figure 290, showing details of D and D′. The diameter of the particles and filaments is approximately 130 Å. × 55,000. *From* G. C. Faith and B. F. Trump. The glomerular capillary wall in human kidney disease: acute glomerulonephritis, systemic lupus erythematosus, and preeclampsia-eclampsia. Comparative electron microscopic observations and a review. *Lab. Invest.* **15:** 1682–1718 (1966).

REFERENCES (In addition to an increase—Figure 290a)

1. Altcheck, A. Electron microscopy of renal biopsies in toxemia of pregnancy. *JAMA* **175:** 791 (1961).
2. Altcheck, A. Renal biopsy and its clinical correlation in toxemia of pregnancy. *Circulation* **30** (Suppl. 2): 43 (1964).
3. Mautner, W., J. Churg, E. Grishman, and S. Dachs. Preeclamptic nephropathy—an electron microscopic study. *Lab. Invest.* **11:** 518 (1962).
4. Pirani, C. L., V. E. Pollack, R. Lannigan, and G. Folli. The renal glomerular lesions of pre-eclampsia: electron microscopic studies. *Am. J. Obstet. Gynecol.* **87:** 1047 (1963).
5. Faith, G. C. and B. F. Trump. The glomerular capillary wall in human kidney disease: acute glomerulonephritis, systemic lupus erythematosus, and preeclampsia- eclampsia. Comparative electron microscopic observations and a review. *Lab. Invest.* **15:** 1682 (1966).
6. Altcheck, A., N. L. Albright, and S. C. Sommers. The renal pathology of toxemia of pregnancy. *Obstet. Gynecol.* **31:** 595 (1968).
7. Fisher, E. R., V. Pardo, R. Paul, and T. T. Hayashi. Ultrastructural studies in hypertension. *Am. J. Pathol.* **55:** 109 (1969).
8. Thompson, D., W. G. Paterson, G. E. Smart, M. K. MacDonald, and J. S. Robson. The renal lesions of toxemia and abruptio placentae studied by light and electron microscopy. *J. Obstet. Gynaecol. Brit. Commonw.* **79:** 311 (1972).
9. Morris, R. H., P. Vassali, F. K. Beller, and R. T. McCluskey. Immunofluorescent studies of renal biopsies in the diagnosis of toxemia of pregnancy. *Obstet. Gynecol.* **24:** 32 (1964).
10. Vassali, P., G. Simon, and C. Rouiller. Production of ultra-structural glomerular lesions resembling those of toxemia of pregnancy of thromboplastin infusion in rabbits. *Nature (London)* **199:** 1105 (1963).

85

Kidney in Abruptio Placentae

Both histologically and ultrastructurally,[1] the glomerular involvement in *abruptio placentae* is similar to that of gestational preeclampsia-eclampsia.

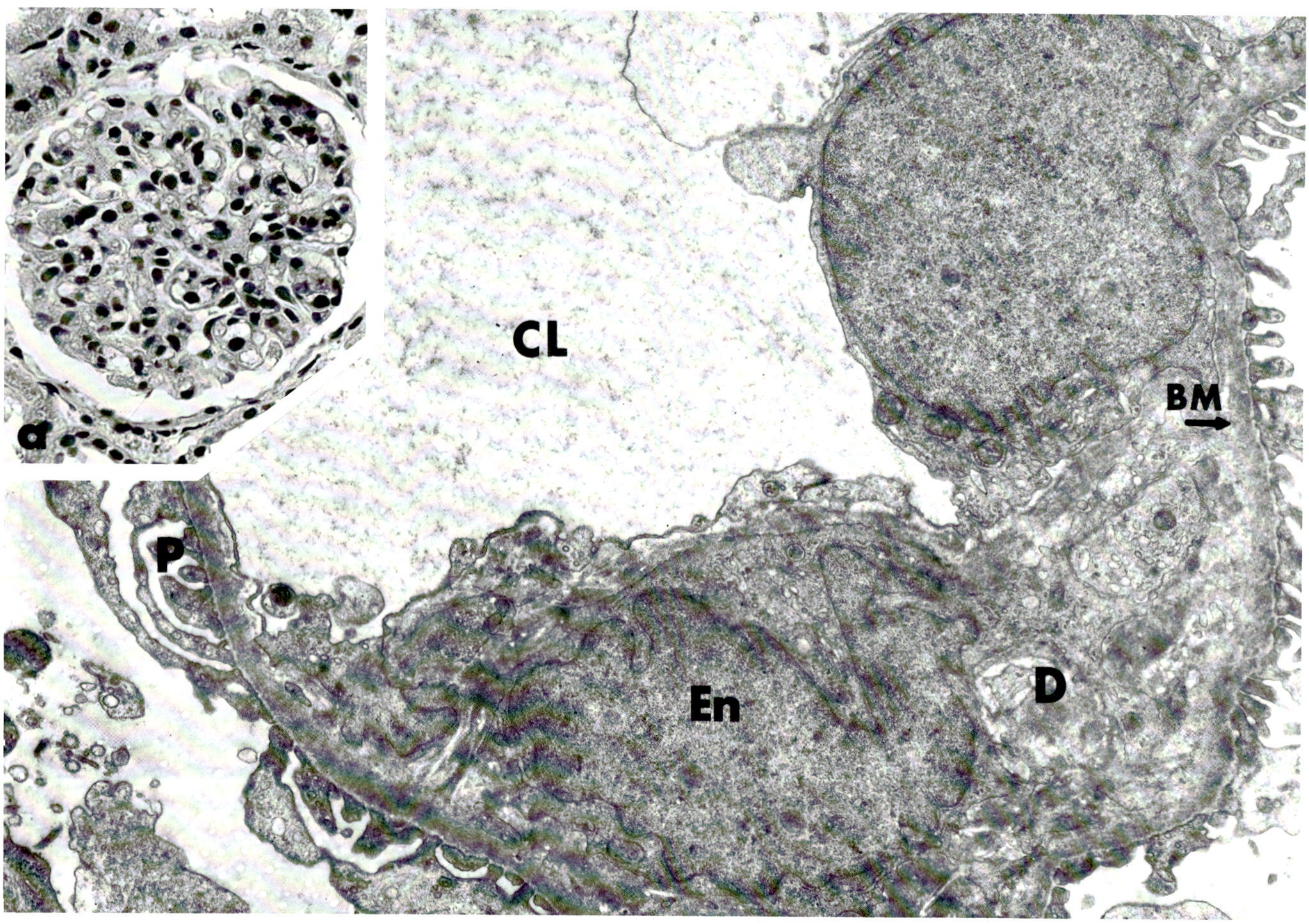

Figure 291a. *Abruptio placentate.* There is an increase in the number of endothelial and mesangial cells, and the mesangial matrix and endothelial cytoplasm are swollen, resulting in a considerable reduction of capillary lumina. (H & E stain, × 300.) *From* D. Thompson, W. G. Paterson, G. E. Smart, M. K. MacDonald, and P. S. Robson. The renal lesions of toxemia and abruptio placentae studied by light and electron microscopy. *J. Obstet. Gynaecol. Brit. Commonw.* **79:** 311–320 (1972).

Figure 291. *Abruptio placentae.* The abundant granular deposit (D) in the subendothelial situation is consistent with the electron microscopic appearance of fibrin. × 6000. En: endothelium; CL: capillary lumen; BM: endothelial basement membrane; P: foot processes of podocytes. *From* D. Thompson, W. G. Paterson, G. E. Smart, M. K. MacDonald, and P. S. Robson. The renal lesions of toxemia and abruptio placentae studied by light and electron microscopy. *J. Obstet. Gynaecol. Brit. Commonw.* **79:** 311–320 (1972).

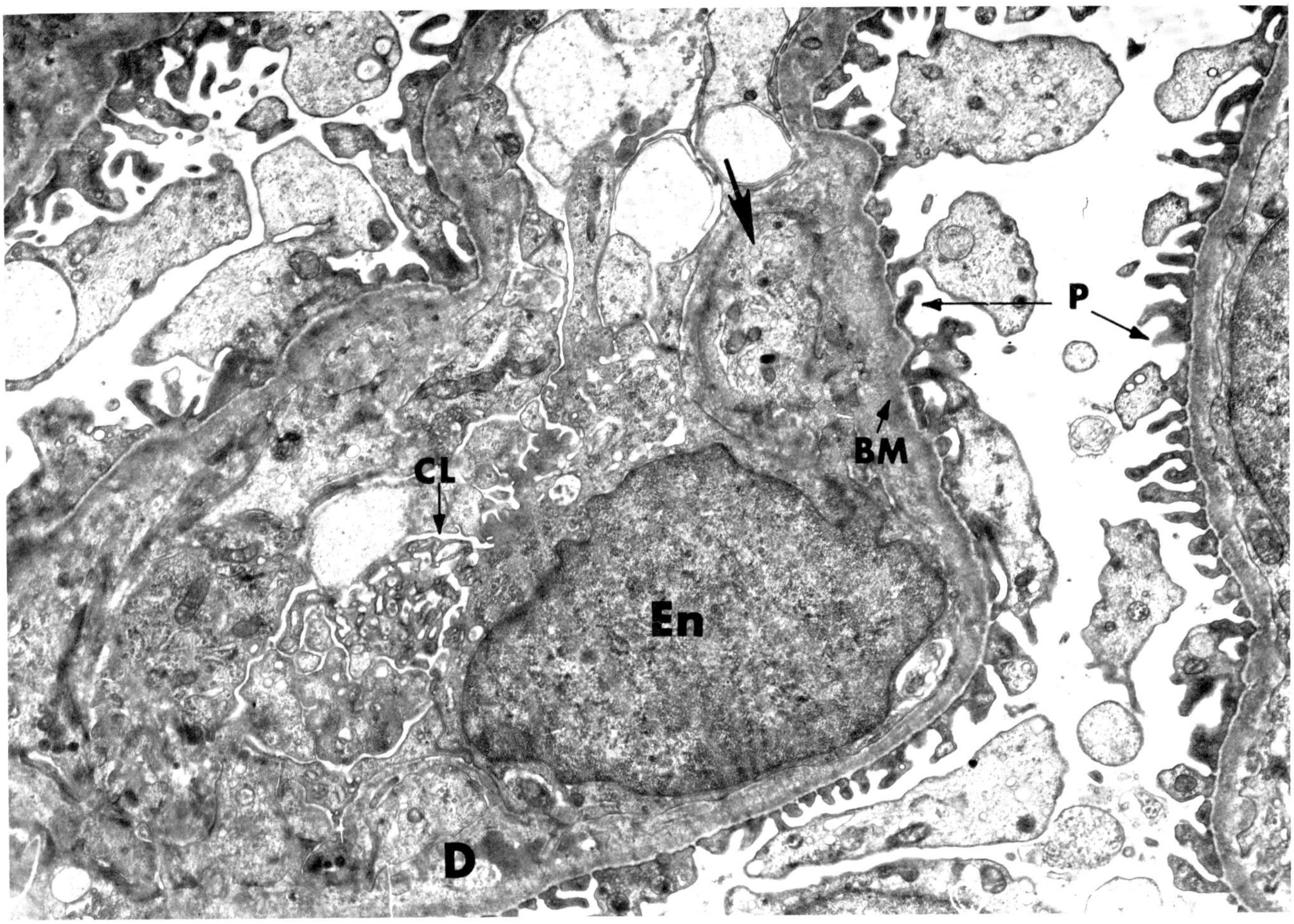

Figure 292. *Abruptio placentae.* Reactive endothelial (En) and mesangial elements all but occlude the capillary lumen (CL). Granular deposit (D) can readily be identified, while loops of "organized" deposit (arrow) enclose fragments of cytoplasm. × 6000. P: foot processes of podocytes; BM: endothelial basement membrane. *From* D. Thompson, W. G. Paterson, G. E. Smart, M. K. MacDonald, and P. S. Robson. The renal lesions of toxemia and abruptio placentae studied by light and electron microscopy. *J. Obstet. Gynaecol. Brit. Commomw.* **79:** 311–320 (1972).

REFERENCE (Both histologically and sultratructurally—Figure 292)

1. Thompson, D., W. G. Paterson, G. E. Smart, M. K. MacDonald, and J. S. Robson. The renal lesions of toxemia and abruptio placentae studied by light and electron microscopy. *J. Obstet. Gynaecol. Brit. Commonw.* **79:** 311 (1972).

86

Trophoblastic Disease

The term *trophoblastic disease* is used in a generic sense to include the hydatidiform mole, invasive hydatidiform mole (chorioadenoma destruens), and choriocarcinoma, lesions that represent parts in the continuum of trophoblastic neoplasms. The clinical and histologic features of trophoblastic neoplasia have been extensively reviewed by Benirschke and Driscoll[1] and by Ober et al.[2]

HYDATIDIFORM MOLE

The hydatidiform mole is composed of vesicles of different sizes containing an edematous (hydropic) villous mesenchyme that is usually devoid of capillaries. Trophoblastic hyperplasia and anaplasia are prominent. The electron microscopic aspects of hydatidiform moles have been inconsistently described,[3-13] probably because of the great morphological variability observed in chorionic tissues. Most observers agree, however, that the organellar pattern and cytoplasmic organization in molar trophoblastic cells are similar to those of the normal immature placenta and are capable of active chorionic gonadotropin production.

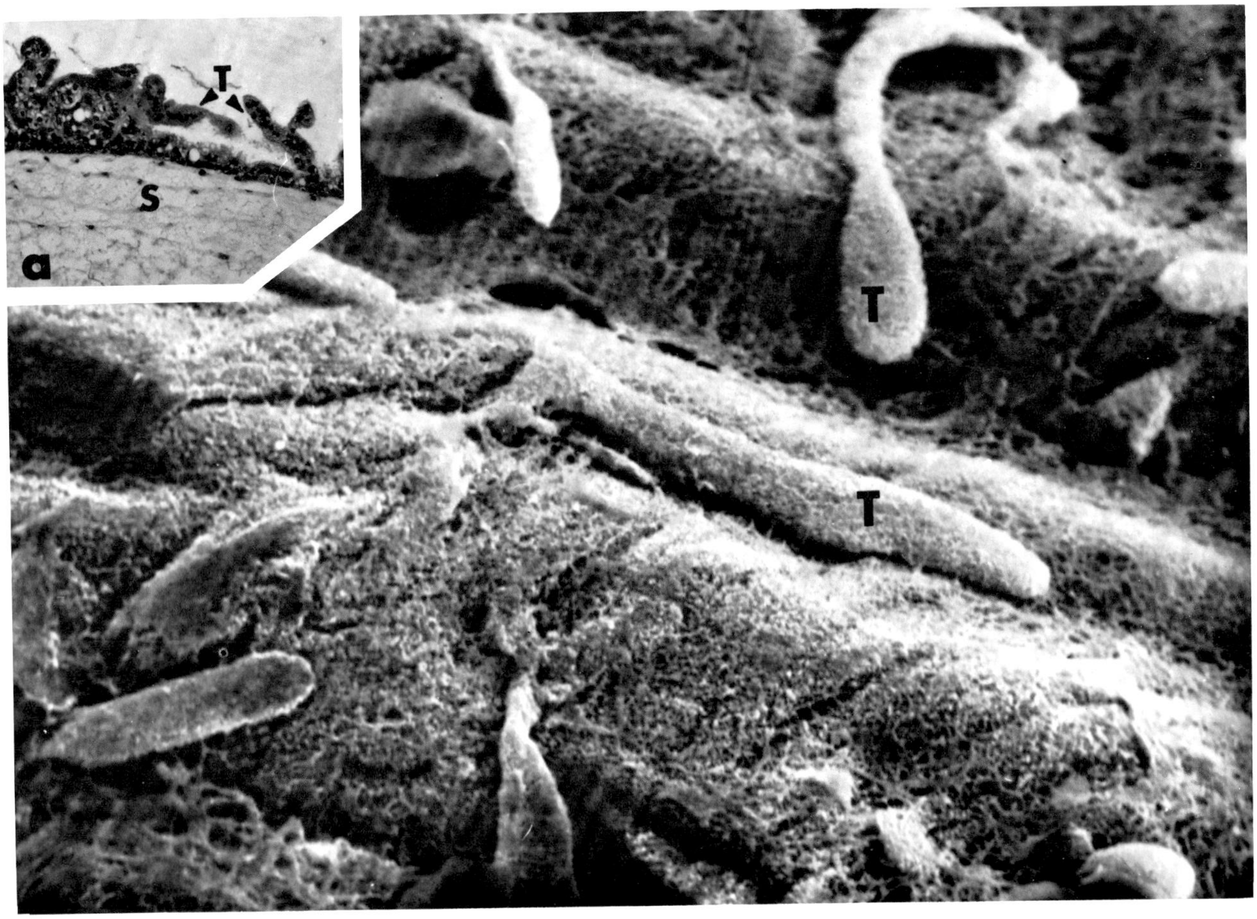

Figure 293a. *Hydatidiform mole.* Portion of a molar vesicle in which the covering trophoblastic membrane contains nodules of cytotrophoblast (left) and villuslike (T) syncytial extensions. The vesicular stroma (S) is markedly edematous, myxoid, and avascular. (H & E stain, × 30.)

Figure 293. *Hydatidiform mole.* The trophoblastic membrane of molar vesicles is slightly undulative and contains numerous, varying-sized trophoblastic buddings (T), which appear as flat, rather than cylindrical, syncytial protrusions and correspond to the villuslike extensions seen in Figure 293*a*. Most of the trophoblastic sprouts that occur in trophoblastic disease lack morphologic evidence of maturation, and they are considerably more abundant in moles than in the normal immature placenta. The abundance of these trophoblastic buddings in the early placenta, as well as in hydatidiform moles, reflects accelerated trophoblastic proliferation.[9,14] × 640. *From* A. Ferenczy and R. M. Richart. Scanning electron microscopic study of normal and molar trophoblast. *Gynecol. Oncol.* **1:** 95–110 (1972).

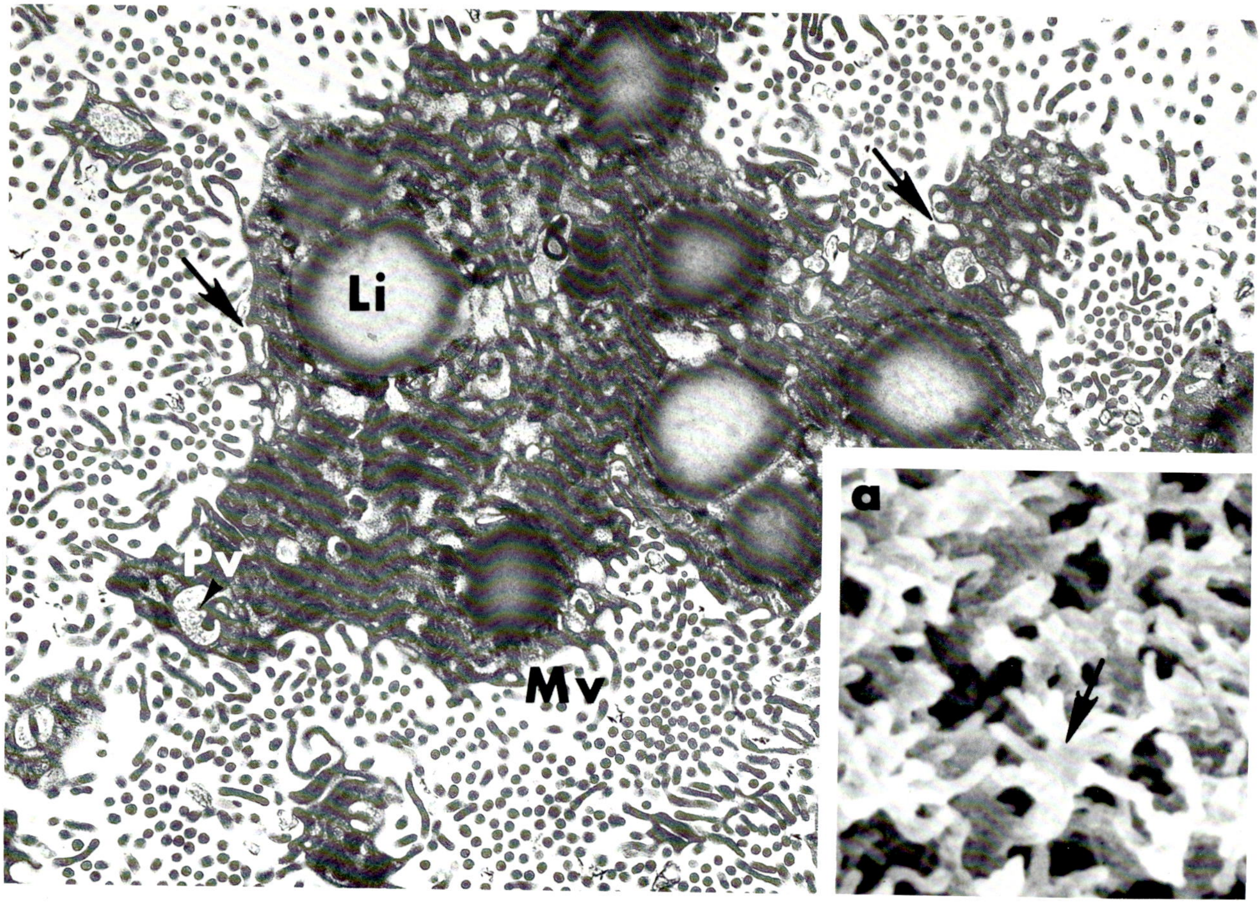

Figure 294a. *Hydatidiform mole.* Although the molar syncytial microvilli show geographical differences in number and configuration, they are generally arranged in complexly branching cytoplasmic processes, and the degree of microvillous arborization (arrow) exceeds that found in either the mature or the immature trophoblast. × 16,000. *From* A. Ferenczy and R. M. Richart. Scanning electron microscopic study of normal and molar trophoblast. *Gynecol. Oncol.* **1**: 95–110 (1972).

Figure 294. *Hydatidiform mole.* Electron micrograph of tangentially sectioned surface of a syncytial extension. Note the abundant, hairlike, microvillous processes (Mv) associated with numerous pinocytic invaginations (arrow) and pinocytic vesicles (Pv). The conspicuous accumulation of lipid droplets (Li) in molar tissues[10,12,13] suggests a lack of utilization of lipid precursors for steroid hormone synthesis. Channels of granular endoplasmic reticulum and clusters of membrane-bound dense bodies are scattered throughout the cytoplasm. × 15,600.

REFERENCES (The term trophoblastic disease—Figure 294a)

1. Benirshcke, K. and S. E. Driscoll. *The Pathology of the Placenta*. Springer-Verlag, New York, 1967, pp. 348–430.
2. Ober, W. B., J. H. Edgcomb, and E. B. Price, Jr. The pathology of choriocarcinoma. *Ann. N.Y. Acad. Sci.* **172:** 299 (1971).
3. Mori, Y., M. Hashimoto, A. Komori, T. Shimoyama, and K. Akashi. Electron microscopic studies of the hydatidiform mole. *Proc. Jap. Cancer Res.* **50:** 222, 1959 (Suppl.).
4. Bargmann, W. and A. Knoop. Electron microscopic studies on the placental villi in man (remarks on the syncytium problem). *Z. Zellforsch.* **50:** 472 (1959).
5. Geller, H. F. Electron microscope findings on the syncytium of the human placenta. *Geburtsch. Frauenheilkd.* **22:** 1234 (1962).
6. Rigano, A. and R. Serman. Prime osservazioni sull'ultrastruttura del villo coriale nella degenerazione vesicolomolare. *Riv. Ostet. Ginecol.* **18:** 12 (1963).
7. Larsen, J. F. Electron microscopy of the human placenta. *Transcript of the Second Rochester Trophoblast Conference,* C. J. Lund and H. A. Thiede (Eds.). University of Rochester School of Medicine and Dentistry, Rochester, New York, 1963, p. 280.
8. Wakitani, T. Electron microscopic observation on the hydatidiform mole. *Mie Med. J.* **13:** 123 (1964).
9. Wynn, R. M. and J. Davies. Ultrastructure of hydatidiform mole. Correlative electron microscopic and functional aspects. *Am. J. Obstet. Gynecol.* **90:** 293 (1964).
10. Gonzalez-Angulo, A., H. Marquez-Monter, B. J. Zavala, E. Yabur, and H. Salazar. Electron microscopic observations in hydatidiform mole. *Obstet. Gynecol.* **27:** 455 (1966).
11. Cesarini, J. P., M. Berebbi, Y. Ayme, H. Ruf, and H. Bonneau. Some aspects of the ultrastructure of a case of hydatidiform mole and of a case of chorioepithelioma. *Gynécol. Obstét. (Paris)* **66:** 303 (1967).
12. Okudaira, Y. and L. Strauss. Ultrastructure of molar trophoblast. Observations on hydatidiform mole and chorioadenoma destruens. *Obstet. Gynecol.* **30:** 172 (1967).
13. Merkow, L. P., H. F. Acevedo, and J. Gilmore. Trophoblastic disease. A correlative ultrastructural and biochemical study. *Obstet. Gynecol.* **37:** 348 (1971).
14. Ferenczy, A. and R. M. Richart. Scanning electron microscopic study of normal and molar trophoblast. *Gynecol. Oncol.* **1:** 95 (1972).

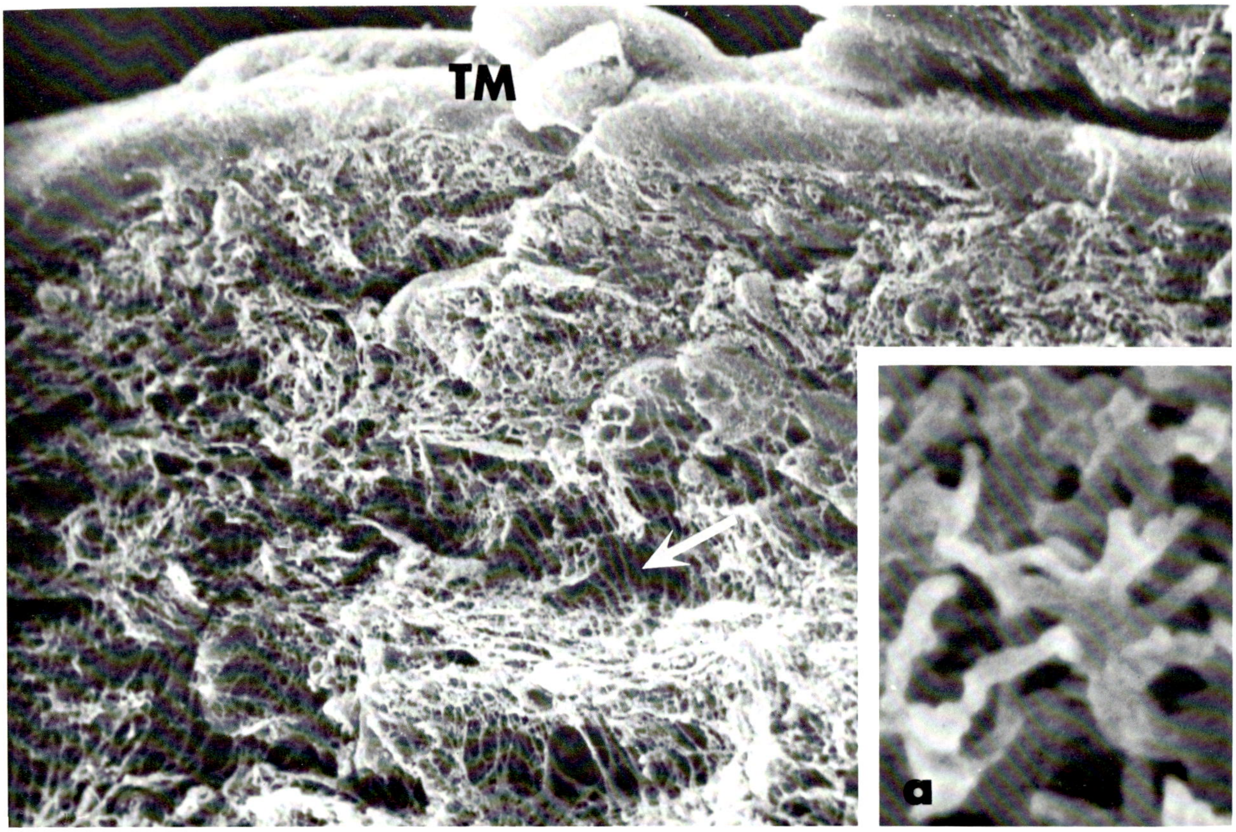

Figure 295. *Hydatidiform mole.* Scanning electron micrograph of an intentionally fractured molar vesicle, illustrating the fine rhythmic pattern (arrow) of the supporting reticulum network, after dehydration by the freeze-drying technique. × 1280. TM: trophoblastic membrane. *From* A. Ferenczy and R. M. Richart. Scanning electron microscopic study of normal and molar trophoblast. *Gynecol. Oncol.* **1:** 95–110 (1972).

Figure 295a. *Higher magnification of Figure 294a.* Note the complex arborization of molar syncytial microvilli. × 25,000.

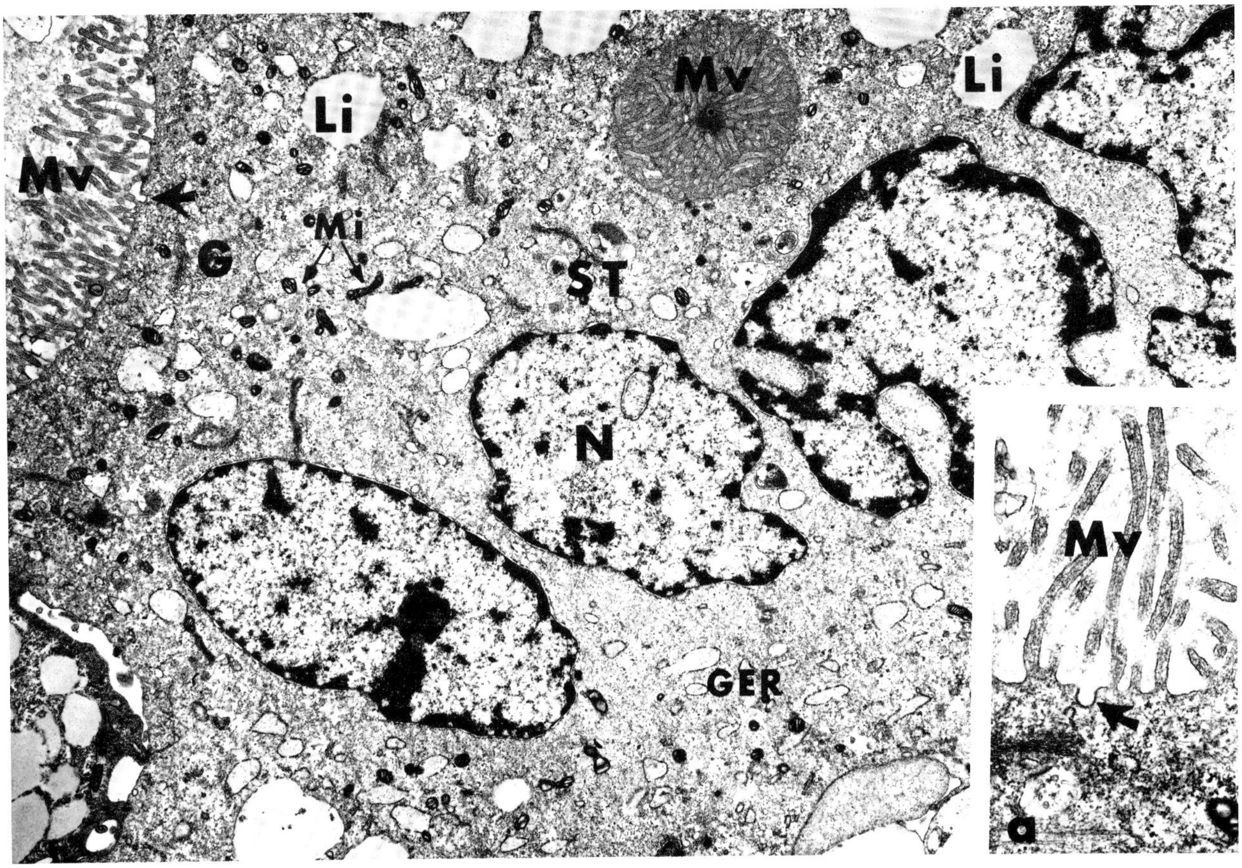

Figure 296. *Hydatidiform mole.* A multinucleated (N) molar syncytiotrophoblast (ST) has an intracytoplasmic lacuna, the lumen of which is obliterated by numerous interdigitating microvilli (Mv). The cytoplasm is rich in free ribosomes, lipid droplets (Li), vesicles of granular endoplasmic reticulum (GER), and Golgi (G). Characteristically, the cigar-shaped mitochondria are small and are concentrated near the surface plasma membrane. The latter contains a myriad of well-developed microvillous projections (Mv) associated with pinocytic invaginations (arrow). The abundant surface microvilli (the function of which is apparently to increase the cell surface and therefore its absorptive area), the pinocytic activity, and the dissimilar osmotic pressure and amino acid concentration between molar vesicular stroma and maternal plasma[1] indicate that accumulation of intravesicular fluid occurs by absorptive phenomena (imbibition). Whether these morphologic changes in molar tissue are a reflection of a hyperplastic, rather than a neoplastic, process is still a matter of discussion, but the aneuploid nuclear DNA content of molar trophoblast suggests that the lesions are malignant neoplasms or precursors thereto.[2] × 5600.

Figure 296a. *Cellular detail of Figure 296.* Note the typical pinocytotic invagination (arrow) of the surface plasma membrane and the slender microvilli (Mv) supported by a filamentous matrix. × 20,600.

REFERENCES (Figures 295–296a)

1. McKay, D. G., M. V. Richardson, and A. T. Hertig. Studies of the formation of early human trophoblast. III. A study of the protein structure of mole fluid, chorionic and amniotic fluids by paper electrophoresis. *Am. J. Obstet. Gynecol.* **75:** 699 (1958).
2. Goldfarb, S., R. M. Richart, and T. Okagaki. A cytophotometric study of nuclear DNA content of cyto- and syncytiotrophoblast in trophoblastic disease. *Cancer* **27:** 83 (1971).

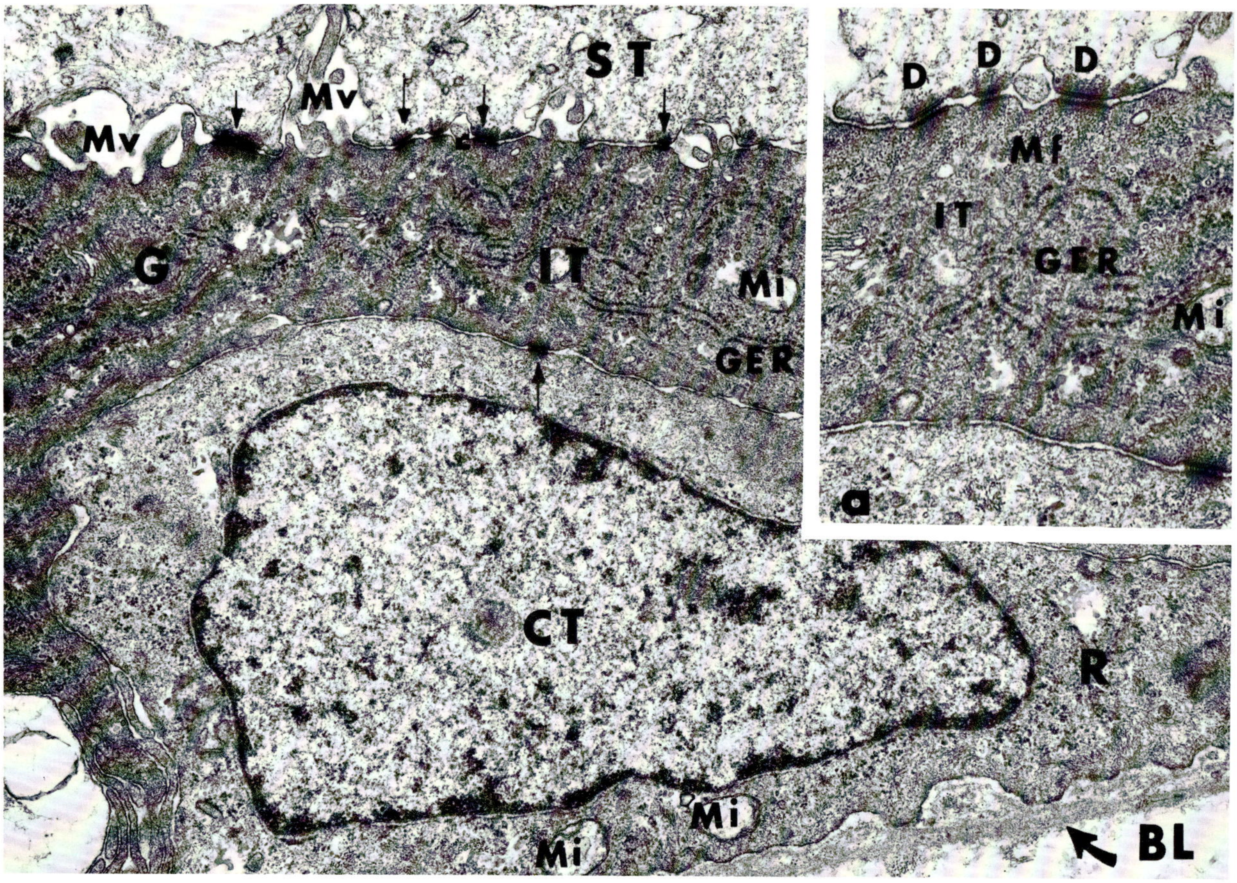

Figure 297. *Hydatidiform mole.* Electron micrograph of a transitional or intermediary (IT) trophoblast, attached by numerous desmosomal belts (arrows) to both the underlying cytotrophoblast (CT) and the overlying syncytial cell (ST). This cell type differs from the cytotrophoblast by its comparatively rich organellar content, including free ribosomes, granular endoplasmic reticulum (GER), and Golgi (G). These organelles, however, are even better developed in the syncytial cells. Since intermediary cells are regarded as precursor elements for the formation of new syncytium,[1] their great number in molar tissue is indicative of the increased proliferative activity of the molar trophoblast. × 20,600. Mv: microvilli of intermediary trophoblast; Mi: mitochondria, larger in both intermediary trophoblast and cytotrophoblast than in syncytiotrophoblast; R: ribosome in cytotrophoblast; BL: basal lamina.

Figure 297a. *Cellular detail of Figure 297,* illustrating the well-developed constituents of intermediary trophoblast (IT). × 29,200. GER: membranes of granular endoplasmic reticulum; Mi: mitochondria; Mf: tangentially sectioned microfilaments; D: desmosomes between the intermediary trophoblast and syncytial cell.

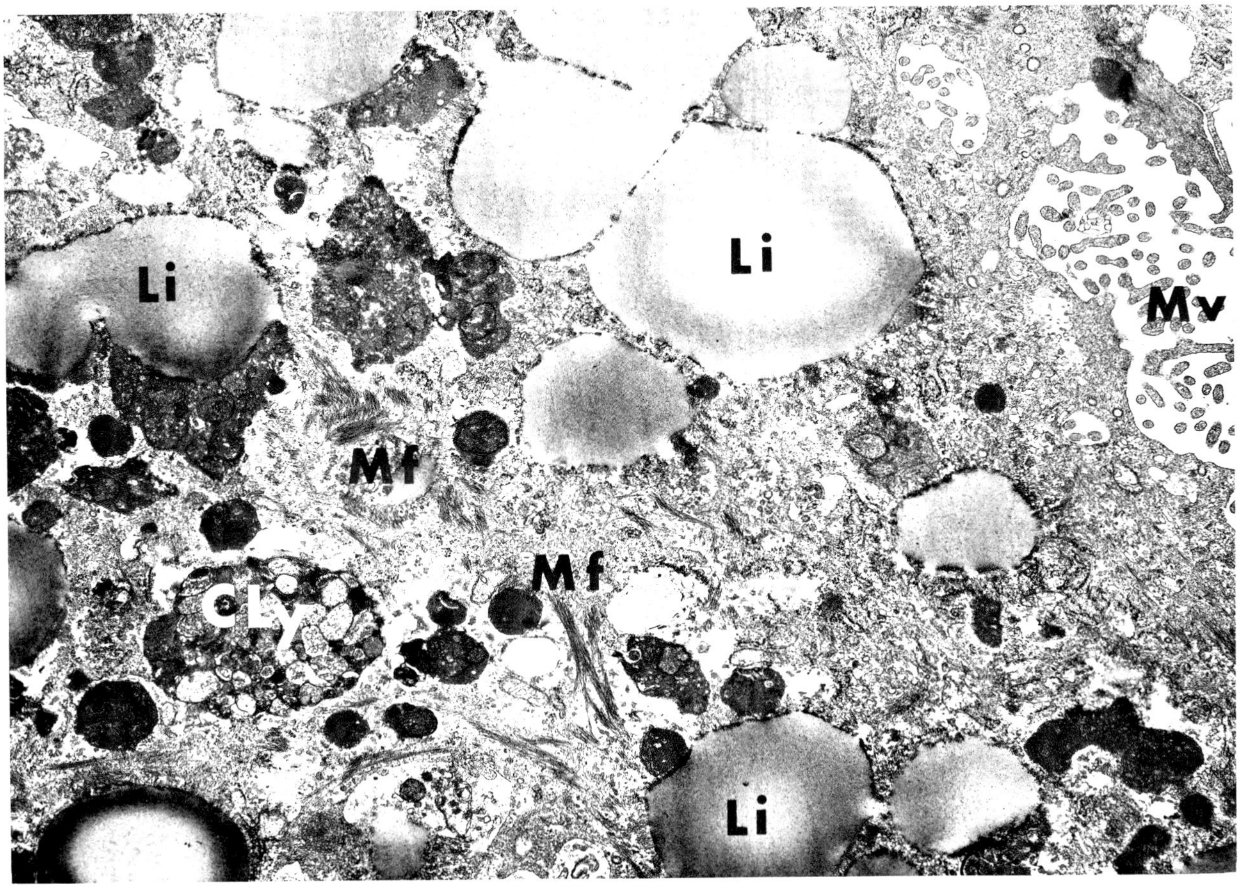

Figure 298. *Hydatidiform mole.* This patient, a 26-year-old nulliparous woman, was given actinomycin-D for 2 days before molar evacuation. Note the prominent accumulation of lipid droplets (Li) and autophagic cytolysosomes (CLy), filled with engulfed cytoplasmic debris associated with focal cytoplasmic degeneration. × 12,600. Mf: bundles of microfilaments; Mv: surface microvilli.

REFERENCE (Figures 297–298)

1. Wynn, R. M. and J. Davies. Ultrastructure of hydatidiform mole. Correlative electron microscopic and functional aspects. *Am. J. Obstet. Gynecol.* **90:** 293 (1964).

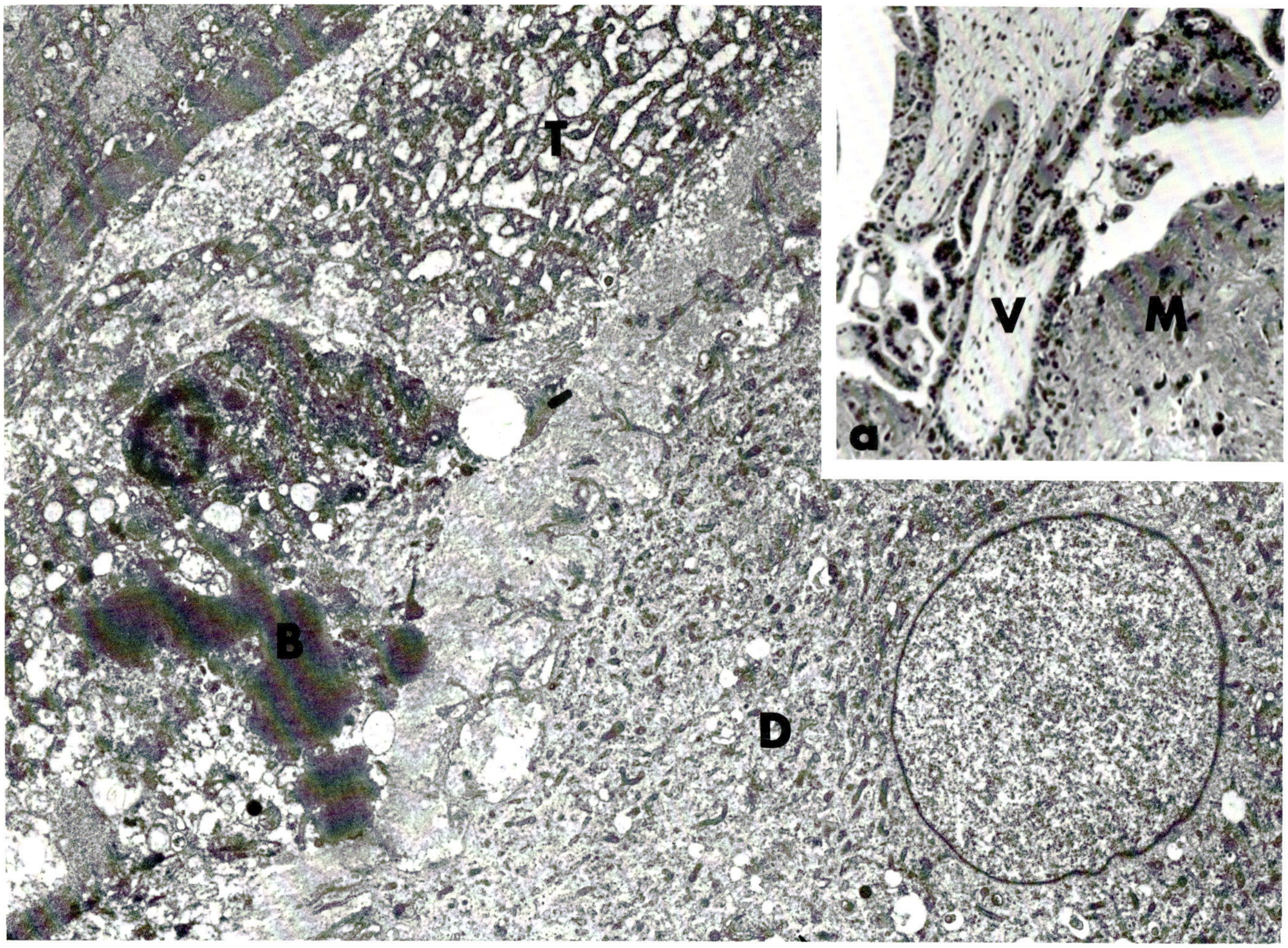

INVASIVE HYDATIDIFORM MOLE (CHORIOADENOMA DESTRUENS)

The invasive hydatidiform mole (chorioadenoma destruens) is a lesion that invades the myometrium, penetrates uterine vasculature, and may present with extrauterine extension or transport. At the ultrastructural level[1,2] the trophoblast of invasive moles is similar to its noninvasive counterpart and to normal immature placental tissue. In contrast to the normal deciduotrophoblastic relationship, however, there is comparatively less junctional necrosis and fibrinoid.[2] Since fetomaternal "fibrinoid" has been linked to the control of trophoblastic invasiveness, it is possible that the decreased cellular reaction may enhance the molar myometrial invasion,[2] a phenomenon morphologically similar to that seen in placenta accreta.

Figure 299a. *Histological section of invasive mole,* illustrating hydropic villi (V), penetrating deep into the myometrium (M). (H & E stain, × 133). *From* R. M. Wynn and J. A. Harris. Ultrastructure of trophoblast and endometrium in invasive hydatidiform mole (chorioadenoma destruens). *Am. J. Obstet. Gynecol.* **99:** 1125–1135 (1967).

Figure 299. *Invasive mole.* A decidual cell (D) is in proximity to a degenerating trophoblast (T) and extravasated red blood cells (B). × 15,000. *From* R. M. Wynn and J. A. Harris. Ultrastructure of trophoblast and endometrium in invasive hydatidiform mole (chorioadenoma destruens). *Am. J. Obstet. Gynecol.* **99:** 1125–1135 (1967).

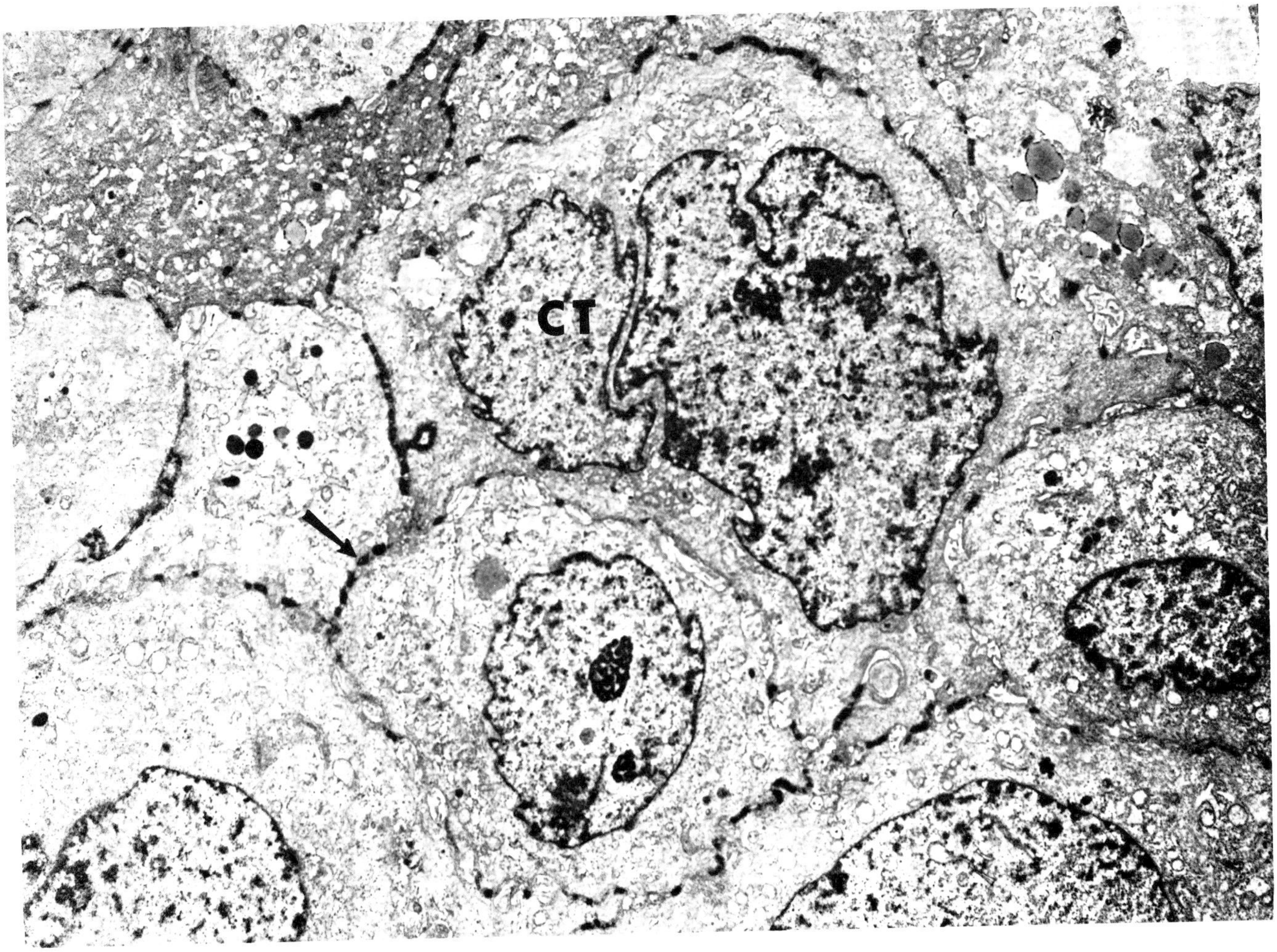

Figure 300. *Invasive mole.* Electron micrograph of well-preserved cytotrophoblast (CT) within the myometrium. Numerous, well-developed desmosomal belts (arrow) are seen between the neoplastic cytotrophoblasts. × 15,000. *From* R. M. Wynn and J. A. Harris. Ultrastructure of trophoblast and endometrium in invasive hydatidiform mole (chorioadenoma destruens). *Am. J. Obstet. Gynecol.* **99:** 1125–1135 (1967).

REFERENCES (The invasive hydatidiform mole—Figure 300)

1. Okudaira, Y. and L. Strauss. Ultrastructure of molar trophoblast. Observation on hydatidiform mole and chorioadenoma destruens. *Obstet. Gynecol.* **30:** 172 (1967).
2. Wynn, R. M. and J. A. Harris. Ultrastructure of trophoblast and endometrium in invasive hydatidiform mole (chorioadenoma destruens). *Am. J. Obstet. Gynecol.* **99:** 1125 (1967).

CHORIOCARCINOMA

Choriocarcinoma is the most primitive and malignant form of trophoblastic disease and shows the greatest deviation from the normal chromosome number and the most widely spread nuclear DNA values.[1] The lesion is usually composed entirely of malignant cyto- and syncytiotrophoblast with extensive vascular invasion. Villi are characteristically lacking. Ultrastructurally,[2-6] except for marked nucleocytoplasmic pleomorphism, the cells of choriocarcinoma resemble those found in the hydatidiform mole and the normal immature placenta, especially the part surrounding the early ovum.[6] The pertinent fine structural features include the presence of a prominent granular endoplasmic reticulum system in the syncytial cells[6] (probably related to the high levels of chorionic gonadotropin), abundant intermediate cytotrophoblast,[6]

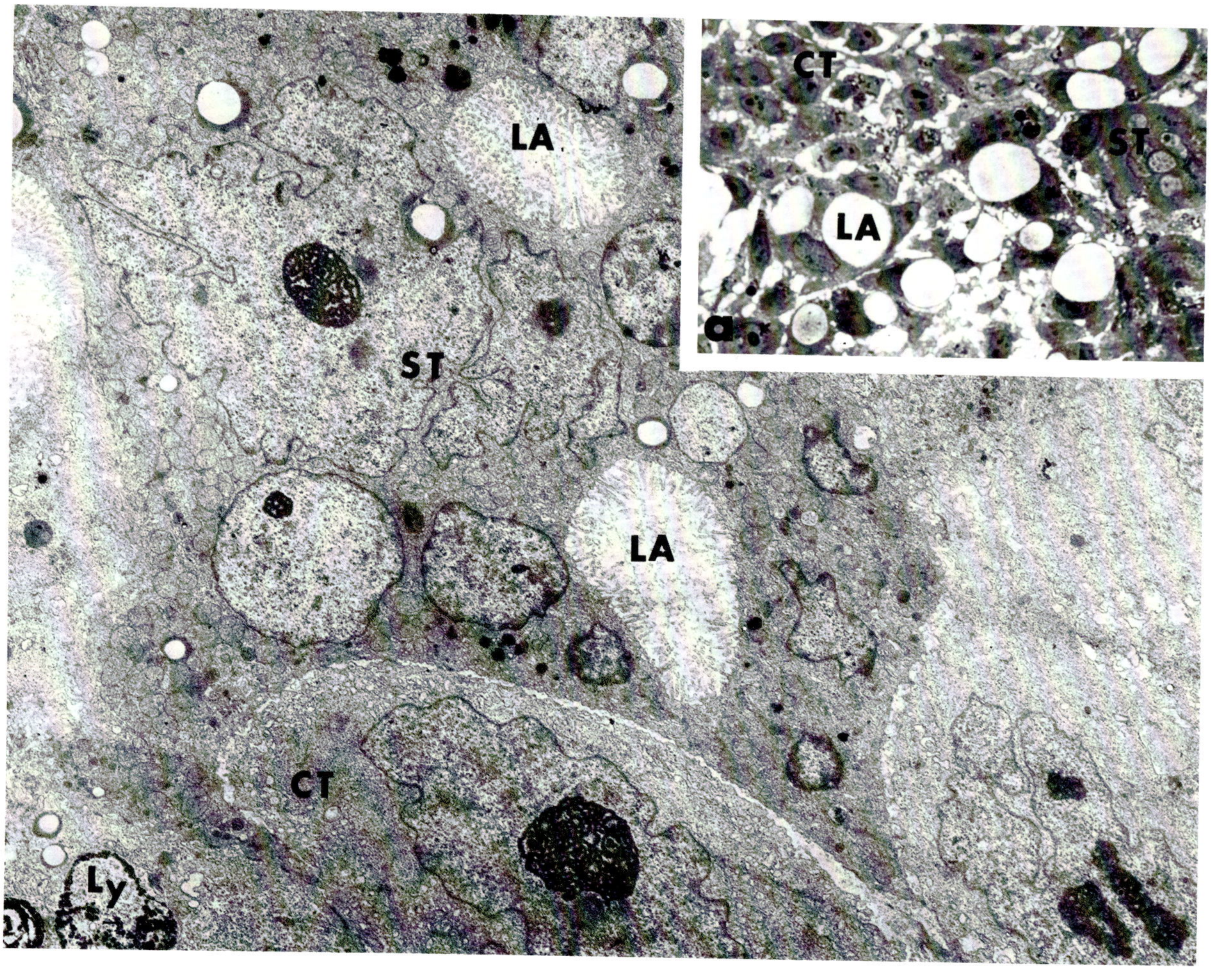

and the abortive formation of intervillous spaces, a characteristic feature of both uterine and extrauterine choriocarcinoma. The syncytiotrophoblast is conspicuously phagocytic in choriocarcinoma,[5] a feature not found in molar trophoblast.

Figure 301a. *Histologically,* the choriocarcinoma contains an admixture of highly pleomorphic malignant cytotrophoblast (CT) and syncytiotrophoblast (ST). Characteristically, intracytoplasmic lacunae (LA) are numerous in the syncytial cells, and chorionic villi are lacking. (Toluidine blue stain, × 150). *From* J. Larsen, E. Falck, L. Robert, and F. Bierring. Electron microscopy of human choriocarcinoma transplanted into hamster liver. *Am. J. Obstet. Gynecol.* **99:** 1109–1124 (1967).

Figure 301. *Electron micrograph of human choriocarcinoma.* In the center a neoplastic syncytial cell (ST) with large irregular nuclei and nucleoli and large lacunae (LA) lined by microvilli is seen. The cytoplasm is dense compared with that of the neoplastic cytotrophoblastic cells (CT), which also have large nuclei and large, skeinlike nucleoli. Many lysosomes (Ly) are found in both types of cells. × 3000. *From* J. Larsen, E. Falck, L. Robert, and F. Bierring. Electron microscopy of human choriocarcinoma transplanted into hamster liver. *Am. J. Obstet. Gynecol.* **99:** 1109–1124 (1967).

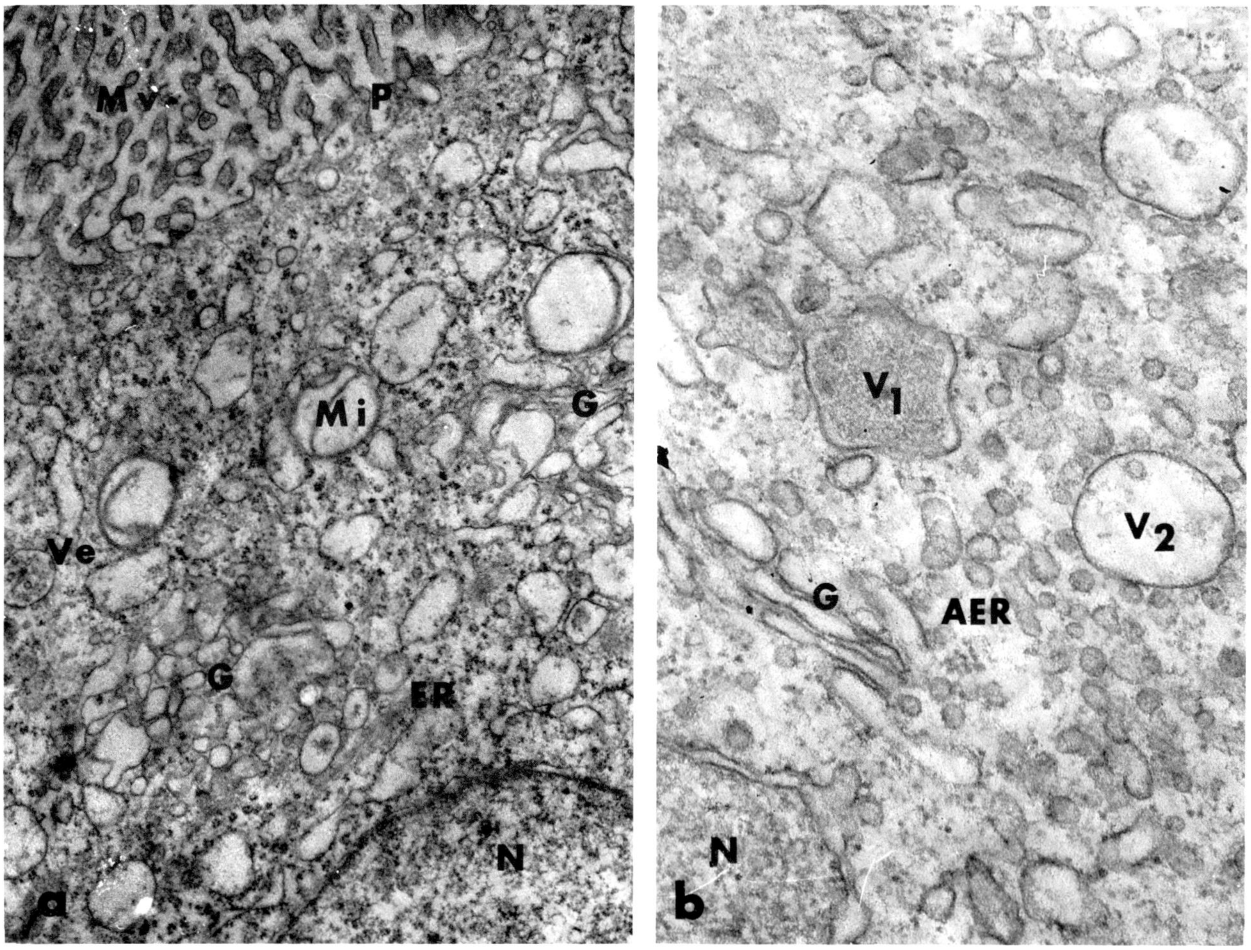

Figure 302a. *Portion of neoplastic syncytial cell.* The cytoplasm contains granular endoplasmic reticulum (ER), Golgi (G), and multivesicular bodies (Ve). The mitochondria (Mi) are regular but have only a few cristae. The cell surface has abundant microvilli (Mv) and vesicles indicating pinocytosis (P). × 30,000. N: nucleus. *From* J. Larsen, E. Falck, L. Robert, and F. Bierring. Electron microscopy of human choriocarcinoma transplanted into hamster liver. *Am. J. Obstet. Gynecol.* **99:** 1109–1124 (1967).

Figure 302. *Portion of neoplastic cytotrophoblastic cell.* The cytoplasm contains elements of agranular endoplasmic reticulum (AER), as well as vacuoles with fine electron-dense particles (V_1) and vesicles that appear empty (V_2). × 30,000. N: nucleus; G: Golgi. *From* J. Larsen, E. Falck, L. Robert, and F. Bierring. Electron microscopy of human choriocarcinoma transplanted into hamster liver. *Am. J. Obstet. Gynecol.* **99:** 1109–1124 (1967).

REFERENCES (Choriocarcinoma–Figure 302)

1. Goldfarb, S., R. M. Richart, and T. Okagaki. A cytophotometric study of nuclear DNA content of cyto- and syncytiotrophoblast in trophoblastic disease. *Cancer* **27:** 83 (1971).
2. Mori, Y., M. Hashimoto, A. Komori, M. Kosaka, T. Shimoyama, and K. Akashi. Electron microscopic studies on chorioepithelioma. *Proc. Jap. Cancer Res.* **51:** (Suppl). 118 (1960).
3. Pierce, G. B., Jr. and A. R. Midgley, Jr. The origin and function of human syncytiotrophoblastic giant cells. *Am. J. Pathol.* **43:** 153 (1963).
4. Cesarini, J. P., M. Berebbi, Y. Ayme, H. Ruf, and H. Bonneau. Some aspects of the ultrastructure of a case of hydatidiform mole and of a case of chorioepithelioma. *Gynecol. Obstet.* **66:** 303 (1967).
5. Larsen, J. F., R. L. Ehrmann, and F. Bierring. Electron microscopy of human choriocarcinoma transplanted into hamster liver. *Am. J. Obstet. Gynecol.* **99:** 1109 (1967).
6. Wynn, R. M. and J. Davies. Ultrastructure of transplanted choriocarcinoma and its endocrine implications. *Am. J. Obstet. Gynecol.* **88:** 618 (1964).

INDEX